Leadership
&Nursing Care
Management

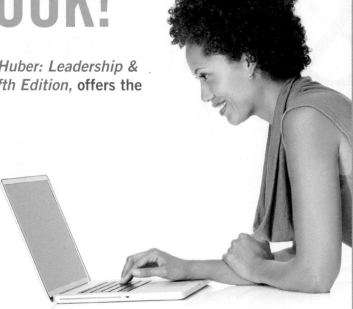

Leadership & Nursing Care Management

Fifth Edition

Diane L. Huber, PhD, RN, NEA-BC, FAAN

Professor
College of Nursing and College of Public Health
The University of Iowa
Iowa City, Iowa

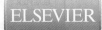
ELSEVIER

3251 Riverport Lane
St. Louis, Missouri 63043

Leadership and Nursing Care Management, Fifth Edition   978-1-4557-4071-0

Notices

Knowledge and best practice in this field are constantly changing. As new research and experience broaden our understanding, changes in research methods, professional practices, or medical treatment may become necessary.

Practitioners and researchers must always rely on their own experience and knowledge in evaluating and using any information, methods, compounds, or experiments described herein. In using such information or methods they should be mindful of their own safety and the safety of others, including parties for whom they have a professional responsibility.

With respect to any drug or pharmaceutical products identified, readers are advised to check the most current information provided (i) on procedures featured or (ii) by the manufacturer of each product to be administered, to verify the recommended dose or formula, the method and duration of administration, and contraindications. It is the responsibility of practitioners, relying on their own experience and knowledge of their patients, to make diagnoses, to determine dosages and the best treatment for each individual patient, and to take all appropriate safety precautions.

To the fullest extent of the law, neither the Publisher nor the authors, contributors, or editors, assume any liability for any injury and/or damage to persons or property as a matter of products liability, negligence or otherwise, or from any use or operation of any methods, products, instructions, or ideas contained in the material herein.

Library of Congress Cataloging-in-Publication Data
Leadership and nursing care management / [edited by] Diane L. Huber. – 5th ed.
       p. ; cm.
   Includes bibliographical references and index.
   ISBN 978-1-4557-4071-0 (pbk.)
   I. Huber, Diane.
   [DNLM: 1. Nursing Services–organization & administration. 2. Leadership. 3. Nursing, Supervisory. WY 105]
   RT89
   362.17'3068–dc23   2013003538

Senior Content Strategist: Yvonne Alexopoulos
Associated Content Development Specialist: Emily Vaughters
Publishing Services Manager: Jeff Patterson
Senior Project Manager: Tracey Schriefer
Designer: Ashley Eberts

Printed in China.
Last digit is the print number: 9   8   7   6   5   4   3   2

CONTRIBUTORS

Jennifer Bellot, PhD, RN, MHSA, CNE
Associate Professor
Jefferson School of Nursing
Thomas Jefferson University
Philadelphia, Pennsylvania

Sharon Eck Birmingham, DNSc, MA, BSN, RN
Chief Nursing Executive
Clairvia Operations, Cerner
Adjunct Faculty, University of
North Carolina, Colorado, Yale,
and Iowa Schools of Nursing
Durham, North Carolina

Alice R. Boyington, PhD, RN
Director of Nursing Research
H. Lee Moffitt Cancer Center &
Research Institute
Tampa, Florida

Jane M. Brokel, PhD, RN, FNI
Assistant Professor
College of Nursing
University of Iowa
Member of the Executive Com-
mittee and Advisory Council
Iowa e-Health Project
Iowa City, Iowa

Lori Carson, MSN, RN
Nurse Executive Consultant
Frisco, Texas

Sean P. Clarke, PhD, RN, FAAN
Professor and Susan E. French
Chair and Director, McGill
Nursing Collaborative
McGill University, Montreal, QC
Status Faculty
Lawrence S. Bloomberg Faculty of
Nursing, University of Toronto

Robert W. Cooper, PhD
Employers Mutual Distinguished
Professor of Insurance
Drake University
Des Moines, Iowa

Karen S. Cox, PhD, RN, FACHE, FAAN
Executive Vice President
Co-Chief Operating Officer
Children's Mercy Hospitals and
Clinics
Kansas City, Missouri

Kathleen B. Cox, PhD
Assistant Professor
University of Virginia School of
Nursing
Charlottesville, Virginia

Laura Cullen, DNP, RN, FAAN
Evidence-Based Practice
Coordinator
Nursing Research &
Evidence-Based Practice
Department of Nursing and
Patient Care Services
University of Iowa Hospitals and
Clinics
Iowa City, Iowa

Cindy J. Dawson, MSN, RN, CORLN
Director, Clinical Functions
Ambulatory Care Nursing
University of Iowa Hospitals and
Clinics
Iowa City, Iowa

Nancy Dole, RN, BSN, BC
Staff Nurse
Ambulatory Care Nursing
Department of Nursing and
Patient Care Services
University of Iowa Hospitals and
Clinics
Iowa City, Iowa

Karen Drenkard, PhD, RN, NEA-BC, FAAN
Executive Director
American Nurses Credentialing
Center
Silver Spring, Maryland

Elizabeth T. Dugan, PhD, RN, NEA-BC
Chief Nurse Executive and AVP
Patient Care Services
Inova Loudoun Hospital
Leesburg, Virginia

Betsy Frank, PhD, RN, ANEF
Professor Emeritus
College of Nursing, Health, and
Human Services
Indiana State University
Terre Haute, Indiana

Jane M. Fusilero, RN, MSN, MBA, NEA-BC
Vice President, Patient Care
Services/Chief Nursing Officer
Moffitt Cancer Center
Tampa, Florida

Maryanne Garon, RN, DNSc
Professor
California State University –
Fullerton
Fullerton, California

Gregory O. Ginn, BA, MEd, MBA, PhD
Associate Professor
University of Nevada, Las Vegas
Las Vegas, Nevada

Caryl Goodyear-Bruch, PhD, RN, NEA-BC
Director of Professional Resources & Leadership Development
Children's Mercy Hospital and Clinics
Kansas City, Missouri

Kirsten Hanrahan, DNP, ARNP
Nurse Scientist
Nursing Research and Evidence-Based Practice
University of Iowa Hospital and Clinics
Iowa City, Iowa

L. Jean Henry, PhD
Associate Professor, Community Health Promotion
Department of Health, Human Performance, and Recreation
University of Arkansas
Fayetteville, Arkansas

Cheryl Hoying, PhD, RN, NEA-BC, FACHE, FAAN
Senior Vice President of Patient Services
Cincinnati Children's Hospital Medical Center
Associate Dean
College of Nursing
University of Cincinnati
Adjunct Instructor
Wright State University–Miami Valley School of Nursing
Cincinnati, Ohio

Lianne Jeffs, PhD, RN
St. Michael's Hospital Volunteer Association Chair in Nursing Research
Scientist, Keenan Research Centre of the Li Ka Shing Knowledge Institute
St. Michael's Hospital Scientific Director, Nursing Health Services Research Unit
Assistant Professor, Bloomberg Faculty of Nursing
University of Toronto

Susan R. Lacey, PhD, RN, MSN
Director, Strategic Collaborations
Director, Nursing Innovation Center
Children's Mercy Hospitals and Clinics
Kansas City, Missouri

Jo Manion, PhD, RN, NEA-BC, FAAN
Owner/Senior Consultant Manion & Associates
The Villages, Florida

Raquel M. Meyer, PhD, RN
Manager
Baycrest Centre for Learning, Research and Innovation in Long-Term Care
Assistant Professor
Lawrence S. Bloomberg Faculty of Nursing
University of Toronto
Toronto, Ontario, Canada

Mary Ellen Murray, PhD, RN
Professor
Associate Dean Academic Affairs
University of Wisconsin – Madison School of Nursing
Madison, Wisconsin

Lynne S. Nemeth, PhD, RN
Associate Professor
College of Nursing
Medical University of South Carolina
Charleston, South Carolina

Adrienne Olney, MS
Research Associate
Children's Mercy Hospitals and Clinics
Kansas City, Missouri

Luc R. Pelletier, MSN, APRN, PMHCNS-BC, FAAN, CPHQ, FNAHQ
Administrative Liaison
Sharp Mesa Vista Hospital
Core Adjunct Faculty
National University
San Diego, California

Beth Pickard, BSN
General Manager
Clairvia Operations, Cerner
Durham, North Carolina

Belinda E. Puetz, PhD, RN
Principal
Puetz Consulting Services, Inc.
Pensacola, Florida

Gene S. Rigotti, MSN, BSN, RN, NEA-BC
Clifton, Virginia

Linda L. Workman, PhD, RN, NEA-BC
VP Center for Professional Excellence
Children's Hospital Medical Center
Cincinnati, Ohio

Stephanie Corder, ND, RN
Associate Professor
Missouri Western State University
St. Joseph, Missouri

Denise Hirst, RN, MSN
Clinical Assistant Professor
School of Nursing
University of North Carolina at Chapel Hill
Chapel Hill, North Carolina

PREFACE

The time is now for strong leadership and care management in nursing. Highlighted by a series of reports from the prestigious Institute of Medicine (IOM), most recently *The Future of Nursing: Leading Change, Advancing Health,* it is clear that nurses matter to health care delivery systems. Yet the United States is in the midst of a continuing and projected nurse shortage. Strong nurse leaders and administrators are important for clients (and their safety), for delivery systems (and their viability), and for payers (and their solvency). Some have called this the Age of the Nurse, but pressures remain to balance cost and quality considerations in a complex, chaotic, and turbulent health care environment. Although society's need for excellent nursing care remains the nurse's constant underlying reason for existence, nursing is in reality much more than that. It is the Age of the Nurse precisely because nurses offer cost-effective expertise in solving problems related to the coordination and delivery of health care to individuals and populations in society. Nurses are well prepared to lead clinical change strategies and to effectively manage the coordination and integration of interdisciplinary teams, population needs, and systems of care across the continuum. This is especially important as implementation of the 2010 Patient Protection and Affordable Care Act rolls forward and nurses are needed to address care coordination and integration.

It can be argued that nursing is a unique profession in which the primary focus is caring—giving and managing the care that clients need. Thus nurses are both health care providers and health care coordinators; that is, they have both clinical and managerial role components. Beginning with the first edition of *Leadership & Nursing Care Management,* it has been this text's philosophy that these two components can be discussed separately but in fact overlap. Because all nurses are involved in coordinating client care, leadership and management principles are a part of the core competencies they need to function in a complex health care environment.

The turbulent swirl of change in this country's health care industry has become a paradigm shift that has provided both challenges and opportunities for nursing. Nurses have needed a stronger background in nursing leadership and client care management to be prepared for contemporary and future nursing practice. As nurses mature in advanced practice roles and as the health care delivery system restructures, nurses will become increasingly pivotal to cost-effective health care delivery. Leadership and management are crucial skills and abilities for complex and integrated community and regional networks that employ and deploy nurses to provide health care services to clients and communities.

Today nurses are expected to be able to lead and manage care across the health care continuum—a radically different approach to nursing than has been the norm for hospital staff nursing practice. In all settings, including both nurse-run and interdisciplinary clinics, nursing leadership and management are complementary skills that add value to solid clinical care and client-oriented practice. Thus there is an urgent need to advance nurses' knowledge and skills in leadership and management. In addition, nurses who are expected to make and implement day-to-day management decisions need to know how these precepts can be practically applied to the organization and delivery of nursing care in a way that conserves scarce resources, reduces costs, and maintains or improves quality of care.

The primary modality for health care in the United States has moved away from acute care hospitalization. As prevention, wellness, and alternative sites for care delivery become more important, nursing's already rich experiential tradition of practice in these settings is emerging. This text reflects this contemporary trend by blending the hospital and nonhospital perspectives when examining and analyzing nursing care, leadership, and management. The reader will notice examples from the wide spectrum of nursing practice settings in the specific applications of nursing leadership and care management principles.

PURPOSE AND AUDIENCE

The intent of this text is to provide both a broad introduction to the field and a synthesis of the knowledge base and skills related to both nursing leadership and nursing management. It is an evidence-based blend of practice and theory. It breaks new ground by explaining the intersection of nursing care with leading people and managing organizations and systems. It highlights the evidence base for care management. It combines traditional management perspectives and theory with contemporary health care trends and issues and consistently integrates leadership and management concepts. These concepts are illustrated and made relevant by practice-based examples.

The impetus for writing this text comes from teaching both undergraduate and graduate students in nursing leadership and management and from perceiving the need for a comprehensive, practice-based textbook that blends and integrates leadership and management into an understandable and applicable whole.

Therefore the main goal of *Leadership and Nursing Care Management* is twofold: (1) to clearly differentiate traditional leadership and management perspectives, and (2) to relate them in an integrated way with contemporary nursing trends and practice applications. This textbook is designed to serve the needs of nurses and nursing students who seek a foundation in the principles of coordinating nursing services. It will serve the need for these principles in relation to client care, peers, superiors, and subordinates.

ORGANIZATION AND COVERAGE

This fifth edition continues the format first used with the third edition. The first two editions were Dr. Huber's single-authored texts. The edited book approach draws together the best thinking of experts in the field—both nurses and non-nurses—to enrich and deepen the presentation of core essential knowledge and skills. Beginning with the first edition, a hallmark of *Leadership and Nursing Care Management* has been its depth of coverage, its comprehensiveness, and its strong evidence-based foundation. This fifth edition continues the emphasis on explaining theory in an easily understandable way to enhance comprehension.

The content of this fifth edition has been reorganized and refreshed to integrate leadership and care management topics with the nurse executive leadership competencies of the 2005 American Organization of Nurse Executives (AONE) while trimming down the content through refocusing and synthesis. As the professional organization that speaks for nurse leaders, managers, and executives, AONE has identified the evidence-based core competencies in the field, and the content of this book has been aligned accordingly to reflect the knowledge underlying quality management of nursing services. This will help the reader develop the crucial skills and knowledge needed for core competencies.

The organizational framework of this book groups the 27 chapters into the following five parts:

Part I: Leadership aligns with the AONE competency category of the same name and provides an orientation to the basic principles of both leadership and management. Part I contains chapters on Leadership and Management Principles, Change and Innovation, and Organizational Climate and Culture.

Part II: Professionalism aligns with the AONE competency category of the same name and addresses the nurse's role and career development. The reader is prompted to examine the role of the nurse leader and manager. Part II discusses the content areas of Critical Thinking and Decision-Making Skills, Managing Time and Stress, and Legal and Ethical Issues.

Part III: Communication and Relationship Building aligns with the AONE competency category of the same name. Part III focuses on Communication Leadership, Team Building and Working with Effective Groups, Delegation, Power and Conflict, and Workplace Diversity. These are essential knowledge and skills areas for nurse leaders and managers as they work with and through others in care delivery.

Part IV: Knowledge of the Health Care Environment covers the AONE competency category of the same name and features a broad array of chapters. Part IV encompasses Case and Population Health Management, Organizational Structure, Decentralization and Shared Governance, Professional Practice Models, Evidence-Based Practice: Strategies for Nursing Leaders, Quality and Safety, and Measuring and Managing Outcomes. This discussion highlights the importance of understanding the health care system and the organizational structures within which nursing care delivery must operate. This section includes information on traditional organizational theory, professional practice models, and the dynamics of decentralized and shared governance.

Part V: Business Skills aligns with the AONE competency category on business skills and principles and contains an extensive grouping of chapters related to Strategic Management; Nursing Shortage; Recruitment and Retention; Staffing and Scheduling; Budgeting, Productivity, and Costing Out Nursing; Performance Appraisal; Prevention of Workplace Violence; All-Hazards Disaster Preparedness; Data Management and Informatics; and Marketing. These chapters discuss the opportunities and challenges for the nurse leader-manager when dealing with the health care workforce. The wide range of human resource responsibilities of nurse managers is reviewed, and resources for further study are provided. The significant share of scarce organization budgets consumed by the human resources of an institution makes this area of management a key challenge that requires intricate skills in leadership and management. This section examines some of the important factors that nurse leader-managers must consider in the nursing and health care environment. Also in this section are chapters that build on organizational theory and demonstrate the importance of integrating organizations and systems with the current technology and theory applications, including data management and informatics, strategic management, and marketing.

The 27 chapters in this text are organized into a consistent format that highlights the following features:
- Concept definitions
- Theoretical and research background
- Leadership and management implications
- Current issues and trends
- Case Study and Critical Thinking Exercise
- Research Note

This format is designed to bridge the gap between theory and practice and to increase the relevance of nursing leadership and management by demonstrating the way in which theory translates into behaviors appropriate to contemporary leadership and nursing care management.

TEXT FEATURES

This book contains several interesting and effective aids to readers' comprehension, critical thinking, and application.

Critical Thinking Exercises

Found at the end of each chapter, this feature challenges readers to inquire and reflect, to analyze critically the knowledge presented, and to apply it to the situation.

Research Notes

These summaries of current research studies are highlighted in every chapter and introduce the reader to the liveliness and applicability of the available literature in nursing leadership and management.

Case Studies

Found at the end of each chapter, these vignettes introduce the reader to the "real world" of nursing leadership and management and demonstrate the ways in which the chapter concepts operate in specific situations. These vignettes show the creativity and energy that characterize expert nurse administrators as they tackle issues in practice.

LEARNING AND TEACHING AIDS

For Students

The Evolve Student Resources for this book include the following:
- NCLEX *Review* Questions, including rationales and page references

For Instructors

The Evolve Instructor Resources for this book include the following:
- *TEACH for Nurses* Lesson Plans, based on textbook chapter Learning Objectives, serve as ready-made, modifiable lesson plans and a complete roadmap to link all parts of the educational package. These concise and straightforward lesson plans can be modified or combined to meet your particular scheduling and teaching needs.
- *Test Bank* in ExamView formats, featuring approximately 250 test items, complete with correct answer, rationale, cognitive level, nursing process

step, appropriate NCLEX label, and corresponding textbook page references. The ExamView program allows instructors to create new tests; edit, add, and delete test questions; sort questions by NCLEX category, cognitive level, and nursing process step; and administer and grade tests online.

- *PowerPoint Presentations* with more than 600 customizable lecture slides.
- *Audience Response Questions* for i-clicker and other systems with 2 to 3 multiple-answer questions per chapter to stimulate class discussion and assess student understanding of key concepts.

ACKNOWLEDGMENTS

This book is dedicated to my husband, Bob Huber. He made this book a reality and was the text and graphics support behind it. For his love, caring, and support, I am eternally grateful. To my children, Brad Gardner and Lisa Witte, and their spouses, Nonalee Gardner and John Witte, I am grateful for their enthusiasm and love. I am forever privileged that they are in my life. I thank them for the gifts of Kathryn Anne Gardner (the Princess), Anthony James Gardner (A.J.), Logan Thomas Witte, and Olivia Morgan Witte. I love being Grandma to these wonderful people. Also special are Chris Huber; Beth and Brad Nau and grandchildren Brandon, Danielle, Creighton, and the late Cameron Nau; and Von and Kirk Danielson and Kory, Ryan, and Sean Danielson.

To my professional colleagues who inspired me and served as examples of excellence in nursing, I am grateful. To my nursing students, past and future, my thanks for being a source of continual intellectual stimulation and challenge.

This book's first two editions evolved under the tender care of Thomas Eoyang, former Editorial Manager at W.B. Saunders Company, whose guidance, support, and caring were invaluable. To the editors in the Elsevier Nursing Division who worked so hard to facilitate everything related to the Fifth Edition, and to the excellent staff at Elsevier, a sincere thank you.

Diane L. Huber

CONTENTS

PART V   BUSINESS SKILLS

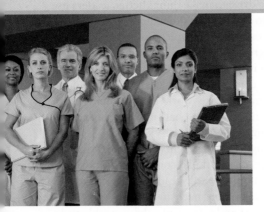

Leadership and Management Principles

Diane L. Huber

WEBSITE

http://evolve.elsevier.com/Huber/leadership/

LEADERSHIP AND CARE MANAGEMENT DIFFERENTIATED

In nursing, leadership is studied as a way of increasing the skills and abilities needed to facilitate clinical outcomes while working with people across a variety of situations and to increase understanding and control of the professional work setting. A long history and rich literature surround leadership theories, much of it from outside of nursing. Nursing has drawn from both classic and contemporary thinkers. Bennis (1994) made a strong argument for leadership, stating that quality of life depends on the quality of leaders. He noted three reasons why leaders are important: the character of change in society, the de-emphasis on integrity in institutions, and the responsibility for the effectiveness of organizations. Fiedler and Garcia (1987) argued that leadership is one of the most important factors that determine the survival and success of groups and organizations. *Effective* leadership is important in nursing for those same reasons, specifically because of its impact on the quality of nurses' work lives, being a stabilizing

influence during constant change, and for nurses' productivity and quality of care.

Leadership theory often is discussed separately from management theory. Some say leadership and management are two very different things. Yet clearly there is overlap in that one can be *both* leading and managing in some cases. The area of overlap may not be clear or explained. Some have seen management as a subset of leadership. The premise of this book is that leadership and management are not identical ideas. This can be seen in their distinct definitions.

If the delivery of nursing services involves the organization and coordination of complex activities in the human services realm, then both leadership and management are important elements. The leader's focus is on people; the manager focuses on systems and structure (Bennis, 1994). Thus although both are used to accomplish goals, each has a different focus. For example, a nurse may use leadership strategies or management strategies to motivate others, but the desired outcome of the motivation is likely to be different. However, leadership and management have some shared characteristics. In this area of overlap, the processes and strategies look similar and may be employed for a similar outcome or blended together to accomplish goals.

Leadership and management are equally important processes. Because they each have a different focus, their importance varies according to what is needed in a specific situation. Hersey and colleagues (2013) thought that leadership was a broader concept than management. They described management as a special kind of leadership. This view would position management as a part of leadership, not as a distinct concept. However, according to the definitions, characteristics, and processes, the concepts of leadership and management are different, but at the area of overlap they look similar. For example, directing occurs in both leadership and management activities (the area of overlap), whereas inspiring a vision is clearly a leadership function. Both leadership and management are necessary. Mintzberg's (1994) idea was that nursing management occurred in an interactive model rather than through a stepwise linear process.

An evidence-based approach to differentiating nursing leadership from management was taken to identify discrete competencies through an integrative content analysis of the literature base (Jennings et al., 2007). In 140 articles reviewed, they found 894 competencies, of which 862 (96%) were common to both leadership and management. Thus the overlap area appeared to be larger than previously thought. However, leadership and management do serve distinct purposes. Perhaps it is time to apply leadership and management concepts and competencies by setting, level of role responsibility, career stage, and social context to more fully apply the evidence base to practice.

The focus of each is different: management is focused on task accomplishment and leadership is focused on human relationship aspects. They may be sequential, and they are interrelated. Clearly, a balance of the two is necessary. There is a "gray area" in which the foci of their outcomes overlap. This overlap occurs where the two processes are integrated or synthesized to accomplish goals and where the same strategies are employed even though the goals may differ.

Leadership is an activity of human engagement and a relationship experience founded in trust, communication, inspiration, action, and "servanthood." The leadership role is so important because it embodies commitment and forward-reaching action. Arising from a drive to make things better, leaders use their power to bring teams together, spark innovation, create positive communication, and drive forward toward group goals.

Leadership is important to study, learn, and practice in today's complex, rapidly changing, turbulent, and chaotic health care work environment. Such an environment generates challenges to the nurse's identity, coping skills, and ability to work with others in harmony. It also presents the opportunity to lead, challenge assumptions, consolidate a purpose, and move a vision forward. Leadership is important for nurses because they need to possess knowledge and skill in the art and science of solving problems in work groups, systems of care, and the environment of care delivery. The effectiveness of an individual nurse depends partly on that individual's competence and partly on the creation of a facilitating environment that contains sufficient resources to accomplish goals. The nurse leader combines clinical, administrative, financial, and operational skills to solve problems in the care environment so that nurses can provide cost-effective care in a way that is satisfying and health promoting for patients and clients. Such an environment does not simply happen; it requires special skills and the courage and motivation to move a vision into action. Thus the study of nursing leadership and care management focuses critical thinking on what it takes to be a nursing "environment architect," transition leader, and manager of care delivery services.

"The nurse leader plays a critical role in the business of the healthcare organization and the quality and safety of the services provided" (O'Connor, 2008, p. 21). Strong evidence for the nurse leader's critical role both in the business of a health care organization and in the quality and safety of service delivery has been laid out by the Institute of Medicine (IOM) (2004), the American Nurses Credentialing Center's (ANCC) Magnet Recognition Program® (ANCC, 2008a, b), and the American Organization of Nurse Executives (AONE) (2005). The IOM focus is on the following five areas of management practice:

- Implementing evidence-based management
- Balancing tensions between efficiency and reliability
- Creating and sustaining trust

- Actively managing the change process through communication, feedback, training, sustained effort and attention, and worker involvement
- Creating a learning environment

The ANCC's magnet program acknowledges excellence in nursing services and leadership based on these five components: transformational leadership, structural empowerment, new knowledge, exemplary professional practice, and empirical outcomes (Wolf et al., 2008). The AONE 2005 nurse executive competencies are described in the following five domains of skill:

- Communication and relationship management
- Leadership
- Business skills and principles
- Knowledge of the health care environment
- Professionalism

Taken together, these source documents overlap and converge on the primary attributes, knowledge domains, and skills that nurse leaders need to lead people and manage organizations in health care.

THE TWO ROLES OF A NURSE

Nursing is a service profession whose core mission is the care and nurturing of human beings in their experiences of health and illness. Nurses have two basic roles: care providers and care coordinators. The first role is more often the role that is recognized. The acute care medical model in hospitals over time came to be the primary focus of attention and jobs for nurses. In this illness-focused model, the nurse's care provider or "doing" role was the most important and valued aspect of nursing. Little reward came from the "thinking" and integrating skills nurses were capable of. With a shift to primary care and care coordination, the nurse's care management role has become more prominent, needed, and valued. The delivery of nursing services involves the organization and coordination of complex activities. Nurses use managerial and leadership skills to facilitate delivery of quality nursing care.

THE LEADERSHIP ROLE

Leadership is a unique role and function. It can be part of a formal organizational managerial position, or it can arise spontaneously in any group. Certain characteristics, such as being motivated by challenge, commitment, and autonomy, are thought to be associated with leadership. Effectiveness is a key outcome of leadership efforts in health care. It has been suggested that there is a scarcity of leaders and a crisis in leadership in nursing. The IOM has raised awareness about patient safety and quality of care issues, and the Magnet Recognition Program® is one evidence-based nursing response. In times of chaos, complexity, and change, leadership is essential to provide the guidance, direction, and sense of stability needed to ensure followers' effectiveness and satisfaction.

The focus on leadership as a crucial need arises from the impact of significant changes that have occurred in the organization, delivery, and financing of health care during this period of time that has been characterized as turbulent and tumultuous because of "waves of chaos." Under such circumstances, nurses are challenged to respond with leadership. Nurses can best respond by demonstrating vision, adapting to changes, seeking new tools for dealing with the new health care environment, and leading the way with client-centered strategies.

Both nurses and the health care delivery systems in which they practice need leaders. Potential health care leaders likely will possess "a passion to make things better, a commitment to values, a focus on creativity and innovation, and the knowledge and skills necessary to identify health care needs and then to mobilize and array the human and other resources necessary to achieve goals and effect outcomes" (Huber & Watson, 2001, p. 29). Exhibiting quiet but respected competence, a leader may be the wise or go-to person within the group, a superior problem solver, a strategic communicator, or someone who is emotionally intelligent and strong in interpersonal relationship skills. Leaders may grow gradually out of a smoldering issue or erupt through a crisis event. Clearly, "something changes as leadership blossoms" (Huber & Watson, 2001, p. 29).

LEADERSHIP OVERVIEW

Leadership is a natural element of nursing practice because the majority of nurses practice in work groups or units. Possessing the license of an RN implies certain leadership skills and requires the ability to delegate and supervise the work of others. Leadership can be understood as the ability to inspire confidence and support among followers, especially in organizations in which competence and commitment produce performance.

Leadership Skills

Leadership is an important issue related to how nurses integrate the various elements of nursing practice to ensure the highest quality of care for clients. Every nurse needs two critical skills to enhance professional practice. One is a skill at interpersonal relationships. This is fundamental to leadership and the work of nursing. The second is skill in applying the problem-solving process. This involves the ability to think critically, to identify problems, and to develop objectivity and a degree of maturity or judgment. Leadership skills build on professional and clinical skills. Hersey and colleagues (2013) identified the following three skills needed for leading or influencing:

1. *Diagnosing:* Diagnosing involves being able to understand the situation and the problem to be solved or resolved. This is a cognitive competency.
2. *Adapting:* Adapting involves being able to adapt behaviors and other resources to match the situation. This is a behavioral competency.
3. *Communicating:* Communicating is used to advance the process in a way that individuals can understand and accept. This is a process competency.

Among the important personal leadership skills is emotional intelligence. Based on the work of Goleman (2007), relational and emotional integrity are hallmarks of good leaders. This is because the leader operates in a crucial cultural and contextual influencing mode. The leader's behavior, patterns of actions, attitude, and performance have a special impact on the team's attitude and behaviors and on the context and character of work life. Followers need to be able to depend on role consistency, balance, and behavioral integrity from the leader. The four skill sets needed by good leaders are as follows:

1. *Self-awareness:* Ability to read one's own emotional state and be aware of one's own mood and how this affects staff relationships
2. *Self-management:* Ability to take corrective action so as not to transfer negative moods to staff relationships
3. *Social awareness:* An intuitive skill of empathy and expressiveness in being sensitive and aware of the emotions and moods of others

4. *Relationship management:* Use of effective communication with others to disarm conflict, and the ability to develop the emotional maturity of team members

Gittell (2009) emphasized the centrality of relationship management because patient care is a coordination challenge. She noted that relational coordination drives quality and efficiency outcomes and health care performance. Relational coordination is defined as "coordinating work through relationships of shared goals, shared knowledge, and mutual respect" (p. xiii). Relational coordination focuses on relationships between roles rather than between individuals.

These interpersonal relationship skills are crucial to the work of leadership. The chaos and complexity of the seismic shifts in health care structure, delivery, form, technology, and content have made visible the urgent need for leaders to emerge, mobilize, and encourage followers. Leaders are pivotal for connecting the efforts of followers to organizational goals. This is both tricky and risky and may be overwhelming (Porter-O'Grady, 2003). However, good leaders are anchors to the vision and the larger mission, guides to coping and being productive, and champions of energy and enthusiasm for the work.

DEFINITIONS

There are a variety of definitions of leadership. **Leadership** is defined here as the process of influencing people to accomplish goals. Key concepts related to leadership are influence, communication, group process, goal attainment, and motivation. Hersey and colleagues (2013) defined leadership as a process of influencing the behavior of either an individual or a group, regardless of the reason, in an effort to achieve goals in a given situation. Burns (1978) noted that leadership occurs when human beings with motives and purposes mobilize in competition or conflict with others to arouse, engage, and satisfy motives.

Most leadership definitions incorporate the two components of an interaction among people and the process of influencing. Thus leadership is a social exchange phenomenon. At its core, leadership is about influencing people. In contrast, management involves influencing employees to meet an organization's goals and is focused primarily on organizational goals and objectives. Bennis (1994) listed a number of distinctions between leadership and management. He noted that the leader focuses on people, whereas the manager focuses on systems and structures. The leader innovates and conquers the context. Another distinction is that a leader innovates, whereas a manager administers. Kotter (2001) noted that managers cope with complexity whereas leaders cope with change.

Management is defined as the coordination and integration of resources through planning, organizing, coordinating, directing, and controlling to accomplish specific institutional goals and objectives. Hersey and colleagues (2013) defined management as the "process of working with and through individuals and groups and other resources (such as equipment, capital, and technology) to accomplish organizational goals" (p. 3). They identified management as a special kind of leadership that concentrates on the achievement of organizational goals. If this idea were visualized, it would appear as concentric circles—not as separate but overlapping circles.

Leadership is a broad concept and a process that can be applied to any group. Grant (1994) noted that leadership, management, and professionalism have different but related meanings, as follows:

- *Leadership:* Guiding, directing, teaching, and motivating to set and achieve goals
- *Management:* Resource coordination and integration to accomplish specific goals
- *Professionalism:* An approach to an occupation that distinguishes it from being merely a job, focuses on service as the highest ideal, follows a code of ethics, and is seen as a lifetime commitment

LEADERSHIP AND MANAGEMENT ROLES

A distinction can be made between leadership and management roles. Management activities are concerned with managing the resources of an organization. The idea of management can generate a negative reaction when it is equated with the "command and control" concept of authoritarian and bureaucratic organizations. These management models do not fit well with an environment that is constantly changing. Certain pressures influence the role of the manager and demand new skill sets to facilitate clinical work. Examples include when technology changes more quickly than clinicians are able to learn and adapt to

it, when management duties extend to include temporary workers employed by others (e.g., outsourced functions and agency nurses), and when a radical organizational shift to an accountable care organization (ACO) is necessary. The demands of management work are increasing in amount, scope, complexity, and intensity and thus increase role stress and leave less time to plan and focus on unit management (Porter-O'Grady, 2003).

BACKGROUND ON LEADERSHIP

Terms related to leadership are *leadership styles, followership*, and *empowerment*. **Leadership styles** are defined as different combinations of task and relationship behaviors used to influence others to accomplish goals. **Followership** is defined as an interpersonal process of participation. **Empowerment** means giving people the authority, responsibility, and freedom to act on their expert knowledge and skills.

Leadership can be best understood as a process. Much attention has been focused on leadership as a group and organizational process because organizational change is heavily influenced by the context or environment. Nurses need to have a solid foundation of knowledge in leadership and care management. This applies at all levels: nurse care provider, nurse manager, and nurse executive. However, the depth and focus of care management roles and skills may vary by level. For example, the nurse care provider concentrates on the coordination of nursing care to individuals or groups. This may include such activities as arranging access to services, providing direct care, doing referrals, and supporting a patient's family. At the next level, the nurse manager concentrates on the day-to-day administration and coordination of services provided by a group of nurses. The nurse executive's role and function concentrate on long-term administration of an institution or program that delivers nursing services, focusing on integrating the system and building a culture (Mintzberg, 1998).

LEADERSHIP: FIVE INTERWOVEN ASPECTS

Hersey and colleagues (2013) noted that the leadership process is a function of the leader, the followers, and other situational variables. The leadership

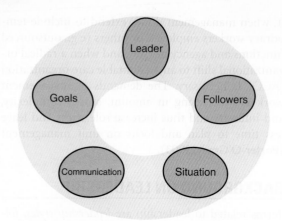

FIGURE 1-1 Components of a leadership moment.

process includes five interwoven aspects: (1) the leader, (2) the follower, (3) the situation, (4) the communication process, and (5) the goals (Kison, 1989). Figure 1-1 shows how these components relate to one another. All five elements interact within any given leadership moment.

Process Part 1: The Leader

The values, skills, and style of leaders are important. Their internalized pattern of basic behaviors influences actions and the ability to lead. Leaders' perceptions of themselves, their roles, and their expectations also have an impact on their followers. Self-awareness is crucial to leadership effectiveness and is the focus for many leadership exercises. Internal forces in leaders that impinge on leadership style are values, confidence in employees, leadership inclinations, and sense of security in uncertainty (Tannenbaum & Schmidt, 1973). Interpersonal, emotional, and social intelligence skills also contribute to the effective leadership of knowledge workers (Goleman, 2007; Porter-O'Grady, 2003).

Process Part 2: The Follower

Followership is the flip side of leadership. It is likely that without followers there is no leadership. Followers are vital because they accept or reject the leader and determine the leader's personal power (Hersey et al., 2013). Followers also need self-awareness to know themselves and their expectations. Situations in which members of a group are not accustomed to working together or do not hold shared expectations frequently lead to conflict. Groups have personalities that include a discernible

level of trust. The wise leader assesses the trust and readiness to change levels of the group. Followership is not as simple as it seems (see Followership section).

Process Part 3: The Situation

The specific circumstances surrounding any given leadership situation will vary. Elements such as work demands, control systems, amount of task structure, degree of interaction, amount of time available for decision making, and external environment shape the differences among situations (Hersey et al., 2013). Organizational culture and ethos also are important factors in the situation. For example, in one setting the culture may resemble one big happy family, with an emphasis on teamwork and morale boosting. The cultural aspects of that leadership situation are different from those of an organization in which there is a fast-paced tempo and people seem very busy. Environmental or cultural differences also cause the leadership situation to vary. The leadership situation in a group that is knowledgeable and experienced in solving problems is very different from the leadership situation in a group that is not experienced at the task or at working together. The personality styles of both superiors and subordinates have an influence on the situation, the work demands, and the amount of time and resources available.

Process Part 4: Communication

Communication processes vary among groups regarding the patterns and channels used and how open or closed the communication flow is. Communicating is basic to the process of influencing and thus to leadership. Almost every issue or problem contains a communication aspect. Through communication, the leader's vision and message are received by the followers. After choosing a channel, the sender transmits a message. However, the message is filtered through the receiver's perception. Communication is transmitted through both verbal and nonverbal modes. Organizations include a variety of communication structures and flows. These may be downward, upward, horizontal, grapevines, or networks. Communication may be formal or informal (Hersey et al., 2013). Certain acts performed by leaders have positive effects and make people feel more respected; listening and informal chatting are prime examples (Alvesson & Sveningsson, 2003).

Process Part 5: Goals

Organizations have goals, and individuals working in organizations also have goals. These goals may or may not be congruent. For example, the goal of the organization may be to decrease costs or increase revenue. In contrast, the goal of the individual nurse may be to spend time counseling and teaching clients because that is what is seen by the nurse as the most important activity. Goals may thus be in conflict, in which case there is tension and a need for leadership.

Clearly, leadership is a complex and multidimensional process. Nurses need to be aware of the interacting elements in any leadership situation. Critical thinking can be applied to:

1. Diagnosing and analyzing the five elements,
2. Adapting to the situation, and
3. Communicating for effectiveness.

For example, if a nurse works in a situation in which there is a high level of frustration, it may be time to step back and analyze the basic five elements. Doing so sets the stage for better decision making about change strategies and strategic management.

LEADERSHIP THEORIES

Hersey and colleagues (2013) have done a thorough overview of leadership and organizational theory through the situational leadership school of thought. From an early awareness of the leader's need to be concerned about both tasks and human relationships (output and people) sprang a long history of leadership theories that can be grouped as *trait, attitudinal,* and *situational* (Hersey et al., 2013). The trait approach focuses on identifying specific characteristics of leaders. The attitudinal approach measures attitudes toward leader behavior. The situational approach focuses on observed behaviors of leaders and how leadership styles can be matched to situations. Leadership theories have evolved away from an early focus on the traits or characteristics of the leader as a person because it was found that it is not possible to predict leadership from clusters of traits. However, several authors have developed lists of traits common to good leaders (Bass, 1985; Bennis & Nanus, 1985), and interest remains in the characteristics to look for in good leaders. Further background on the history of leadership research can be found online (e.g., *www.sedl.org/change/leadership/history.html*).

Trait Theories
Characteristics of Leadership

In the trait approach, theorists have sought to understand leadership by examining the characteristics of leaders. Presumably, leaders could be differentiated from non-leaders. The trait approach has generated multiple lists of traits proposed to be essential to leadership. Bennis (1994) identified a recipe for leadership that contained six ingredients: a guiding vision, passion, integrity (including self-knowledge, candor, and maturity), trust, curiosity, and daring. Leaders arise in a context, and they are said to be made, not born. They appear to learn leadership skills in stages (Bennis, 2004). Thus leadership skills can be both taught and learned. It is important for nurses to recognize that they can learn, practice, and improve their personal leadership competencies.

Drucker (1996) noted that effective leaders know the following four things:

1. The only definition of a leader is someone who has followers.
2. Popularity is not leadership; results are.
3. Leaders are visible and set examples.
4. Leadership is not rank but responsibility.

Leaders need to ask the right questions, such as these: What needs to be done? What can I do to make a difference? What are the goals? What constitutes performance and results?

Leaders are active, not passive. The risk-taking element of leadership involves taking action. Leaders engage their environment with behaviors of doing, influencing, and moving. These are action terms. Pagonis (1992) noted that to lead successfully a leader must demonstrate two active, essential, and interrelated traits: expertise and empathy. Leaders are those who talk about adventures into new territory and take the risks inherent in innovation (Kouzes & Posner, 1995). Leadership means giving guidance and using a focused vision.

A leader may see the need to chart a course that is new or unknown, unpopular, or risky because it challenges those with vested interests who have much to lose. In a way, nursing's struggle for greater economic parity in health care is courageous and risky. Clancy (2003) noted that leaders need to "consistently find the courage to hold true to their beliefs and convictions" (p. 128). Both ethical fitness and moral courage form the backbone of making necessary and hard—but right and unpopular—decisions. Cost containment, patient's rights, safe staffing, stress and anger, and ethical dilemmas all challenge the leader to identify right from wrong and act from his or her sense of conviction. The leadership courage continuum runs from "good coward" (cannot muster courage to make tough choices) to "reckless courage" (shoot from the hip). Leaders need to be willing to make tough choices plus overcome the fear associated with them.

Research by Bennis and Thomas (2002) indicated that extraordinary leaders possess skills required to overcome adversity and emerge stronger and more committed. They suggest that "one of the most reliable indicators and predictors of true leadership is an individual's ability to find meaning in negative events and to learn from even the most trying circumstances" (Bennis & Thomas, 2002, p. 39). "Crucible" experiences shape leaders. These are trials, tests, and transformative experiences that force leaders to question themselves and what matters and to hone their judgment. Consequently, leaders come to a new or altered sense of identity. Crucible experiences can occur from positive or negative triggers, but leaders see them as opportunities for reinvention. Great leaders possess the following four essential skills:

1. The ability to engage others in shared meaning
2. A distinctive and compelling vocal tone
3. A sense of integrity
4. A combination of hardiness and ability to grasp context, called "adaptive capacity"

Characteristics such as knowledge, motivating people to work harder, trust, communication, enthusiasm, vision, courage, ability to see the big picture, and ability to take risks are associated with important leadership qualities in research findings. For example, Bennis and Nanus (1985) studied 90 chief executives from 1978 to 1983 and found that there were two key leadership traits. One is a guiding set of concepts, and the other is the ability to communicate a vision. Kouzes and Posner (1995) defined the following five behaviors that correlated with leadership excellence:

1. *Challenging the process:* Leaders go beyond the status quo to search for opportunities, experiment, and take risks to achieve lofty goals.
2. *Inspiring shared vision:* Leaders envision the future and enlist others in sharing the dream.
3. *Enabling others to act:* Leaders foster collaboration and develop and strengthen others so that the whole team performs well.
4. *Modeling the way:* Leaders set an example and structure events so that incremental progress is celebrated as small wins.
5. *Encouraging the heart:* Leaders appreciate and recognize individual contributions and formally celebrate accomplishments.

These five practices can be seen as the way leaders get extraordinary things done through people in an organization. The practices and qualities of leadership help nurses enrich their own style and contribute to a more productive workplace. This model of leadership has been used in nursing research (Patrick et al., 2011).

One research-based nursing model (Mathena, 2002) identified the following six core behaviors critical for nursing leadership success:

1. Visioning
2. Interdisciplinary team building
3. Workload complexity analysis
4. Work process analysis
5. Stakeholder analysis
6. Interactive planning

Vision and Trust

Although the lists of leadership characteristics and competencies vary somewhat, the functions of visioning, setting the direction, inspiration, motivation, and enabling systems and followers are at the core of leadership activity. Bennis (1994) discussed what has come to be called "the vision thing." The one specific defining quality of leaders is vision—the ability to create a vision and put it into operation.

Leadership is founded on trust: "Trust is the emotional glue that binds leaders and employees together and is a measure of the legitimacy of leadership" (Malloch, 2002, p. 14). Organizations that focus on sustaining a healing culture rebuild organizational trust by focusing on trust in relationships with employees. Behaviors that build trust include sharing relevant information, reducing controls, and meeting expectations. Trust-destroying behaviors include being insensitive to beliefs and values, avoiding discussion of sensitive issues, and encouraging competition via winners and losers. Nurses can be aware of the crucial nature of trust in the leadership and management relationship. Trust goes both ways and needs to be nurtured. Nurses can start by examining their own behaviors and then taking deliberative actions to strengthen trust in the environment.

Followers expect that leaders will provide a sense of vision and a sense of direction with standards for achieving the group's goals. Leaders can create an environment that is positively charged for productivity or that allows followers to languish without direction or mission. It is possible that leaders can create a negative climate that becomes destructive to the group. If the leader plays a major role in creating a group's culture and ethos, then closing down communication, breeding distrust and competition, and neglecting positive motivation can sow the seeds of group disintegration. Thus the characteristics possessed and used by the leader can make a crucial difference in the functioning and effectiveness of any group.

Leadership *Dos* and *Don'ts*

The long history of leadership theory has highlighted the importance of focusing on both of the two basic leadership elements of tasks and relationships. These are core to all leadership in all situations. The Trait Approach has led to long lists of skills and characteristics associated with successful leaders. These can be distilled into leadership *dos* and *don'ts.*

A profile of leaderships *dos* includes honesty, energy, drive, tenacity, creativity, flexibility, visibility, emotional stability, knowledge, conceptual skills, and leadership motivation. Among these characteristics, honesty (defined as trustworthiness) and energy are at the top of the list. Leadership is founded on trust and does not survive without it. Leadership is hard, sustained work that requires a great deal of energy and sputters without it.

A profile of leadership *don'ts* includes untrustworthiness, insensitivity to others, aloofness, over-managing, abrasiveness, inability to think strategically or staff effectively, inability to build a team, and focusing on internal organizational politics (overly ambitious). Among these characteristics, untrustworthiness is a fatal flaw, and insensitivity

to others is a likely cause for ineffective leadership (Hersey et al., 2013).

Leadership Styles

As leadership theories evolved, leadership came to be viewed as a dynamic process and an interaction among the leader, the followers, and the situation. Leadership theory began to move beyond a focus on traits to explore the concept of leadership styles. Styles of leadership range from authoritarian to permissive to democratic and from transactional to transformational. The individual nurse's task is to determine in which environments he or she functions best and is most comfortable or where he or she most likely will succeed. This facilitates placement for success and a better match between leader and follower.

Leadership styles are defined as different combinations of task and relationship behaviors used to influence others to accomplish goals. They are sets or clusters of behaviors used in the process of effecting leadership. Leaders need to be concerned about both tasks to be accomplished and human relationships in groups and organizations. Hersey and colleagues (2013) said that leadership styles are the consistent behavior patterns exhibited in influencing the activities of others by working with and through them, as perceived by those others. Different styles evoke variable responses in different situations. The way people influence others through actions taken and the perspectives of other people is related to leadership efforts and constitutes leadership style. The two major leadership terms are *task behavior* and *relationship behavior,* and a leader's leadership style is some combination of task and relationship behavior. Hersey and colleagues (2013) defined these terms as follows:

- *Task behavior:* The extent to which leaders organize and define roles; explain activities; determine when, where, and how tasks are to be accomplished; and endeavor to get work accomplished
- *Relationship behavior:* The extent to which leaders maintain personal relationships by opening communication and providing psychoemotional support and facilitating behaviors

Tannenbaum and Schmidt (1973) suggested that a leader might select one of many behavior styles arrayed along a continuum. The continuum ranges from democratic to authoritarian (or subordinate-centered

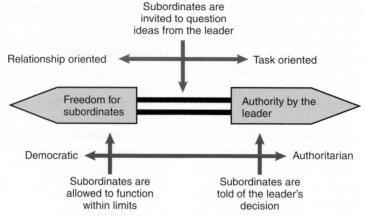

FIGURE 1-2 Continuum of leader behavior.

to leader-centered). Their work suggested that there are a variety of leadership styles (Figure 1-2) or points along the continuum. They discussed three distinct styles: authoritarian, democratic, and laissez-faire. Some individuals are able to integrate styles and flexibly match to the situation at hand, but this is rare.

Authoritarian. The authoritarian leadership style uses primarily directive behaviors. Decisions of policy are made solely by the leader who tends to dictate tasks and techniques to followers. Leaders tell the followers what to do and how to do it. This style emphasizes a high concern for task. Authoritarian leaders are characterized by giving orders. Their style can create hostility and dependency among followers; it may also stifle creativity and innovation. On the other hand, this style can be very efficient, especially in a crisis.

Democratic. This approach implies a relationship and person orientation. Policies are a matter of group discussion and decision. The leader encourages and assists discussion and group decision making. Human relations and teamwork are the focus. The leader shares responsibility with the followers by involving them in decision making. In nursing, interdisciplinary teamwork is a major element in effectiveness. The democratic style makes output appear to move more slowly and is thought to take longer than using an authoritarian style. Group consensus needs time and facilitation to be fostered. Furthermore, the needs of disenfranchised minority groups must be balanced. Intergroup cohesion is a focus with this style. The challenge of the democratic style is to get people with different professional backgrounds, personal biases,

and psychological needs together to focus on the problem and next action steps. Motivating participation is a constant challenge.

Laissez-Faire. This style promotes complete freedom for group or individual decisions. There is a minimum of leader participation. A leader using this style may seem to be apathetic. Because the style is based on noninterference, a clear decision may never be formulated. The laissez-faire style results in a decision, conscious or otherwise, to avoid interference and let events take their own course. The leader is either permissive and fosters freedom or is inept at guiding a group. Followers may need greater structure than the leader gives them. Despite its potential drawbacks, this style has advantages when used with groups of fully independent care providers or professionals working together.

Overall, one style is not necessarily better than another. Each has advantages and disadvantages. There are situational and contextual factors to consider when choosing a style. Styles should vary according to the appropriateness of the situation with reference to an evaluation of effectiveness. Flexibility is important. For example, if a nurse prefers to operate in a democratic style yet suddenly a code situation occurs, then the nurse must rapidly switch from a democratic to an authoritarian style. Some democratic leaders cannot vary their style sufficiently to handle crises. On the other hand, in a staff meeting, an authoritarian leader may be ineffective with a group of professionals and would need to be flexible enough to switch to a democratic or laissez-faire style, depending on the circumstances. The basic needs are for leader self-awareness and knowledge of the group's ability and willingness levels before examining the situational elements and choosing a leadership style. Self-awareness is key to strategically using leadership styles.

Feminist Leadership Perspective

Leadership styles appear to have a gender component. The feminist perspective on leadership was presented by Helgeson (1995a, b). She identified female leadership as a weblike structure—dynamic and continuously expanding and contracting. It is characterized by a concern for family, community, and culture. The inclination is for a democratic power style, and the emphasis is on the importance of establishing relationships, maintaining connections with others, and deriving strength from empowering others. By contrast, leadership approaches described by men tend to be influenced by the military and participating in team sports. Men tend to spend their time on meetings and tasks requiring immediate attention, focusing on completion of tasks and achievement of goals. Women tend to focus on process; men tend to focus on achievement and closure. Women tend to be more flexible and value cooperation, connectedness, and relationships. Exploring the feminist perspective on leadership is valuable in that it provides food for thought as health care organizations and the nurses working in them struggle with not wanting to let go of the familiar hierarchy management style yet needing to reconfigure to the circular or web structure to be effective. It is not known whether gender differences are permanent characteristics or are culturally mediated artifacts that blur with time.

ATTITUDINAL LEADERSHIP THEORIES

Hersey and colleagues (2013) identified a second approach to leadership research that focused on the measurement of attitudes or predispositions toward leader behavior. Occurring mainly between 1945 and the mid-1960s, the attitudinal approaches began with the Ohio State Leadership Studies and included the Michigan Leadership Studies, Group Dynamics Studies, and Blake and McCanse's Leadership Grid.

Leader behavior was described as having two separate dimensions, as follows:

1. Initiating structure and consideration in the Ohio State Leadership Studies
2. Employee orientation and production orientation in the Michigan Leadership Studies

These dimensions are similar to the authoritarian (or task) and democratic (or relationship) ideas of the leader behavior continuum. The Group Dynamics Studies highlighted goal achievement (similar to task) and group maintenance (similar to relationship) elements of leadership behavior (Cartwright & Zander, 1960).

Blake and Mouton (1964) used task and relationship concepts in their grid, which was later modified by Blake and McCanse (1991). The following five types of leadership or management styles, based on concern for production (task) and concern for people (relationship), emerged:

1. *Impoverished:* This style uses minimal effort to get the work done.
2. *Country club:* This approach emphasizes attention to the needs of people to effect satisfying relationships.
3. *Authority-obedience:* This style strives for efficiency in operations.
4. *Organizational man:* This approach works on balancing the necessity to accomplish the task with maintaining morale.
5. *Team:* This style promotes work accomplishment from committed people and interdependence through a common cause, leading to trust and respect.

Hersey and colleagues (2013) noted that Blake and Mouton's (1964) conceptualization tended to be an attitudinal model that measured the values and feelings of managers, whereas the Ohio State model included both attitudes and behaviors and focused on leadership. Both the leadership style (task versus relationship) and the attitude of the leader about leadership behaviors are important. However, attitudinal theories still did not fully capture the leadership experience because the environment and its complexity were not factored in.

Situational Theories

A third phase of leadership theories grew out of a group of contingency theories whose central idea was that organizational behavior is contingent on the situation or environment. This means that which theory or style is the best all depends on the situation at hand. What is needed by the leader is diagnostic ability. The leader observes and analyzes which abilities and motives are present in the followers. With sensitivity, cues in the environment can be identified and used to make choices regarding leadership style. One choice a leader has is to alter his or her own behavior and the leadership style used. Personal flexibility and leadership skills are needed to vary one's style when the followers' needs and motives change or vary. The ability to diagnose, choose, and alter behavior to implement a leadership style best matched to the situation is a critical skill needed for effective leadership. Thus no one leadership style is optimal in all situations. The nature of the situation needs to be considered. Styles can be chosen to match the situation (Hersey et al., 2013).

Fiedler's Contingency Theory

As situations become more complex, leadership becomes more difficult. Fiedler (1967) developed a Leadership Contingency Model to explain how to apply this idea. He classified group situational variables of leader-member relations, task structure, and position power into eight possible combinations, ranging from high to low on these three major variables. *Leader-member relations* refers to the type and quality of the leader's personal relationships with followers. *Task structure* means how structured the group's assigned task is. *Position power* refers to power that is conferred on the leader by the organization as a result of the assigned job. Fiedler examined the favorableness of the situation from the perspective of the leader's influence over the group. The most favorable situation occurs with good leader-member relations, high task structure, and high position power. The least favorable situation occurs when the leader is disliked, has an unstructured task, and has little position power. With Fiedler's model, group situations can be analyzed to determine the most effective leadership style.

Fiedler (1967) examined which style (task-oriented versus relationship-oriented) would be most effective for each of eight situations. A key general principle is that the need for task-oriented leaders occurs when the situation is either highly favorable or very unfavorable. A task-oriented style is needed for situations on the extremes, whereas a relationship-oriented style is needed when the situation is moderately favorable.

For example, a staff nurse goes into a nursing unit meeting not wanting any extra assignments but hoping that some of the ongoing problems will be solved. If the nurse has a reasonably good relationship with the leader, the leader should use a high-relationship style with the nurse. The leader should use selling, convincing, encouraging, and motivating strategies. The leader should make the nurse feel good about his or her ability to accomplish a task, provide something of quality, and work with other people. If, however, the staff nurse's mind is closed about any changes or if passive-aggressive or subversive actions occur, then the leader needs be more directive. A possible reaction might be to give the nurse an assigned task. On the extremes of highly favorable or highly unfavorable situations, leaders need to use task-oriented behavior to get the work moving. In the middle of the continuum, a high-relationship style is needed, again to foster productivity.

In Situational Leadership® theory,* leadership in groups is never a static circumstance. The situation is dynamic and subject to change. In a very difficult situation, relationships may be the leader's preferred emphasis. However, if interpersonal relationships are not an immediate problem or if the group is on the verge of collapse, then strong authoritative direction is needed to get the group moving and accomplishing. For this situation, the task-oriented leader is a more effective match between leader and job. However, groups do not remain static; they move back and forth through stages. When the problem no longer is just the need to get the group moving but also includes solving numerous interpersonal conflicts, a relationship-oriented leader is better matched to the situation. Eventually, as the situation progresses, a relationship-oriented leader can become less effective. This occurs because once the group has less conflict, individuals may begin to coast along and positive motivation may be lost as individuals become apathetic. Once again, a task-oriented style is called for—challenging individuals by using the motivation they need to continue to produce. Because of the factor of constant change, maintaining good leadership is complicated for

---

any group. One way to foster effective leadership is to evaluate leaders according to Fiedler's contingency model (1967) and then use this information to increase leaders' awareness of their natural style tendency: relationship-oriented or task-oriented. Fiedler's measure for leadership style is the Least Preferred Coworker (LPC) scale (Fiedler & Chemers, 1984). The LPC is an 18-item semantic differential scale that is the personality measure of Fiedler's contingency model (Fiedler & Garcia, 1987).

Favorable or unfavorable situations are determined in part by the receptivity of the followers, but they are also determined by whether the larger environment is positive or negative. An example of an unfavorable situation in nursing is the following:

> *A nurse's job is to lead and manage a hospital's critical care area, which has serious morale problems. The nurse is new and has a master's degree but soon discovers that a majority of the followers have long tenure on the unit and both educational and experiential backgrounds that are very different. There may be values clashes between the leader and the followers. The task is to change the environment, but the nurse discovers that this work group has maintained its traditions over a long period.*

This is an unfavorable situation and a leadership challenge. Fiedler's theory (1967) suggests that the best leadership style under unfavorable circumstances is task-oriented.

Hersey and Blanchard's Tri-Dimensional Leader Effectiveness Model

Hersey and colleagues (2013) described the Tri-Dimensional Leader Effectiveness Model first developed by Hersey and Blanchard. First, a two-dimensional model was constructed, in which task behavior and relationship behavior were displayed on a grid from high to low and were divided into four quadrants: (1) high task, low relationship; (2) high task, high relationship; (3) high relationship, low task; and (4) low task, low relationship (Figure 1-3). These quadrants represent four basic leadership styles: telling, selling, participating, and delegating. As applied to the continuum of authoritarian versus democratic styles, telling would be authoritarian and participating would be democratic. The two most common

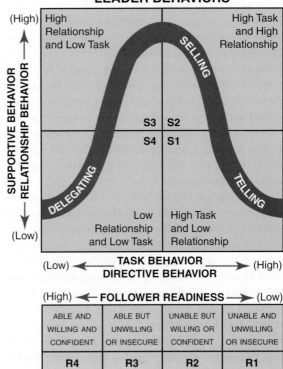

FIGURE 1-3 Expanded Situational Leadership® model. (© Copyright 2006. Reprinted with permission of the Center for Leadership Studies, Inc., Escondido, CA 92025. All rights reserved.)

leadership styles are selling and participating. Selling requires the most from a leader, who must provide high amounts of guidance and support. Movement into a participative leadership style requires much less structure and task-directive behavior from the leader because the individual or group is performing but is not quite confident enough in its own ability for the leader to completely let go. The individual or group wants to talk about things.

To choose an appropriate style, the leader needs to be knowledgeable about the readiness of the followers. This leads to the third dimension of effectiveness. *Effectiveness* is defined as how appropriately a given leader's style interrelates with a given situation. The third dimension is the environment in which a leader operates and which interacts with the leader's style.

Overlaid on the basic grid is a continuum of readiness ranging from low to high. *Readiness* has two aspects: ability and willingness. Job *ability* is based on the amount of past job experience, job knowledge, ability to solve problems, ability to take responsibility, and ability to meet deadlines. This forms a composite of the ability to do the job. The other part of readiness is psychological *willingness,* which means being willing to take responsibility and have a positive attitude toward accepting the obligation to complete a task. Psychological readiness is manifested by willingness to take some risk and by accepting the job requirements. It includes achievement motivation, wanting to do well, persistence, a work attitude, and a sense of independence. These factors create a willingness to take on and complete a job. Hersey and colleagues (2013) combined ability and willingness into four levels of readiness. Level 1 is unable and unwilling or insecure. Level 2 is unable but willing or confident. Level 3 is able but unwilling or insecure. Level 4 is able and willing or confident. These readiness levels can be matched with the corresponding leadership styles of level 1 with telling, level 2 with selling, level 3 with participating, and level 4 with delegating. Thus readiness assessment can help predict appropriate leadership style selection.

Hersey and colleagues (2013) emphasized the importance of the readiness of followers. Readiness can be applied to a work group. Have the members worked together for a long time in the job, or are they new employees? The culture is more solidified in a work group that has worked together for many years on a particular unit. The leader's leadership style would have to take into account where the followers are in terms of their readiness as a critical factor for determining the style to choose. Using leadership theory, leaders assess themselves, look at the followers' readiness, and assess the situation to determine whether it is favorable or unfavorable. Then a telling, selling, participating, or delegating style is selected.

For example, telling is an appropriate leadership style to use with followers who are at the novice level and with followers who are not able or willing. For example, a nurse is appointed as chair of a committee. First, the nurse might undertake a leadership analysis to determine whether this group needs high-relationship behaviors. If they do not know each other and the situation is politically charged, the nurse leader needs to help people become comfortable with each other. If the nurse leader is a task-oriented person, a high-relationship person may need to be called on to assist the group process so that it is facilitated and becomes effective.

One currently accepted view of organizational behavior describes leadership as situational or contingent and concerned with what produces effectiveness. Hersey and colleagues (2013) noted that the common themes include the following: the leader needs to be flexible in behavior, able to diagnose the leadership style appropriate to the situation, and able to apply the appropriate style. Thus there is no one best way to influence others or one best style. Their Situational Leadership® is a synthesis of the interplay among task behavior, relationship behavior, and the readiness of the followers.

TRANSACTIONAL AND TRANSFORMATIONAL LEADERSHIP

After the eras of trait, attitudinal, and Situational Leadership® theories, an interest arose in how leaders produced quantum results. Burns (1978) and Dunham and Klafehn (1990) broadened the concept of leadership styles to include two types of leaders: the transactional leader and the transformational leader.

A *transactional leader* is defined as a leader or manager who functions in a caregiver role and is focused on day-to-day operations. Such leaders survey their followers' needs and set goals for them based on what can be expected from the followers. A transactional leader is focused on the maintenance and management of ongoing and routine work.

A *transformational leader* is defined as a leader who motivates followers to perform to their full potential over time by influencing a change in perceptions and by providing a sense of direction. Transformational leaders use charisma, individualized consideration, and intellectual stimulation to produce greater effort, effectiveness, and satisfaction in followers (Bass & Avolio, 1990). Figure 1-4 distinguishes between transactional and transformational leadership.

The transactional leader is more common. This type of leader approaches followers in an exchange posture, with the purpose of exchanging one thing for another, such as a politician who promises jobs for votes. Burns (1978) said that transactional leadership

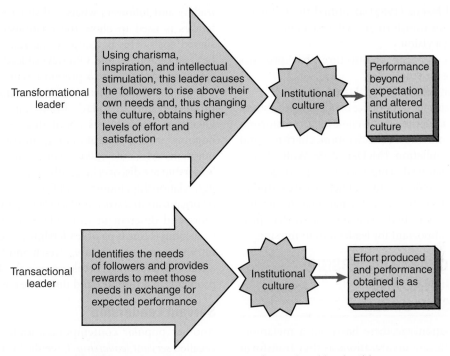

FIGURE 1-4 Transactional and transformational leadership.

occurs when the leader takes the initiative in contacting others for the exchange of valued things. Therefore transactional leadership is comparable to a bargain or contract for mutual benefits that aids the individual differences of both the leader and the follower. Key characteristics are contingent rewards and management-by-exception. Expected effort and expected performance are the outcomes. The transactional leader works within the existing organizational culture and is an essential component of effective leadership (Bass & Avolio, 1990). Examples would be the exchange of a salary for the services of a nurse to provide care or when a leader offers release time or paid time to entice staff members to do project or committee work. Continuous or incremental change, the first order of change, can be handled well at the transactional level.

Transformational leadership occurs when persons engage with others so that leaders and followers raise each other to higher levels of motivation and ethical decision making (Burns, 1978). Instead of emphasizing differences between the leader and the followers, transformational leadership focuses on collective purpose and mutual growth and development.

Transformational leadership augments transactional leadership by being committed, having a vision, and empowering others to heighten motivation in a way that attains extra effort beyond performance expectations. Transformational leadership is used for higher-order change and to change the organization's culture. Circumstances of growth, change, and crisis call forth transformational leaders (Bass & Avolio, 1990).

The American Nurses Credentialing Center's (ANCC) Magnet Recognition Program® has emphasized transformational leadership. A transformational leadership style has been shown to generate greater follower commitment, follower satisfaction, and overall effectiveness (Kleinman, 2004). In nursing homes, the most transformative style of top managers (consensus managers) was found to be associated with better quality outcomes (Castle & Decker, 2011). As health care is transforming, so too must nurse leaders transform organizational values, beliefs, and behaviors to lead people to where they need to be for the future. The ANCC (2008a, p. 52) noted: "Such leadership requires vision, influence, clinical knowledge, and expertise as well as an understanding that transformation may require atypical solutions and create turbulence."

Bennis and Nanus (1985) identified the following four activities for transformational leadership:

1. Creating a vision
2. Building a social architecture that provides meaning for employees
3. Sustaining organizational trust
4. Recognizing the importance of building self-esteem

Three factors underlie effectiveness as a transformational leader: individual consideration, charisma, and intellectual stimulation (McDaniel & Wolf, 1992). Transformational leadership was the type of leadership most often reported in magnet research studies (Upenieks, 2003a, b). Transformational leadership qualities appear to be better suited to the work of professionals and important for leadership in nursing.

CONTEMPORARY LEADERSHIP: INTERACTIONAL AND RELATIONSHIP-BASED

In the information age there has been a metamorphosis in health care organizations as they transform into knowledge or learning organizations. Nurses are knowledge workers who use expertise and specialized knowledge in the care of patients. They need matching organizations that will value, nurture, and foster the acquisition of the data, information, and knowledge needed for effectiveness. Today's health care environments demand that frontline workers such as nurses have and maintain the expertise and the information necessary to take action to solve problems, and they need leadership that is interactional, relational, and transformational at all levels.

Arising in conjunction with the application of complexity theory and chaos theory, leadership was described by Wheatley (1992) as being simpler, less stressful, and more appropriate to complex organizations in the midst of chaos. Her view of leadership emphasized the importance of connectedness and relationships within self-organizing systems. Nursing has a natural niche within interactional and relationship leadership theories. Optimal health care delivery is truly interdisciplinary and holistic. When connections and relationships are strong, patients benefit.

Quantum Leadership

Contemporary definitions of leadership describe leadership as being the result of a relationship between leaders and followers where a distinct set of competencies is used to allow the relationship to achieve shared goals. This is complex and requires nurses to be creative and flexible. Old ways of leading and managing are insufficient to present circumstances. Thus it is proposed that "quantum" leadership is needed to produce results in today's health care environment. Quantum leadership is about discovering—it is an ongoing process of exploration, curiosity, and asking questions (McCauley, 2005). The elements of quantum leadership are discovering, authenticity, passion, creating, relationship, inquiry, and fiscal astuteness. Driven by organizational stress and the feeling that something more and different in work life is needed, quantum leadership is one type of leadership strategy that helps nurses focus on the future, stretch and break boundaries, and encourage breakthrough thinking to solve problems in a complex and fluid care environment.

Servant Leadership

Another popular contemporary leadership concept is called *servant leadership.* Greenleaf (2002) used the term to describe leaders who choose first to serve others and then to be a leader, as opposed to those who are leaders first (often because of a power drive or need to acquire material possessions) and later choose to serve. Servant-leaders put others first. They choose to make sure that other people's highest-priority needs are being served in a way that promotes personal growth and helps others become freer and more autonomous. When applied to health care, servant leadership is an attractive alternative to the traditional bureaucratic environment experienced by nurses. The servant leadership model draws attention to the necessity for leaders to be attentive to the needs of others and is a model that enhances the personal growth of nurses, improves the quality of care, values teamwork, and promotes personal involvement and caring behavior.

CLINICAL LEADERSHIP

There is a renewed focus on clinical leadership models at the point of care. Typically aimed at a hospital unit where care is delivered, the crucial role played by nurses in quality, safety, care coordination and related aims of the IOM are the centerpiece. Clinical leadership is defined as "staff nurse behaviours that provide direction and support to clients and the health care team in the delivery of patient care" (Patrick et al., 2011, p. 450). Patrick and colleagues (2011) viewed every registered staff nurse as a clinical leader and used Kouzes and Posner's (1995) model of transformational leadership as a framework to describe and measure clinical leadership practices. Their review of literature identified five key aspects of clinical leadership: clinical expertise, effective communication, collaboration, coordination, and interpersonal understanding. Empowering work environments create support for staff nurses as clinical leaders to achieve the best outcomes of care.

EFFECTIVE LEADERSHIP

Effective leadership is an integrated blend of leadership principles and characteristics with management principles and techniques. Tornabeni (2001) outlined practical leadership techniques for the nurse leader. Table 1-1 displays practical actions for nurses to take to improve leadership skills. Nurses can grow such skills by knowledge and awareness (e.g., through assessment tools) and then may put knowledge and skills to work through guided exercises and mentored experiences.

Leadership research in nursing has revealed the following factors central to successful nursing leadership (Upenieks, 2003a, b):

- Formal and informal power
- Access to information and resources
- Opportunity to grow from new challenges
- Supportive organizational cultures in which nurses are valued for their expertise
- Visibility, responsiveness, a passion for nursing, and business astuteness shown by nurse leaders
- Respectful and collaborative teamwork
- Adequate compensation representing value

In 2005, the American Organization of Nurse Executives identified five core nurse executive competency domains: (1) leadership, (2) communication and relationship management, (3) professionalism, (4) knowledge of the health care environment, and

TABLE 1-1	**TORNABENI'S PRACTICAL ADVICE**
LONGEST'S CATEGORY	**TORNABENI'S ADVICE**
Conceptual	Have a vision. Gather information. Broaden your scope. Take risks.
Technical managerial/clinical	Devise a step-by-step approach and plan. Generate buy-in. Delegate tasks. Motivate continuously by recruiting competent people; developing them; giving them appropriate tools, authority, and resources; holding them accountable; and rewarding "right" behavior.
Interpersonal/collaborative	Build your team. Look for talent within. Pick the cream of the crop. Establish a sense of collegiality. Help your people cope with change.
Political	Understand the politics. Build an internal network.
Commercial	Build an external network. Exchange ideas and challenges with outside colleagues.
Governance	Trust your intuition. Have a sense of purpose. Do the hard work (perspiration). Have passion.

Data from Tornabeni, J. (2001). The competency game: My take on what it really takes to lead. *Nursing Administration Quarterly, 25*(4), 1-13.

(5) business skills and principles. Each domain was further elaborated with specific skill categories. This conceptualization provides a road map for curriculum and continuing education and a blueprint for nurse executive self-assessment and evaluation. Leadership effectiveness theories and skills can be explored by nurses who seek to learn and improve their personal leadership competency.

Leadership effectiveness is based on the ability to adapt in a complex and chaotic environment. Adaptive problems arise from change and chaos and often are systems problems that affect people, planning, institutional operations, or work processes. Effective leaders have a grasp of themselves, their team, their goals, nursing and health care, and important evaluative data for "dashboards." They use their personal style, vision, and energy to focus on goal attainment and group satisfaction. Starting with whatever natural talent a nurse possesses, essential leadership skills can be practiced over time for greater effectiveness. Effective leadership uses empowerment. For nurses, empowering means that the power over clinical practice decisions is invested in staff nurses, enabling them to do what they do best. This process is similar to nurses empowering clients. Leadership involves elements of vigor and vision and can be understood as a dynamic combination of competence, willingness to take responsibility, and strength of character to do what is right because it is the right thing to do.

FOLLOWERSHIP

Pagonis (1992) noted that, by definition, leaders do not operate in isolation. Instead, leadership involves cooperation and collaboration. The basic nature of leadership is interactive; it revolves around the interpersonal relationships among leaders and followers. Therefore cooperation and collaboration between leader and followers and between followers and the leader enhance the group's effectiveness. Although it may seem obvious, followership quality is important.

Kellerman (2008) defined followers as "subordinates who have less power, authority, and influence than do their superiors and who therefore usually, but not invariably, fall into line" (p. xix). She noted that followership "implies a relationship (rank), between subordinates and superiors, and a response (behavior), of the former to the latter" (p. xx). There is a dynamic relationship between leaders and followers, and both are important.

Followership is an interpersonal process of participation. It implies an engagement of the follower with the leader, and possibly a group, by which the follower takes guidance and direction from the leader to accomplish group goals. The importance of followership is emphasized because leadership requires the presence of followers. The relationship between the leader and the followers defines leadership. The corollary to leadership is followership, or helping to get the job done. A good leader clearly needs good followers (Brakey, 1991). Bennis (1994) noted that followers need three things from leaders: direction, trust, and hope. With these three elements in place, followers are empowered in their participation efforts.

Types of Followers

There are several typologies that distinguish types of followers. Kelley (1992) explored followership style and plotted styles along the two axes of passive to active and dependent to independent. The five styles of followership are alienated, exemplary, conformist, passive, and pragmatist. Chaleff's (2003) grid used axes of low to high challenge and low to high support, resulting in four quadrants: implementer, partner, individualist, and resource. Kellerman (2008) aligned followers on the single dimension of engagement and divided them into five types: isolate, bystander, participant, activist, and diehard. Isolates are completely detached/not engaged. Bystanders, participants, activists, and diehards are engaged to some degree with leaders, other followers, the group or the organization. Bystanders observe, participants engage, activists feel strongly and act, and diehards are prepared to die for the cause. Understanding types of followers is as important as understanding types of leaders: it creates the ability to match style to effectiveness in care delivery. Effective followers are an asset to be nurtured, developed, and valued. Effective followers contribute to success in organizations. Nurses can and should examine their own behavior and ask themselves the question, "In this situation, what kind of follower am I?"

Self-awareness is an important aspect of both leadership and followership. This means that nurses can assess themselves to better understand their own style and leadership characteristics. Self-assessment tools are available to assist nurses in awareness of both leadership and followership behaviors. One example is the LEAD instruments developed by Hersey and colleagues (2013). Leadership self-assessment instruments can be found online (e.g., *www.nwlink. com/~donclark/leader/survlead.html*). Other instruments include the Leader Behavior Description Questionnaire, or LBDQ-12 (Stodgill, 1963), the Least Preferred Coworker Scale (Fiedler & Chemers, 1984; Fiedler & Garcia, 1987), the Leadership Practices Inventory (Kouzes & Posner, 1988), the Multifactor Leadership Questionnaire (MLQ) (Bass & Avolio, 1990), the Self-Assessment Leadership Instrument (Smola, 1988), and multiple training instruments. Leadership-related research instruments were identified, compared, and evaluated by Huber and colleagues (2000). Some instruments are useful for research and others for leadership training or self-diagnosis. A wide variety of tools are available. Individuals can increase their effectiveness through greater awareness and subsequent honing of both their leadership and followership skills.

LEADERSHIP AND MANAGEMENT IMPLICATIONS

As nurses work in a rapidly changing practice environment, leadership is important because it affects the climate and work environment of the organization. It affects how nurses feel about themselves at work and about their jobs. By extension, leadership is thought to affect organizational and individual productivity. For example, if nurses feel goal-directed and think that their contributions are important, they are more motivated to do the work. Important for the professional practice of nurses is how they feel about themselves and how satisfied they are with their jobs. Both aspects have implications for how well nurses are retained and recruited. Leadership cannot be overlooked because leaders function as problem finders and problem solvers. They are people who help everyone else overcome obstacles. The leadership role is one of bridging, integrating, motivating, and creating organizational "glue."

Leadership in nursing is crucial. *First*, it is important to nurses because of the size of the profession. Nurses make up the largest single health care occupation and one that is experiencing critical shortages.

Pressures, including costs, in the health care environment are rapidly thrusting nurses into leadership roles in highly complex and stressful work situations.

Nurses are the largest group of health care professionals in most settings of service delivery and represent the largest human resource expenditure in most care settings (O'Neil et al., 2008). Besides volume, nurses also are distributed both horizontally and vertically and in leadership roles throughout care delivery systems. Nurses are found at the first level of caregiving process management and on up to executive level of leadership and strategic decision making. Given the challenges of cost containment, an aging population needing more health care services, and issues of access and quality of care, nurse leaders are experiencing greater pressure to perform and produce more effective alignment of key processes, functions, and resources. Organizations have underinvested in nursing leadership skill development, leaving them at risk of underperforming, especially in the three strategic challenges of finance, workforce, and patient safety (O'Neil et al., 2008).

Recent research has brought to light the gaps, barriers, and needs related to developing nursing leaders as a human capital asset (O'Neil et al., 2008). The top five competencies identified by nurse leaders were the following (O'Neil et al., 2008):
- Building effective teams
- Translating vision into strategy
- Communicating vision and strategy internally
- Managing conflict
- Managing focus on patient and customer

Barriers to expanding leadership training for nurses were the inability to get release time away to attend and the budget to fund attendance. Thus "budget and release time were rate-limiting realities" (O'Neil et al., 2008, p. 182).

Second, nursing's work is complex, often conducted in complex settings. Tremendous changes in nursing have occurred in the past 25 years. These are changes in philosophy, knowledge base, technological complexity, ethical dilemmas, and impacts from constant change and societal pressures. Thus leadership is needed to guide and motivate the nurses and health care delivery systems toward positive achievements for better patient care. Leadership in nursing is needed to influence the organizational context of care for greater effectiveness and productivity.

Contextual aspects include culture, leadership, and organizational infrastructure (Marchionni & Ritchie, 2008). Leaders establish norms and values, define expectations, reward behaviors, and reinforce culture (Shirey, 2007). Authenticity and caring are valued in nurse leaders and are exhibited by people who are genuine, trustworthy, reliable, and believable and who create a positive environment (Pipe, 2008; Shirey, 2006).

Third, nurses enter the practice of nursing by licensure, but they come from a variety of educational backgrounds. A baccalaureate degree or certification as a clinical nurse leader (CNL) does not automatically confer advanced leadership skills. However, without a baccalaureate degree at minimum, nursing as a profession is disadvantaged when compared with other professions whose minimum preparation is uniformly baccalaureate or above. In addition, the evidence-based recommendations of the IOM (2011) for 80% BSN workforce by 2020 speaks to the need for educational preparation for the complexities of health care. Thus nurses will need strong leadership to resolve the interprofessional dilemmas derived from educational diversity and issues related to professionalization and employment.

Nurses are knowledge workers in an information age. Knowledge workers respond to inspiration, not supervision. Although professionals require little direction and supervision, what they do need is protection and support (Mintzberg, 1998). This is best manifested in the covert leadership of the unobtrusive actions that permeate all the things the leader does. Inspiration also can come from a focus on results. Leaders need to model what they want. The good news is that leadership can be taught and learned. Nurses can read, learn, and practice effective leadership and followership.

CURRENT ISSUES AND TRENDS

Current issues and trends that have significance for leadership in nursing include the dramatic U.S. demographic data related to the aging of the baby boom generation and the demographic profile of nursing in the United States. A major societal and public policy issue related to the aging of a large demographic bulge of baby boomers is beginning to reach a critical point. Called the "2030 problem" (Knickman & Snell, 2002), this socioeconomic and demographic phenomenon is real, looming, urgent, and fraught with health care challenges. Statistics show that there are approximately 40.3 million Americans ages 65 years and older, representing 13% of the population, or 1 in 8 Americans (U.S. Census Bureau, 2012). The percentage of Americans 65 years of age and older has tripled since 1900. Issues related to health burdens and chronic illness are characteristic of older adults. In fact, persons 85 years of age and older may spend up to half of their remaining lives inactive or dependent.

U.S. population and health trends are assessed and monitored by governmental agencies such as the U.S. Census Bureau, Centers for Disease Control and Prevention, Bureau of Labor Statistics, and Health Resources and Services Administration. The statistics related to the baby boom generation are impressive. Born between 1946 and 1964, baby boomers in 2030 will be between the ages of 66 and 84 years and are projected to number 61 million people. In addition to baby boomers, the U.S. population in 2030 is projected also to include 9 million people born before 1946. The projected population of people 65 years and older in 2050 is 88.5 million (U.S. Census, 2012). This predictable tidal wave will make chronic illness and long-term care a huge economic burden. Knickman and Snell (2002) suggested that there are four key "aging shocks": (1) uncovered costs of prescription medications, (2) uncovered medical care costs, (3) private insurance costs for the Medigap, and (4) costs of long-term care. They projected that there will be an overwhelming economic burden if tax rates need to be raised dramatically, economic growth is retarded because of high service costs, or future generations of workers have worse general well-being because of service costs or income transfers. Nurses and the health care system will be challenged to find evidence-based care delivery and service systems models and strategies that address the projected growth industry in chronic illness.

Examining the demographic profile of nursing in the United States offers a clue about nursing followership. The median age of a licensed, registered professional nurse in the United States was 46 years in 2008 (Bureau of Health Professions [BHPr], 2010). The Ninth National Sample Survey of Registered Nurses was conducted in 2008 and published in 2010

(BHPr, 2010). There were an estimated 3,063,162 licensed RNs in the United States, and 84.8% were employed in nursing. The ADN was the most commonly reported initial nursing education. There has been a slowdown in the aging trend in nursing, due to an increase in 2008 in the number of employed RNs who are less than 30 years of age. This was the first such increase since the initial RN Sample Survey was conducted in 1977 (BHPr, 2010).

Leadership is considered key to the success of health care organizations. Nurses are pressed to demonstrate the outcomes of their care and provide evidence of the effectiveness of their service delivery. The link between leadership style and staff satisfaction highlights the importance of leadership in times of chaos. A nurse leader needs to be dynamic, show interpersonal skills, and be a visionary for the organization and the profession. The ability to inspire and motivate followers to carry out the vision is crucial.

MANAGEMENT OVERVIEW

The global information age has engulfed our society, yet challenges to health care management linger. Along with an array of opportunities, such as instantaneous communication across vast distances, health care organizations and the people in them struggle with an ever-accelerating rate of change, knowledge explosion, and information flow. The recruitment, development, deployment, motivation, and leveraging of human capital (nurses) as scarce resources and prime assets are critical management issues for service industries in general and nursing and health care

specifically. At the core, managers manage people and organizations. People's time and effort, as well as organizations' money, facilities, and supplies, need to be directed in a coordinated effort to achieve best results and meet objectives.

DEFINITIONS

Management is defined as the process of coordination and integration of resources through activities of planning, organizing, coordinating, directing, and controlling to accomplish specific institutional goals and objectives. Management has been viewed as an art and a science related to planning and directing human effort and scarce resources to attain established objectives. Management has been viewed in a variety of ways. Another definition of management is a process by which organizational goals are met through the application of skills and the use of resources. Hersey and colleagues (2013) defined management as "the process of working with and through individuals and groups and other resources (such as equipment, capital, and technology) to accomplish organizational goals" (p. 3).

Management, then, applies to organizations. The definition of leadership emphasizes actions that influence toward group goals; the definition of management focuses on organizational goals. The achievement of organizational goals through leadership and manipulation of the environment is management. In a systems approach to management, the inputs would be represented by human resources and physical and technical resources. The outputs would be the realization of goals (Figure 1-5). Koontz

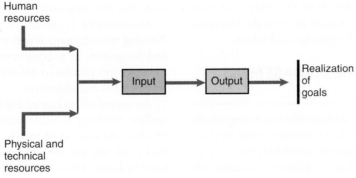

FIGURE 1-5 Systems view of management.

(1961) concluded that management is the art of the following:

- Getting things done through and with people in formally organized groups
- Creating an environment in an organized group in which people can perform as individuals yet cooperate to attain group goals
- Removing barriers and roadblocks to performance
- Optimizing efficiency in effectively reaching goals

Thus management is a separate function with a specific purpose and related roles but one that is focused on organizations. It is associated with important day-to-day functions and operations geared toward maintenance and stability and associated with transactional leadership or "doing things right" via task accomplishment. To achieve organizational goals, managers are involved in activities such as analyzing issues, establishing goals and objectives, mapping out work plans, organizing assets and supplies, developing and motivating people, communicating, managing technology, handling change and conflict, measurement, analysis, and evaluation. Without talent and attention to these functions, effectiveness and morale drop.

Effective managers are thought to be those who can weave strategy, execution, discipline, inspiration, and leadership together as they unite an organization toward achieving its goals. Sull (2003) found that successful managers may vary in personal attributes but all excel at managing commitments. Managerial commitments may be capital investments, hiring or firing decisions, public statements, or other strategy decisions. A commitment is defined as "any action taken in the present that binds an organization to a future course of action" (Sull, 2003, p. 84). Commitments give employees a clear sense of focus for prioritization and motivation; however, they limit flexibility. The most enduring commitments tend to be strategic directions, resources, processes, relationships, and values.

BACKGROUND: THE MANAGEMENT PROCESS

Drucker (2004) suggested that effective executives do not need to be leaders. "Great managers may be charismatic or dull, generous or tightfisted, visionary or numbers oriented. But every effective executive follows eight simple practices" (Drucker, 2004, p. 59).

These eight practices are divided into the following three categories:

Practices That Give Executives the Knowledge They Need

1. They asked: "What needs to be done?"
2. They asked: "What is right for the enterprise?"

Practices That Help Executives Convert Knowledge to Action

1. They developed action plans.
2. They took responsibility for decisions.
3. They took responsibility for communicating.
4. They were focused on opportunities, not problems.

Practices That Ensure That the Whole Organization Feels Responsible and Accountable

1. They ran productive meetings.
2. They thought and said "we," not "I."

Effective management also appears to be a result of artful balancing. Managers need to function at the point at which reflective thinking combines with practical doing (Gosling & Mintzberg, 2003). Described as managerial mind-sets within the bounds of management, managers interpret and deal with their world from the following five perspectives (Gosling & Mintzberg, 2003):

1. *Reflective mind-set:* Managing self
2. *Analytic mind-set:* Managing organizations
3. *Worldly mind-set:* Managing context
4. *Collaborative mind-set:* Managing relationships
5. *Action mind-set:* Managing change

These five mind-sets were described as being like threads for the manager to weave. The process is as follows: analyze, act, reflect, act, collaborate, reanalyze, articulate new insights, and act again.

Management is central to the work of nursing. **Nursing management** is defined as the coordination and integration of nursing resources by applying the management process to accomplish nursing care and service goals and objectives.

An organization can be any institution, agency, or facility. Working to achieve an organization's goals involves the process of management. The principles that guide the process of management were formulated by Fayol (1949). He said that managers perform unique and discrete functions: they plan, organize, coordinate, and control. Fayol's ideas were revolutionary in that, for the first time, management was seen as a unique and separate activity from the work of producing a product. Workers labor to produce the product; managers labor to manage organizations toward goal achievement. Someone needs to monitor financial indicators; hire, train, and evaluate personnel; improve quality; coordinate work and effort; fix systems problems; and ensure that goals are met. In nursing, this means that nurses do the work of providing nursing care while nurse managers coordinate and integrate the work of individual nurses with the larger system.

The four steps of the management process are as follows (Fayol, 1949; Figure 1-6):

1. Planning
2. Organizing
3. Coordinating or directing
4. Controlling

These functions make up the scope of a manager's major effort. Planning involves determining the long-term and short-term objectives and the corresponding actions that must be taken. Organizing means mobilizing human and material resources to accomplish what is needed. Directing relates to methods of motivating, guiding, and leading people through work processes. Controlling has a specific meaning closer to the monitoring and evaluating actions that are familiar to nurses. The management process can be compared to an orchestra performing a concert or a team playing a football game. There is a plan and an organized group of players. A director manages the performance and controls the outcome by making corrections and adjustments along the way but does not play an instrument or a position. Management is discrete and separate work. The management

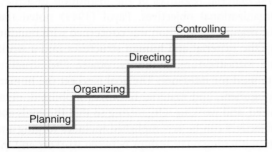

FIGURE 1-6 Four steps of the management process.

process is a rational, logical process based on problem-solving principles. Fayol's classic management process idea remains the core framework around discussions about what management is and does.

Planning

Planning is the managerial function of selecting priorities, results, and methods to achieve results (McNamara, 1999a). It is setting the direction for a system and then guiding the system to follow the direction (McNamara, 1999b). **Planning** is defined as determining the long-term and short-term objectives and the corresponding actions that must be taken to achieve these objectives. Planning can be detailed, specific, and rigid, or it can be broad, general, and flexible. Planning is deciding in advance what is to be done and when, by whom, and how it is to be done. It is traditionally thought of as a linear process. Hersey and colleagues (2013) described planning as involving the setting of goals and objectives and developing "work maps" to show how they are to be accomplished. Planning activities include identifying goals, objectives, methods, resources, responsible parties, and due dates. There are two types of planning: strategic and tactical.

Strategic planning: More broad-ranged, this approach means determining the overall purposes and directions of the organization. This is often focused on mission, vision, and major goal identification.

Tactical planning: More short-ranged, this type means determining the specific details of implementing broader goals. Examples are project planning, staffing planning, and marketing plans.

Three types of errors can create planning flaws: (1) errors of fact: the plan is based on misinformation; (2) errors in assumption: the plan is based on incorrect assumptions; and (3) errors of logic: the plan is based on faulty reasoning. Planning flaws carry over into organizing, directing, and controlling activities.

Planning is a process that heavily depends on the decision-making process. Part of planning is choosing among a number of alternatives. Thus in nursing, the manager often must balance the needs of clients, staff, administrators, and physicians under conditions of limited resources.

Planning involves considering systems inputs, processes, outputs, and outcomes. The process of planning in its larger context means that planners work backwards through the system. Starting with the results, outcomes, or outputs desired, they then identify the processes needed to produce the results and then identify the inputs or resources needed to carry out the processes (McNamara, 1999b). Typical planning phases include the following:

- Identify the mission.
- Conduct an environmental scan.
- Analyze the situation (e.g., SWOT analysis of strengths, weaknesses, opportunities, and threats).
- Establish goals.
- Identify strategies to reach goals.
- Set objectives to achieve goals.
- Assign responsibilities and timelines.
- Write a planning document.
- Celebrate success and completion.

Many plans fail because of incompletion; thus it is important to focus on ensuring that the plan is carried out or that deviations are recognized and managed. Recommended guidelines are as follows (McNamara, 1999b):

- Involve the right people in planning.
- Do a written plan, and communicate it widely.
- Establish goals and objectives that are specific, measurable, acceptable, placed in a time frame, stretching, and rewarding.
- Build in accountability (regular review).
- Note deviations, and replan.
- Evaluate the planning process and the plan.
- Conduct ongoing communications.
- Make the planning process compatible with the preferences of the planners.
- Acknowledge and celebrate results.

The planning process is intimately involved with establishing objectives. Fayol (1949) identified planning as examining the future and drawing up a plan of action. Activities involved include laying out of the work to be done, determining the use of resources, and establishing the standards for evaluation. The nurse is engaged in a constant mental planning operation when deciding what specific things are to be accomplished for the client. The same is true for the nurse manager who is deciding how to devise, implement, and maintain a positive and productive work environment for nurses.

An alternative conceptualization to the model of planning that views it as an orderly, top-down, linear sequence is the model proposed by Hayes-Roth and Hayes-Roth (1979). Their idea was that opportunistic planning approaches are used to face complex planning tasks. Planners, under conditions of complexity, pursue whatever seems opportune or promising at the time. A plan becomes multidirectional and develops by increments. This approach may appear chaotic compared with systematic planning, but it leads to better plans in complex task situations. Similar to the interactive planning that nurses do with patients, interactive planning between nurses and nurse managers also is the best strategy for effective planning. This may be due in part to the phenomenon of an environment of chaos and complexity.

Planning is a function that assumes stability and the ability to predict and project into the future. Yet the current environment is turbulent, making planning difficult. Learning and adapting are important abilities in a changeable environment. Interactive planning has been suggested as an approach to planning in complex situations and changing environments (Foust, 1994). Interactive planning takes a developmental approach. Problems are viewed as interrelated. Interactive planning principles emphasize the importance of participation among participants, a nonlinear view of relationships called *systems thinking,* and a focus on creating a desired future outcome. Interactive planning can contribute to effective care planning and to effective care management by nurses (Foust, 1994).

Organizing

Organizing is a management function related to allocating and configuring resources to accomplish preferred goals and objectives. It is the activities done to collect and configure resources to effectively and efficiently implement plans (McNamara, 1999a, c). **Organizing** can be defined as mobilizing the human and material resources of the institution to achieve organizational objectives. Fayol (1949) noted that the organizing function was concerned with building up the material and human structures into a working infrastructure. Authority, power, and structure are used for influence. The goal is to get the human, equipment, and material resources mobilized, organized, and working. Organizing so that the goals and objectives can be accomplished includes forging and strengthening relationships between workers and the environment. The first step is to organize the work;

then the people are organized; finally the environment is organized.

Organizing closely follows the planning process. In fact, these terms are often referred to together: *planning* and *organizing*. Organizing encompasses activities designed to bring together an array of various resources including personnel, money, and equipment in a manner that is the most effective for accomplishing organizational goals. There are a variety of ways to do this, but the essence of organizing is the integration and coordination of resources (Hersey et al., 2013).

There are a wide variety of topics related to organizing, which is considered to be one of the major functions of management. Lack of organization can be a major source of stress. McNamara (1999a, c) identified the following categories under managerial organizing:

- Organizing yourself, your office, your files
- Organizing a task, job, or role through task and job analysis, job descriptions, and time management
- Organizing various groups of people such as staff, committees, meetings, and teams
- Organizing human resources through benefits, compensation, staffing and deployment, and training and development
- Organizing facilities and technology

Organizing can be thought of also as a process of identifying roles in relationship to one another. Thus organizing involves activities related to establishing a structure and hierarchy of jobs and positions within a unit or department. Responsibilities are assigned to each job. The complexity of this aspect of organizing is related to the size of the organization and the number of employees and jobs. Organizing in nursing also relates to the activities of budget management, staffing, and scheduling and to other human resources and personnel functions such as developing committees and bylaws, orientation, and staff in-service. Organizations organize by establishing a structure, such as a hierarchy with divisions or departments, and by developing some method for division of labor and subsequent coordination among subunits.

Directing

Directing is the managerial function of establishing direction and then influencing people to follow that direction. Directing can also be called *leading* (McNamara, 1999a) or *coordinating*. **Coordinating** is defined as motivating and leading personnel to carry out the desired actions. Fayol (1949) identified coordination as including activities of binding together, unifying, and harmonizing the activity and effort of various personnel.

Along with communicating and leading, motivation often is included with the description of the activities of directing others. Motivating is a major strategy related to determining the followers' level of performance and thereby to influencing how effectively the goals of the organization will be met. The amount of employee effort that can be influenced by motivation is thought to be from 20% to 30% at the low end and as high as 80% to 90% for highly motivated people (Hersey et al., 2013). A wide range of effort can be influenced through motivation. Motivation is a complex activity, but it is a critical managerial function.

On a day-to-day basis, coaching is used as a technique to direct and motivate followers. The manager delegates activities and responsibilities when making assignments. The function of directing involves actions of supervising and guiding others within their assigned duties. The use of interpersonal skills is required to delicately balance the need to direct and supervise for task accomplishment with the need to create and maintain a motivational climate with high participation and positive outcomes.

Within nursing there is a legal aspect to the managerial directing function. In some state licensing laws, supervision is a defined and regulated legal element of nursing practice. Delegation and supervision are viewed legally as a part of the practice of nursing. Thus nurses have a specific need to know and understand this area of nursing responsibility within their scope of practice. Nurses carry responsibility and accountability for the quality and quantity of their supervision, as well as for the quality and quantity of their own actions in regard to care provision. Nurses also are being tapped for their important role as care coordinators. Nurse managers carry the added responsibility and accountability for the coordination of groups of nurse providers and assistive or ancillary personnel, sometimes across settings and sites of care. Nurse managers also have an overall responsibility to monitor and provide surveillance or vigilance regarding situations that can lead to failure to rescue, patient safety errors, or negligence. Too many hours worked, nurse fatigue from stress, too heavy a patient workload, and other systems problems are situations to monitor with regard to legal accountability.

Controlling

Controlling is the management function of monitoring and adjusting the plan, processes, and resources to effectively and efficiently achieve goals. It is a way of coordinating activities within organizations by systematically figuring out whether what is occurring is what is wanted (McNamara, 1999a, d). The controlling aspect of the managerial process may seem at first to carry a negative connotation. However, when used in reference to management, the word *control* does not mean being negatively manipulative or punitive toward others. Managerial controlling means ensuring that the proper processes are followed. Fayol (1949) called this the activity of seeing that everything occurs in conformity with established rules. In nursing, the term *evaluation* is used to refer to similar actions and activities. Control or evaluation means ensuring that the flow and processes of work, as well as goal accomplishment, proceed as planned. **Controlling** is defined as comparing the results of work with predetermined standards of performance and taking corrective action when needed. This means ensuring that the results are as desired and, if they are not up to standards, then taking some action to modify, remediate, or reverse variances.

The coordination of activities of a system is one aspect of managerial control, along with financial management, compliance, quality and risk management, feedback mechanisms, performance management, policies and procedures, and research and trend analysis. These control activities are used by managers to communicate to reach a goal, track activities toward the goal, guide behaviors, and coordinate efforts and decide what to do. Managerial coordination and control are important to the success of any organization (McNamara, 1999a, d). Ongoing, careful review using standardized documents, informatics systems, and standardized measures prevents drift and the waste of time and resources that occur when direction is vague. Well-exercised, managerial control is flexible enough to allow innovation yet present enough to effectively structure groups and organizations toward goal attainment.

The management function of controlling involves feeding back information about the results and outcomes of work activities, combined with activities to follow up and compare outcomes with plans. Appropriate adjustments need to be made wherever outcomes vary or deviate from expectations (Hersey et al., 2013). In nursing, when a critical path is used to track client care, the variances are analyzed and corrected as a function of managerial control. The controlling function of management is a constant process of internal reevaluation.

MANAGEMENT IN NURSING PRACTICE

Two Roles of the Nurse

Nurses have two major components to their role: care provider and care integrator. McClure (1991) called these the *caregiver* and *integrator* roles. The image of the "bedside nurse" emphasizes the care provider aspect of nursing. The integrator role is a complementary function that arises from nursing's central positioning in the day-to-day coordination of service delivery and central location at the hub of information flow regarding care and service delivery. This linkage relationship is depicted visually in Figure 1-7. Although the coordination of care has always been a key nursing function, it is becoming more visible and valued in health care and as nurses assume case management roles that

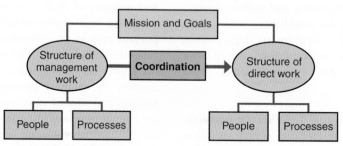

FIGURE 1-7 Linkage of clinical and management domains.

focus on integrating clinical care. However, the relative proportion of the nurse's role that is devoted to management and coordination functions varies within nursing according to the job category. One way to analyze nursing jobs is to assess the relative balance of the two role components in any job.

There is value in investing in infrastructure that organizes and supports the work that nurses do. Managers in nursing perform discrete and important functions that provide an environment and climate to facilitate delivery of client services. Mintzberg (1994) described this managing as *blended care.*

One part of managing people and relationships in organization is to manage the expression of emotion. The management of emotions, called *emotional intelligence (EI)*, has come to be recognized as foundational for organizational health and its four components of strategy, capability, viability, and spirit (Metts, 2008). Emotional intelligence is the intersection of thinking and emotion. Skill building and training in positive thinking and a focus on positive emotions assist nurses to better listen, encourage, motivate, and create connections. The goal is to achieve optimal outcomes. EI is thus both a leadership and a management competency.

In nursing, the management process is directed primarily toward the human element, or the management of human resources. It is through this dynamic and interactive process that the work of nursing is accomplished. Nurse managers balance two competing needs: the needs of the staff related to growth, efficiency, motivation, morale, and accomplishment with the outcome of staff satisfaction; and the needs of the employer for productivity, quality, and cost-effectiveness with the outcome of productivity.

MANAGEMENT IN ORGANIZATIONS
The Nature of Managerial Work

Lewin (1947) said that the behavior of human beings is a function of individual psychology, the needs patterns of people, and the environment in which they work. Behavioral theory and its applications to the management of people focuses on organizing and processing work and accomplishing organizational objectives at a targeted minimum cost and minimum waste. The responsibility for doing that lies with management. Managers manage people and the environment. One view of management suggests that the manager's

behavior, the role, and the situation created for people to work in actually trigger or cause followers' behavior. Thus the manager's role is distinct and important for individual and organizational outcomes because of its direct impact on how and what gets done.

Mintzberg (1973, 1975) reformulated Fayol's (1949) ideas about the nature of managerial work. Mintzberg's synthesis of research findings about managers in general revealed the following:

- Managers work at an unrelenting pace at activities characterized by brevity, variety, and discontinuity. Managers are strongly action-oriented.
- Managers handle exceptions and perform regular work, such as ritual and ceremonial duties, negotiation, and processing of soft information linking the organization to its environment.
- Managers prefer oral communication.
- "Judgment" and "intuition" describe the procedures managers use to schedule time, process information, and make decisions.

Mintzberg (1975) described the manager's job in terms of ten roles or sets of behaviors. Derived from the formal authority and status of the position are three interpersonal roles: figurehead, leader, and liaison. As the nerve center of the organizational unit, information processing is a key part of the role. Informational roles are monitor, disseminator, and spokesperson. Information is the basic input to decision making. The decisional roles are entrepreneur, disturbance handler, resource allocator, and negotiator (Figure 1-8). Mintzberg suggested a number of important managerial skills, as follows:

- Developing peer relationships
- Carrying out negotiations
- Motivating subordinates
- Resolving conflicts
- Establishing information networks and disseminating information
- Making decisions in conditions of extreme ambiguity
- Allocating resources

If management is important to achieving organizational goals, then the skills, abilities, functions, actions, and strategies used by managers to manage are important to know and understand. Mintzberg (1994) elaborated his earlier work on the nature of managerial work by expanding it to an interactive model (Figure 1-9). The model uses concentric circles. At the

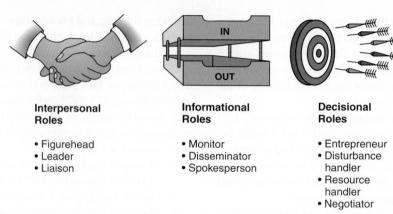

Interpersonal Roles

- Figurehead
- Leader
- Liaison

Informational Roles

- Monitor
- Disseminator
- Spokesperson

Decisional Roles

- Entrepreneur
- Disturbance handler
- Resource handler
- Negotiator

FIGURE 1-8 Mintzberg's 10 managerial roles. (Data from Mintzberg, H. [1975]. The manager's job: Folklore and fact. In M. Matteson, & J. Ivancevich [Eds.], *Management classics* [3rd ed., pp. 63-85]. Plano, TX: Business Publications.)

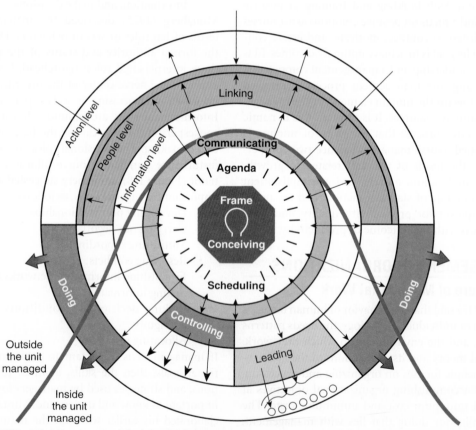

FIGURE 1-9 Mintzberg's Model of Managerial Work. (Redrawn from Mintzberg, H. [1994]. Managing as blended care. *Journal of Nursing Administration, 24*[9], 30.)

core is a person who is in a job. The person has some unique set of values, experiences, knowledge, and competencies. The combination of the person and the job creates a frame composed of the job's purpose, the person's perspective about what needs to be done, and selected strategies for doing the job. The frame can range across two continua: from vague to very specific and from person-selected to externally imposed. The frame results in an agenda of work issues and time scheduling. Placed at the center of the figure, these elements form the core of the job of a manager. Managerial roles and behaviors at this level include conceiving the frame and scheduling the agenda.

Growing out of the core are three concentric circles—from abstract to concrete. These are called the *information, people,* and *action levels* of managerial work. At the most abstract level, the manager processes information and uses it to drive the action. At the next level, the manager works with people to encourage work activities. At the most concrete level, the manager manages the action.

At the information level, the associated managerial roles are communicating information and controlling by using information to control the work of others. At the people level, the managerial roles are leading and linking. Leading involves encouraging and enabling individuals (by mentoring and rewarding), groups (by team building and conflict resolution), and the whole organization (by building a culture). The linking roles have the manager relating to the external environment by building networks of contacts and acquiring information from the environment to transmit back to the unit. At the action level, the associated managerial role is called *doing* or *supervising.* Behaviors include doing, handling disturbances, and negotiating (Mintzberg, 1994).

Mintzberg's (1994) interactive model provides a visual display of a way of thinking about managerial work and associated roles and activities. The model could be used as a basis for self-assessment and can be applied to specific managerial jobs. Nurses who strive to apply the concepts to their managerial work could use the model to examine and analyze managerial styles, behaviors, and roles. As managers, nurses manage both people (clients, themselves, and other staff or providers) and the environment of client care delivery. An understanding of the management process and the roles

related to the work of a manager can assist nurses to improve their personal effectiveness and their organization's productivity.

Contemporary Management Theories

Human organizations are complex in nature. It is tricky to provide overall direction for an organization in times of rapid environmental change. The recent focus of leadership theory has been on interactional, relational, and transformational leadership to guide organizations through successful change and chaos. However, less attention has been focused on how to advise managers who are working toward the organization's goals and trying to use resources effectively and efficiently under conditions of change, scarcity, and complexity. It is thought that the nature of how the four managerial functions of planning, organizing, coordinating or directing, and controlling are carried out needs to change to accommodate a new management paradigm. Because of forces such as technology, the Internet, increasing diversity, and a global marketplace, organizations have experienced pressure to be more sensitive, flexible, and adaptable to stakeholders' expectations and demands (McNamara, 1999e, f).

The result has been a reconfiguration or restructuring of many organizations from the classic hierarchical, top-down, rigid form to a more fluid, organic, team-based, collaborative structure. This has had an impact on how managers manage. Managers cannot control continued rapid change. Old familiar plans and behaviors no longer provide clear direction for the future. Managers now need to focus on two major aspects of management: managing change through constant assessment, guidance, and adaptation; and managing employees through worker-centered teams and other self-organizing and self-designing group structures (McNamara, 1999f). Bureaucratic management is out; organic and virtual management is in.

A variety of contemporary theories of management have arisen to help organize management thought. Four major management theories now predominate: contingency theory, systems theory, complexity theory, and chaos theory. Each one contributes principles useful for nursing management and administration and for nurse managers working to coordinate and integrate health care delivery.

Contingency Theory

Contingency theory is considered to be a leadership theory, but it also applies to management. The basic principle is that managers need to consider the situation and all its elements when making a decision. Managers need to act on the key situational aspects with which they are confronted. Sometimes described as "it all depends" decision making, contingency theory is most often used for choosing a leadership or management style. The "best" style depends on the situation (McNamara, 1999g).

Systems Theory

Systems theory has helped managers to recognize their work as being embedded within a system and to better understand what a system is. Managers have learned that changing one part of a system inevitably affects the whole system. General systems theory is a way of thinking about studying organizational wholes. General systems theory uses the following concepts:

- Organization
- Wholeness
- Control
- Self-regulation
- Purposiveness
- Environment
- Boundaries
- Equilibrium
- Steady state
- Feedback

A system is a set of interrelated and interdependent parts that are designed to achieve common goals. Systems contain a collection of elements that interact with each other in some environment. The elements of an open system and related examples in health care are shown in Table 1-2.

A key principle of systems theory is that changes in one part of the system affect other parts, creating a ripple effect within the whole. Using systems theory implies a rational approach to common goals, a global view of the whole, and an emphasis on order rather than chaos. The input-throughput-output model exemplifies this linear thinking aspect of general systems theory.

Systems theory is easy to understand but difficult to apply in bureaucratic systems or organizations with

TABLE 1-2	OPEN SYSTEM ELEMENTS AND HEALTH CARE EXAMPLES
OPEN SYSTEM ELEMENTS	**HEALTH CARE EXAMPLES**
Inputs to the system (resources)	Money, people, technology
Transforming processes and interactions (throughputs)	Nursing services, management
Outputs of the system	Clinical outcomes, better quality of life
Feedback	Customer and nurse satisfaction, government regulation, accreditation, lawsuits

strong departmental "silos." This is because coordinators and integrators with sufficient organizational power to cross the system are needed but often not deployed. Without integrators, systems parts tend to make changes without consideration of the whole system. Shifting to systems theory thinking helps managers view, analyze, and interpret patterns and events through the lens of interrelationships of the parts and coordination of the whole (McNamara, 1999g).

In health care, concepts such as interrelatedness and interdependence fit well with multidisciplinary teamwork and shared governance professional models. However, concepts of attaining a steady state and equilibrium are difficult to reconcile with the reality of uncertainty, risk, change, and ambiguity that characterize the turbulence of the change occurring in the health care delivery environment. Previously, managers were advised to draw up 5-year and even 10-year plans; managers today have seriously shortened their strategic planning and other related time lines in response to the rapidity of change. An example of the use of systems theory is basing an analysis of a planned change, such as implementing a new program, on systems concepts by identifying inputs, throughputs, outputs, and feedback loops to more effectively plan how the new program fits into the existing system. Sometimes this process is used for short time frame rapid response team projects.

Complexity Theory

Arising in scientific fields such as astronomy, chemistry, biology, geology, and meteorology and involving disciplines such as engineering, mathematics, physics, psychology, and economics, literature is growing since the late 1980s on the behavior of complex adaptive systems (Rosenhead, 1998). Complexity theory is a more general umbrella theory that encompasses chaos theory. The focus of complexity theory is the behavior over time of certain complex and dynamically changing systems. The concern is about the predictability of the behavior of systems that under certain conditions perform in regular and predictable ways but in other conditions change in irregular and unpredictable ways, are unstable, and move further away from starting conditions unless stopped by an overriding constraint. What is most intriguing is that almost undetectable differences in initial conditions will lead to diverging reactions in these systems until the evolution of their behavior is highly dissimilar. Thus stable and unstable behavior is the focus of interest (Rosenhead, 1998).

Stable and unstable behavior can be thought of as two zones. In the stable zone, a disturbed system returns to its initial state. In the unstable zone, any small disturbance leads to movement away from the starting point and further divergence. Which subsequent type of behavior will occur depends on environmental conditions. The area between starting and divergence is called *chaotic behavior*. This refers to systems that have behavior with certain regularity yet defy prediction based on that regularity. The classic example of this is weather prediction (Rosenhead, 1998).

Before the formulation of complexity theory, the unpredictability of systems was attributed to randomness that was measured by statistical probability. It is now understood that a small difference in starting conditions can result in apparently random, quite different trajectories that are highly irregular but not without some form. Plotted over time, the apparently random meanderings of these systems can show a pattern to the movements; but the variation stays within a pattern that repeats itself (Rosenhead, 1998).

Complexity theory has informed classical management theories. Previous management theories heavily emphasized rationality, predictability, stability, setting a mission, determining strategy, and eliminating deviation. Discoveries from complexity and chaos theories include the fact that the natural world does not operate like clockwork machinery. Key findings of complexity theory are the "effective unknowability" of the future and an understanding of the role of creative disorder. Managers need to alter their reflexive behaviors, put an emphasis on "double-loop learning" that also examines the appropriateness of operating assumptions, foster diversity, be open to strategy based on serendipity, welcome disorder as a partner, use instability positively, provoke a controlled ferment of ideas, release creativity, and seek the edge of chaos in the complex interactions that occur among people. Change management takes on a very different form when complexity theory is used (Rosenhead, 1998).

Chaos Theory

Most would agree that one characteristic of nursing is its unpredictability, its chaos and complexity. To use a theory about chaos and complexity is intuitively attractive. Sometimes, no matter how hard nursing leaders try to maintain consistency and control, things do become chaotic. Projects seem to take off "on their own" and defy direction. Chaos is commonly known as disorganization and disorderliness, but the meaning for this concept in chaos theory is quite different. It refers to behavior that is unpredictable in spite of certain regularities. As described by Lorenz (1993), the chaos phenomenon differs from the predictable swinging of a pendulum of a clock. Instead, it is more like the unpredictable random patterns of weather. A meteorologist, Lorenz was preparing for presenting the weather report when he decided to run the numbers through the computer once more to update the information. He initiated the program a short time later than his original run, and the outcome was quite different. This illustrates a fundamental observation of chaos theory: changing the starting point of a computer analysis of the weather can result in a change in the

RESEARCH NOTE

Source

Ebright, P.R., Patterson, E.S., Chalko, B.A., & Render, M.L. (2003). Understanding the complexity of registered nurse work in acute care settings. *Journal of Nursing Administration, 33*(12), 630-638.

Purpose

Complexity in nursing comes from multiple goals, obstacles, hazards, missing data, and behaviors surrounding care situations. To keep things from going wrong, nurses make decisions to adapt and manage complexity in the midst of a changing environment. The purpose of this research was to investigate RN work complexity in an acute care setting using a human performance framework. Field observations followed by semistructured interviews were the methods used with a purposive sample of eight expert RNs. The research question was this: "What human and environmental factors affect decision making by expert RNs on medical-surgical acute care units?"

Discussion

Content analysis resulted in the emergence of 22 patterns across participants that were grouped into the following three main categories:

1. Patterns of work complexity (n=8) that are human and environmental factors affecting work, such as disjointed supply sources, repetitive travel, and interruptions
2. Patterns of cognitive factors driving performance and decisions (n=8), such as maintaining patient safety and knowing unit routines and work flow
3. Patterns of care management strategies (n=6), such as stacking and stabilizing and moving on. The results revealed multiple patterns that characterize RN work on medical/surgical acute care units and how RNs cope and adapt to manage workload demands.

Application to Practice

This study examined the actual work of RNs in the context of patient assignments within conditions of unpredictability, missing information, and unreliable access to resources and processes. The rich data suggested ways to redesign systems to decrease or better manage work complexity. The human performance framework helped uncover routine aspects of the daily management of work that came to be seen as a series of gaps and discontinuities that serve to distract RNs from focusing on critical role functions such as clinical reasoning about patient care. Managerial actions to fix these systems gaps support the work of nursing and avoid wasting large amounts of valuable time.

outcome. Lorenz (1993) presented a paper entitled "Does the Flap of a Butterfly's Wing in Brazil Set Off a Tornado in Texas?" in which he described this phenomenon of chaos. This "butterfly wing flap" label is often referred to in the literature when discussing chaos theory.

Chaos has become a concept of complexity theory. Over the past three or four decades, complexity theory has been the focus of scientific disciplines such as astronomy, chemistry, physics, evolutionary biology, geology, and meteorology. Systems studied in these disciplines have phenomena in common, which seem to pass from an organized state through a chaotic phase, and then emerge or evolve into a higher level of organization. Examples of this emergence is not unlike Darwin's evolutionary theory of natural selection. The theory originated at the Santa Fe Institute, a think tank involving the top 10 percent of scientists from numerous countries and of diverse disciplines. The institute, incorporated in 1984, has been funded by a large number of individuals as well as private foundations to study the "emerging synthesis of science" (Waldrop, 1992, p. 79).

Pediani (1996) pointed to examples from the sciences, such as pharmacology, in which chaos theory and complexity theory seem relevant to some patients' responses to drugs. This newer theory may have broad application in relation to clinical cases.

In management, the traditional focus for leaders is to identify organizational goals and to make decisions facilitating goal achievement. Control is central to logical management processes. However, in complexity theory, the idea of control is considered a delusion because uncertainty and deviations are denied and disregarded. The natural world, according to this theory, does not operate this way and is continually evolving to a higher level of complexity. In complexity theory, the future is so unpredictable that long-term planning is not helpful. Rather, it is suggested that managers need to look for instability and complex interactions between people so that learning occurs and the best result "emerges." Management needs to be alert to creative approaches and allow some ambiguity among ideas (Waldrop, 1992). The idea of the interconnectedness of the parts (people) of the whole suggests that communication among the parts (people) is a key feature of complexity theory.

However, for nursing leaders to consider this approach when initiating a new program may be risky. The way to incorporate this new theory is not yet supported by solid research and "emerged" intelligent practices. The idea of interconnectedness of things does fit the concept of holistic care, and it can also "make important contributions toward restructuring and reorganizing nursing" (Walsh, 2000, p. 39).

Chaos is seen as a particular mode of behavior within the more general field of complexity theory (Rosenhead, 1998). Sometimes the two are used together: chaos and complexity. Chaos, as used in complexity theory, is not utter confusion and disorder but rather a system that defies prediction despite certain regularities. Chaos is the boundary zone between stability and instability, and systems in chaos exhibit bounded instability and unpredictability of specific behavior within a predictable general structure of behavior. They may pass through randomness to evolve to a higher order of self-organized complex adaptive structures (Rosenhead, 1998). At first, this seems to make no sense. However, chaos theory principles can be applied in health care.

As many health care organizations move away from bureaucratic models and recognize organizations as whole systems, more organic and fluid structures are replacing the older ones. Sometimes referred to as "learning organizations," these structures are tapping into the inherent capacity for individuals to exhibit self-organization. In the transition, experiences of change, information overload, entrenched behaviors, and chaos reflect human reactions to organizations as living systems that are adapting and growing (Wheatley, 1999). Complexity and a sense of things being beyond one's control create a search for a simpler way of understanding and leading organizations.

Randomness and complexity are two principal characteristics of chaos. There is a paradox in the fact that even in the simplest of systems, it is extraordinarily difficult to accurately predict the course of events; yet some order arises spontaneously even in these simple systems. Patterns form in nature—some are orderly, and some are not orderly. Concepts of nonlinearity and feedback help explain situations of complexity without randomness (with order). Chaos theory suggests that simple systems may give rise to complex behavior, and complex systems may exhibit simple behavior. At the essence of chaos is a fine balance between forces of stability and those of instability. Two examples are snowflake formation and the behavior of the weather.

It is difficult for minds trained in linear thinking to grasp chaos theory. In the past, the effects of nonlinearity were discounted. Much of scientific thought was based on assumptions of linearity and beliefs that small differences averaged out, slight variances converged toward a point, and approximations could give a relatively accurate picture of what could happen. It was assumed that predictability would come from learning how to account for all variables and a greater level of detail. However, the wholeness of systems resists being studied in parts. Both chaos and order are important elements in the powerful and unpredictable effects created by iteration in nonlinear systems (Wheatley, 1999). An example of chaos theory in action is when a seemingly small change, such as using assistive personnel instead of professionals, in effect creates ripples and larger impacts on the system than preplanning would seem to indicate.

There are many implications of chaos theory for health care delivery systems. The slightest variation can have enormous results in a dynamic and changing system. What is important is the quality of the system, its complexity, its distinguishing shapes, how it develops and changes, and how it differs from or compares with another system. In many ways, this highlights what nurses have known: the whole of nursing is complex and crucial to health care delivery systems in which nurses are major care coordinators.

A search for ever finer measures for discrete parts of the system probably is futile. Looking for themes or patterns rather than isolated causes is encouraged. Clearly, predictability still exists. However, for nonlinear variables and systems, randomness plays a key role in the creation of patterns of complexity and harmony of form (Wheatley, 1999).

Chaos theory can be applied to management in health care organizations. Viewing the organization as similar to a living organism, taking a holistic approach, and trusting in a natural organizing phenomenon, the manager combines expressed expectations of acceptable behavior and the grant of the freedom to individuals to assert themselves in nondeterministic ways. Guiding principles or values create powerful motivation. The manager's job is to reveal and handle the mostly hidden dynamics of the system and forge a direction for the organization as a complex adaptive system. The goal is for a self-managed system with people capable of engaging in cooperative behavior, using feedback to learn and adapt, self-organizing, and operating with flexibility.

LEADERSHIP AND MANAGEMENT IMPLICATIONS

It can be argued that all nurses are managers. Staff nurses are the employees at the most critical point in fulfilling the purpose of health care organizations: they are in close and frequent contact with the client at the point of care, and they coordinate the delivery of health care services.

The American Nurses Association (2009) defined the administration of nursing services as divided into two basic levels: the nurse manager and the nurse executive. Both have the responsibility to create a work environment that facilitates and encourages nursing staff and nursing practice. The nurse manager manages one or more defined areas of nursing services and is responsible to a nurse executive. Nurse managers allocate available resources, coordinate activities, facilitate interactive management, and have major responsibility for implementing the vision, mission, philosophy, goals, plans, and standards of the organization and nursing services. The nurse executive is responsible for managing organized nursing services from the perspective of the organization as a whole and for transforming values into daily operations to produce an efficient, effective, and caring organization. The nurse executive is accountable for the environment in which clinical nursing practice occurs.

The nurse executive provides leadership and direction for all aspects of nursing care.

The work of nursing is complex, and the role of the nurse manager is influenced by human and environmental factors in complex organizations. Being on the front lines of health care, nurse managers collaborate with others and carry out activities such as the following:

- Managing clinical nursing practice and care delivery
- Coordinating care with other disciplines to integrate services
- Managing the budget
- Managing human resources
- Being responsible for staffing and scheduling
- Evaluating the quality and appropriateness of care
- Orienting and developing employees
- Ensuring compliance with regulatory and professional standards
- Maintaining patient safety

Because of chaos, complexity, and change, client care management has needed new structures and managerial behaviors. Predicated on trust and cooperation in human relations, managers are challenged to promote consistency and stability and be anchors in an unstable world. Curtin (2000) suggested the following 10 ethical principles that might help managers reconcile perspectives and interests while centering on mission and core values:

1. Frugality and sophisticated therapeutic skill (doing the most with the least resource expenditure)
2. Clinical credibility through organizational competence
3. Presence (visibility)
4. Responsible representation at highest levels
5. Loyal service
6. Deliberate delegation
7. Responsible innovation
8. Fiduciary accountability
9. Self-discipline
10. Continuous learning

Clearly, both nurse managers and executives need a background and ability in the day-to-day fundamentals of management to achieve goals. Beyond this, skill and ability in "extraordinary management" will serve to enhance individual and collective competence.

Balancing day-to-day operations with transformative management and leadership is a creative synthesis of the best of the old with the best of the new management theories.

CURRENT ISSUES AND TRENDS

The classic notions of management and managerial work were developed in a sociopolitical era of industrialization and bureaucratization. Competitive pressures and economic forces now are compelling organizations to adopt new flexible strategies and structures. Organizations are being urged to become leaner, more entrepreneurial, and less bureaucratic. This trend has created levels of complexity and interdependency.

The result has altered conventional ideas and realities of managerial work, including shifts in roles and tasks. Traditional sources of power are eroding, and some motivational tools are less effective than they used to be. The erosion of power from hierarchical positions is perceived as a loss of authority and may create confusion about how to mobilize and motivate staff (Kanter, 1989). Kanter noted that in a leaner and flatter corporation there are many more channels for action, and managers need to work synergistically with other departments. Managers' strategic and collaborative roles become more important as they serve as integrators and facilitators, not as watchdogs and interventionists.

Current and emerging issues in health care are complex and ethically challenging for managers. The "big three" issues of access, cost, and quality continue to be organizing themes that affect any organization's internal operations. Insurance coverage is an issue of access, as is the geographic location of facilities, providers, and services. Increased complexity and technology prompt provider specialization and affect cost. Consumer preferences and increased health care awareness affect both cost and quality.

Critical medical errors and patient safety issues create pressure related to the need for quality. Complexity, randomness, and chaos created by change all call for new management and leadership strategies.

Within health care delivery systems, issues and trends facing today's managers include the following:
- Management of populations with chronic illnesses
- Resources to acquire technology on an ongoing basis
- The need for primary and preventive services and programs, including complementary and alternative programs
- Integration and seamlessness of clinical and financial services and information
- Protection of consumers' privacy
- Shortages of key personnel, especially registered nurses
- Financing structures such as accountable care organizations
- Care delivery and process management
- Management of knowledge workers and personal accountability
- Pressures for quality and sustainable outcomes
- Leadership skills related to change management

Drucker (1988) used the hospital, the university, and a symphony orchestra as models for organizations evolving in today's society. As health care reconfigures, health care delivery settings will likely be knowledge-based organizations composed primarily of specialists whose performance is directed by organized feedback from colleagues, clients, and headquarters. Nurses are positioned at the care coordination intersection and have needed skills for facilitating flow and integrating care delivery. Nurses' roles may change, but their need for managerial competence will remain. Nurses are well prepared to serve as integrators and facilitators of client care. Thus nurses appear to move easily into management and blend care into management for effectiveness (Mintzberg, 1994).

CASE STUDY

Nurse Anthony Kaufman is the director of Ambulatory Clinic A. Last year he participated in strategic planning for all the ambulatory clinics. A plan for Clinic A also was developed and approved. This year Nurse Kaufman concentrated on fine-tuning the management of the clinic. He developed a data tracking system, and trend data are now in. One disturbing trend is the rise in visit cancellations. Although the rate of cancellations is not a threat to clinic management, the increase needs to be evaluated. He does further analysis and discovers that the increase has been occurring mostly among adult females of the Muslim religion. Nurse Kaufman needs to determine the root cause: Is this an issue of individual staff cultural sensitivity, a systems problem, or some other cause?

The data are shared with the staff, and a brainstorming session occurs. One of the staff has a terrific idea: to use community contacts and internal group leaders to help inform the clinic staff as to the problem(s). The marketing and social services departments are enlisted to help. They set up roundtable gatherings, champi-

oned by the local leaders among Muslim women. One major concern emerges from these meetings: the traditional hospital gown is too revealing, unacceptable, and embarrassing. Many Muslim women had cancelled appointments for this very reason. The information is eye-opening for Nurse Kaufman. First, he is glad that it was not a staff performance issue. Second, it had never occurred to him. Hospital gowns have been the same for a very long time, and no one questions them. He calls another meeting, explores the results with staff, and asks for creative solutions. This seems like a simple managerial move. However, as the mostly female staff members begin to analyze the issue, they become excited about the possibility of a needed change. Nurse Kaufman is afraid that things might spin out of control as nurses discuss hospital gown redesign options, such as contacting New York name-brand designers. Eventually the process is worked through, using multidisciplinary collaboration, and a new gown design with extra coverage is approved and ordered.

CRITICAL THINKING EXERCISE

Nurse Victoria Munoz has been reading leadership theory. She had hoped to be inspired by this new knowledge and discover better ways to solve some problems in the nursing work environment. Instead, Nurse Munoz is puzzled. The real work environment is dramatically different from what the theory says it should be. Many articles call for strong, motivating leadership in nursing with shared leadership and empowerment of staff nurses. However, in the health care environment in which Nurse Munoz works, nursing units have been consolidated and reorganized. The inpatient nurse managers are now responsible for multiple nursing units. The nurse managers of the ambulatory clinics have been realigned to report to a physician Director of Clinics. Everyone has a new role, position, boss, and followers.

Furthermore, the nurses of the inpatient clinical departments have been exhausted from work overload and now feel angry and devalued because of the effects on the Department of Nursing. The final straw comes when they realize that the new directors of the nonclinical departments have been promoted within 3 months of the organizational changes, whereas the nurse managers remain at their previous level.

1. What is the problem?
2. What are the key issues?
3. How should Nurse Munoz handle the situation?
4. What should Nurse Munoz do first to demonstrate leadership?
5. What leadership style would be most appropriate in this situation?
6. What leadership and management strategies might be helpful?

Change and Innovation

Maryanne Garon

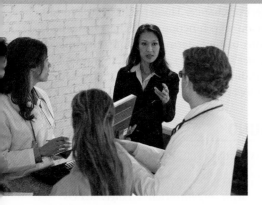

⊖volve WEBSITE

http://evolve.elsevier.com/Huber/leadership/

Change is a pervasive element of society, of today's health care environment, and of life. Many words are used to describe change, including *constant, inevitable, pervasive, universal,* and *powerful.*

> *We participate in a world where change is all there is. We sit in the midst of continuous creation, in a universe whose creativity and adaptability are beyond comprehension. Nothing is ever the same twice, really. (Wheatley, 2007, p. 84)*

Change is inevitable in health care, just as it is in life. Nurses today are accustomed to change in their environments. Many have seen changes in the acuity of patients, changes in practice models and skill mixes, a change to evidence-based practice, changes in educational requirements, and changes within their own roles. Some nurses report that changes in practice are so frequent that they are taken for granted (Copnell & Bruni, 2006). Yet they also indicate that the very basis of nursing, providing care and support for patients, has not changed (Copnell & Bruni, 2006).

Within the past few years, health care has undergone tremendous change. Health care reform, the Human Genome Project, aging baby boomers, "never events," pay for performance, and nurse shortages followed by a flood of new nurses have all impacted and led to changes in the health care system over the last decade. Still, the pace of change is only accelerating, and continuous change is becoming the new normal. The Institute of Medicine (IOM) in its 2010 report, *The Future of Nursing: Leading Change, Advancing Health,* has called upon nurses to use their numbers and adaptive capacity to take leading roles in health care change. All these changes demand the time and attention of nurses, who can choose to resist and ignore or who can decided to participate actively in the change process.

Within organizations, change can be initiated in response to external pressures, or it may come from within. In health care, change has often been externally imposed because of changes in reimbursement, regulatory changes, requirements of accrediting bodies, and marketplace demands. Changes in health care organization can also originate internally. Examples of internally initiated changes might include a unit that wants to change its practice model or a nursing service that wants to incorporate evidence-based practice.

Change is seldom easy. It can be complex and irrational. Even when it is the individual's own decision to make a change, it can be difficult. When someone makes a change, such as deciding to stop smoking, to lose weight, or to go back to school, initiating, following through, and sustaining that change is challenging. Initiating and sustaining organizational change adds unique challenges. When change is seen as unnecessary, imposed from above, or threatening workers' sense of security, the process is even more difficult. To guide the change process, nurse managers and leaders need a thorough understanding of change grounded in theory, applicable research, and reports of successful change processes.

Two approaches or models of change are found in the literature: planned change theories or models and emergent models (Shanley, 2007). Critiques of the planned approach highlight the prominence of its top-down approach and overemphasis on the role of managers in the process. In addition, the emphasis on cookbook-like approaches portrays change itself as linear rather than complex and multidimensional.

In emergent approaches, the complex and multidimensional view of change is central. The emphasis is on principles or processes of change because there is little support for one particular strategy or number of steps being more effective than another (Shanley, 2007). Emerging views of change also emphasize the importance of the participatory process in change. Therefore, in this model, it is essential for nurse leaders to understand the role of the recipients in creating and sustaining change. Viewing change and resistance as two opposing forces can result in *stereotyping* one group as irrational resisters, rather than as partners in and co-creators of change.

DEFINITIONS

Concepts related to change and innovation include change, planned change, innovation, transformation, resistance, and change agent.

Change is an alteration to make something different; a complex process that occurs over time and is influenced by any number of unpredictable variables. **Planned change** is a decision to make a deliberate effort to improve the system. Innovation is the use of a new idea or method. **Transformation** means the use of new ideas, innovation, and creativity to change fundamental properties or the state of a system. **Resistance** means to refuse to accept or be changed by something.

Change agent is a person or thing that produces a particular effect or change. The term has come to be used for a person who functions as a change facilitator. (Definitions of these terms are from *Cambridge Advanced Learner's Dictionary* (2008); Pettigrew, A.M. (1990). Longitudinal field research on change: Theory and practice. *Organizational Science, 3*(1), 267-292.)

BACKGROUND

According to Wheatley (2007):

> In the 1990s, surveys began reporting disappointing failures with organization change. CEOs reported that up to 75 percent of their organizational change efforts did not yield the promised results. These change efforts fail to produce what had been hoped for yet always produce a stream of unintended and unhelpful consequences. Leaders end up managing the impact of unwanted effects rather than the planned results that do not materialize. (p. 83)

Change has long been a topic of interest to individuals and organizations. In the past, writings on organizational change emphasized a top-down planned change strategy. In most of these, the focus was on the role of administrators and top managers in the change process. Change was seen as initiated by administrators who formulate a plan for the change and communicate it to middle managers and others. Strategies for disseminating the change, informing staff, and dealing with resisters (often viewed as stubborn and irrational) are developed and implemented (Table 2-1 displays contrasting views of change).

Alternative views emerged that promoted the idea that top-down change is not just undesirable; it does not work (Balogun, 2006). Staff and other "recipients" of change must be viewed as integral to the process rather than as potential obstructions to be influenced and acted upon (Porter-O'Grady & Malloch, 2011). All levels need to be involved in planning for and sustaining change, and ideas for change can come from all levels. In addition, when considering the processes of change, issues of power and how individuals make sense of the change are essential.

Evidence supports this emergent view of change (Shanley, 2007). There is little evidence in the literature showing whether any of the specific approaches

TABLE 2-1   CONTRASTING VIEWS OF CHANGE

	PLANNED CHANGE (TRADITIONAL VIEW)	EMERGENT VIEW
Direction	Top-down, linear	Multidirectional, multidimensional
Initiator	Leader initiated	Diffuse
Process	Planned, step-by-step process	Principles to guide process
Organizational culture	May be considered	Essential to consider
Power issues	Not considered, or not spoken	Essential to consider
Role of staff/recipients of change	Resisters	Participants in change process
View of the change recipients	May be assessed so they can be changed or manipulated	Essential to process

to planned change actually work. There is evidence about what *does* work (Balogun, 2006). The literature points to the decreased importance of executives and increased importance of those affected by any change. The planned approach is too simplistic, takes too much for granted, and does not allow the analysis of the complex aspects of change over time.

Theories of change that focus on the human side of change are important to consider. The leader-collaborator relationship needs to be central to the process. In addition, leaders must assess and understand the participants' response to change, political and power issues that affect initiation of change, and how to develop organizational or unit cultures that facilitate and sustain change.

Along with communication, change management is a critical leadership competency. The Nurse Executive Competencies developed in 2005 by the American Organization of Nurse Executives (AONE) emphasize the need for change management knowledge, skills, and abilities.

PERSPECTIVES ON CHANGE

Types of Change

Two major types of change are applicable both to individuals and to organizations. They are first-order and second-order change. A classic book by Watzlawick and colleagues (1974) popularized the terms. In their definitions, a first-order change is one within a given system in which the system itself is unchanged. The terms *first-order change* and *second-order change* can be applied to individuals, small systems, and organizations.

First-order change occurs in a stable system and is characterized by rational stepwise processes. It is seen as a method for maintaining stability in a system while making small incremental adjustments. First-order change is not seen as a vehicle for innovation, nor would it achieve organizational transformation (Alas, 2007). For an organization, it is adaptation based on monitoring the environment and making purposeful adjustments. At the industry level, this is evolution as a response to external forces such as markets. An example in nursing is when a new evidence-based protocol is developed and put into use in clinical practice. This is adaptation and adjustment.

Second-order change is discontinuous and radical and occurs when fundamental properties or states of systems are changed. Second-order change calls for transformation, using innovation, new ideas, and creativity. In a second-order change, however, the occurrence changes the system itself. Watzlawick and colleagues (1974) found that second-order change often appears strange, unexpected, and even nonsensical.

At the organization level, second-order change is described as *metamorphosis*. The entire organization is transformed, reconfigured, or moved along its life cycle. At the industry level, second-order change occurs when an entire industry is revolutionized or experiences quantum change such as emergence, transformation, or decline. An example in health care is the widespread implementation of computerized physician order entry (CPOE) technology in response to the Institute of Medicine's recommendations for patient safety reforms.

Organizational Change

Organizational change has been defined as any modification in organizational composition, structure, or behavior (Bowditch & Buono, 2001). Most often, it refers to management efforts to move an organization from a current state to "some desired future state to increase organizational functioning" (Weimer et al., 2008, p. 381). These efforts are often described as planned change and involve top-down conception, communication, and implementation. Literature on organizational change is extensive. Lewin's (1947, 1951) unfreezing, moving, and refreezing three stages of change theory is the classic model. In addition, newer approaches to organizational change, consistent with the emergent views, and can be found in the literature. In the 1990s, Senge (1990) introduced the idea of learning organizations. Learning organizations are ones that learn to adapt to change (Alas, 2007). How organizations adapt is related to their ability to be open, dynamic, and responsive to changes in the environment. The success of the learning organization is directly related to the people within the organization and their own learning. Workers need to be empowered themselves to be open and responsive to changes and to become "lifelong learners" (Senge et al., 1994).

Within the learning organizations, Senge (1990) described the following five learning disciplines:

- **Personal mastery:** Refers both to individual capacity to create desired results and to the creation of an environment or culture in which others can do the same
- **Mental models:** How individuals develop, create, and project the personal vision they have of the world and understand how these personal views affect their decisions and actions
- **Shared vision:** Sharing preferred future visions within a group for developing plans to get to that preferred future
- **Team learning:** A sharing of learning skills and conversations so that the group can develop skills and learning greater than the individual parts
- **Systems thinking:** Envisioning the organization as an interrelated system rather than unrelated parts

Learning organizations are about change and helping people embrace change. Although Senge and colleagues (1994) noted that change and learning are certainly not synonymous, they believe they are clearly linked. Senge (1990) also emphasized that developing learning organizations equal to the challenges of today's societal issues will require moving away from hierarchical leadership models and towards a new evolving idea of leadership.

Anderson and Anderson (2009) also challenged hierarchical approaches to organizational change. They described how organizational leaders realized that traditional top-down, manager-driven approaches were no longer working. On encountering obstacles and resistance, leaders learned that they had to focus more on the process of change and human relationship aspects. Anderson and Anderson (2009) call the old way of viewing change as the industrial mind-set, and that organizational leaders need to move towards an emerging mindset. The industrial mindset is a mechanistic world view, relying on power and control, certainty and predictability. Anderson and Anderson (2009) identified the emerging mindset, like other complexity views, as one grounded in wholeness and relationship, embracing co-creation and participation. A component of this emerging mindset is that leaders need to move to what they call *conscious change* leadership. Conscious change leaders are aware of the dynamics of change and learn to lead from the principles of the emerging mindset. Conscious change leaders must be willing to look internally to transform their own mind-set, expand their thinking about process, and evolve their own leadership style.

Like learning organizations and conscious change leadership, systems theory, complexity theory, and chaos theory are all models or worldviews that influence organizational change. These models suggest that the behaviors of complex systems are nonlinear, spontaneous, and self-organizing. Small changes can often produce larger dynamic (and sometimes unintended) effects. These models help us promote different understandings of changes in complex systems and how systems adapt to change (Porter-O'Grady & Malloch, 2011). However, these are not prescriptive models; instead, the focus is on interrelationships, processes, and systemic behavior.

CHANGE THEORIES

Nurse leaders, from the bedside to the executive suite, need to understand and be able to apply a variety of change theories. The majority of change theories

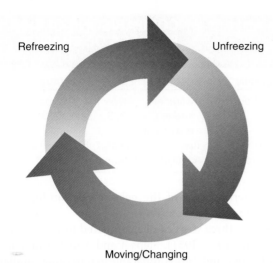

Refreezing   Unfreezing

Moving/Changing

FIGURE 2-1 Elements of a successful change. (Data from Lewin, K. [1947]. *Frontiers in group dynamics: Concept, method, and reality in social science; social equilibrium and social change. Human Relations, 1*[1], 5-41; Lewin, K. [1951]. *Field theory in social science: Selected theoretical papers.* New York: Harper & Row.)

originate from the work of Kurt Lewin. Most nurses have heard of Lewin and his three elements for a successful change: (1) unfreezing, (2) moving, and (3) refreezing (Figure 2-1). Since his work outlining the basic concepts of the change process was first published in 1947, it has been influential to those interested in change. It might be tempting to consider his ideas more consistent with the older, more traditional views of planned change (Burnes, 2004). However, Lewin was not only a remarkable thinker but also a humanitarian who believed that it was essential for democratic values to permeate all aspects of society. His model is also meant to help increase understanding about how groups and organizations change, and not as a rigid strategy to impose change. Lewin's basic change process is still useful and applicable today and is the basis for many newer theories.

Lewin's Change Process

Lewin coined the term *planned change* to distinguish the process from accidental or imposed change (Burnes, 2004). Lewin's (1947, 1951) theory of change used ideas of equilibrium within systems. *Unfreezing,* the first stage of change, can be characterized as a process of "thawing out" the system and creating the motivation or readiness for change. An awareness of

the need for change occurs. This first stage is cognitive exposure to the change idea, diagnosis of the problem, and work to generate alternative solutions. The unfreezing stage is considered to be finalized when those involved in the change process understand and generally accept the necessity of change.

The second change stage is *moving*. This means proceeding to a new level of behavior, which implies that the actual visible change occurs in this stage. When the individuals involved collect enough information to clarify and identify the problem, the change itself can be planned and initiated. Lewin (1951) observed that a process of "cognitive redefinition," or looking at the problem from a new perspective, happens. As a first step to launch a change, a pilot test may be done so that the change can be pretested and a transition period launched.

The final change stage is *refreezing*. In this stage, new changes are integrated and stabilized. Reinforcement of behavior is crucial as individuals integrate the change into their own value systems. It is important to reward change behavior. Leadership strategies of *positive feedback, encouragement,* and *constructive criticism* reinforce new behavior. Leaders point the way throughout the process of change.

Lewin's (1947, 1951) planned change process stages can be compared to the nursing process and the generic problem-solving process (Table 2-2). Unfreezing is like assessing in the nursing process and

TABLE 2-2	SIMILARITIES OF CHANGE, NURSING PROCESS, AND PROBLEM SOLVING	
CHANGE	**NURSING PROCESS**	**PROBLEM SOLVING**
Unfreezing	Assessing	Problem identification and definition
Moving	Planning and implementing	Problem analysis and seeking alternatives
Refreezing	Evaluation	Implementation and evaluation

Data from Workman, R., & Kenney, M. (1988). The change experience. In S. Pinkerton, & P. Schroeder (Eds.), *Commitment to excellence: Developing a professional nursing staff* (pp. 17-25). Rockville, MD: Aspen.

like problem identification and definition in the problem-solving process. Moving is similar to planning and implementing in the nursing process and similar to problem analysis and seeking alternative solutions in the problem-solving process. Refreezing is like evaluation in the nursing process and like implementation and evaluation in the problem-solving process.

Individuals and systems naturally strive for equilibrium. Lewin (1951) saw this as a balance between driving forces that promote change and restraining forces that inhibit change. Both driving and restraining forces impinge on any situation. The relative strengths of these forces can be analyzed. To create change, the equilibrium is broken by altering the relative strengths of driving and restraining forces. A force field analysis facilitates the identification and analysis of driving and restraining forces in any situation. Unfreezing occurs when disequilibrium is introduced into the system to disrupt the status quo. Moving is the change to a new status quo. Refreezing occurs when the change becomes the new status quo and new behaviors are frozen.

The process of change may flow back and forth among stages. It is not a simple linear process in which one step follows the preceding one. The process may move rapidly, or it may stall in any one phase. The goal of planned change is to plan, control, and evaluate the change.

Lewin's (1947, 1951) work forms the classic foundation for change theory. Other change theorists have elaborated further understanding and application of change theory. Bennis and colleagues (1961) assembled a book of readings on planned change that emphasized planner-adopter cooperation and high levels of adopter participation. Because actually implementing planned change is more dynamic and complex than Lewin's model, Lippitt (1973) refined and expanded Lewin's (1947, 1951) work on unfreezing, moving, and refreezing to identify the following seven phases of the change process that more fully describe planned change:

1. Diagnosis of the problem
2. Assessment of motivation and capacity to change
3. Assessment of the change agent's motivation and resources
4. Selecting progressive change objectives
5. Choosing an appropriate role for the change agent
6. Maintaining the change once it is started

TABLE 2-3 COMPARISONS OF THE PROCESS OF CHANGE THEORIES

LEWIN	ROGERS	LIPPITT	HAVELOCK
Unfreezing	Awareness, interest, evaluation	Steps 1, 2, 3	Steps 1, 2, 3
Moving	Trial	Steps 4, 5	Steps 4, 5
Refreezing	Adoption	Steps 6, 7	Step 6

7. Termination of the helping relationship with the change agent

The first three steps can be compared to Lewin's unfreezing (1947, 1951). Steps 4 and 5 match moving, and steps 6 and 7 are comparable to refreezing. Similar to Lippitt (1973), Havelock (1973) listed the following six elements in the process of planned change:

1. Building a relationship
2. Diagnosing the problem
3. Acquiring relevant resources
4. Choosing the solution
5. Gaining acceptance
6. Stabilization and self-renewal

The first three steps correspond to the unfreezing stage of change, the fourth and fifth are similar to the moving stage, and the last relates to refreezing. The various conceptualizations of the stages of the process of change bear similarity to one another but vary in emphasis (Table 2-3).

Innovation Theory

Change and *innovation* are companion terms, but innovation has been differentiated from change by many authors over time. Change is a disruption; innovation is the use of change to provide some new product or service (Romano, 1990). An innovation is defined as something new—the introduction of a new process or new way of doing something. Innovation also has been viewed as the use of a new idea to solve a problem (Kanter, 1983).

Kanter (1983) said that innovation refers to the process of bringing any new or problem-solving idea into use. Innovation is often linked with creativity. Organizations need to promote environments that encourage creativity and opportunities for innovation (Hughes, 2006). Leaders are essential to innovation because they must help create the environment and opportunities for innovation.

Innovation is a complex phenomenon. It is of interest in many fields from business to science, and, of course, in health care. In some views, innovation is considered a radical act, such as the introduction of a new product or process (Aranda & Molina-Fernandez, 2002). Others, such as Drucker (1992), believe that it can be a purposeful and systematic use of opportunity from changes in the economy, technology, and demographics. In this view, innovation is systematic, takes hard work, and has little to do with genius and inspiration. A purposeful and organized search for change is the basis for systematic innovation. A careful analysis of the opportunities for change is the best hope for successful economic or social innovation. This occurs because successful innovations exploit change. Drucker noted that the challenge is to make institutions capable of innovation; innovation depends on "organized abandonment" (1992, p. 340). This is a process of eliminating the obsolete and the no longer productive efforts of the past. A willingness to view change as an opportunity is needed.

Rogers (2003) described a cognitive innovation-decision process through which individuals and groups pass. The five stages of innovation-decision are as follows (Rogers, 2003):

1. First knowledge of an innovation's existence and functions
2. Persuasion to form an attitude toward the innovation
3. Decision to adopt or reject
4. Implementation of the new idea
5. Confirmation to reinforce or reverse the innovation decision

The innovation-decision process is a series of actions, behaviors, and choices over time as a new idea is evaluated and a decision is made whether to incorporate this into practice. The perceived newness and associated uncertainty are distinctive aspects of the innovation.

According to Rogers (2003), most change agents concentrate on creating awareness-knowledge. However, a more important role could be played by concentrating on how-to knowledge, which adopters need to test out an innovation. Using Hersey and colleagues' (2008) four levels of change concept, the change agent would first work on awareness-knowledge, then address attitudes and emotions, and then work on how-to skills to create a change in individual behavior.

Individual members of a group or social system will adopt an innovation at different rates. This time element of the adoption of an innovation usually follows a normal, bell-shaped curve when plotted over time on a frequency basis. However, if the cumulative number of adopters is plotted, an S-shaped curve appears (Rogers, 2003). The normal adopter frequency distribution was segmented into the following five categories (Rogers, 2003):

1. Innovators
2. Early adopters
3. Early majority
4. Late majority
5. Laggards

Change agents can anticipate these five categories as an expected phenomenon, identify followers as to likely adopter category, and target interventions accordingly. This means that for effective change, nurse leaders can recognize that there will be individual variance in "warming up" to an innovation, plan for this with targeted strategies to decrease resistance, and capitalize on the power of innovations and early adopters.

Individuals need to be interested in the innovation and committed to making change occur. The outcomes of change are either that the change is accepted or adopted or that the change is rejected. If the change is accepted, it can be either continued or eventually dropped. If the change is rejected, it can remain rejected or be adopted later in some other form. Rogers' theory (2003) described change as more complex than Lewin's (1947, 1951) three stages. The following five factors determine successful planned change (Rogers, 2003):

1. *Relative advantage:* The degree to which the change is thought to be better than the status quo
2. *Compatibility:* The degree to which the change is compatible with existing values of the individuals or group
3. *Complexity:* The degree to which a change is perceived as difficult to use and understand
4. *"Trialability":* The degree to which a change can be tested out on a limited basis
5. *"Observability":* The degree to which the results of a change are visible to others

The *diffusion of innovations* is a term derived from Rogers' work (2003) that is used to discuss the adoption of a new idea or process. Innovations create consequences. To move a new idea to the level of dissemination and adoption requires information, enthusiasm, and authority (Romano, 1990). Four elements to consider in an innovation diffusion are the innovation itself, communication channels, time, and the members of the social system (Romano, 1990).

Hughes (2006) presented a review of innovations developed by nurses worldwide. The examples given were grouped in categories of historical examples, research, clinical practice, business, education, technology, public health, and policy. The following are some examples:

- Development of hospital-based coaches, MSN prepared nurses, to assist nurses in developing process improvement projects to enhance geriatric care (AHRQ, 2012). Adapting an evidence-based "bundle", reducing ventilator-acquired pneumonia and lowering costs (AHRQ)
- Multidisciplinary team–generated interventions to improve medication reconciliation and patient safety (AHRQ).
- An Interdisciplinary Neighborhood Team project, which developed teams of public health nurses and community outreach workers to mobilize community-driven, population-based projects (Hughes, 2006).

Hughes (2006) found that nurse innovators share some common characteristics. They are self-confident, conscientious, and ambitious. Furthermore, these nurses demonstrated the following:

- A strong desire to acquire recognized qualifications
- Motivation to learn
- Perseverance
- Initiative
- Tenacity
- Determination
- A willingness to take risks

Hughes also found that innovation is both achievable and cost-effective. She believed that reporting the number of innovations that nurses have created worldwide will help demonstrate a better understanding of the role that nurses take in creating innovation.

In contrast to system-related views of innovation, Professor Clayton M. Christensen of the Harvard Business School described "disruptive innovation." Disruptive innovation describes a process wherein a simplifying technology takes root and displaces more established technologies or business practices that are slower to change, rooted in tradition, or constrained by regulation and the status quo (Christensen et al., 2000). As an example, he described a portable low intensity x-ray machine that can be used in clinics, doctors' offices, and in the field. This new technology was said to cost 10% of traditional x-rays, but it never gained acceptance or a market. In Christensen's view, this is because it threatened current business models. Regulators would hold approval of the technology, insurance companies might not pay for these x-rays, and hospitals, already invested in more expensive equipment, would also join in resisting this innovation. Christensen and colleagues (2000) also identified other disruptive innovations that could positively improve health care in the United States, including increasing the use of nurse practitioners for primary care and moving more care from acute care hospitals to clinics and homes (already occurring). An example of a disruptive innovation is shown in Box 2-1. In his opinion, health care needs creative leaders and flexible organizations to incorporate new ideas and innovations and to move forward.

BOX 2-1   EXAMPLE OF DISRUPTIVE INNOVATION IN HEALTH CARE

Disruptive innovations were described by Christensen and colleagues (2000) as simplifying "technology" that takes root. One such innovation that fits his definition was a barber-based blood pressure control program for African-American men (AHRQ, 2012). In this innovation, "trained barbers in African-American owned shops provided ongoing monitoring of blood pressure to African American male patrons during each haircut, along with printed educational materials and feedback designed to encourage those with elevated blood pressure to visit the doctor." African-American men suffer higher rates of hypertension than the rest of the population and often have higher rates of disability due to it. By providing this screening and educational materials at every haircut, the program significantly improved treatment rates and blood pressure control in hypertensive patrons. This outside-the-box innovation was a low cost approach that was successful in meeting a community health need.

THE PROCESS OF CHANGE

Change in health care has been shown to be continuous and rapid. It may appear to be like a continuum from haphazard drift at one end to a structured, planned change at the other. Van Woerkum and colleagues (2011) acknowledged that "change happens" (p. 148), and that there are three ways it happens:

1. The emergence of events: essentially change by chance
2. The use of language: how we arrive at new interpretations and ideas, by talking with one another about them
3. The development of practices: the result of a chain of activities; purposeful and planned

Within nursing and health care, change is sometimes forced upon us by events, whether it be changing disaster policies because of lessons learned from a hurricane or changing the way patient records are handled after the **Health Insurance Portability and Accountability Act of 1996 (HIPAA)** was passed. Through language, which may include meetings, journal stories, and interpretations of reports, nurses make conscious efforts to change to meet latest accreditation requirements or safety standards. The development of new practices, due to new evidence or best practices, occur regularly and fall under planned change. One example is the broad adoption of evidence-based protocols and practices as a way of making sure that desirable outcomes are achieved.

Planned Change

The amount of change and the rapidity of change can disrupt and disorganize people. Because of the rapidity of change in areas such as technology, it is easy to slip into the perception that history is what occurred 2 years ago and ancient history refers to 5 years ago. Obsolescence occurs before people have had a chance to adapt to the last round of changes. The inevitable result is stress on individuals as they try to cope. These dynamics affect nurses in their roles as care providers and care managers and profoundly influence the profession of nursing through employment and compensation fluctuations. One method to enhance nurses' productivity and decrease stress from turbulence in the environment is to strategically use planned change.

The use of planned change is a nursing management intervention strategy. The nurse uses diagnosis and intervention in clinical practice: the nurse assesses, diagnoses, develops a plan for the client's care needs, and selects an intervention that is matched to that assessment and diagnosis. Managers also assess, diagnose, and plan interventions to meet organizational needs and goals. They look at resource allocation and deployment of people in using planned change as a management intervention. Planned change theories are engineering theories in that they use social science principles to plan change (Tiffany & Lutjens, 1998). Planning and managing the change process may focus on any or all of the following situational elements: organizational structure, people, or resources. *Planned change* refers to deliberately engineered change in groups. A planned change theory is a set of logically interrelated concepts that explain how change occurs, predict forces and effects, and help planners control variables in a change process. In their review and analysis of the change theory literature, Tiffany and Lutjens (1998) identified three theories popular in nursing and one in a non-nursing model. The three main theories used in nursing are Lewin's (1947, 1951) planned change theory, writings by Bennis and colleagues (1961, 1976), and Rogers' (2003) theory of diffusion of innovations. One model not used in nursing is Bhola's (1994) **c**onfigurations, **l**inkages, **e**nvironment, and **r**esources (CLER) systems model. Lewin's (1947, 1951) theory ranks as the most popular change theory among nurses (Tiffany & Lutjens, 1998).

Change Management

To ensure that the process of change is effective, it is important to understand how unintended consequences can result from top-down planning or ineffective communication. Based on her extensive research on organizational change, Balogun (2006) noted the following implications for leaders managing the process of change:

- Executives and administrators do not direct change, but they do initiate and influence the direction of change.
- The recipients of change (middle managers and staff) translate and edit plans for change.
- The main method by which recipients interpret what the change is all about is through informal

communication with peers (not top-down or official information channels).

- Senior managers need to monitor these communications and learn to engage in lateral, informal communications. Some of this can be accomplished using "management by walking about."
- More explicit attention must be given to open discussions and storytelling in communication about change.
- The recipients of change will mediate the outcomes, so senior managers need to acknowledge this and actively engage with them.
- In large organizations, using change ambassadors to help with the engagement/discussion process may be helpful.
- Finally, senior managers need to "live the changes" they want others to adopt. The recipients of change are quick to notice inconsistencies between the actions, words, and deeds of the leaders.

Balogun (2006) asserted that the meaning of "managing" change needs to be reconsidered. The idea needs to change from one of top-down control to one of participation and communication.

Another useful strategy for preplanning the management of change is to assess readiness for organizational change. One inventory is the Organizational Change-Readiness Scale (OCRS) (Jones & Bearley, 1996). This 76-item inventory was designed to analyze the ability of an organization to manage change effectively. The five dimensions of structure, technology, climate, system, and people are assessed for barriers and supportive conditions. The five dimensions tend to influence each other. A Lewin-type force field analysis is applied to the results. A structured assessment tool is helpful for comprehensive data gathering.

Change Management: Small Scale

In today's health care environment, with the emphasis on patient safety and quality goals, there is a need to make small rapid changes to improve care. Two related models can be used to make these small rapid changes. They are rapid cycle change and Transforming Care at the Bedside (TCAB) (Robert Wood Johnson Foundation [RWJF], 2008). Both use the plan-do-study-act model as a basis. Rapid cycle change is based on the idea that changes should first be tried on a small scale, to see how they work. TCAB was a program created by RWJF with the idea of improving quality and safety on medical-surgical acute care units by engaging in changes to improve practice. The idea is to create a small test, evolve the idea, get feedback, and proceed. RWJF has a downloadable toolkit on its website to help organizations implement TCAB. Numerous projects have been implemented since its initiation in 2003, such as creation of rapid response teams, initiating multidisciplinary rounds at the bedside, and planning inventions to decrease patient falls.

Rapid-cycle change, a methodology adapted from Toyota Production System principles, uses a small, focused, rapid process to make process improvements (AHRQ, 2012). The idea is that, rather than initiating long research studies, staff are encouraged to brainstorm new ideas, try a potential change, and test its effectiveness. This can be done with one nurse, one shift, and one patient. Demonstrating the effectiveness of small change encourages nurses to try others. Rapid cycle change is often discussed and used in conjunction with TCAB (Valente, 2011).

The Human Factor: Resistance

Resistance to change should be expected as integral to the whole process of change. Like the Peanuts© cartoon character Linus, human beings need something to hang on to. The old ways may indeed need to be changed, but the natural fear of what will replace them may cause people to cling to the old. People may fear being disorganized or having their routines interrupted. Some may have a vested interest in the status quo. Others may believe that a change may diminish their own status or disrupt their network of interpersonal relationships.

Almost all changes encounter some resistance as a natural phenomenon. Resistance may be rooted in anxiety or fear. For example, some individuals fear expenditure of the energy needed to cope with change. Some fear a loss of status, power, control, money, or employment. Misconceptions and inaccurate information about what the change might mean and individuals' emotional reactions create resistance to change. Although resistance is characterized as a challenge, a negative behavior, or something to be overcome, not all resistance is bad. It may be a warning to the change agent to reevaluate the change, clarify the purpose, or increase communication. The leader or change agent may need to re-conceptualize his or her approach to the change, anticipate resistance, determine why it is occurring, and better understand the perspective of the resisters.

To fully understand the concept of resistance, it is helpful to re-conceptualize staff nurses as the solution in initiating change rather than as the problem. Too often, nurses have been characterized as the targets of change, irrational resisters, and problems to overcome rather than as co-creators of change. Nurses are central to change within health care. They are the largest group of health care providers. They play a key role in the initiation, planning, and sustenance of change (Leeman et al., 2007). In fact, because of their numbers and their key role in the process, nurses were found to be the only viable agents of sustaining change (Balfour & Clarke, 2001).

Resistance Reframed

One way to reframe perceptions of resistance is to consider the positive effect that resisters and resistance have played in history and in the development of the United States. From the actions of the rebels in the Boston Tea Party to the antislavery abolitionists in the nineteenth century to the civil rights activists of the 1960s, resistance has shaped our history. Furthermore, some individuals have contributed to our views on resistance. They include Thoreau, who in 1849 wrote his classic essay, "Civil Disobedience," and contributed the underlying idea that acting from principle, on the belief of what is right, is above the law. John Woolman, a Quaker, spent his life convincing other Quakers to give up slavery by personally visiting them one by one and discussing their views of morality. Sojourner Truth, an African-American woman born as a slave, worked tirelessly for the rights of African Americans. Martin Luther King, Jr., led the Civil Rights Movement in the 1960s and inspired with his words on passive resistance. All of these resisters were leaders who inspired others to work for change. So, as leaders, how do we inspire others to work for change rather than impose organizational change from above? This is the challenge.

Re-conceptualizing staff and others as the co-creators of change instead of resisters not only provides an alternative view of change and resistance but also can point to new strategies for moving organizations toward change. In viewing resistance from the emergent view, it is important not to dichotomize initiators and recipients of change. Involving everyone is essential to the change process. The success and sustainability of the change depends on the commitment to the change by those at the level of the change.

Nurses live with change daily. The common belief that nurses resist change is just not accurate. Instead, nurses have reported that changes occur so frequently that they could not remember all of them (Copnell & Bruni, 2006). Falk-Rafael (2000) found that the nurses in her qualitative study had six different orientations to change. Three of these were ways they ended up accepting change: critical approval, insidious assimilation, wounded acquiescence. She found that nurses used judicious circumvention and constructive opposition when they believed that changes could jeopardize their clients' health (Falk-Rafael, 2000). The final orientation was nurses initiating change themselves through what she labeled "visionary transformation" (Falk-Rafael, 2000, p. 336). Her findings countered some commonly held beliefs about nurses' resistance to change.

EMOTIONAL RESPONSES TO CHANGE

Dealing with change evokes emotional responses for all involved. Although individuals must devote personal resources and energy to accomplish change, organizations tend to overlook the human emotions associated with an organizational change. Change is more successful as the intellectual and emotional issues involved in change phases are recognized and addressed.

Managers often find it difficult to manage change, and as noted earlier, experience a host of negative emotions themselves (Shanley, 2007). Employees also exhibit emotional responses to change, ranging from fear, sadness, outrage, stress, and disorientation to eroded loyalty, lack of commitment, and low risk taking (Shanley, 2007). Organizational leaders need to be aware of the potential fallout of these emotional responses when undertaking change.

Managers can provide emotional support to staff in periods of stress and change. Some of the effective strategies are:

1. Active listening
2. Promoting action steps and solutions
3. Keeping staff informed of decisions
4. Soliciting input and encouraging participation
5. Reframing difficult messages

The meaning that a change has for the individual is important and influences how they view that change. The meaning that the initiator of change intends is not always what the recipient of change perceives. For example, Bartunek and colleagues (2006) studied those on the receiving end of change in a hospital implementing shared governance. Although the change agents saw shared governance as an opportunity for increased empowerment for the staff, many of those on the receiving end saw it as an increase in workload. Any perceived positive gain was negated by the personal feelings of added work. Additional factors influencing this implementation were the role of emotional contagion and "inadequate, infrequent and poorly time education about it" (Bartunek et al., 2006, p. 203). These researchers noted that emotion did play a strong role in this change effort, and the associated emotions differed between units. The emotional contagion was due to the staff influencing one another.

Although most people inherently distrust change, change can be viewed either positively or negatively. To facilitate the change process, leaders or change agents need to actively involve the recipients of change, work to understand their view, and plan adequate, timely education on the change. An additional intervention might be to monitor unit level reactions and understanding, because it appears that individuals who understand the change better view it more positively.

Like so much in leadership, learning to lead and manage change must be a mutual process between leaders and followers. Leaders need to listen, understand, validate feelings, instruct, and encourage… and then go back and do it again. Followers need to engage with the change in good faith, allowing for a reasonable chance for success.

EFFECTIVE CHANGE

A decisive factor in how change proceeds is how it is managed (Savcik et al., 2007). Ineffective implementation of or responses to change do not allow the change process to go forward. Responses can include inadequate preparation, being defensive, not listening, and prematurely persuading. The way to deal with emotionality is to allow people to express themselves while avoiding action based on the emotionality. Trying to immediately persuade people cuts off their ability to vent emotions. Without venting, they may not be able to work through the stages.

Censuring, controlling, or punishing likely drives resistance underground. The more that a planned change is driven by authoritarian actions, the more that the seeds of future discontent are sown. The most effective managers possess self-confidence, knowledge of the change process, and the interpersonal skill to help participants accept, allow, and see the process of change as natural, thereby enhancing coping while facilitating planned change.

Change cycles can be either participative or directive. In a participative change, new knowledge is made available to participants to trigger change. Personal power is used to trigger knowledge, attitude, individual behavior, and group behavior change. Directive change occurs when a change is imposed by some external force. Position power is used to trigger group behavior, individual behavior, attitudes, and knowledge change (Hersey et al., 2008).

The probability of effectiveness of the change process can be increased through several techniques, as follows:

- Explain the rationale for a change so that individuals understand it.
- Allow emotions to be worked out.
- Give participants all the information they need.
- Help individuals cope with change.

The following actions should be avoided when implementing a change within an organization:

- Simply announce a change without bothering to lay a foundation.
- Ignore or offend powerful people in the organization.
- Violate the authority and communication lines in the existing organization.
- Rely only on formal authority in implementing a change.
- Overestimate your formal authority.
- Make a poor decision about what change is needed and be closed to people critiquing the decision.
- Communicate ineffectively.
- Put people on the defensive.
- Underestimate the perceived magnitude of the change.
- Do not deal with the people's fears about insecurity or change of status.

Concerns, insecurities, and resistance are predictable as a part of change. Effectiveness and success are increased as these reactions are anticipated and strategies to cope are developed. The leader's role is to recognize, accept, and help followers process, adapt, and cope with these emotional stages to deal effectively with change. The leader's behaviors are crucial to helping followers with the disruption and reintegration that occur during any change. Thus leaders need to focus on people, considering factors such as the following:

- The time and effort it takes to adjust
- The possibility of less desirable outcomes
- Fear of the unknown
- Tolerance for change capacity
- Trust levels
- Needs for security
- Leadership skills
- Vested interests and "sacred cows"
- Opposing group values
- How coalitions form
- Strongly held views
- Existing relationship-dynamics disruptions

How is change effective? A positive and constructive group process needs to be established. Interpersonal relationships are very important. Given the number of changes going on in the environment, empowerment involves using change successfully. Successful change empowers participants. Nurses are empowered when change increases their responsibility, authority, and accountability and gives them the mechanisms to make decisions to be able to affect client care.

LEADERSHIP AND CHANGE

Never doubt that a small group of thoughtful, committed citizens can change the world. Indeed, it is the only thing that ever has.

-Margaret Mead

Leaders are an essential part of the change process. The approach, skills, and values that individual leaders bring to change efforts are integral to its success. Some authors have even used change as part of the definition for leadership. Burns (1978), credited with introducing the idea of transformational leadership, emphasized that leadership is about transformation. Transformational leadership is a model of leadership that embodies change. Rost (1994) conceived leadership not as positional but as a process that moves people to work together to make real change in their lives

or in organizations. The value of Rost's definition is that leaders do not depend on an organizational position, and the leader role may rotate depending on the change desired and the approach taken. Despite their earlier formulation, these views of leadership are more consistent with the emergent view of change.

Within health care, with the continuous and rapid rate of change, nurse leaders need knowledge, skills, and abilities in working with the change process. In the Nurse Executive Competencies from the AONE (2005), understanding change and innovation and how to manage it is an essential leadership competency for nurses. Shirey (2007) presented 10 tips for expert, effective leadership based on the AONE's competencies. Number four was *"Be a change agent and advocate for innovation"* (p. 169).

Despite the fact that change is ever-present and necessary, leaders/managers still find it one of the most difficult aspects of their role. In fact, managers often report that their reactions to change and the need to initiate change are emotions similar to and as strong as those associated with disasters, catastrophes, and even abuse (Shanley, 2007). Change can be positive but also have multiple negative outcomes, including low morale, stress, and low self-esteem. The key lies in the management of change and human reactions through the process.

Leadership Roles in Change

Nurse leaders may take a number of roles in the process of change. Nurse executives and administrators are essential for providing the vision of a preferred future, initiating change, and helping guide the direction of change. Middle-level and first-level managers and staff, as the recipients of change, may also take roles in initiating and sustaining change. In addition, nurses in a variety of roles, from educators to clinical specialists to staff nurses, may take on roles of change agents, opinion leaders, and early adopters of innovations. This often resembles a brokering or buffering role.

Leaders as Change Agents

Change agents can follow a number of steps in the process of change, as follows:

- Articulate a clear need for the change.
- Have the group participate by leaving details to those who have to implement the change.

- Provide reliable information and details to those who are to implement the change.
- Motivate through rewards and benefits to help the change along.
- Do not promise anything that cannot be delivered.

For example, when implementing a planned change to a new care delivery system, the change agent would need to be clear about the need for and the benefits of the change. This might include greater autonomy for nurses, greater safety and quality or improved effectiveness. The details of implementation should be left to the group, but only after reliable and detailed information is communicated to them. Rewards and benefits, not threats about performance scrutiny, should be the basis of the motivation to change. Participation itself may be motivating. Promised benefits from the change should be limited to what the change agent can reasonably deliver.

POWER AND POLITICS

Power issues and politics are central in considering change and have often been overlooked. Leaders need to consider power issues when planning for change. Shanley (2007) suggested that change initiators ask, "Whose needs are being met by the change, and whose interests are being served by the change?" In addition, many of the usual approaches to planned change reinforce hierarchical managerial practices and top-down control, thus making change more difficult to implement. Powerful change can occur through shared governance mechanisms that enhance sustainability.

Some past changes in health care, such as the restructuring efforts of the 1990s, created change that was negative for nurses and, eventually, organizations and patients. These changes were externally imposed, reportedly for cost-containment because of reimbursement changes. The top-down destructive influences of those changes were demoralizing to nurses and had long-term, unintended consequences, including changed staffing ratios, increased usage of unlicensed personnel, and possibly even contributed to the nursing shortage of the early 2000s.

In implementing change, considerations of power may be one of the most difficult areas for nurse leaders. Powerful economic or political interests may pressure nurse leaders to make organizational changes or enact restructuring to alleviate immediate problems.

Unfortunately, the long-term effects of these changes may be difficult to foresee or to quantify. Nurses, at all levels, must learn to speak up, articulate, and support the value of their role and evaluate change for the long term. As nurses become more involved in leadership roles in the health care system, as suggested in the IOM report, *The Future of Nursing* (2011), they can use their own positional influence to chart nursing's own destiny and, hopefully, prevent destructive practices like those that emerged in the 1990s.

LEADERSHIP AND MANAGEMENT IMPLICATIONS

Because of the complexity and extent of change, knowledge and skill in applying systems principles are needed by nurses who are leading and managing change. An organization that is committed to changing itself needs continuous learning and adaptation as a systems value. As described earlier, this is a *learning organization*. These innovative and creative organizations need to foster their commitment to change and innovation. Porter-O'Grady and Malloch (2011) moved away from discussion of structural components of change and emphasized the following four practices for current workplaces that foster learning organizations:

1. Empowerment
2. Shared decision making
3. Self-direction
4. Shared governance

Change is implied in the definition of leadership. If leadership is defined as influencing others, then the activity of influencing is directed toward some change. The ability to envision and communicate a changed future is part of the definition of leadership. Numerous authors have noted that change is an inevitable fact of life, but leaders and managers can cope by developing processes that allow them to initiate and influence change. The essentials of leadership that are needed are an ability to envision the change needed, reflection on the issues inherent in the change, positive communication skills, an ability to promote cultures that encourage creativity and change, and showing that they actually "walk the talk."

Transformational change is a part of organizational transformation. To produce strategic change, transformational leaders work with others to ignite a

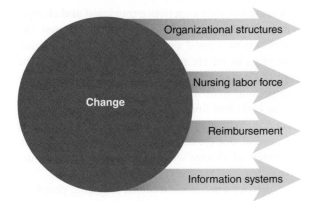

FIGURE 2-2 Areas of major change in health care and nursing.

vision, change structure and culture, change mindsets and power structures, and empower others (Robbins & Davidhizar, 2007). Both leaders and managers can be effective in initiating and influencing organizational change. Anyone in the organization can be the focal point for making appropriate and effective change, but the employees in staff positions need to enlist the cooperation and support of the administrative hierarchy.

Because of constant change, nurses and health care systems have had to learn and adapt. To view the scope of change surrounding nursing in perspective, four areas of major change can be identified: organizational structures, nursing labor force, reimbursement, and information systems (Figure 2-2). First, organizational structures have been changing and reconfiguring in response to the environment and financial pressures. For example, population-based care, case management, patient-centered care, and patient safety initiatives are elements reflecting change in regard to the redesign of client care systems. In health care, bureaucratic systems endured for a long time but were not well suited to the work of professionals. The empowerment of staff to result in outcomes of quality is the goal. Clearly, the Affordable Care Act (ACA) of 2010 is an issue creating uncertainty and change throughout the health care delivery system and its organizations because it has triggered a change process that is ongoing and possibly transformative. Changes also are occurring in health care as integrated networks form and care increasingly is moved into community settings.

Changing organizational structures are occurring in the midst of a nurse shortage. The complexion of the nurse workforce is changing; and recruitment and retention, education, and staff deployment alternatives are being explored.

Another area of important change in health care is reimbursement. For example, reimbursement (payment) for physicians has been changing, driven previously by the federal government's relative value units determinations and now pay-for-performance and pay based on outcomes. Reimbursement for nurse practitioners currently is allowed under Medicare/Medicaid. However, managed care, with its capitated reimbursement structure, has changed payment to all forms of health care providers. Payment reforms are likely to continue and change. The cost areas include physician payment, already being ratcheted down; pharmaceutical costs; and equipment and technology costs. The government will continue to review and explore the amount of dollars spent and the way those dollars are spent in an effort to reduce a huge national budget deficit fueled partly by health care costs. An increase in governmental intervention and regulatory control can be predicted in health care.

Present and future changes will bring an increasing use of computerized information systems. A massive increase in computerization is underway with the electronic health record (EHR) and meaningful use initiatives. Powerful computers and sophisticated software programs have a pattern of undergoing updates and generational changes frequently, creating challenges of compatibility, archival retrieval, maintaining currency, and staff training. Compatibility among systems, such as relational databases, remains challenging.

CURRENT ISSUES AND TRENDS

At the end of the last century, multiple authors identified future trends in health care. They predicted that these amounted to major paradigm shifts. In 1996, Issel and Anderson identified the following six interconnected transformations that are major areas of change still influencing health care today:

1. From person-as-customer to the population-as-customer
2. From illness care to wellness care and prevention

3. From revenue management to cost management
4. From autonomy of professionals to their interdependence
5. From client as nonconsumer to consumer of cost and quality information
6. From continuity of provider to continuity of information

Although the transformations they identified have not all yet been incorporated within health care as the authors may have imagined, there have been slow shifts toward those changes. For example, the ACA (2010) is not just a payment or insurance program; its aims are to guide the United States to shift health care priorities to wellness and prevention. The IOM report on the *Future of Nursing* (2011) emphasized the need for professionals to increase interdependence and collaboration. Attempts to increase utilization of electronic health records (and make them portable) are a way to improve continuity of information. Other trends that will impact health care in the United States include:

- Increased emphasis on evidence-based interventions
- Rising rates of obesity
- Aging population
- Advances in genomics
- Advances in technology and electronic health records
- Increased numbers of veterans with PTSD and traumatic brain injury
- Telehealth
- Integrative medicine
- Pay-for-performance
- Focus on safety and quality
- Medical homes, Accountable Care Organizations, and patient-centered care.

These changes have and will continue to alter the health care delivery system. They present both opportunities and challenges, and nurses need to be able to anticipate and monitor trends for their immediate and long-term effects on practice. Nurses can participate in and even lead some of these trends, as they create new environments or establish new organizational forms to shape the direction of health care. It is a question of which are the best courses of action and what is the best way to direct the transformations.

It is a new era for leadership with new rules (Porter-O'Grady & Malloch, 2011). This means that leaders need to be able to guide others through this new reality as they experience transition and change. Porter-O'Grady and Malloch (2011) said that the leader acts as a good signpost reader in a transition time (e.g., as we are now living); they anticipate the path of change and guide others in the direction of change so as to be able to continue to work and survive in turbulent times when the environment is ever-changing. Wheatley (2007) suggested that principles are needed, not techniques or models. The four core principles of change she proposes are the following (Wheatley, 2007):

- *Participation is not a choice:* Engaging people in the change from the beginning can prevent unintended consequences in the end.
- *Life always reacts to directives; it does not obey them:* This principle suggests offering invitations for others to work with us, rather than issuing directives or orders or even giving "visionary" messages.
- *We do not see "reality"; we create our own interpretation of what is real:* This principle stresses the importance about not arguing who is right or who is wrong, but rather understanding that each one of us filters reality through our own lenses.
- *To create living health in a living system; connect it to more of itself:* This principle is based on a strong respect for systems, and it supports the leader's task of strengthening communication and connections within the system.

The health care environment has been described as turbulent because of the rapid rate of change and the perceived constancy of change. However, change can be growth-producing, renewing, and invigorating for individuals and organizations. This occurs as individuals and organizations enlist creativity to derive an innovation that improves the environment or client care delivery. "Leadership *is* the leading of creativity which leads to creative change" (Kerfoot, 1998, p. 99).

An investment in creativity and innovation, with resulting change, provides strategic advantage. Creativity withers in hostile environments in which all of the time is spent thinking about survival. Strategies to develop a culture that fosters creativity and change include the following (Kerfoot, 1998):

- Promoting conversations and dialogue
- Providing access to information
- Building relationships

- Teaching rethinking, questioning, and innovation
- Creating a culture of innovation
- Orchestrating and executing

In an organizational context, creativity means producing novel and useful ideas by an individual or a group. It is the basis of invention and innovation. Creativity in organizations is influenced by management practices and creativity-relevant work group skills. Creativity is one important aspect of organizational innovation (Gilmartin, 1999).

RESEARCH NOTE

Source

Grant, B., Colello, S., Reihle, M., & Dende, D. (2010). An evaluation of the nursing practice environment and successful change management using the new generation Magnet Model. *Journal of Nursing Management, 18*, 326-331.

Purpose

The authors discussed a successful implementation of a practice change that was evaluated using the ANCC Magnet Model's success factors. A group of staff nurses working on an orthopedic and neuro-trauma unit wanted to initiate a change in shift-to-shift reporting by moving it to the bedside to engage the patients and families as partners. The goals for the change, the engagement of the staff nurses and the partnership with patients and families, were consistent with the hospital's Magnet environment and supported by the nursing management team.

Discussion

Because of the Magnet culture and the management team's commitment to an empowered, engaged staff, the staff took on the leadership roles and were essential to the success of this new practice, called Partnership Rounding.

The authors discussed how the staff leaders of this effort considered the complexity of the culture change and group dynamics and utilized Lewin's change theory. The result was a highly successful change, with many benefits for patients, families, and staff. For outcomes, it was found that 1 year after implementation, 100% of patients and 97.5% of staff had experienced Partnership Rounding. The change studied in this case was initiated by the staff and supported by leadership. This provided additional support for the literature that attests to the success of change when it is participatory rather than imposed top-down.

Application to Practice

The health care environment has been described as turbulent because of the rapid rate of change and the perceived constancy of change. However, change can be growth producing, renewing, and empowering for individuals and organizations. This occurs as individuals and organizations enlist creativity to derive an innovation that improves the environment or client care delivery. Additionally, the Magnet Model in this case provided an important and useful framework to develop both the work environment that is receptive of change and the dynamic and empowered workforce to engage in change.

CASE STUDY

Nurse Sara Lopez works as the director of the medical surgical (med-surg) unit at a regional medical center that is currently undergoing extensive organizational change. The medical center is in the midst of a large construction project with a new patient care tower. In planning for the transition to the new tower, the current med-surg unit will be splitting into two separate units, one medical unit and one surgical unit. As a result, this means staff must be divided between two units.

The nursing management team is committed to a participatory management style and wants to plan for the changes and the move, with participation from the staff and by being as fair as possible.

With the approval of Human Resources, the management team first approached key stakeholders, such as the medical teams involved, surgeons, hospital supervisors, and executive team members, to inform them of the pending change. They then informed the staff of the split and took the time to talk to each staff member one-on-one. Some staff reacted emotionally and with a lot of apprehension.

Once Sara and her management team had informed the staff nurses, they gave them 3 weeks to think about and come to a decision about their unit preference. Sara also met with the clinical practice council (shared governance), which included a patient representative, to get input on what they considered to be a fair process of dividing the staff. The council requested that job descriptions be posted to help with the nursing staff with their decisions. The council also suggested a float pool for staff who were unsure or undecided, so they could go between the two units until they figure their personal preferences.

Continued

CASE STUDY—cont'd

Sara and team also consulted with the executive team and human resources for further advice, including how best to develop the future policies for major changes involving a selection process, such as a policy for layoffs. This helped them to prioritize how best to divide the staff to the different units.

Sara and the team also talked to managers and staff from other units who had split in the past, to learn what worked well and what did not. The move to the new units will proceed in 2 months, and Sara believes they have good groundwork for this change to proceed smoothly.

The process for change utilized by Nurse Lopez included the following:

1. An assessment of the change, including needs of each new unit, position descriptions, space, and patient needs, including a review of the health care system's policies to ensure that they were consistent
2. A change process that incorporated the governance structure and consensus decision-making style of the department
3. New role descriptions for RNs, consistent with their current positions
4. Continuing to build trust and relationships within the staff and to reassure all stakeholders, physicians, administration, patients, and families that the changes will result in improved patient care
5. Keeping changes consistent with need to balance staffing levels, skills, and unit needs
6. Efficient and effective infrastructure and operating processes
7. Recognition that the need for staff acceptance and participation will aid the transition process
8. Keeping within budget, resources, and staffing needs allotted for the two units

Using these eight points as a guideline, Nurse Lopez and the staff together began to implement their plan for organizational change and transformation.

▌ CRITICAL THINKING EXERCISE

Nurse Jim Chen has been the nurse manager of the primary care clinics within a large health care organization for over 10 years. Jim is considered an excellent communicator and is well regarded by the physicians, nurses, and auxiliary staff. The health care system has been converting the acute care areas to electronic health care records (EHR) and is now ready to introduce them to the outpatient clinics. Jim has been appointed a "champion" of EHR for the clinics, and is charged with gathering a committee for implementation. He knows that members of the staff have differing views on the EHR, but most view it as a necessary change. However, some of the older staff feel very threatened (that jobs must be in danger), because they are uncomfortable with computers and new technology and have limited keyboarding skills.

1. What are some of the issues that Jim must plan for?
2. What theory or model might be useful?
3. Who should be involved in the committee to plan this change?
4. What might be Jim's first step in planning for this innovation?
5. How might he or the committee prevent or decrease resistance of other staff?

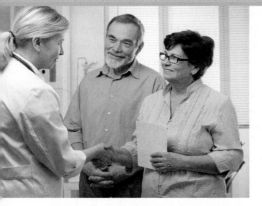

Organizational Climate and Culture

Jennifer Bellot

⊖volve WEBSITE

http://evolve.elsevier.com/Huber/leadership/

Since the 1960s, health care organizations have systematically responded to economic, social, and financial challenges that have ultimately caused a transformation in health care delivery. Health care organizations now compete in a marketplace based on their ability to demonstrate lean performance, increased efficiency, and quality health outcomes. The payment structure for health care has shifted from fee-for-service to prospective payment to pay-for-performance and outcomes. Further, the landmark Institute of Medicine (IOM) report, *Crossing the Quality Chasm* (IOM, 2001) described the challenge of care provision in the twenty-first century and detailed the shift that includes moving from provider-centered care to patient-centered care. Inclusion of patient and family values, norms, customs, and need for participation is now a dominant force in treatment decisions. Furthermore, recent inquiry regarding patient safety has emphasized not only patient outcomes, but also the processes and behaviors that lead to safe care. An explosion in information technology capacity is altering the speed and transparency of communication and information delivery. Interdisciplinary care and teamwork are gaining prominence, showing better care outcomes

Photo used with permission from Photos.com.

(Stock et al., 2008). The impact of an impending nurse shortage, the increasing demand for nursing care, and the drive to incorporate evidence-based practice are changing the face of nursing care. Taken together, these issues have transformed health care structure and delivery, creating a fast-paced and ever-changing practice environment for nurses to negotiate.

An appreciation for workplace culture is critical for today's nurse leader. In the perfect storm, nurses may wonder how these factors link with culture and their role as nurses and leaders. Nurses' insight into culture enables them to better understand staff behaviors and relationships, norms, change processes, expectations, and communications. This holds true for all levels of nurses from novice to expert practitioner, direct care provider to administrator. This chapter provides an overview of culture, focusing on the factors that affect the culture within an organization also discusses organizational culture and climate and their relationship to the nursing work environment, workforce, and practice.

DEFINITIONS

Culture

Organizational culture is rooted in anthropology, psychology, sociology, and management theory and first appeared in the academic literature in 1952

(Scott et al., 2003). **Culture** is the set of values, beliefs, and assumptions that are shared by members of an organization. An organization's culture provides a common belief system among its members. The purpose of culture is to provide a common bond so that members know how to relate to one another and to show others who are outside of the organization what is valued. Culture is sometimes likened to an iceberg in that only the top of the iceberg is visible and the invisible part of the iceberg runs deep into the ocean (Daft, 2001). The top of the iceberg can be thought of as being the mission statement, policies, procedures, organizational charts, the way people dress, and the language they use. The invisible part of the iceberg can be what is implicit in the organization, such as the unwritten rules and customs that pervade the work environment (most are easily missed, yet critical to know). Collectively, these variables define the character and norms of the organization.

Culture is represented in several ways. For example, the care delivery model that guides nursing practice helps interpret the culture. For example, when a relationship-based nursing care model is used, it represents an underlying belief in patient-centered care. Open visiting hours in the ICU convey the importance of family as partners in care delivery. How new nurses are oriented expresses values about the socialization of new nurses. Many visible aspects of culture reflect the underlying values of the organization.

Culture is a multifaceted phenomenon, difficult to comprehend and unravel. The health care system is incredibly complex. High quality health care delivery is dependent upon good communication and collaboration between providers, patients and their families. One way to better understand such relationships is to appreciate how the hospital culture affects nursing units, nursing practice, and patient outcomes. For a nurse to function effectively in an organization, a solid grasp of organizational culture, characteristics, and operations is essential.

Culture has been measured both quantitatively and qualitatively. Initially, it was thought that something as diffuse and intangible as culture could only be measured using qualitative techniques. Bellot (2011, p. 33) stated that "early culture researchers believed that standardized, quantitative instruments were inappropriate for cultural assessment because they would be unable to capture the subjective and unique aspects of each culture." A strictly qualitative approach of cultural assessment can be time-consuming, expensive, and difficult to interpret. Thus various quantitative tools have been developed to more quickly assess culture and allow for comparison across different work environments. In reality, it is likely that a combination of qualitative and quantitative measures are best for capturing organizational culture (Bellot, 2011). The choice of a measurement instrument should be directed by definition, purpose, and context for cultural assessment (Scott et al., 2003).

Climate

Organizational climate is a concept that is closely linked to the organization's culture and is sometimes confused with it. Although many people use *culture* and *climate* interchangeably, the terms are not the same. **Climate** is an individual perception of what it feels like to work in an environment (Snow, 2002). It is how nurses perceive and feel about practices, procedures, and rewards (Sleutel, 2000). People form perceptions of the work environment because they focus on what is important and meaningful to them. This explains why some aspects of culture may be interpreted differently. Climate can be easier to identify than culture, and so climate refers to the aspects of the work environment that can be measured. Researchers who study climate describe various components of the work environment that influence behaviors (Sleutel, 2000). Some characteristics that are used to study climate are decision making, leadership, supervisor support, peer cohesion, autonomy, conflict, work pressure, rewards, feeling of warmth, and risk (Litwin & Stringer, 1968; Stone et al., 2005). Within organizations, it is common to identify subclimates that focus on very specific aspects of the organizations (e.g., climates related to patient safety, ethics, and learning).

Culture-Climate Link

Climate research has formed the basis for the definition and research surrounding organizational culture, and the two are closely linked (Bellot, 2011). Regardless of the practice setting, a link exists between culture and climate; and that link is what is important to understanding attitudes, motivations, and behavior among nurses (Stone et al., 2005). The common links between culture and climate can be described as the interaction of shared values about what things are important, beliefs about how things work, and behaviors about how things get done (Uttal, 1983). Research has shown that, among nurses, culture or climate affects job satisfaction (Hart & Moore, 1989), intent to turnover (Hemingway & Smith, 1999), needlestick injuries and near misses (Clarke, Rockett, Sloane, & Aiken, 2002; Clarke, Sloane, & Aiken, 2002), surgical outcomes (Friese et al., 2008), and patient mortality (Aiken et al., 2008).

Nursing Work Group or Nurse Practice Environment

Although organizations usually have a single, overarching culture, many climates can exist within that culture, for instance, floor to floor. Groups and organizations exist within society and develop a culture that has a significant effect on how members think, feel, and act. Culture becomes a learned product of the group experience. In general, nurses work together in a group such as on a nursing unit, in home care, in long-term care, or in communities. The nursing unit, or **nursing work group,** is a small geographic area within the larger hospital system where nurses work interdependently to care for a group of patients. On units, groups of nurses work together, spend time together, and set up their own norms and values and ways to communicate with each other (Brennan & Anthony, 2000). These factors contribute to that unit having its own climate, or perception of what it feels like to work on that unit. Climate is evident in staff perceptions of policies, practices, and goal achievement. Some authors describe this as a work group subculture (Coeling & Simms, 1993). Understanding culture from the unit perspective offers an unprecedented view of nurses' work. The importance of creating an environment with a culture and climate that empowers nurses to practice in ways that support a positive practice environment can maximize nurse and patient outcomes.

BACKGROUND

Organizational culture has been studied as both something an organization *has* and something an organization *is* (Mark, 1996). Peters and Waterman's *In Search of Excellence* fueled a renewed business focus on culture as the means to achieve organizational

success and competitive advantage (Peters & Waterman, 1982). Industry leaders in the corporate world quickly realized that the philosophy and values of an organization could determine success and secure market advantage (Wooten & Crane, 2003). The health care industry has been slower than the corporate world to embrace culture as a means to optimize organizational performance.

Schein (1996), a renowned sociologist, has defined organizational culture as a shared value system, developed over time, that guides members on how to problem solve, adapt to the external environment, and manage relationships. The mission statement for an organization offers a snapshot of strategic priorities and is an important way to get a sense of organizational values. Schein suggested that a deeper understanding of cultural issues in organizations is necessary not only to understand what goes on but also, more important, to affect outcomes.

Organizational culture affects the quality of nursing care and patient outcomes. Shared meanings, the taken-for-granted practice and assumptions of a work unit group, can exert a significant effect on performance and outcomes. Basic underlying assumptions are those that are never questioned and make up an integral part of the fabric of an organization that extends to the unit work level, such as a commitment to excellence and to the surrounding community. Each organizational unit has cultural norms and values that blend the social realities and features that shape interactions among staff, patients, and families. The manner in which the staff perceives organizational culture, manages boundaries, and translates implied values to the unit level has a direct effect on the production of patient care (Alderfer, 1980).

RESEARCH

A growing body of research confirms that the relationship between nurse staffing and patient outcomes is influenced by culture or climate and the organizational characteristics of the structure in which nurses practice (Aiken, Sochalski, & Lake, 1997; Mitchell & Shortell, 1997; Needleman et al., 2001; Seago, 2001; Sovie & Jawad, 2001). More recently, studying the impact of culture has shifted from the organizational level to the unit level where caregiver relationships, communication, and autonomy intersect to inform care decisions that affect individual outcomes. Boyle (2004) found that nurse autonomy/collaboration, practice control, manager support, or continuity/specialization was significantly related to adverse events. To understand how the culture of the organization and climate of a unit are related to professional practice, three contemporary trends in achieving a culture/climate of quality are discussed here: Magnet Recognition Program®, patient safety climate, and learning climate.

Magnet Recognition Program®

In 1983, the American Academy of Nursing's Task Force on Nursing Practice in Hospitals studied nursing service best practices by surveying 163 hospitals. The goal was to identify and describe those factors that, when present, created an environment that attracted and retained qualified RNs who delivered quality care. The 41 best hospitals were called "Magnet hospitals" because of their clear ability to attract professional nurses. The 14 characteristics they displayed were identified and called "Forces of Magnetism." Since 1983, the Magnet Recognition Program has become the gold standard for excellence in nursing. In Magnet-designated hospitals, a strong visionary nurse leader nurtures a professional nursing environment and advocates for, and is supportive of, excellence in nursing practice. Magnet-designated hospitals have been recognized over the years for excellence in patient care, strong nursing practice environments and the ability to attract and retain nurses (ANA, 1997; Kramer & Hafner, 1989).

Aiken and colleagues (1994) transformed the initial Magnet hospital work into a program of research congruent with quality of care and organizational effectiveness through study of the links between hospital organizational culture and care outcomes. Magnet hospitals were conceptualized as those institutions that have a specific organizational culture with characteristics of autonomy, practice control, and collaboration. Aiken and colleagues (1994) examined mortality rates in 39 Magnet hospitals and 195 control hospitals using multivariate matched control sampling. Magnet hospitals had a significantly lower mortality rate (4.6% lower) for Medicare patients than that of control hospitals. The Magnet-designated hospitals' cultures provided higher levels of autonomy and control of practice and fostered stronger professional

relationships among nurses and physicians than did non-Magnet-designated hospitals.

Magnet research and an organizational framework developed by Aiken, Lake, Sochalski, and Sloane (1997) provide the means to better understand the link between the unit culture characteristics and adverse events. A nursing unit culture that supports and values nurse autonomy and the provision of adequate resources and effective communication among providers most likely constitutes an environment where practice excellence is the norm. Effects of nursing interventions are mediated by such organizational characteristics at the unit level (Aiken & Fagin, 1997). Magnet hospitals are an example of a positive culture that affects nurse and patient outcomes. Today, Magnet recognition is considered the gold standard for excellence in nursing, although at this time it largely applies only to the acute care, hospital environment (Wolf, 2006).

Hospitals wanting to achieve Magnet status must meet the 14 Forces of Magnetism identified by the American Nurses Credentialing Center (ANCC, 2004, 2008). Research that measures the Magnet hospital standards focuses on eight characteristics of an excellent work environment: clinically competent peers, collaborative nurse-MD relationships, clinical autonomy, support for education, perception of adequate staffing, nurse manager support, control of nursing practice, and patient-centered values (Schmalenberg & Kramer, 2008). From a broader perspective, Stone and colleagues (2005) developed an integrated structure-process-outcome model of relationships among factors describing organizational climate and its effect on outcomes. They identified leadership values, strategy and style, and organizational structure aspects such as communication, governance, and technology as the structural components of climate. Likewise, the process elements of climate include supervision, work design, group behavior, and emphasis on quality that is driven by patient centeredness, safety, innovation, and evidence-based practice. Taken together, these components are likely to have an effect on nurse and patient outcomes.

Further, in the journey toward Magnet designation, research and evidence-based practice become important in meeting the core criteria and representing a culture and climate of learning. In a learning culture, the norms and assumptions for learning lead to behaviors that support continuous learning (Daft, 2001). A learning climate is characterized by a shared and positive perception of the value of learning to enhance practice, quality, and outcomes.

Cultures in which continuous learning is valued are less likely to become outdated and stale. In the past, it was not unusual to hear nurses say in relation to their practice, "We have always done it this way." Today, a learning environment encourages nurses to propose new ideas. Moving new research findings into practice has historically taken many years. In a continuous learning culture nurses are challenged to ask, "How can this be done better?" Nurses interact with many patients on a daily basis. Patients are experts about themselves, and nurses are experts about nursing practice. Blending these areas of expertise best positions nurses to ask the question, "How can practice and the environment in which practice occurs be improved?" Nursing practice then becomes a vehicle for generating questions that are important to practice.

Culture and group norms can have a profound impact on the shared values that are expressed by nursing staff on individual work units in the hospital setting (Koerner, 1996). The formation of the team at the unit level holds a collective vision for continuous learning. In turn, the norm for learning intersects with the desire for good practice and forms a cohesive unit that shares a value for learning that generates excitement for moving beyond traditional practice. Cultures and climates in which knowledge is freely shared can have a groundswell effect. Examples of outward and visible signs that support nurses' shared values for inquiry include journal clubs, unit presentations, poster displays, and participation in evidence-based research teams.

Patient Safety Culture and Climate

Since the publication of the Institute of Medicine report *To Err is Human: Building a Safer Health System* suggesting that 98,000 persons die annually in hospitals because of errors, an emphasis on an organization's patient safety culture and climate has driven both research and change in hospital practices (Kohn et al., 2000). A safety culture is an outgrowth of the larger organizational culture and emphasizes the deeper assumptions and values of the organization toward safety, whereas the safety climate is the shared perception of employees about the importance of safety within the organization (DeJoy et al., 2004). Like organizational climate, the safety climate has a number of different components including leadership, involvement, blameless culture, communication, teamwork, commitment to safety, beliefs about errors and their cause, and others (Blegen et al., 2005).

Safety climate refers to keeping both patients and nurses safe. Strong surveillance skills regarding patients is at the heart of safety. Nurses, who are on the front line of patient care, are in an optimal position to monitor patients to prevent adverse events or near misses of adverse events. The ability of nurses to understand a patient's baseline status and recognize early, critical warning signs or changes in health status is a skill derived from having a strong nursing knowledge base. It is not simply task application. Astute recognition of deviations from normal and timely intervention signify that nurses understand patient baseline status and are capable of intervening to prevent or remediate an adverse event. Knowledge of the patient and the patient's baseline status is derived through subjective, objective, and intuitive observations that are honed as nurses develop a level of expertise in working with specific patient populations. Factors that influence a nurse's ability to watch over patients to avoid errors and adverse events include staffing levels, excess fatigue, and lack of education and experience (Hinshaw, 2008).

Included in the concept of a safety climate is a focus on nurses' health and safety. Nurses working in hospitals have one of the highest rates of work-related injuries, especially back injuries and needlesticks (Mark et al., 2007). When fewer nurses are working, less help is available to provide care to patients. This results in more work needing to be done in a shorter time and can lead to taking shortcuts, which can result in injury.

Regardless of whether the focus of safety is on the patient or the nurse, the likelihood of injury can be lessened where there is a cohesive team. When there is a shared perception among a group of care providers about the value and importance of safety, they are more likely to work together effectively toward common goals. Espousing the values of a safety climate and endeavoring to prevent, detect, and mitigate the effect of errors and injuries increases the likelihood of improved outcomes. As nurses work together as a team, they share information, can anticipate events, and are more likely to respond positively to unanticipated events.

One major shift in an organization's safety climate is the move from a punitive and reactive culture to a fair and just culture. Marx (2001) suggested that in a just culture, organizational, individual, and interpersonal learning are balanced with personal accountability and discipline. In a fair and just culture, expectations for system and individual learning and accountability are transparent. Underlying these beliefs, the overall organizational strategy must effectively implement a fair and just culture. When an organization can freely discuss mistakes with the intention of learning from them and when it takes the time and resources needed to understand the mistakes (e.g., root cause analysis), the organizational culture changes from a "blame game" to an environment that is respectful and open to learning (Connor et al., 2007). Within a systems-oriented approach, learning from adverse events can lead to new wisdom and improved ways of doing things.

Culture Change in Long-Term Care

Following the passage of the Nursing Home Reform Act legislation (OBRA, 1987), a series of quality improvement programs were implemented in nursing homes. By the mid-1990s, the culture change movement had begun to gain popularity. Culture change is distinguished from typical quality improvement activities in its attempt to simultaneously alter multiple aspects of care and caregiving in the nursing home. Culture change is so named because of its aim to adopt an entirely new philosophy in long term elder care; there is no universal operational definition of what specific elements constitute culture change programming. Culture change refers to the movement to reorganize nursing home care completely. Included under this umbrella are several different initiatives that address staff, resident, environmental, or behavioral outcomes or some combination of these factors. Most culture change initiatives are focused upon resident-directed care, providing services that are directed by the strengths and preferences of the individual resident.

Some research has been done to evaluate various culture change initiatives; however, some models have been promulgated and replicated more than others. Lustbader (2001) noted that early culture change initiatives, although generally dedicated to the same principles of resident-directed care and homelike social structures, were unique from nursing home to nursing home. Despite the wide range of programming, Shields (2004) stated that nursing homes that have engaged in culture change activities report less staff turnover, a stable administration and full occupancy.

In 1995, at a meeting of the National Citizens' Coalition for Nursing Home Reform (NCCNHR), a panel of administrators whose nursing homes were engaged in culture change initiatives was convened. This group grew in size and strength and became known as the Pioneer Network. Today, the Pioneer Network is an organization of facilities engaged in many diverse culture change initiatives, dedicated to a common set of values. These values include returning the locus of control to residents, enhancing the capacity of frontline staff to be responsive, and establishing a homelike environment (Lustbader, 2001). Some of the most prominent culture change models include the Eden Alternative, The Green House Project, and the Wellspring Program.

Development of a new model or culture change must be preceded by comprehensive assessment of the unit culture, an understanding of the patient population, what members of the staff need to care for them, and what roles are required to form the unit team. There is no one right model, nor does one size fit all settings. The work entails a deliberative process to facilitate change that will improve outcomes. Culture development must be an essential component of any new culture change. Transparency and frequency of clear communication is critical for cultural transformation and buy-in from all staff.

LEADERSHIP AND MANAGEMENT IMPLICATIONS

Culture is characterized by complexity and is relatively enduring, making it hard to change. Climate, on the other hand, can be easier to change. Regardless, the basic elements that constitute culture and climate must be understood before any change. Change that begins at the unit level may be most influenced by nursing leadership. Nurses have the ability to create or change a work culture or climate to accomplish a change that may affect productivity, satisfaction, and safe, high quality, patient-centered care.

The role of a nursing leader is to influence culture and the climate. A primary task of the leader is to create a convincing vision that inspires and engages the entire team to move it forward. Values drive behaviors. The leader communicates this vision by influencing norms and values and creating a shared perception through role modeling and ensuring role clarity, accountability, and a nurse practice environment that promotes safe, patient-centered care.

Nursing unit leadership is key to creating a positive unit climate that promotes effective unit functioning and quality care (Sorrentino et al., 1992). Unit-based nurse managers serve as bridges between the senior nursing leadership and direct care nursing staff. By virtue of their position, nurse managers are instrumental in shaping and managing the core values of their staff (Anthony et al., 2005). "Nurse managers have multiple and competing demands that they must balance in defining, prioritizing, and implementing their role responsibilities to meet the goals of the organization as well as those of the profession" (Anthony et al., 2005, p. 146). Increasingly, studies are showing that the nurse manager is important in retention (Anthony et al., 2005; Boyle et al., 1999; Taunton et al., 1997), professional practice (Manojlovich, 2005), and work environments (Upenieks, 2003). However, this influence is diluted when nurse managers are managing too many units or across too many areas and need to create and support a climate unique to each practice environment (Kimball & O'Neill, 2002).

Key areas within the leader's scope of control are recruiting and retaining staff, welcoming new staff, providing orientation, celebrating and recognizing staff accomplishments, facilitating change, and promoting a learning environment. Climate is evident in how policies are enacted, unit norms, dress code and appearance, environment, communication, and teamwork. The nurse manager can articulate the vision, mission, and goals of the organization and work with staff to translate them into unit-level values for performance, thus linking the context of the organization to clinical practice.

Values drive the way resources are distributed. They contribute to a general attitude and sense about the quality of working life and reflect the organization's core goals. Clues can be gleaned from organizational documents such as philosophy statements and meeting minutes. Caring values of the organization are reflected in the way the organization treats its staff. Organizational values may not mirror professional values. The leader's role is to bridge such values with the values of individual team members to construct individual unit climate. Values support the mission and the related vision, which, in turn, support strategies and action plans. The key platform is shared values. Given the complexity and diversity of the nursing workforce, developing and sustaining a set of shared values is no easy task and requires leadership skill.

Leaders are expected to chart a clear course for change and mobilize staff to accomplish organizational goals. This means implementing change effectively. Effective cultural change requires communication, passion, and sense of the whole. The nurse manager can create such opportunities through using focus groups, holding team meetings, coaching and mentoring, posting minutes from staff meetings, consulting communication books, and empowering staff by soliciting their input. The value of communication cannot be overstated. Much of the work is common sense, but the importance of doing this work lies in carefully attending to the basic change process as a way to avoid the need for damage control later.

Peters and Waterman (1982) stressed that the greatest professional need people have is to find meaning in their work life. The job of managers is to help create meaning through the use of stories, slogans, symbols, rituals, legends, and myths that convey the values, beliefs, and meanings shared among the staff. Managers should function as passionate leaders to motivate staff.

The challenges of leadership belong to every nurse, not just those in formal administrative or management roles. Leadership at the staff level may simply take a different form. For example, a staff nurse adapting to a challenging patient assignment, taking initiative to change practice through performance improvement, or challenging the status quo is participating in unit culture construction. Further, staff nurses are critical to founding and maintaining a Magnet-designated organization.

Implications

Nurse leaders with an accurate and comprehensive assessment of culture and climate can identify strategic target areas for change. A thorough understanding of organizational culture and climate is a powerful diagnostic tool that may be used to identify both troubled and high-performance areas. An effective organizational culture empowers nurses to practice fully within the scope of their knowledge and education. The culture of a nursing unit practice environment may exert a significant and independent effect beyond that of staffing and skill mix by enhancing or impeding interventions once problems are detected. Nurses serve as the surveillance system for early detection of adverse events. The number of nurses may have less influence on patient outcomes than the organization and structure of the work environment itself, including the perceived level of autonomy, the amount of control over their practice, and effective collaboration with physicians (Aiken et al., 2001; Sochalski et al., 1999; Sovie & Jawad, 2001).

CURRENT ISSUES AND TRENDS

At the beginning of the chapter, a number of forces were identified that have had significant influence in changing the culture of health care delivery. Several of these forces have particular impact on nursing care, and a brief discussion of patient- and family-centered care, generational diversity and the Quality and Safety Education for Nurses (QSEN) initiative follows to exemplify current issues and trends related to organizational climate and culture.

Patient-Centered and Family-Centered Care

The Institute of Medicine's *Crossing the Quality Chasm* (2001) has identified that the culture of patient care must transition from care that is driven by providers to care that is patient-centered and family-centered in which patient and family norms, values, and preferences are respected. The National Healthcare Quality Report from the Agency for Healthcare Research and Quality (2002) defined two aspects of patient-centered care: the patient experience and patient partnerships. The patient's experience of care includes communication, care, and understanding of the meaning of his or her illness. This approach changes the focus from a patient with a disease to that of an individual with an experience.

Patient partnerships, the second dimension of patient-centered care, are formed when nurses are responsive to patient needs, values, and preferences and then customize the care to the patient. For example, when performing discharge teaching, information that is of high importance and value to the patient is addressed first in a patient-centered model of care. As patient advocates, nurses can be leaders in transitioning an organizational culture from provider-driven care to care that is truly patient-centered.

Generational Diversity and the Nursing Shortage

The importance of a positive work climate on organizational, patient, and nurse outcomes is firmly established and evidence-based. However, creating a work environment for nurses that meets their personal and professional values can be a challenge. In 2008, for the first time since the inaugural National Sample Survey of Registered Nurses, the number of nurses working who were under age 30 years and over age 60 years were almost equal (U.S. Department of Health and Human Services, 2008). Because nurses from each of these generations were raised with a different set of priorities and values, a work environment supportive to each generation is an important retention strategy. For example, baby boomer nurses value rewards. Recognition and pay may be motivators for them. In contrast, Generation X nurses are concerned with a better balance of work and life (Duchscher & Cowin, 2004). Tailoring the work environment to meet generational and life-stage needs is a recurrent theme in being able to successfully address the impending nursing shortage.

Quality and Safety Education for Nurses (QSEN)

In 2005, a joint project of the Robert Wood Johnson Foundation and the National League for Nursing, called the Quality and Safety Education for Nurses (QSEN), was announced. The purpose of QSEN is "to address the challenge of preparing future nurses with the knowledge, skills and attitudes necessary to continuously improve the quality and safety of the healthcare systems in which they work" (QSEN, 2012, p. 1). Widespread rollout of the QSEN program has resulted in extensive nursing faculty education that is designed to create nursing curriculum that emphasizes organizational culture attributes such as the implementation of patient-centered care, emphasis on teamwork and collaboration, integration of evidence-based practice and creation of a culture that supports quality improvement, safety, and informatics. To this end, QSEN key tenets are geared toward teaching nursing students the competencies they will need to affect organizational culture and create an environment that maximizes patient safety and health outcomes. By incorporating these elements into nursing education, it is believed that nurses will enter the workforce with the tools necessary to help create an organizational culture that fosters high quality nursing care. QSEN has now expanded to target nurses both prelicensure and at the advanced practice level. This initiative is an example of how to make large-scale cultural change in nursing.

RESEARCH NOTE

Source

Stone, P.W., et al. (2006). Organizational climate and intensive care nurses' intention to leave. *Critical Care Medicine, 34,* 1907-1912.

Background

The shortage of nurses is particularly evident in a critical care unit where nurses with specialized knowledge and skills are needed to meet the care requirements of complex patients. A work environment that is satisfying to the needs of nurses promotes retention of nurses in these units with traditionally high turnover rates.

Study Methods and Design

Purpose: The purpose of the study was to evaluate the incidence of nurses working in an ICU who intended to leave their unit because of working conditions and then to identify factors that could be used to predict intention to leave.

Design: This descriptive study was part of a larger study to evaluate ICU nosocomial infections. *Sample:* The sample was composed of 2323 registered nurses working in 110 ICUs across 66 hospitals. On average, nurses were 39.5 years old, had a total of 15.6 years of experience, and worked in their current position for 8.0 years.

Instruments: The Perceived Nurse Working Environment Scale, developed from the Nursing Work Index Revised (NWI-R), had seven subscales measuring unit climate and included the following: professional practice, staffing/resource adequacy, nurse management, nursing process, nurse-physician collaboration, clinical competence, and positive scheduling climate. Nurses were asked to respond to the item "Do you plan to leave your current position in the coming year?" If they responded positively, they were asked to describe their reasons. For nurses who indicated their intention to leave, their responses were analyzed and divided into two groups: those leaving because of retirement or promotion and those intending to leave because of working conditions.

Results: Seventeen percent of nurses (n=391) indicated they were intending to leave within the next year. Of those 391, 202 (52%) gave their reason for leaving as being related to working conditions. The other 48% of nurses indicated their reason for leaving was associated with a career opportunity, personal or family, retirement, or no reason given. In general, nurses who were intending to leave because of the work environment rated all of the organizational climate dimensions lower than all other responding nurses. Three of the climate factors were statistically significant in predicting nurses' intention to leave. Professional practice (measured as nurses' involvement in hospital decision governance and opportunities to advance), nurses' perception of the competence of other nurses, and experience were found to decrease the likelihood of intention to leave by 48%, 39%, and 3%, respectively.

Application to Practice

In a time when hospitals struggled to fill RN vacancies, the findings strengthened the premise that the climate of the work environment is an important predictor of nurses' intention to leave the unit. Although response rates were low, in ICUs, which are noted for their difficulty in recruiting and retaining nurses, these findings validate the importance of creating a unit climate in which nurses have opportunities to participate in practice decisions, can professionally develop, and value the contributions of their peers.

In response to an anticipated workforce shortage, the patient service leadership team of one organization elected to collaborate with human resources to develop a strategy for future success. It quickly became clear that planning for the shortage translated to crafting a plan for the future and was far greater than recruitment and retention. The work evolved into a broad initiative with a vision, guiding principles, core strategies, expected outcomes, and development of a leadership infrastructure. This work, called *Striving for Excellence,* was intended to change the culture. The work plan included extensive communication of the vision, identification of key stakeholders, assessment of the current and desired future state, gap analysis, and implementation plan. The vision was translated into actionable concrete steps that engaged nurse managers and direct care nurses in the change process.

A nurse manager identified patient safety as a high-risk issue for the population of children on an inpatient psychiatric unit. A review of the literature substantiated that traumatic sequelae resulted from the use of restraints. Furthermore, regulatory agencies mandated a reduction in the use of restraints.

Challenges facing this manager were cultural resistance, knowledge deficits, and a changing patient population. The *Striving for Excellence* vision served as a unifying concept, and change theory provided the framework for mobilizing staff commitment. Psychodynamic concepts helped ensure that the change was integrated into clinical practice. Use of restraints was viewed as a treatment failure, and staff experienced a shift in thinking. Interventions moved from stopping aberrant behavior through use of restraints to reflection about what the behavior meant. Outcomes demonstrated a 60% reduction in the use of restraints. This also resulted in a sustained change in practice for that nursing unit and has been recognized as a best-practice model. The nurse manager astutely summarized the implementation as culture change.

CRITICAL THINKING EXERCISE

Helping Hands Hospital made a strategic decision to transform a 12-bed rehabilitation unit that had operated for 30 years and was a recognized leader in excellent multidisciplinary care for patients and families to meet emergency patient care needs. The experienced nursing staff had low turnover and enjoyed strong partnerships with physicians, social workers, physical therapists, and occupational therapists.

The new unit was designed to meet the acute care needs of older patients with medical diagnoses. The change introduced an entirely new patient population and called for development of a new model of care for acutely ill older patients who would experience a significantly shorter length of stay than would a rehabilitation patient population. Subsequently, a new team of caregivers had to be identified to create new processes of care to ensure effective outcomes.

1. What is the problem?
2. Identify challenges faced by the manager and staff.
3. What steps would you take to define the new model of care?
4. How will the culture of this unit change?
5. What can the staff do?

Critical Thinking and Decision-Making Skills

Betsy Frank

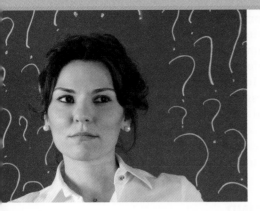

evolve WEBSITE

http://evolve.elsevier.com/Huber/leadership/

In an era of changing reimbursements, value based purchasing, and expanded roles for nursing in the health care delivery system, critical thinking and decision making are important skills for nurses caring for patients and for nurse leaders and managers. Both the American Nurses Association's (2009) and American Association of Nurse Executives' (2005) standards for practice for nurse administrators and executives support the fact that in a fast-paced health care delivery environment, staff nurses, leaders, and managers must be able to analyze and synthesize a large array of information, use critical thinking and decision making skills to deliver effective day to day patient care, and solve complex problems that occur in complex health care delivery systems (see Figure 4-1). Furthermore, the Magnet Hospital initiative and the Institute of Medicine's (Committee on the Robert Wood Johnson Foundation, 2011) *Future of Nursing* report highlight the need for nurses to be able to be fully involved and even take the lead in decision making from the unit level to the larger health care delivery system.

Nurses are a cadre of knowledge workers within the health care system. As such, they need information, resources, and support from their environment. In fact, the nurse manager's expertise in critical thinking and shared decision making are essential for creating healthy work environments where quality and effective care can be delivered (Kramer et al., 2010; Zori et al., 2010).

Critical thinking and decision-making competences include analytical skills as well as intuition. Just as intuition is part of expert clinical practice (Benner, 1984), intuition plays an important role in developing managerial and leadership expertise (Shirey, 2007).

DEFINITIONS

Critical thinking can be defined as a set of cognitive skills including "interpretation, analysis, evaluation, inference, explanation, and self-regulation" (Facione, 2007, p. 1). Using these skills, nurses in direct patient care and leaders and managers can reflect analytically, reconceptualize events, and avoid the tendency to make decisions and problem solve hastily or on the basis of inadequate information. Facione also pointed out that critical thinking is not only a skill but also a disposition that is grounded in a strong ethical component.

65

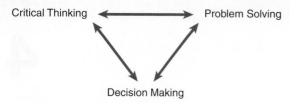

FIGURE 4-1 Differences and interactions among critical thinking, problem solving, and decision making.

Critical thinking in nursing can be defined as "purposeful, informed, outcomes focused thinking…[that] applies logic, intuition, creativity and is grounded in specific knowledge, skills, and experience" (Alfaro-LeFevre, 2009, p. 7). Alfaro-LeFevre noted that outcomes-focused thinking helps to prevent, control, and solve problems. Tanner (2000) noted that critical thinking is much more than just the five steps of the nursing process.

Problem solving involves moving from an undesirable to a desirable state (Chambers, 2009). Problem solving occurs in a variety of nursing contexts, including direct client care, team-level leadership, and systems-level leadership. Nurses and nurse managers are challenged to move from step-by-step problem-solving techniques to incorporating creative thinking, which involves considering the context when meeting current and future challenges in health care delivery (Chambers, 2009; Rubenfeld & Scheffer, 2006).

Decision making is the process of making choices that will provide maximum benefit (Drummond, 2001). Decision making can also be defined as a behavior exhibited in selecting and implementing a course of action from alternative courses of action for dealing with a situation or problem. It may or may not be the result of an immediate problem. Critical thinking and effective decision making are the foundation of effective problem solving. If problems require urgent action, then decisions must be made rapidly; if solutions do not need to be identified immediately, decision making can occur in a more deliberative way. Because problems change over time, decisions made at one point in time may need to be changed (Choo, 2006). For example, decisions about how to staff a unit when a nurse calls in sick have to be made immediately. However, if a unit is chronically short-staffed, a decision regarding long-term solutions will have to be made.

The process of selecting one course of action from alternatives forms the basic core of the definition of decision making. Choo (2006) noted that all decisions are bounded by cognitive and mental limits, how much information is processed, and values and assumptions. In other words, no matter the decision-making process, all decisions are limited by a variety of known and unknown factors. In a chaotic health care delivery environment, where regulations and standards of care are always changing, any decision may cause an unanticipated future problem.

BACKGROUND

Critical Thinking

Critical thinking is both an attitude toward handling issues and a reasoning process. Critical thinking is not synonymous with problem solving and decision making (Figure 4-1), but it is the foundation for effective decision making that helps to solve problems (Fioratou et al., 2011). Figure 4-2 illustrates the way obstacles such as poor judgment or biased thinking create detours to good judgment and effective decision making. Critical thinking helps overcome these obstacles. Critical thinking skills may not come naturally. The nurse who is a critical thinker has to be open-minded and have the ability to reflect on present and past actions and to analyze complex information. Nurses who are critical thinkers also have a keen awareness of their surroundings (Fioratou et al., 2011).

Critical thinking is a skill that is developed for clarity of thought and improvement in decision-making effectiveness. The roots of the concept of critical thinking can be traced to Socrates, who developed a method of questioning as a way of thinking more clearly and with greater logical consistency. He demonstrated that people often cannot rationally justify confident claims to knowledge. Confused meanings, inadequate evidence, or self-contradictory beliefs may lie below the surface of rhetoric. Therefore it is important to ask deep questions and probe into thinking sequences, seek evidence, closely examine reasoning and assumptions, analyze basic concepts, and trace out implications. Other thinkers, such as Plato, Aristotle, Thomas Aquinas, Francis Bacon, and Descartes, emphasized the importance of

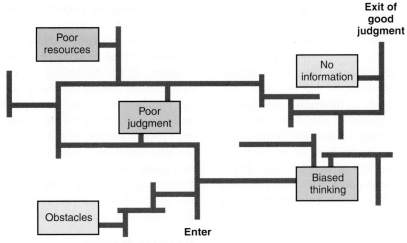

FIGURE 4-2 Decision-making maze.

systematic critical thinking and the need for a systematic disciplining of the mind to guide it in clarity and precision of thinking. In the early 1900s, Dewey equated critical thinking with reflective thought (The Critical Thinking Community, 2008). Critical thinking, then, is characterized by thinking that has a purpose, is systematic, considers alternative viewpoints, occurs within a frame of reference, and is grounded in information (The Critical Thinking Community, 2008).

Questioning is implicit in the critical thinking process. The following are some of the questions to be asked when thinking critically about a problem or issue (Elder & Paul, n.d.):

- What is the question being asked?
- Is this the right question?
- Is there another question that must be answered first?
- What information is needed?
- Given the information, what conclusions are justified?
- Are there alternative viewpoints?

No matter what questions are asked, critical thinkers need to know the "why" of the thinking, the mode of reasoning (inductive or deductive), what the source and accuracy of the information is, what the underlying assumptions and concepts are, and what might be the outcome of the thinking (The Critical Thinking Community, 2008).

Critical Thinking in Nursing

Nurses in clinical practice continually make judgments and decisions based on the assessment and diagnosis of client needs and practice problems or situations. Clinical judgment is a complex skill grounded in critical thinking. Clinical judgment results in nursing actions directed toward achieving health outcomes (Alfaro-LeFevre, 2009). Scheffer and Rubenfeld (2000) have stated that habits of the mind that are characteristic of critical thinking by nurses include confidence, contextual perspective, creativity, flexibility, inquisitiveness, intellectual integrity, open-mindedness, perseverance, and reflection. Emphasizing the value of expert experience and holistic judgment ability, Benner (2003) cautioned that clinical judgments must not rely too heavily on technology and that the economic incentives to use technology must not come at the expense of human critical thinking and reasoning in individual cases.

Critical thinkers have been distinguished from traditional thinkers in nursing. A traditional thinker, thought to be the norm in nursing, preserves status quo. Critical thinkers go beyond the step-by-step processes outlined in the nursing process and traditional problem solving. A critical thinker challenges and questions the norm and considers in the context of decision making potential unintended consequences. Unlike traditional thinkers, critical thinkers are creative in their thinking and anticipate the consequences of their thinking (Rubenfeld & Scheffer, 2006). Creativity is necessary to deal with the complex twenty-first century health care delivery environment.

Nurse leaders and managers have an obligation to create care delivery climates that promote critical thinking, which leads to innovative solutions to problems within the system of care (Committee on the Robert Wood Johnson Foundation Initiative on the Future of Nursing, at the Institute of Medicine; Institute of Medicine, 2011; Porter-O'Grady, 2011). Such a climate encourages deep reflection, especially so that nurses feel safe to learn from mistakes, and encourages nurses to ask questions and consider a variety of viewpoints and alternative solutions to problems.

What specific strategies can be used to promote a climate in which critical thinking is fostered? First and foremost, the nurse manager/leader, in the role of mentor, coach, or preceptor, should encourage questions such as "Is what you are doing or proposing based on sound evidence?" (Ignatavicius, 2008). However, Snowden and Boone (2007) cautioned that "best practice, by definition is past practice" (p. 71). Therefore use of best practices needs to be examined carefully in order to use them appropriately. Staff nurses and managers must use critical thinking skills in order to determine the appropriateness of implementing recommended practice protocols.

As managers, allowing staff and self "think time" is essential for reflection and is a key component of critical thinking (Zori & Morrison, 2009). Nurse managers' critical thinking abilities promotes a positive practice environment which can lead to better patient outcomes (Zori, Nosek, & Musil, 2010).

Coaching new and experienced nurses to develop expertise in clinical judgment is critically important. Many new nurses, in particular, need to further develop their critical thinking skills (Fero et al., 2008; Forneris & Peden-McAlpine, 2009). In addition to having preceptors and others ask questions of new nurses, nurse managers and leaders can use other strategies to enhance critical thinking in nursing staff.

Developing concept maps is another useful strategy to promote critical thinking. Although typically used in prelicensure programs (Ellermann et al., 2006), nurse managers can encourage their preceptors to use concept maps with orientees (Toofany,

2008). Developing concept maps in concert with others further develops a nurse's critical thinking through the process of dialogue. Simulations also promote critical thinking or "thinking like a nurse" (Tanner, 2006). According to Tanner, simulations can promote clinical reasoning, which leads to making conclusions in the form of clinical judgments and, thus, effective problem solving. The use of human patient simulators is well known in educational settings. Simulators may also be useful in orienting new graduates to the acute care setting (Leigh, 2011). Pulman and colleagues (2009) have reported on the use of simulators to promote critical thinking role development in inter-professional environments.

Decision Making

Decision making is the essence of leadership and management. It is what leaders and managers are expected to do (Keynes, 2008). Thus decisions are visible outcomes of the leadership and management process. The effectiveness of decision making is one criterion for evaluating a leader or manager. Yet staff nurses and nurse managers and leaders must make decisions in uncertain and complex environments (Clancy & Delaney, 2005).

Within a climate of uncertainty and complexity, nurse managers and leaders must also understand that all decision making involves high-stakes risk taking (Clancy & Delaney, 2005; Keynes, 2008). If poor decisions are made, progress can be impeded, resources wasted, harm caused, and a career adversely affected. The results of poor decisions may be subtle and not appear until years later. Take, for instance, a decision to reduce expenses by decreasing the ratio of registered nurses to nurses' aides. There may be a short-term cost savings, but if not implemented appropriately, this tactic may result in the gradual erosion of patient care over time (Kane et al., 2007). Unintended effects may include higher turnover of experienced nurses, increased adverse events such as medication errors, decreased staff morale, and lower patient satisfaction scores. The long-term outcome of this decision may actually result in increased expenses not reduced expenses. Thus it is vital for nurses to understand decision making and explore styles and strategies to enhance decision-making skills.

Decision making, like traditional problem solving, has been traditionally thought of as a process with identifiable steps yet influenced by the context and by whether there is an intuitive grasp of the situation. However, Effken and colleagues (2010) stated that decision making is much more.

> *Expert decision making is a constructive process in which the outcomes are not preplanned or simply pulled out of a memory bank. Instead, expert decision-making activities are creative, innovative, and adapted to uncertainty and the context of the current problem, using learning from prior experience (p. 189).*

Nurses make decisions in personal, clinical, and organizational situations and under conditions of certainty, uncertainty, and risk. Various decision-making models and strategies exist. Nurses' control over decision making may vary as to amount of control and where in the process they can influence decisions. Although decision-making is more than a step-by-step process as noted by Effken and colleagues (2010), awareness of the components, process, and strategies of decision making contributes to effectiveness in nursing leadership and management decision making. The basic elements of decision making, which enhances day to day activities, contributes to strategic planning and solves problems can be summarized into the following two parts: (1) identifying the goal for decision-making, and (2) making the decision. According to Guo (2008, p. 120), the steps of the decision-making process can be illustrated as follows, using DECIDE:

- **D**efine the problem and determine why anything should be done about it and explore what could be happening.
- **E**stablish desirable criteria for what you want to accomplish. What should stay the same and what can be done to avoid future problems?
- **C**onsider all possible alternative choices that will accomplish the desired goal or criteria for problem solution.
- **I**dentify the best choice or alternative based on experience, intuition, experimentation.
- **D**evelop and implement an action plan for problem solution.
- **E**valuate decision through monitoring, troubleshooting, and feedback.

Notice how these steps are analogous to the traditional problem-solving process or nursing process

well-known by nurses and nurse managers. Thus decision making is used to solve problems.

However, decision making is *more* than just problem solving. Decision making may also be the result of opportunities, challenges, or more long-term leadership initiatives as opposed to being triggered by an immediate problem. In any case, the processes are virtually the same, but their purposes may be slightly different. Nurse managers use decision making in managing resources and the environment of care delivery. Decision making involves an evaluation of the effectiveness of the outcomes that result from the decision-making process itself.

Whether nurse managers are the sole decision makers or facilitate group decision making, all the factors that influence the problem-solving process also impact how decisions are made: who owns the problem that will result in a decision, what is the context of the decision to be made, and what lenses or perspectives influence the decision to be made? For example, the chief executive officer may frame issues as a competitive struggle not unlike a sports event. The marketing staff may interpret problems as military battles that need to be won. Nurse executives may view concerns from a care or family frame that emphasizes collaboration and working together. Learning and understanding which analogies and perspectives offer the best view of a problem or issue are vital to effective decision making. It may be necessary for nurse managers to expand their frame of reference and be willing to consider even the most outlandish ideas. Obviously, it is important to begin the goal definition phase with staff members who are closest to the issue. That includes staff nurses in concert with their managers. Often, decisions can originate within the confines of the shared governance system that may be in place within an organization (Dunbar et al., 2007). It is wise, also, to consider adding individuals who have no connection with the issue whatsoever. Often it is these "unconnected" staff members who bring new decision frames to the meeting and have the most unbiased view of the problem. One of the core competencies for all health professionals is working in interprofessional teams (Interprofessional Education Collaborative Expert Panel, 2011). Therefore using interprofessional teams for problem solving and decision making can be assumed to be more effective than working in disciplinary silos. No matter who is involved in the decision-making process, the basic steps to arrive at a decision to resolve problems remain the same. One critical aspect to note, however, is that in making decisions, nurse managers must have situational awareness (Sharma & Ivancevic, 2010). That is, decision makers must always consider the context in which the outcome of the decision is to occur. A decision that leads to a desired outcome on one patient care unit may lead to undesirable outcomes on another unit because the patient care environment and personnel are different.

DECISION OUTCOMES

When looking at outcomes, one critical aspect of decision making is to determine the desired outcome. The desired outcome may vary, according to Guo (2008), from an ideal or short-term resolution to covering up a situation. What is desired may be (1) for a problem to go away forever, (2) to make sure that all involved in this problem are satisfied with the solution and gain some benefit from it, or (3) to obtain an ideal solution. Sometimes a quick decision is desired, and researching different aspects of the problem or allowing for participation in decision making is not appropriate. For example, in disaster management, the nurse leader will use predetermined procedures for determining roles of the various personnel involved (Coyle et al., 2007).

Desired decisions can be categorized into two end points: minimal and optimal. A minimal decision results in an outcome that is sufficient, satisfies basic requirements, and minimally meets desired objectives. This is sometimes called a *"satisficing"* decision. An *optimizing decision* includes comparing all possible solutions with desired objectives and then selecting the optimal solution that best meets objectives (Choo, 2006; Guo, 2008). In addition to these two strategies, Layman (2011) drawing from Etzioni (1986), discussed two other strategies: mixed scanning and incrementalism. *Incrementalism* is slow progress toward an optimal course of action. *Mixed scanning* combines the stringent rationalism of optimizing with the "muddling through" approach of incrementalism to form substrategies. *Optimizing* has the goal of selecting the course of action with the highest payoff (maximization). Limitations of time, money, or people may

prevent the decision maker from selecting the more deliberative and slower process of optimizing. Still, the decision maker needs to focus on techniques that will enhance effectiveness in decision-making situations.

Barriers to effective decision making exist and, once identified, can lead to going back through the decision-making process. Flaws in thinking can create hidden traps in decision making. These are common psychological tendencies that create barriers or biases in cognitive reflection and appraisal. Six common distortions are as follows (Hammond et al., 1998; 2006):

1. *Anchoring trap:* When a decision is being considered, the mind gives a disproportionate weight to the first information it receives. Past events, trends, and numbers outweigh current and future realities. All individuals have preconceived notions and biases that influence decisions in a variety of ways. For instance the Institute of Medicine (IOM, 2001) endorsed the use of **c**omputerized **p**hysician **o**rder **e**ntry (CPOE) as one solution to reduce medication errors. Furthermore, The Centers for Medicare and Medicaid Services has set forth meaningful use criteria for implementation of CPOE as well as electronic health records (EHR). Despite incentive payments for implementing EHR (HFMA P & P Board, 2012), the financial costs involved, human-factor errors and work-flow issues can hamper successful implementation (Campbell et al., 2006).

2. *Status-quo trap:* Decision makers display a strong bias toward alternatives that perpetuate the status quo. In the face or rapid change in the environment, past practices that exhibit any sense of permanence provide managers with a feeling of security.

3. *Sunk-cost trap:* Past decisions become sunk costs, and new choices are often made in a way that justifies past choices. This may result in becoming trapped by an escalation of commitment. Because of rapid, ongoing advances in medical technology, managers are frequently pressured to replace existing equipment before it is fully depreciated. If the new equipment provides a higher level of quality at a lower cost, the sunk cost of the existing equipment is irrelevant to the decision-making process. However, managers may delay purchasing new equipment and forgo subsequent savings because the equipment has yet to reach the end of its useful life.

4. *Confirming-evidence trap:* Kahneman and colleagues (2011) noted that decision makers also fall into the trap of confirmation bias where contradictory data are ignored. This bias leads people to seek out information that supports an existing instinct or point of view while avoiding contradictory evidence. A typical example is favoring new technology over less glamorous alternatives. A decision maker may become so enamored by technological solutions (and slick vendor demonstrations) that he or she may unconsciously decide in favor of these systems even though strong evidence supports implementing less costly solutions first.

5. *Framing trap:* The way a problem is initially framed profoundly influences the choices made. Different framing of the same problem can lead to different decision responses. A decision frame can be viewed as a window into the varied reasons a problem exists. As implied by the word *frame*, individuals may perceive problems only within the boundaries of their own frame. The human resources director may perceive a staffing shortage as a compensation problem, the chief financial officer as an insurance reimbursement issue, the director of education as a training issue, and the chief nursing officer as a work environment problem. Obviously all these issues may contribute, in part, to the problem; however, each person, in looking through his or her individual frame, sees only that portion with which he or she is most familiar (Layman, 2011).

6. *Estimating and forecasting traps:* People make estimates or forecasts about uncertain events, but their minds are not calibrated for making estimates in the face of uncertainty. The notion that experience is the parent of wisdom suggests that mature managers, over the course of their careers, learn from their mistakes. It is reasonable to assume that the knowledge gained from a manager's failed projects would be applied to future decisions. Whether right or wrong, humans tend to take credit for successful projects and find ways to blame external factors on failed ones. Unfortunately, this form of overconfidence often results in overly optimistic projections in project planning. This optimism is usually buried in the analysis done before ranking alternatives and recommendations. Conversely, excessive cautiousness or prudence may also result in faulty decisions. This is called aversion bias (Kahneman et al., 2011).

Dramatic events may overly influence decisions because of recall and memory, exaggerating the probability of rare but catastrophic occurrences. It is important that managers objectively examine project planning assumptions in the decision-making process to ensure accurate projections. Because misperceptions, biases, and flaws in thinking can influence choices, actions related to awareness, testing, and mental discipline can be employed to ferret out errors in thinking before the stage of decision making (Hammond et al., 1998).

Data-driven decision making is important (Dexter et al., 2011; Lamont, 2010; Mick, 2011). The electronic health record can be mined for valuable data, upon which fiscal, human resource, and patient care decisions can be made. However, the data derived can be overwhelming and cause decision makers to make less than optimal decisions.

Shared decision making can help ameliorate decision traps (Kahneman et al., 2011) because dissent within the group may help those accountable for the decision to prevent errors that are "motivated by self-interest" (p. 54). More alternatives can be generated by a group and more data can be gathered upon which to base the decision, rather than just using data that is more readily apparent.

DECISION-MAKING SITUATIONS

The situations in which decisions are made may be personal, clinical, or organizational (Figure 4-3). Personal decision making is a familiar part of everyday life. Personal decisions range from multiple small daily choices to time management and career or life choices.

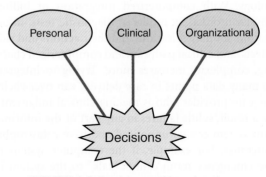

FIGURE 4-3 Decision-making situations.

Clinical decision making in nursing relates to quality of care and competency issues. According to Tanner (2006), decision making in the clinical arena is called *clinical judgment*. In nursing, as with all health professions, clinical judgments should be patient-centered, use available evidence from research and other sources, and use available informatics tools (IOM, 2003). These crucial judgments should take place within the context of interprofessional collaboration. Within a hospital or other health care agency, a social network forms that is interprofessional (Tan et al., 2005). This social network has to collaborate for positive change within the organization and to make clinical decisions of the highest quality.

Nurses manage care and make decisions under conditions of certainty, uncertainty, and risk. For example, if research has shown that, under prescribed conditions, the selection of a specific nursing intervention is highly likely to produce a certain outcome, then the nurse in that situation faces a condition of relative certainty. An example would be the prevention of decubitus ulcers by frequent repositioning. If little knowledge is available or if the specific situation is more complex or variant from the usual, then the nurse faces uncertainty. Risk situations occur when a threat of harm to patients exists. Conditions of risk occur commonly relative to the administration of medications, crisis events, infection control, invasive procedures, and the use of technology in nursing practice. Furthermore, these conditions also apply to the administration of nursing care delivery, in which decision making is a critical function.

Conditions of uncertainty and complexity are common in nursing care management. Over time, the complexity of health care processes has increased as a natural outgrowth of innovation and new technology. With computerized integration of billing, physician ordering, results of diagnostic tests, information about medications and their actions and side effects, and critical pathways and computerized charting, complexity increases more. Trying to integrate so many data points in care delivery can overwhelm the care provider who is making clinical judgments. As a result, subtle failures in any part of the information system can go unnoticed and have catastrophic outcomes. For example, if the computer system in the emergency room cannot "talk" to the system in the operating room, then errors in care management,

such as giving cephalexin to patient who has an allergy can occur. If a provider fails to input critical information, such as a medication that a patient is taking, a fatal drug interaction could occur when another provider prescribes a new medication. Ready access to the Internet and online library sources can further create complexity in the decision-making process as care providers have access to more information upon which to make decisions.

Readily accessible information related to evidence-based practice and information gleaned from human resources records and clinical systems can overwhelm nurse managers and leaders. Nurse leaders are coming to understand that innovation and new technology are the driving forces behind the discovery of new knowledge and improvements in patient care. Overlapping, unclear, and changing roles for nurses as a result of new technology and services create complex decision-making situations and impact the quality of care delivered (IOM, 2003). In addition, workflow interruptions can inhibit critical thinking, particularly in a chaotic environment (Cornell et al., 2011; Sitterding et al., 2012).

ADMINISTRATIVE AND ORGANIZATIONAL DECISION MAKING

According to Choo (2006), organizations use information to "make decisions that commit resources and capabilities to purposeful action" (p. 1). Nurse managers, for example, make staffing decisions and thus commit financial resources for the purpose of delivering patient care. Hospital administrators may decide to add additional services to keep up with external forces. These decisions subsequently have financial implications related to reimbursement, staffing, and the like.

Etzioni (1989) noted that the traditional model for business decisions was rationalism. However, he further asserted that as information flow became more complex and faster-paced, a new decision-making model based on the use of partial information that has not been fully analyzed had begun to evolve. He called this model "humble decision making."

This approach arises in response to the need to make a decision when the amount of data exceeds the time available to analyze it. For instance, predicting the outcome of clinical and administrative decisions in health care is problematic because such processes are collectively defined as complex adaptive systems (CASs). A CAS is characterized by groups of individuals who act in unpredictable, nonlinear (not cause and effect) ways, such that one person's actions affect all the others (Holden, 2005).

In CASs, humans do behave in unpredictable ways (Tan et al., 2005). Critical thinking can help all health care personnel to examine these complex systems, wherein groups solve problems through complex, continually altering interactions between the environment and all involved in the decision making (Fioratou et al., 2011). Situations within the environment constantly change and decision makers need to reframe their thinking as they broaden their awareness of the context of their decisions (Sharma & Ivancevic, 2010). Having situation awareness is a must (Fioratou et al., 2011; Sitterding et al., 2012).

Decision makers need to make every effort to forecast unanticipated consequences of their decisions. For example if staffing is cut, what adverse events might occur (Kane et al., 2007)?

Decision making is also influenced by the manager's leadership style. A democratic/collaborative style of leadership and decision making works best in a complex adaptive system, such as a hospital, which is characterized by a large array of social relationships that can have an economic impact on an organization. Staff nurses who are not engaged in shared decision making may experience less job satisfaction and subsequently may leave an organization, leading to loss of expertise in patient care (Gromley, 2011).

However, the full array of leadership styles may at some time be used in the decision-making process. Vroom and Yetton (1973) proposed a classic managerial decision-making model that identified five managerial decision styles on a continuum from minimal subordinate involvement to delegation. Their model uses a contingency approach, which assumes that situational variables and personal attributes of the leader influence leader behavior and thus can affect organizational effectiveness. To diagnose the situation, the decision maker examines the following seven problem attributes:

1. The importance of the quality of the decision
2. Whether there is sufficient information/expertise
3. The amount of structure to the problem

4. The extent to which acceptance/commitment of followers is critical to implementation
5. The probability that an autocratic decision will be accepted
6. The motivation of followers to achieve organizational goals
7. The extent to which conflict over preferred solutions is likely

The nurse manager has a full range of decision-making styles available. The choice of style depends on the context for the decision to be made. The decision style should be matched to situational needs so the probability of effective decision making increases.

DECISION-MAKING TOOLS AND STRATEGIES USED TO SOLVE PROBLEMS

Various strategies are used for decision making aimed at solving problems. These strategies are based on time and mental structure variations (e.g., fast, slow, impulsive, intuitive, or logical) and the context of the decision. Some formal decision-making strategies are as follows.

Trial and Error

In using trial and error, a shoot-from-the-hip or dart-throw type of solution is put into effect. A solution that seems attractive is chosen and simply tried out. Those managers who use trial and error as the usual strategy for decision making often are seen as ineffective. They are perceived as poor problem solvers. Evidence-based practice protocols have largely replaced trial-and-error decision making at the bedside as the standard of practice (Cannon et al., 2007).

Pilot Projects

Pilot projects involve experimentation with limited trials. Pilot projects or carefully defined trials are used to experiment by trying out a solution alternative on a small or restricted basis to see whether major problems will occur and to reduce risk. Pilot project strategies may resemble research projects. These projects may also be linked to quality improvement initiatives.

Creativity Techniques

Creativity techniques include brainstorming sessions, the Delphi process, and nominal group techniques, in which a group gathers for free-thinking exercises. They have been used with varying success in the decision-making process. For example, brainstorming was once highly touted as a primary strategy for creative decision making. However, more recent research suggests that group brainstorming can often limit ideas because collaborative fixation or focusing on a few ideas occurs (Kohn & Smith, 2011). Generating ideas individually before bringing ideas to a group setting may generate more ideas than group brainstorming alone (Castaldo, 2010).

Decision Tree

A decision tree, or algorithm, is a graphic model that visually displays the options, outcomes, and risks to be anticipated (see the Case Study at the end of this chapter). A decision tree starts to the left and flows to the right or starts at the top and flows to the bottom. A question or problem is posed, and the possible options become branching nodes. Thus decision paths can be traced through option points and beyond. For example, a very simple decision tree might start with the question "Are you committed to becoming a nurse?" The answer to that question is *yes* or *no*. Depending on the answer, the corresponding path is followed as mapped out on the decision tree. The tree enables visualization of the alternatives and their consequences. It helps with decision making through analysis and clarity (Pidgeon & Gregory, 2004). For example, one hospital, which was a part of the Transforming Care at the Bedside (TCAB) (Robert Wood Johnson Foundation, 2008) initiative, developed an algorithm to assist nurses in making the decision about whether or not a patient on the telemetry unit needed to be accompanied by a nurse during transportation to a place where a procedure such as angiography was to take place (Mayer, 2009).

Critical paths are similar to decision trees. Critical pathways are descriptions of the specific protocol steps needed for critical or key incidents that must occur in a predictable or timely order to keep the expected outcomes, length of stay, and overall costs appropriate. They are designed to be used with a defined patient population and are grounded within evidence-based practice (De Bleser et al., 2006). Critical pathways are designed to incorporate multidisciplinary perspectives and to display and track the client's entire expected course of treatment and expected outcomes.

Variances are identified immediately and managed by the health care provider. A recent Cochrane review (Rotter et al, 2010) revealed that critical pathways do shorten hospital stays and in some instances decrease complications.

As health care evolves in sophistication and knowledge base, with better identification of patient diagnoses and the array of matching multidisciplinary interventions, standardized languages might be incorporated into decision trees that are readily accessible to the entire health care team.

Shared Decision Making

In the group problem-solving and decision-making technique, the leader calls the group together to discuss and participate in solving a problem. The leader invites participation, either in the problem-identification or the problem-resolution part of the decision-making process. A transformative leadership style appears to influence the effectiveness of group decision making (Shoemaker et al., 2010). There are a number of models of group decision making. The four general models are as follows:

1. The rational model, based on an economic perspective of decision making and maximum utility
2. The political model, based on power, influence, negotiation, bargaining, and interest group influence
3. The process model, which uses standard operating procedures and guidelines
4. The "garbage can" model, characterized by difficult problem identification and difficult problem resolution under circumstances of ambiguity, complexity, and non-rationality

All these models can be used at one time or another, either singly or in combination, depending on the nature of the issue at hand. For example, when a problem involves budgetary allocations, the political model might be used. After an evidence-based practice guideline has been agreed upon, the process model might be used to implement the guideline.

Scenario Planning

Scenario planning is a problem-solving and decision-making strategy given an uncertain and changing future. It is a group process strategy that encourages group participants to create "possible future" stories. Thus it is forward-looking and appropriate for fluid and changing environments in which there are many possible futures. This technique asks the question "What if …?"; then different stories of the future are described (scenarios). In this way, a wide array of perspectives is gathered, and the entrenched mindset is overcome. Stories of the future are constructed in a way that highlights pathways, driving forces, turning points, and deep behavioral forces. Scenario planning helps illuminate early warning signs, trigger new opportunity ideas, and may protect from some risks.

Worst-Case Scenario

Worst-case scenario is especially helpful in making decisions that involve risk. Risky decisions frequently, but not always, relate to the use of money or prestige. In this technique, the "worst case" (i.e., everything that could go wrong does go wrong) is determined. The worst case is outlined for each known alternative. Then the alternative with the best result—when, or if, everything possible does go wrong—is selected. So if value-based reimbursement is on the line, the "least of all the evils" is chosen. For instance, CPOE systems, if used correctly, have been shown to significantly reduce medication errors. However, because of the enormous cost and social change required to implement such systems, establishing an adequate return on the investment has been difficult. Unfortunately, documented savings from avoidable and unavoidable adverse drug events may be thought of as "soft" numbers and open to speculation. By determining the absolute worst that could happen and working backward from that scenario, the decision maker chooses the best alternative

for the situation to minimize potential anticipated risk or damage and in turn maximize reimbursement.

In their book *Smart Choices*, Hammond and colleagues (1999) recommended creating a "consequences table" for addressing multiple alternatives. To develop such a table, list the problem consequences objectives along the left side of a page and the various alternatives along the top. To rate the ability of each alternative to meet the desired objective, create a standardized key that ranks each alternative. For example, consider the following problem statement regarding medication errors:

The rate of adverse drug events has exceeded the benchmark rate for three consecutive quarters. This has coincided with two sentinel events that required extended patient hospitalization and potential litigation.

After a period of analysis, a cross-functional team lists the following alternatives as potential solutions to the medication error problem:

- Add robot technology to current system of CPOE and bar coding.
- Standardize all medication abbreviations on order sheets.
- Remove high-risk drugs such as potassium chloride from ward stock, and place pharmacists on the floor to assist with medication orders.
- Have two nurses check high-risk medications before giving to patient.

Table 4-1 displays the desired objectives and a standardized key to analyze and rank them.

TABLE 4-1	**DESIRED OBJECTIVES ANALYSIS**			
OBJECTIVE	**ALTERNATIVE A**	**ALTERNATIVE B**	**ALTERNATIVE C**	**ALTERNATIVE D**
1. Reduces the number of medication transactions	5	4	2	3
2. Enables medication administration through automation	5	4	2	2
3. Meets or exceeds net present value target	3	2	5	3
4. Meets regulatory standards	3	3	3	3
5. Improves accuracy	4	4	5	4
Total Score	20	17	17	15

1, Does not meet objective; *2*, meets some aspects of objective; *3*, meets objective; *4*, exceeds objective; *5*, significantly exceeds objective.

By ranking the various alternatives through a standardized key, a fair comparison among alternatives can assist managers eliminate undesirable choices. When developing a consequences table, it is important to view the long-term or downstream effects of implementing specific alternatives. Make sure to "play out" different scenarios and the tactics needed to overcome them. For instance, in evaluating which system to purchase when implementing CPOE, several scenarios may result and need to be evaluated in planning and management. As shown in Table 4-2, identifying how one action can lead to another makes it possible to preempt significant barriers to implementation.

Computerized Decision Making

In the arena of decision-making strategies and analytical tools, there are also sophisticated and computerized forecasting techniques, such as linear programming models, and mathematical techniques, such as predictive modeling, that assign a probability to each possible outcome and then run multiple analyses on multiple combinations. However, traditional statistical analysis may fail to capture the dynamic and nonlinear aspects of complex systems such as hospitals. As a result, complex system problems quickly become intractable using standard statistical analysis tools. One tactic suggested in the IOM (2001) report to overcome this problem was to increase the use of simulation (computational modeling) as a decision tool in designing safer processes within complex hospital systems (IOM, 2001). Electronic Health Records (EHRs) have great potential in helping health care providers in assisting with clinical decision making

and billing appropriately (Lamont, 2010). Data also can be used in dashboard analysis wherein the manager can analyze computerized data to evaluate how nurses are using evidence-based practice resources to change practice (Mick, 2011).

Computational Modeling

A computational modeling approach views organizations (hospitals and other community agencies) as a collection of computer-simulated agents that are both intelligent and adaptive. By conducting "virtual experiments," computational models can provide a "what-if" analysis of various tactics aimed at decision making. Although a variety of methods may be used, the general process for computational modeling begins with encoding a series of statements in propositional calculus, or "if …, then …" format, into a computer program. Using a series of computer algorithms, these statements can represent various theories and be analyzed to produce output that simulates corresponding social behavior. A computer modeling simulation has been used to demonstrate how a smallpox epidemic could be contained under various projected scenarios (Burke et al., 2006).

Six Sigma

Another group problem-solving and decision-making approach is *Six Sigma* (Frings & Grant, 2005; Morgan & Cooper, 2004). This statistical approach to problem solving reduces actions that can lead to errors and that have an adverse impact on patient outcomes and organizational financial outcomes. Precise data are gathered and analyzed statistically. Based on the data,

TABLE 4-2	SCENARIO ANALYSIS: IMPLEMENT CPOE ON ALL INPATIENT UNITS BY A GIVEN DATE	
RESULT PERIOD #1	**RESULT PERIOD #2**	**RESULT PERIOD #3**
Physician response to training is poor, resulting in …	Difficulty in operating the system, resulting in …	The nursing staff having to use both a paper and an online record, leading to …
There are many computer interface problems, resulting in …	A slow, unreliable, and cumbersome system, leading to …	Refusal of the staff to use the system, leading to …
Physicians have to change their medication ordering practice, leading to …	Longer patient rounding time, resulting in …	A perception of less physician productivity, leading to …

CPOE, Computerized physician order entry.

process improvements are made. With this approach, the goal is a virtually error-free health care delivery environment. By way of example, hospital discharge processes could be improved based on a *Six Sigma* approach (Frings & Grant, 2005).

LEADERSHIP AND MANAGEMENT IMPLICATIONS

Critical thinking skills enhance the quality of clinical judgment, problem solving, and decision making. Furthermore, nurse managers must consider the ethical consequences when using critical thinking as a foundation for decision making (Toren & Wagner, 2010). Critical thinking skills are one of the top-rated competencies required for staff nurses (del Bueno, 2005) and nurse leaders and managers (Hawkins et al., 2009) within this chaotic health care delivery system. Within a complex and high-risk health care delivery environment, decision making requires deliberation and some creativity. Decisions made using a variety of tools and strategies can lead to safer care delivery environments. The focus of leadership and management decision making is more closely related to the nurse's role as care coordinator and systems problem solver. Some decisions, such as those requiring disciplinary action, do require the manager's *direct intervention.* In conflicts between staff members or between family and staff members, the manager might use negotiation and other forms of conflict management that could be viewed as *indirect intervention* because the manager does not actually solve the problem but, rather, persuades others to solve the problem themselves. The nurse manager might *delegate* the problem solving to others. For example, a unit manager might ask a team of staff nurses and the unit secretary to figure out when is the best time to order supplies for the unit.

Sometimes, the nurse manager might choose *watchful waiting.* A particular staff member might be causing some interpersonal difficulties. If the staff member has submitted his or her resignation, dealing with the behavior might not be worth the energy.

Most problem solving and decision making should take place within the confines of *collaboration and consultation.* Shared governance initiatives have shown that collaboration and consultation result in high-quality patient care delivery systems. Therefore a critical role for nurse managers and leaders is *facilitation* by fostering a climate that encourages creativity and interdependence.

Modeling desired critical thinking behaviors is also important. For example, in hospitals, nurse leaders and managers can use change-of-shift reports to promote critical thinking and subsequent problem solving by using the Socratic method and asking who, what, when, and where questions such as "What nursing interventions have been effective?" or "What will happen if this course of action is chosen?" Another strategy for promoting critical thinking is to create a climate where mistakes can be made and then analyzed without fear of punishment (Cohen, 2002). Figure 4-4 summarizes the strategies used for decision making that leads to problem solving.

Nurse managers and leaders have many competing demands on their time. Deciding which problems need immediate attention and which can wait involves the ability to prioritize one's actions. Clinical decision-making skills can be focused and enhanced by the use of critical thinking. Nurses can and do use decision making in all aspects of care management, but the nurse manager deals more with system-level issues rather than the day-to-day direct patient care decisions (Sherman et al., 2007).

Clearly, all nurses are on information overload. Ways to capture the available data and use it for effective problem solving and decision making are critical. Hospital information systems can be used to capture data such as length of stay, skill mix, case mix, patient and employee job satisfaction, and other variables that can be important when decisions need to be made (Junttila et al., 2007).

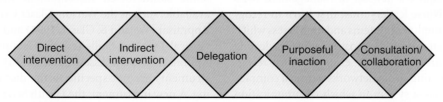

FIGURE 4-4 Strategies for decision-making that leads to problem solving.

Complexity and Chaos

Nurse managers and leaders solve problems in complex systems in which all decisions carry some amount of risk. Complexity and chaos theory has application to leadership and management decision making. The behavior of nurses is governed, to some extent, by the rules (formal and informal), information flow, diversity, and interconnectedness of the organization (Chu et al., 2003). This complex web of interdependence and mutual causality among nurses, physicians, and support staff results in a complex adaptive system characterized by open boundaries, multiple levels of organization, and rule sets that serve as the organization's operating procedures. The system changes over time as it adapts to changes in external and internal environments. Multiple feedback loops exist, and new ways of organizational behavior emerge (Minas, 2005). One example of this type of complex adaptive system is how hospitals have adapted to a changing reimbursement environment such that the majority of surgeries, in many places, are done on an outpatient basis. For hospitals and other health care organizations to survive, nurse managers and leaders must use critical thinking skills when considering the vast array of choices that can be made when determining an organization's growth (or shrinkage) and subsequent future.

The "good old days," when life was more predictable and less chaotic and patients routinely stayed 3 to 5 days as inpatients, have disappeared. Coordination of care must begin at the first patient encounter into a system for care. For example, discharge teaching must now begin *before* admission, not after the patient is admitted for surgery. Patients may be at the hospital or surgery center for only 1 to 2 hours after the surgery has ended; thus they are still under the influence of anesthetics or analgesics and cannot comprehend or remember the instructions that were given. Because change is occurring so rapidly, past practices that exhibit any sense of permanence may provide managers with a feeling of security. Leading in a world of complexity does require a new set of management tools (Ford, 2009). Nurse leaders must first learn to recognize complex, nonlinear systems and then assess which management strategies are most effective in dealing with them. Nurse leaders, for example, must recognize the intersecting social networks within a complex adaptive system—a system in which communication network changes in one part can occur independently,

interdependently, and dependently upon other parts of the system (Benham-Hutchins & Clancy, 2010).

Just like complex patient care scenarios, complex social organizations, like hospitals, produce patterns that can be difficult to recognize (Wheatley, 1999) unless one is an expert critical thinker (Benner, 1984; Shirey, 2007). Expert nurse leaders can quickly and intuitively grasp organizational patterns without going through a step-by-step analysis of a situation.

Inevitably, some mistakes will be made; but nurse managers and leaders who look upon mistakes as learning opportunities help promote adaptive systems. However, if leaders foster a climate wherein new communication patterns emerge, bottom-up communication changes the organization, and differences in talents, structures, and communication networks come forth, organizations can adapt to increasing complexity (Ford, 2009). Leaders must transform their workplaces so that shared decision making can take place (MacPhee et al., 2010).

CURRENT ISSUES AND TRENDS

More than 10 years ago the Pew Health Professions Commissions (1998) identified that critical thinking was an essential skill for health care providers in the twenty-first century. The American Association of Colleges of Nursing (2008) has endorsed critical thinking and decision making as key skills for baccalaureate-prepared nurses. Nurse leaders and managers are essential to promoting a climate that encourages critical thinking and innovative problem solving and decision making (Currie et al., 2007). New staff nurses, in particular, need support to develop confidence in learning to think like nurses (Etheridge, 2007; Forneris & Pedin-McAlpin, 2009; Swinny, 2010). Promoting critical thinking is critical to thinking like a nurse.

Since critical thinking is the basis for sound clinical and managerial decision making, getting some sense of nurses' critical thinking abilities is important. Some standardized measurement instruments are available, such as the Watson-Glaser Critical Thinking Appraisal (Watson & Glaser, 1994) and the California Critical Thinking Skills Test, the California Reasoning Appraisal (Insight Assessment, 2008a). But these instruments are not specific to the discipline of nursing. A new instrument, the Health Sciences Reasoning Test (Insight Assessment, 2008b) has potential for more accurately appraising critical thinking skills in nurses (Sullivan-Mann et al., 2009). Measurement issues aside, the use of critical-thinking and decision-making skills is essential for nurse managers who deal with interpreting complex data in order to ensure safe patient care (Hawkins, et al., 2009).

Clearly, more research needs to be done in order to demonstrate that educational and managerial actions do promote critical thinking. Nevertheless, nurturing, developing, and demonstrating evidence of critical thinking skills remain important issues in nursing education and practice. Nurse managers and staff nurses must form partnerships (Kerfoot, 2006) and create a climate in which critical thinking can occur. Such a climate encourages creativity and innovation (Albarran, 2004).

Creativity and innovation will be the cornerstone of nurses' participation in the health care system of the future. A recent IOM report (Committee on the Robert Wood Johnson Foundation, 2011) noted that nurses should and must take the lead in providing care for patients in a complex, rapidly changing health care system. New roles such as the Clinical Nurse Leader, who is a bedside leader and coordinator of complex care, have emerged (Porter-O'Grady et al., 2011). Accountable care organizations (ACOs), which will coordinate primary care for groups of patients, provide many opportunities for nurses to demonstrate their advanced critical-thinking and decision-making skills (Hart, 2012).

Nurse leaders and managers must be on the forefront of providing safe, cost-effective care. Several recent initiatives, including the 5 Million Lives campaign (McCannon et al., 2007) to save patient lives caused by errors, require full nursing participation to prevent adverse events. Value-based purchasing initiatives put forth by the Centers for Medicare and Medicaid Services will require health care systems to deliver safe and cost efficient care or see their reimbursements adversely affected (Shoemaker, 2011). Certainly nurse managers and leaders will be on the forefront of improving such measures as patient satisfaction and hospital-acquired infections. Through analysis for electronic health records and other data sources, nurse managers and leaders will have to engage their staff in critical thinking and shared decision making in order to positively impact financial reimbursements.

Despite the need for creativity, a certain amount of standardization must occur if safe patient care is to be delivered (Clancy et al., 2005; Kerfoot, 2006).

Decision-making activities in nursing include standardization of care and improving quality and safety through evidence-based protocols. The standardization of care, through adoption of standardized languages, is one strategy nurse administrators can use to reduce the complexity of care and enable health care providers to make better decisions (Clancy et al., 2005). Linking standardized care procedures to patient safety initiatives is vital if health care providers and patients are to safely navigate complex care environments. Such procedures are characteristic of a complex system self-organizing (Tan et al., 2005).

Nurse leaders need to advocate for a preferred future for nursing and evaluate the effectiveness of decision making in practice. Both are aimed at making careful projections about what decisions to make, given uncertainty, to improve organizational and system performance. In times of change, nursing has an opportunity to make decisions that proactively direct the future. Nursing has demonstrated its value to the health care system. Therefore nurse leaders must be a party to all decisions regarding how care is delivered in health care organizations via shared governance arrangements.

Many hospitals are applying for Magnet recognition from the American Nurses Credentialing Center. One of the 14 Forces of Magnetism involves management style and another promotes interdisciplinary collaboration. These two elements of a management style that is collaborative and the promotion of interdisciplinary staff input in decision making are evidence-based "best practices" (Thomas & Herrin, 2008).

The efficiency, efficacy, and effectiveness of health care decisions will continue to enjoy a strong focus in nursing, with shifts toward outcomes specification. As performance improvement specialists, nurses will be challenged to make decisions that directly affect quality, access, cost, productivity, and the "bottom line." Effective approaches to decision making are needed when care is delivered in a complex system in which multiple stakeholders need to be served, time is constrained, and the amount of information is overwhelming. Thus multiple solutions for decision making and subsequent problem solving might be needed (Porter-O'Grady, 2011). Furthermore, all nurses must have leadership competencies, including the ability to make effective decisions (Committee on the Robert Wood Johnson Foundation Initiative on the Future of Nursing, Institute of Medicine, 2011).

RESEARCH NOTE

Source

Wilson, D.S., Talsma, A., & Martyn, K. (2011). Mindful staffing: A qualitative description of charge nurses' decision-making behaviors. *Western Journal of Nursing Research*, *33*(6), 805-824.

Purpose

The aim of this qualitative study was to describe effective staffing decision behaviors of shift charge nurses.

Discussion

Eleven charges nurses, seven nurse managers, and six staff nurses were interviewed in order to get a complete picture of staffing decisions made by charge nurses. Results showed that charge nurses needed to be resourceful and knowledgeable about the patients. In addition, for the necessity of tactful communication, charge nurses needed to be flexible and be decisive while keeping budgetary and safe patient care concerns in the forefront of their decision-making process. Being aware of the big picture, or having situation awareness was also crucial.

Application to Practice

Effective decision making with regard to staff is vital to safe and cost efficient patient care. Those in shift managerial and leadership roles must have the decision-making and critical-thinking skills and situation awareness in order to function in their roles. They need to think beyond the immediate situation at hand in order to anticipate the consequences of their actions. Therefore these frontline managers should have the education necessary to function in their roles.

CASE STUDY

Effective decision making relies, in part, on analyzing alternative levels of uncertainty or risk. In addition to making "apples to apples" comparisons through such tools as staffing matrices recommended by professional bodies, daily and monthly patient census data can guide unit managers in their analysis, which might precede a request for more staffing. In addition, the nurse manager must have an awareness of the environment in which care is delivered in order to make the analysis complete. Figure 4-5 is an example of a decision tree. A nurse manager from the emergency room could use such a decision tree to justify an increase in staffing. The tree has several branches, and, depending on the end point, an increase in needed personnel could be handled in several ways. Diagrams such as decision trees can be invaluable in understanding complicated alternative solutions. These diagrams are useful in the assessment and problem definition and in considering the available alternatives for dealing with a problem. Once the alternative is chosen, a plan must be formulated for implementing the approach chosen. The choice implemented must be evaluated. Note, however, the decision tree in Figure 4-5 only lists three alternatives. A more complex tree could be constructed that includes more alternatives based on a different combination of tree branches.

New research into knowledge representation has shown that human cognition is more effective through visualization rather than text. Decision trees, fishbone diagrams, problem continuums, and flowcharts are frequently used as visualization tools in problem analysis. To assist in visualization techniques, managers should consider placing a large grease board, dry-erase board, or flip chart in their office to quickly map out various alternatives.

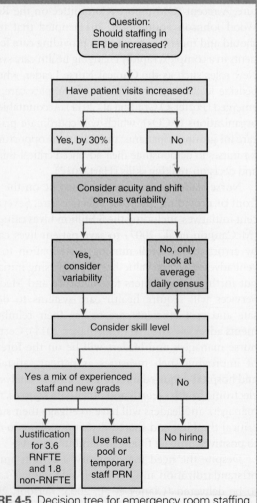

FIGURE 4-5 Decision tree for emergency room staffing.

CRITICAL THINKING EXERCISE

Scenario 1

John Hildebrand is emergency room charge nurse. During an evening shift, four victims come in from a major automobile accident. Two were critically injured, and two had minor injuries. All the other staff nurses were caring for these victims when a 55-year-old female came to the ER complaining of severe epigastric pain and some abdominal pain. John attended to this patient and, per protocol, gave her a GI cocktail (antacid, lidocaine, and phenobarbital [Donnatal]). Her pain level decreased shortly from 6 out of 10 to 3 out of 10. John also did an ECG to rule out any cardiac causes. Because her pain did not completely resolve, John and one of the physicians discussed possible causes. Although the patient did not present with any nausea, vomiting, or fever of any kind, her symptoms overall were vague. The doctor decided that blood work should be done "for the heck of it." The patient was then sent home because she was stable and feeling a bit better. Thirty minutes later John called her with the results of her amylase and lipase levels and told her to go immediately to the ED. In the end, she had pancreatitis.

1. When an additional patient came into the ER, what choices did John have with regard to assigning a nurse the new patient?
2. What are the shift staffing issues in a busy ER?
3. Whose responsibility is it to make the staff assignments during the shift?
4. What decision-making strategies should be used when deciding who should take care of which patients in the ER?
5. How did the use of a clinical protocol help or hinder the care of the new patient with epigastric pain?
6. Who should be involved in patient care decisions?
7. What might have been the consequences of not drawing blood work on the female patient?

Scenario 2

Primary and specialty patient care in multispecialty outpatient clinical settings meets many of the characteristics of a complex adaptive system. Numerous agents (nurses) interact in a diverse social network (patients, physicians, therapists) that overlaps multiple systems (lab, specialty clinics, x-ray, social work) to provide care for patients who have a variety of health care issues. Care is often constrained by the time allowed for each appointment and the type of insurance a patient holds.

Multiple referrals to specialists may occur without coordination by any one person, despite the fact that a patient may be assigned a primary health care provider.

In complex systems such as multispecialty clinics, any disturbance in a positively reinforcing feedback loop may amplify in a "nonlinear" fashion throughout the system. Examples of a disturbance may include changes in a patient's insurance during the course of treatment and miscommunication between nurses and physicians, between physicians, or even the receptionist and the patient. The cascading effect of disturbances within the complex social network of staff and patients may result in unanticipated outcomes. For example, a new insurance carrier may cause the patient delay in treatment because referrals to specialists may require approval from the insurance company. Regardless of its pattern, the emergence of new insurance requirements results in new patterns of care as the appointment system and care providers adapt to new requirements.

Complex systems are nonlinear and unpredictable. However, by altering or "tuning" system parameters, care coordination can lead to desired patient outcomes (Minas, 2005). For instance, if done correctly, adding a care coordinator to the system could facilitate timely and appropriate care for the patients.

In the change of insurance example, the following system changes could make care more efficient and effective for all patients, whether or not insurance changes:

1. Assign each patient a medical home, which is a system of primary care that coordinates all the patient's health care needs (Kuraitis, 2007).
2. The care coordinator in the medical home takes a complete history upon initial entry into the clinic system and monitors patient's health each time a patient has an encounter with a care provider.
3. The care coordinator ensures that referral to specialists and requests for diagnostic tests and treatments are preapproved, if needed, by the insurance carrier.
4. The care coordinator ensures that all test results are communicated to the providers and to the patient and ensures that any needed follow-up takes place.

To ensure effective care coordination, charts would be audited monthly to identify the gaps in communication and appropriate follow-up. By tuning the information flow and communication parameters, care coordinators can steer the system toward a positively reinforcing feedback loop that facilitates continuity

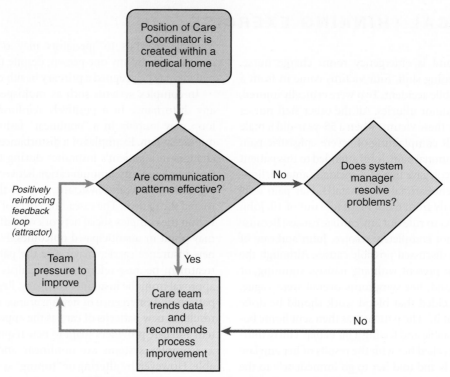

FIGURE 4-6 Decision tree for effective medical home.

of care. The result, demonstrated in Figure 4-6, is an effective medical home. Care teams that consistently score poorly on identified criteria for effective and efficient care self-organize to improve their image and prevent being labeled as uncoordinated and yielding less than optimal patient outcomes. Eventually a new culture will "emerge" throughout the organization as units naturally compete among themselves to improve.

Although seemingly simple, medical home, including care coordination, illustrates an alternative strategy for managing in a CAS environment. Rather than using management strategies that concentrate on enforcing top-down complicated policies and procedures, the CAS organizes according to defined communication patterns to enable naturally occurring, bottom-up self-organization and emergence. Instead of attempts to force system elements directionally, emphasis is on creating a climate for positive change but with an understanding that the final outcome could be uncertain.

1. For what undesirable patterns should system managers be on the alert when implementing change in a complex process such as a medical home system of care?
2. What key parameters within the care coordination process can managers adjust to move the system in a desirable direction?
3. Describe examples of tactics that could be employed to control parameters surrounding the use of care coordination within a medical home.
4. How might managers create positively reinforcing feedback loops that enable staff to self-organize around attractive solutions to such problems as lack of communication regarding diagnostic test results?
5. What computerized data might be available to evaluate the outcome of the medical home effectiveness?

Thanks to Stephanie Laws, RN, MS; Jeffrey Heist, RN, BS; and Jennifer Dalton, RN, BS for assistance in developing the case and scenarios.

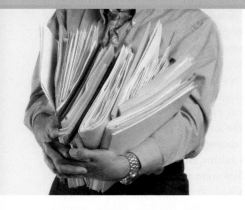

Managing Time and Stress

Caryl Goodyear-Bruch, Adrienne Olney,
Susan R. Lacey, Karen S. Cox

WEBSITE

http://evolve.elsevier.com/Huber/leadership/

We trained hard but it seemed that every time we were beginning to form into teams, we would be reorganized. I was to learn later in life that we tend to meet any new situation by reorganizing. And what a wonderful method it can be for creating the illusion of progress while producing confusion, inefficiency, and demoralization.
Gaius Petronius, Arbiter, First Century A.D.
(as cited in Curtin, 1994, p. 7)

It would be fun to imagine a health care industry that has made enormous strides from when the original contemporary approach for health care reform led by Hillary Clinton was defeated September 27, 1992, but that is not exactly the case (Langner, 1995). Not only is health care reform in a massive state of flux, the entire U.S. economy is only now recovering from the devastation caused by nefarious financial deals and mismanagement by multiple industries. These issues do have a connection with time management and stress. Rosabeth Moss Kanter, the unequivocal leading social scientist in the study of the connections between our professional and personal lives, explained in her seminal book that most of

Photo used with permission from Photos.com.

us cannot fully compartmentalize what is going on at work and home so that neither enters the other domain (Kanter, 1977). Each of us embodies both the world of work, our professional life, and the world outside of work, our personal life. Kanter described this as "spillover," and it is further explicated by Small and Riley (1990). It was then expanded on by others (O'Driscoll, 1996; O'Driscoll et al., 2006).

At a time when our health care industry is at a crossroads with health care reform ever morphing and the uncertain fiscal health of the United States, it is easy to see that all of these things are connected in a way that affects people in all professions. Both reform and the economic downturn are forever changing the way people view their livelihood and employment, as well as their ability to maintain that which they worked hard to achieve in their personal lives. Nurses are no exception.

DEFINITIONS

Stress is defined as a negative emotional experience that is associated with biological changes that trigger the body to make adaptations (Rosenthal, 2002). This means that stress can be a physical, mental, psychological, or spiritual response to a stressor experience that is evaluated by the individual as taxing or exceeding resources and threatening to one's sense of well-being. It was originally conceptualized as a syndrome having a variety of induced changes, including measurable physiological components, such as an increase in heart rate or a rise in blood sugar levels, as well as emotional ones. Chronic stress can lead to acute and chronic health problems. Job stress is a tension that arises related to the person-in-environment demands of a person's role or job. Job stress, or "disquieting influences," can accumulate into levels that are too high, reach the point of burnout, and manifest as emotional and/or physical exhaustion and lowered job productivity. Levels of job stress that are too low or too high decrease individual productivity.

Time management is a deliberative process of identifying and focusing on the activities needed to accomplish tasks and goals. Individuals cannot control time itself; therefore, they need to learn to manage the available time more efficiently and effectively. This may be difficult, especially when comfortable habits need to be changed. However, time management is a major strategy for managing stress. **Time management** is defined as the accomplishment of specified activities during the time available. It is the process of managing the things an individual does with his or her available time. At its core, time management is self-management.

CURRENT ISSUES AND TRENDS

Understanding current trends and issues in the larger sense is critical. Managers who fail to appreciate spillover will render themselves less able to lead and manage stress and time management both for themselves and for direct reports. The following is a chronological synopsis of major events in our recent history that cause great uncertainty for all of us, including over 3 million registered nurses. These historical trends and issues create uncertain times; and uncertainty, regardless of the source, can cause a person to fall somewhere on the continuum from slightly stressed to depressed, finally finding themselves unable to cope with activities of daily living.

Bailouts, Bankruptcies, and Unemployment

In 2008, our nation faced an economic challenge. Although not at the level of the Great Depression, it was serious enough that the financial system teetered on the brink of disaster. The banking and mortgage industries had engaged in making loans to citizens who believed home ownership was the gold standard for success (Office of the Press Secretary, 2002). The problem was a very large number of these loans were made to individuals who would subsequently face adjustable interest rates that would balloon to two or three times the original payment (referred to as adjustable-rate mortgages [ARMs]). The housing market was in a boom, but when these ARMs came due, many families were not able to make their payments and defaulted on their loans. When a tipping point was reached in the market, banks, some of which were thought to be the strongest in the country, began to clamor for a federal infusion of funds to stay solvent (Levitin & Wachter, 2011). Not only did banks want bailouts, but the automotive industry also sought relief from the federal government. This led to one of the largest bailouts in our nation's history, with Congress passing the Troubled Asset Relief Program (TARP) and authorizing up to $700 billion to stop the financial crisis, although the full $700 billion was never completely tapped (The New York Times, 2010).

Health Care Reform

Simultaneously, health care reform once again took center stage. Campaigning on a platform that basic health care is a right not a privilege, President Obama moved forward with this reform, which was met with pushback from Congress and also began what is now a quagmire of bills, state lawsuits, and monikers for health care rationing from those who did not want health care for all. All industrialized nations, except for the United States, have health care for all citizens in some form or another.

Meanwhile, stocks crashed and middle class Americans saw retirement accounts, accumulated after decades of hard work, vanish or become severely diminished. People stopped buying goods and services, leading to more layoffs in manufacturing and other industries. This ripple effect caused unemployment rates to rise to new levels, at one time reaching 10% (Bureau of Labor Statistics, 2012). As the unemployment rate climbed, the economy continued to face monumental challenges in recovery. Faced with chronic unemployment, many filed for bankruptcy, further exacerbating the financial crisis, moving it from industry to a more personal issue and generating more uncertainty. In 2010, bankruptcies were at a high of 1,593,081 business and nonbusiness filings (American Bankruptcy Institute, 2011).

Although the health care industry remains one of the strongest in our country, it too has been met with severe challenges in decreased reimbursements and uncertainty about how health care reform will affect all aspects of daily operations and budgets. It is as if the industry is frozen in time, waiting to see what will happen next before it is willing to make significant moves in one direction or another. As other countries around the world enter what has been called austerity measures, so too has the United States and the health care industry, without naming it as such.

Nurse Employment During the Last Four Years

Once thought of as a recession-proof profession, nursing has also experienced a roller coaster ride in employment. As more partners and spouses lost their jobs, scores of nurses, who were working either part-time or not at all, reentered the workforce, pushing aside those who were new to the profession. As recently as 2011, Peter Buerhaus and colleagues published a paper in *Health Affairs* indicating that the nursing shortage may be over for now (Auerbach et al., 2011). However, for decades there has been a push for more nurses from a wide range of key stakeholders, which includes but is not limited to the following:

- American Association of Retired Persons (AARP)
- American Hospital Association (AHA)
- National League for Nursing (NLN)
- American Association of Colleges of Nursing (AACN)
- The Robert Wood Johnson Foundation, the largest philanthropic foundation that supports health care initiatives, including building human capital.

Central to the common message is that a sufficient number of nurses, the linchpin of the industry, must be ready to meet the impending demand when baby boomers (over 77 million strong) will reach the age at which they will consume the greatest amount of health care goods and services in their lifetime.

There is a significant movement for a more humane approach to managing and leading people in nursing through these difficult times. One such way is for Healthy Work Environment (HWE) standards to

be put in place in health care organizations (American Association of Critical Care Nurses [AACN], 2005). In addition, since the Institute of Medicine's *Future of Nursing* report was published (Institute of Medicine [IOM], 2010), 48 Action Coalitions have been launched to improve the state of nursing and the health care industry by utilizing nurses and their skills more wisely (Robert Wood Johnson Foundation [RWJF], 2011).

The Link to Stress and Time Management

It is clear that uncertainty is the status quo in health care. Managers trying to lead staff nurses to deliver quality care when constantly being pressured to "do more with less" can cause great professional and personal stress on even the strongest leader. Staff nurses are also facing the daily consequences of doing more with less at a time when cost of living raises have all but disappeared, support staff have been cut, jobs are fewer, and even staffing levels fluctuate widely. These issues are facing not only the industry but also the largest group of providers in the country—registered nurses. At the same time, more people are becoming uninsured, which causes them to wait to seek care until they are far sicker than if they had been able to get proper care. Emergency departments are becoming destinations for these uninsured, as they use this far more expensive portal of entry, given they have no other way to access care. What staff nurses see every day are what has been characterized as the "sicker quicker" syndrome, meaning that people who might typically have met the criteria for a critical care bed in the past, are now on a general floor where the nurse-to-patient ratio is far greater than a critical care ratio. This day-to-day grind makes it extremely difficult to feel good about nursing or encourage others to become nurses, and may even cause roots of hostility to form toward the system that seems to constantly be letting nurses down.

Although challenging, these stressors are transient and cyclical. With sound tools prepared to use, nurses and their work environment can stay healthy when these issues recycle.

Stress As We Live It

With all the uncertainty in the nation and world today, it comes as no surprise that stress levels are high. A recent report found that 39% of Americans reported that their stress levels had increased over the past year, whereas only 17% reported decreasing levels (American Psychological Association [APA], 2012). Because stress can be a negative emotional experience that has measurable biological manifestations, stress management techniques must target both aspects.

The most frequency cited sources of stress for Americans today are money, the economy, and work (APA, 2012). Nursing's work is often particularly stressful. In addition to long hours, nurses have the added emotional burden of dealing with human illness and suffering, life-and-death situations, making critical judgments, and balancing work and family (McNeely, 2005). People may be aware when they are stressed but are often unable to determine what coping strategies will help. Only 29% of adults reported that they do an "excellent" or "very good" job at managing stress (APA, 2012). Fortunately, it is possible to learn good stress management techniques.

Personal Management of Stress

One of the most important parts of stress management is self-care. Though everyone needs to spend time on themselves, those in caring professions such as nursing often put the needs of others ahead of their own (Fischer & Keenan, 2010). However, it is difficult to care for patients or families if the nurse is not caring for himself/herself. What constitutes self-care is unique to each person, and each will have to find what works best for him/her. However, the following tips are a good starting point (Fischer & Keenan, 2010):

- Taking personal "downtime" each day
- Getting enough sleep and eating right
- Exercising (even taking a 30-minute walk)
- Having a strong support network of friends and family to make sure there is someone who will occasionally take care of you

Another important step in managing stress in daily life is creating healthy boundaries. A boundary in its most basic sense is a limit, and it can be physical, emotional, or mental (Katherine, 2000). One of the causes of too much stress is that people do not set or enforce their own personal boundaries. Rather than being able to set a limit on how they spend their time, they feel the need to please other people, often at the expense of themselves. In order to change this, nurses need to be aware of what their boundaries are and how to enforce them with other people. Boundaries

on your time allow you to know when to alter commitments, say no when favors are asked by others, and attend to your own needs (Katherine, 2000). Often, people do not give themselves permission to say no and find that all their personal time is spent on other people. This is not to say that boundaries cannot be flexible at times. In fact, it is also unhealthy to have too rigid of boundaries and to never make an exception. However, in general, it is important to maintain consistency with personal boundaries and to not overaccommodate others at the expense of personal mental and physical health (Gionta, 2009).

Because stress is not only emotional, but also physical, it is important to learn to relax the body. There are many relaxation techniques that can be effective in calming the body, such as imagining a peaceful scene or event or breathing deeply (Mind Tools, 2010). By calming the body's physiological response to stress, a person will be able to think more clearly about what needs to be accomplished. One example of a relaxation exercise is known as the relaxation response, and it includes the following steps: (1) sit quietly and comfortably; (2) close your eyes; (3) relax all your muscles, beginning with your feet and moving up the body; and (4) breathe deeply through your nose, concentrating on the breathing. It is recommended that a person continue this exercise for 10 to 20 minutes, once or twice a day (Benson & Klipper, 1976). However, this can still be a beneficial exercise in shorter time periods.

If the person is still feeling stressed but unsure about what is causing it, keeping a stress journal can help the person to focus. In the journal, record times when you felt stressed, the causes, the levels of stress, and your reaction to it. Once collected, this information can show how you best manage stress and highlight areas where you need to improve (Mind Tools, 2010).

Moral Distress

Nurses work within health care systems that are dynamic and complex, with a myriad of regulations, technical advances, and uncertainty. The unpredictable nature of the work, along with its complexity, can be contrasted with the essence of caring, where nurses establish patient/family relationships by synergistically framing meaning and knowledge (Fairchild, 2010). Confronting and resolving the conflicts experienced when caring for patients is intimately tied to the nurse-patient meaningful relationship. Unresolved ethical issues add emotional fracture to the already stressful work within complex systems. This may lead to moral distress, burnout, and intent to leave either the current position or the profession (Redman & Fry, 2000).

Moral distress occurs when clinicians know what ethical action should be taken, but they are prevented from doing so by either internal or external obstacles (Rushton, 2006). Internal obstacles include such personal characteristics as fear or lack of resolve, whereas external ones are more typically a lack of resources or a hierarchy preventing the nurse from taking the desired action (McCarthy & Deady, 2011). The American Association of Critical Care Nurses (AACN) has taken the position that moral distress is very serious problem in nursing today. It is a significant cause of emotional suffering and is a contributing cause to nurses leaving the workplace and the profession (AACN, 2008). In response to this important issue, the AACN has released a paper describing how nurses can deal with moral distress.

The AACN's (2004) *The 4 A's to Rise Above Moral Distress* details the response to moral distress as a change process, consisting of a four-part cycle: ask, affirm, assess, and act. In the first stage *(ask)*, nurses must become aware of their moral distress. The nurse is to ask himself/herself if what he/she is feeling is moral distress. Only by first becoming aware of internal distress, can the nurse then begin to address it.

The next step is to *affirm* the distress by validating feelings and making a commitment to take care of oneself. At this time, commitment to addressing moral distress as part of professional responsibility to oneself is suggested.

Assessing involves identifying the sources of the distress. Take time to understand when and under what circumstances this moral distress is occurring. For instance, it might be related to a particular patient or situation, or it might be a more broad issue with a unit practice. Next assess the severity by rating your distress on a scale of 0 (not distressed) to 5 (very distressed). Use this same scale to assess your readiness to act by determining how important the issue is to you and how strongly you feel about making a change. If you are having difficulty determining if you want to address the issue, it may be helpful to list the benefits and risks of taking a particular action.

The final stage of the cycle involves *acting*. Here the strategy is to address internal and external barriers. When preparing to act, first develop a plan and find sources of support. These support systems can be co-workers, supervisors, or outside resources, such the ANA Code of Ethics or a literature search for relevant information. Finally the plan is put into action. This will start the cycle again, so it is important to monitor the change to see that it has succeeded in eliminating or reducing moral distress.

A Strategy to Decrease Stress: Time Management

One of the most effective ways of managing stress is to efficiently manage time. Stress often occurs when deadlines are not met or tasks begin to pile up. Learning ways to be more productive given the constant bombardment of competing demands for limited time is critical to managing stress. This is particularly important in the Internet age. It is not unusual to open up work or personal e-mail accounts and have hundreds of e-mails that await attention. However, do they need to be immediately answered? Although there could be an expectation that you process an e-mail as soon as it arrives, this may be negotiable to some extent. One of the simplest rules for effectively managing e-mail is to only check e-mails two to three times a day rather than constantly on a mobile device. Also, sorting e-mails by subject and flagging ones that need follow-up can also help in sorting through the often overwhelming number of e-mails and create a manageable system of information (Atwood & Uttley, 2011). For more time on an item, a quick reply can be sent that lets the sender know when he or she will have a more thorough response. Then close the e-mail. Personal contact about more emergent issues can be handled through other devices, such as a pager.

As with the stress journal, one of the best ways to improve time management is a time journal. People are often unaware of exactly how they are spending their time, and a time journal allows you to see precisely where all your time is going. In 30-minute increments, write down how you spend your time. This log can then be analyzed by day, week, month, or year, depending on the circumstances. Recording time use makes the abstract idea of time into a concrete reality and allows for finding opportunities to eliminate time wasters (Randel, 2010). These can be short blocks of time in a given day, but how much does it add up to in a week? What about in a month?

Another important component of effective time management is creating to-do lists. Although this seems like a simple step, working from a list can actually increase productivity by 25% (Tracy, 2007). Prioritization is an essential skill in creating these lists. There are many ways to prioritize, including time constraints, profitability or value, or the pressure to complete the job (Mind Tools, 2010). One way to approach this is to analyze what needs to be done immediately and what can wait. Although it may be tempting to do simple, unimportant tasks first, a more effective way is to complete the most important jobs first (Mind Tools, 2010). It is also helpful to have different lists for different purposes. Many people find that keeping monthly, weekly, and daily lists can dramatically increase their productivity. Items from the monthly list are transferred to the weekly lists, and so forth (Tracy, 2007). Keeping track of all completed tasks and starting a daily planner to log all tasks that need to be completed focuses an individual on personal time management reality.

When confronted with a workload that is overwhelming, a nurse may not create an actual to-do list, but the idea of planning first is still important. It is crucial to take 15 to 20 minutes to plan the day. Skipping this will cost time throughout the day because of the downtime that occurs from doing extra steps that could have been economized by planning ahead. Time is also lost when tasks require redoing.

Analyzing and managing time takes a concentrated effort and an openness to rethinking habits and routines. Often a small amount of effort yields large returns, so changes are important. Assessing personal strengths and weaknesses might help focus personal choices for projects or job duties, such as joining a team. Fundamental motivation, such as doing what you enjoy, also helps time management decisions. Balance is a final consideration. Setting realistic goals, preserving contingency time for the unexpected, and carefully identifying essential tasks in the right order are strategies that help achieve balanced time management.

LEADERSHIP AND MANAGEMENT IMPLICATIONS

Stress and the Nurse Manager

Stress in nurses' work life is a given. There are aspects of caring for patients that can significantly alter anyone's day. Many times, the best laid plans must be adjusted depending on changes in the workplace, as well as changes in each patient's illness. When managing any unit or department, all of these work-flow modifications creep into the routines of the manager's day, creating chaos in a well-planned day. The manager has one of the most difficult jobs in meeting the challenges of managing and leading employees, as well as meeting priorities that flow from higher management. The challenge of meeting the expectations of the multiple roles of the nurse manager can produce stress that reveals itself as role strain, which is an unpleasant feeling of frustration and intense labile emotional state (Richmond et al., 2009). This may lead to communication breakdowns, the sense of failing, and intense anxiety about job performance.

There is a scarcity of evidence on how stress affects the nurse manager role. However, Shirey and colleagues (2010) have provided a rich source of qualitative evidence about sources and factors related to stress, outcomes of this stress, and coping strategies used to decrease stress. In their study, nurse manager participants reported key sources of stress to include dealing with people, specifically related to people with negative attitudes or employees with subpar work performance; patient and family complaints; physician interactions; and working within the political nature of the hospital with a lack of transparency and collaboration. Staffing was noted as the most stressful part of their role. High stress is experienced by nurse managers (Kath et al., 2012) and stems from the challenges of a multifaceted job with myriad sources of stress. However, nurse managers are likely to stay in their positions (Kath et al., 2012; Shirey et al., 2010). Although there is a relationship between job satisfaction and intent to quit, when stress is high for nurse managers, other factors show strong relationships with stress (Kath et al., 2012). Having support from others (e.g., supervisors, co-managers, co-workers) is a factor that decreased stress (Kath et al., 2012; Shirey et al., 2010).

The amount of autonomy and predictability in the job mitigates the negative effects of stress as well (Kath et al., 2012).

Certain nurse manager characteristics may impact the stress levels of employees. Transformational leaders, by transcending their own self-interest, improve work environments by empowering staff to own their practice through innovative efforts (Weberg, 2010). These leaders act in authentic ways to inspire and create a culture of trust. Cummings and colleagues (2010) brought attention to this leadership excellence in the 53 studies they used for their systematic review, reporting that transformational leaders enhance staff satisfaction and a culture of a healthy workplace. The actions of the transformational leader decrease burnout and exhaustion and increase staff well-being (Weberg, 2010). Giving "voice," listening to employees, and considering each individual are key demonstrations of the "people-focused" approach that improves environment and staff satisfaction (Lewis & Malecha, 2011).

On a personal level, both psychological and physiological outcomes of stress are found. Dealing with the complexities and constant change in nurses' environments, coupled with working long hours, can be exhausting mentally and physically, which leads to decreased mental clarity, depression, irritability, and anxiety (Han et al., 2011; Shirey et al., 2010). High blood pressure, sleep disturbances, and obesity are just a few of the many outward physical signs of stress outcomes (Han et al., 2011).

On the unit level, stress can be played out synergistically in the close relationships and interactions we all must have in order to work together as a team on a unit or in a department. Each shares in teamwork, collaborative actions, and in creating necessary energy to get the work done. So, the emotional state of each nurse is highly subject to influencing everyone else in the workplace. Any bullies within the group have perhaps the most negative influence in nurses' environments, and there is evidence to suggest that bullying behavior is related to increased stress (Lindy & Schaefer, 2010). The incivility of acting out creates a negative workplace, leading to work limitation expressed as lost productivity (Lewis & Malecha, 2011). Nurse managers specifically experience a decrease in personal productivity and procrastination in stressful situations (Shirey et al, 2010).

Strategies to Mitigate Stress in the Workplace

Mitigating stress can be challenging within the complexity of nurses' environments. Strategies to decrease stress can be framed with personal and institutional actions. We all have the power to handle workplace stress—tapping into our potential by acknowledgement and awareness is key. Health care institutions in the business of ensuring quality care for patients can be served well by the same acknowledgement, awareness, and assessment of workplace stress. Several key institutional actions are noted in Box 5-1, and personal actions are noted in Box 5-2.

There is a wealth of evidence linking healthy work environments to increased patient satisfaction, better patient outcomes, and fewer errors (AACN, 2005). One of the best institutional strategies to decrease stress at the workplace is the adoption of the six AACN Healthy Work Environment Standards (Table 5-1) as the imperative in setting expectations of behavior for all health care professionals. Implementing these is one way to create positivity for the workplace, thus decreasing stress for everyone. Celebrating successes as a team creates the positive energy needed to push forward in the complex health care environment. Caring

---

BOX 5-1   INSTITUTIONAL STRATEGIES TO DECREASE STRESS AT THE WORKPLACE

- Assess stress levels and stress management strategies of employees.
- Institute the AACN Standards of Establishing and Sustaining Healthy Work Environments.
- Ensure that management and leadership education include vital behaviors and competencies.
- Structure evaluations of managers, directors, supervisors, and senior level management with leadership and management behaviors that provide stress management strategies.
- Ensure transparency of information and set effective communication patterns.
- Implement a top-down approach to sharing and owning quality improvement and outcomes.

BOX 5-2   PERSONAL STRATEGIES TO DECREASE STRESS AT THE WORKPLACE

- Learn chair exercises and complete them while catching up on e-mails or talking on the phone.
- When possible, take the stairs to reenergize yourself.
- Get a de-stress buddy at work and contact them when you need to vent—this is someone you completely trust and ideally someone outside of your unit.
- Have a "getaway" place at work in order to spend a few minutes in silence and thought.
- Get off the unit for at least your lunch break. Do not eat at your desk.
- Schedule lunches with other people outside your unit. This commitment ensures your escape and has the added bonus of putting yourself with another person not associated with your own unit.
- Schedule "think time" appointments at least once a week for a block of time; get out of your office for these times.
- Have a fruit bowl instead of chocolate or candy on your desk
- Bring a water bottle to work, and refill as needed to keep hydrated.

TABLE 5-1   AACN STANDARDS FOR ESTABLISHING AND SUSTAINING HEALTHY WORK ENVIRONMENTS

STANDARD	STATEMENT
Skilled Communication	Nurses must be as proficient in communication skills as they are in clinical skills.
True Collaboration	Nurses must be relentless in pursuing and fostering true collaboration.
Effective Decision Making	Nurses must be valued and committed partners in making policy, directing and evaluating clinical care and leading organizational operations.
Appropriate Staffing	Staffing must ensure the effective match between patient needs and nurse competencies.
Meaningful Recognition	Nurses must be recognized and must recognize others for the value each brings to the work of the organization.
Authentic Leadership	Nurse leaders must fully embrace the imperative of a healthy work environment, authentically live it, and engage others in its achievement.

for others includes recognition of their contributions; celebrating contribution is meaningful to all. There are many ways to celebrate and recognize nurses; however, expanding the search for sources outside of the nursing profession may prove to be valuable.

One of the more unusual sources is a deck of cards called, "52 Ways to Deal Recognition." Made by Gemaco and available online at *www.baudville.com*, this handy reference provides hints, tips, and insights to bring recognition to life and emphasize its importance. If using shared decision making with staff, the nurse manager could consider requesting a "care for yourself" staff-driven group to create positive energy and celebration. This interdisciplinary committee would spread the cheer throughout the whole team and use positive energy to drive a healthy work environment. One interesting concept, workplace spirituality, connects to creating a healthy work environment. This is not about religion; it is about enjoyment at work and organizational commitment and alignment. The ability of the nurse manager to promote workplace spirituality is intimately connected to his/her emotional intelligence (Rego & Cunha, 2008).

To support the nurse manager, the supervisor's supportive behaviors are vital to job satisfaction and organizational commitment (Kath et al., 2012). Nurse managers need a level of decisional authority to be effective at supporting their units or departments. This autonomy is also related to a certain amount of predictability in the experience of the manager. Transparency, sharing information, and then allowing the manager to make informed decisions will enhance a predictable nature to the work flow.

In complex environments, it very difficult to set priorities, and often nurses get caught up in priorities set by others. Setting priorities is a key time management technique. Knowing what is and what is not a priority is the first step. Nurses may think they know what the boss wants as a priority, but often just asking brings relief when true priorities are revealed.

In the business of management, people should always be the priority. Patients and their families need nurses and rely on them to assure their safe passage through the health care system. As managers, staff are the priority; caring for staff means caring for patients, although indirectly. In a qualitative study, Lewis and Malecha (2010) found 14 vital nurse manager behaviors that decreased staff stress. Among the positive and negative behaviors are people-focused actions, such as following through with employees, providing mentoring and coaching, taking an interest in employees' lives, having a positive approach with others, and providing opportunities to voice opinions and views.

Being people-focused sometimes means readjusting tasks and duties. If possible, the chief nurse executive can hire out tasks such as the many aspects associated with the human resource department or other tasks that do not need the skill set of the chief nurse executive for setting vision and creating a healthy work place. Part of using leadership skills to manage the job includes knowing when to delegate and using the skill of empowering others to take responsibility for different aspects of unit functioning. Tackling what can be delegated is an important step. Sharing the load of unit management is key to helping nurses and other health care professionals feel engaged about their contribution to the unit or department. Shared decision-making requires different skills as managers; coaching and mentoring others in aspects of decisions and actions become priorities and are important in creating an environment that is healthy. Some of this requires that the manager updates his or her own skills and becomes the leader who empowers others to become accountable for unit functioning.

One question that should be asked is "Do I really need to go to all those meetings?" Some of them are important, but could staff nurses attend a few of the meetings on the calendar? All staff should be intimately involved in quality improvement (QI) and optimal outcomes. In order for the staff to optimally contribute, they need to have the data about QI and outcomes of their patient population. In order for nurse managers to work effectively and efficiently, they need to have data in real time, including HPPD, significant never events outcomes, and QI initiatives.

Time Management in the Unit

One time management technique is to set self deadlines for completion of tasks. With big projects, dividing up the project into manageable parts and setting deadlines for each part is helpful. Sticking to your deadlines may seem overwhelming, because things do come up and interfere with completion of tasks. It is certainly within an individual's power to renegotiate deadlines, but it should not become a habit. Having a calendar system, whether online or on paper, is vital for meeting deadlines and tracking project progression. Becoming skillful with technology is worth the time and effort, but struggling with the learning curve is inevitable.

A key survival technique in this transparent information-giving/seeking culture where timeliness is of the essence for many, carving time to think is vital. This much needed time reenergizes people and enables them to handle the activities of workplace and decrease the stress response. Creating the time, planning for it, and committing to it are essential. One technique is to send yourself an appointment and keep it as a priority. If needed, when that appointment time arrives, leave your office and find another place to be, such as the library or someone else's office. Take your laptop if you need to actually work on e-mail or other projects, but also make sure you have "think time" during this self-energizing appointment. Ideally these appointments should be for a block of time, at least 2 hours. If possible, have someone else take the beeper or phone to answer those vital questions from staff and charge nurses.

Stress and Time Management with Staff

One of the most important ways to help staff with stress and time management is role modeling all the aspects of stress reducing strategies and managing time. So "walking the talk" is, in essence, a vital component of ensuring unit personnel handle their stress and time as well as possible. If you value these stress reduction strategies, if you value the essence of your overall life as more than being a nurse, then you will teach this to others. "Buying in" creates the base to being an authentic role model. Being the leader requires being true to oneself, which spills over into being true to others. Setting the bar and expectations are key.

Can nurse managers create this type of "getting away" for direct care nurses and others who report to them? Importance should be placed on employees taking breaks and getting away from the unit for those breaks. Giving permission to leave is a key aspect in this strategy. Ensuring continuity of care is vital to help the direct care nurses feel like they can leave the unit to reenergize themselves in a way that will help them cope with their job responsibilities.

Since nurses are in the business of people, blocking "people time" is vitally important as well. There are a variety of ways to ensure that people time is met. The important aspect is creating the culture of caring for patients by creating a culture of caring for staff. A few suggestions for blocking people time are found in Box 5-3. Using the management team (assistants, charge nurses, clinical nurse specialists, educators) to strategize timing for all team members gives a powerful message to schedule people time.

As a manager, an important aspect of creating the environment whereby nurses utilize strategies to decrease stress and manage their own time well is setting expectations for behavior, attitude, and actions.

Sticking with these expectations can set the tone for changing culture to one that is healthy for both staff, patients, and families. The creation of positive energy is vital to the goal of having happy nurses and thus satisfied patients and families.

Given the current tremendous and unprecedented transformation in health care, preparation is the key. A trusted leader is one who prepares for the worst with a steady hand but still looks to the future with passion and great expectations. Our future is in our hands. Let those hands be steady and prepared to traverse the expected and unexpected challenges that lie ahead.

BOX 5-3   STRATEGIES FOR PEOPLE TIME

- Block time for daily rounds for both patients, families, and staff; some days will have longer blocks of time.
- Schedule blocks of time to tackle e-mail. Consider this for the end of your day, not the beginning.
- Prioritize e-mails to address people first—staff issues, patients, and family issues.
- Schedule blocks of time for an "open" door to your office; invite staff to visit.
- Post your daily schedule on your office door with beeper number and/or cell.
- Take note cards to meetings where only listening is required; write personal notes to recognize staff for their contributions and recognize birthdays.
- Schedule periodic "lunch with the manager" sessions for both night and day shifts.
- Set realistic follow-up deadlines for staff issues, questions, and concerns.

RESEARCH NOTE

Source

Hoolahan, S.E., Greenhouse, P.K., Hoffmann, R.L., & Lehman, L.A. (2012). Energy capacity model for nurses: The impact of relaxation and restoration. *The Journal of Nursing Administration, 42*(2), 103-109.

Purpose

This study examined the effect of stress management techniques, in particular a restoration room on the unit, on nurses' levels of stress. The investigators also assessed whether the restoration room had an effect on unplanned absences and nursing turnover.

Discussion

A restoration room was created on the study unit, and health coaches taught a 6-week stress reduction workshop. On average the nurses used the restoration room five times during the study period. Stress levels were measured using the Nursing Stress Scale both before and after the intervention. This scale showed an overall reduction in stress; however, it was not statistically significant. Because of attrition by study participants, not enough nurses completed the study to adequately measure reductions in unplanned time off or turnover. However, anecdotally, the nurses appreciated the restoration room and continued to use it after the study period ended.

Application to Practice

This study considered the importance of stress reduction on a nursing unit. Although the sample size was not large enough to detect statistically significant differences, it did support the idea that a restoration room and a stress management program were useful in helping nurses to manage their stress. It is important that staff nurses find ways to deal with their daily stress on the unit.

CASE STUDY

Nurse Maria Vasquez is thrilled with the results of creating a new unit council and implementing AACN's Healthy Work Environment (HWE) Standards. A year ago, when she became manager of an inpatient unit, she felt as though everything was crashing in on her. The unit was struggling with many issues, including poor patient outcomes, decreased morale, stressed staff nurses, and a high nurse turnover rate. Nurse Vasquez knew that changes had to be made on the unit, so she decided to establish a unit council to address some of the practice issues.

The new unit council and Nurse Vasquez decided to use AACN's HWE Standards. The first standard they wanted to tackle was Skilled Communication. They first created several workshops to teach this skill, and were very pleased with the response. All staff, including physicians and respiratory therapists, attended. Follow-up workshops were then scheduled to be completed every year.

The unit council decided to track whether the workshops had any effect on the nurses' stress and burnout. So they decided to use the Nursing Stress Scale (NSS) to measure the stress levels of the unit nurses both before and after the workshop.

Nurse Vasquez was very pleased to see that not only did patient outcomes improve on the unit, but nurses' stress scores on the NSS significantly improved as well. She was also happy to find that turnover on the unit had also decreased.

■ CRITICAL THINKING EXERCISE

Nurse Whitney Gould was initially very excited about her new job as nurse manager of a 50-bed regional intensive care nursery. She has experience in both leadership and management; however, she is not a clinical expert in this area. The director to whom she reports *is* an expert in the field, and was the nurse manager of this unit for many years before Nurse Gould. The staff nurses are skeptical about Nurse Gould not having the practical experience, but do realize her leadership skills are refreshing. However, they continue to go to the director for practice issues.

The director and Nurse Gould have significant differences about a leadership versus management focus on the unit. The director wants management tasks completed, whereas Nurse Gould believes that the unit needs a strong focus on leadership, role modeling, coaching, and mentoring in order to empower the nurses to own their own practices.

Nurse Gould has established a unit council as well as "Lunch with the Manager" sessions for both the day and night shifts. She hopes this will give the staff opportunities to voice their issues, concerns, and visions for the unit.

The director is constantly on Nurse Gould's case about being behind on e-mails, HR issues, and budget variances. Recently, meetings have been held with the director regarding education issues on the unit, yet Nurse Gould has not been invited.

1. What problem(s) do you see for Nurse Gould in this scenario?
2. Why is it a problem?
3. What sources of stress are present?
4. How does Nurse Gould's stress affect the stress of the nurses on the unit?
5. What should Nurse Gould do first?
6. What factors should Nurse Gould assess and analyze?
7. What strategies could be employed to help control stress and enhance coping?

CHAPTER

6

Legal and Ethical Issues

Robert W. Cooper

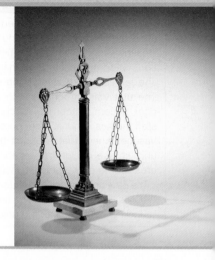

℮volve WEBSITE

http://evolve.elsevier.com/Huber/leadership/

A major advantage of being viewed as a profession is the societal grant of autonomy in practice. In professional terms, *autonomy* means that the occupational group has control over its own practice. The American Nurses Association's (ANA's) *Nursing's Social Policy Statement: The Essence of the Profession* (2010, p. 25) indicates "competence is foundational to autonomy" with the profession ensuring nursing competence to society through professional regulation of nursing practice via standards and ethical codes of practice, legal regulation of nursing practice via state licensure requirements and law pertaining to criminal and civil wrongdoing, and self-regulation in which all nurses retain personal accountability for their own practice.

Although some laws can be unethical, laws generally provide minimum standards of acceptable conduct that are binding on individuals, groups, and businesses in dealing with other members of society. Many situations, however, are either not covered by specific laws or involve issues so complicated that, although the law can provide general guidelines for conduct, the issues cannot be fully resolved by the legal system alone. In these cases, ethical codes for a

profession provide standards of conduct that serve as guidelines for decision making by the members of the profession.

By the very nature of their work, nurses and nurse managers are decision makers constantly faced with making choices in personal, clinical, and organizational situations. These decision-making situations are commonly fraught with legal and ethical issues that often become entwined. As members of a profession, nurses and nurse managers are guided by both legal and ethical considerations in making decisions.

LEGAL ASPECTS

There are extensive legal aspects to both nursing practice and nursing management. For example, nurse practice acts exist for each state and govern the legal practice of nursing, including delegation and supervision. The legal regulation of nursing via nurse practice acts and related administrative rules arises because society needs to have safeguards that protect the health and safety of citizens. In regard to health care, the public demands assurance that health care providers, including nurses, are properly prepared and competent to deliver needed services. Thus to practice nursing, the person must hold a valid license issued by the

Photo used with permission from Photos.com.

state. Therefore it is illegal to practice nursing without a license. State licensure confers autonomy on nurses to the limit of legal standards of practice.

Autonomy involves accountability, as well as authority, for one's decisions and actions. As professional autonomy and responsibility increase, so does the level of accountability and liability. To the extent that nurses are subject to malpractice lawsuits and carry malpractice insurance, nurses are held accountable (Aiken, 2004).

The legal aspects of nursing management center around decision making and supervision. Because all nurses retain personal accountability for their own acts and the use of knowledge and skills in the provision of care, personal accountability cannot be assumed by another. Nurse managers keep their own personal accountability for their own specific acts, but they are accountable also for their acts of delegation and supervision. Nurse managers carry the major responsibility for developing and upholding the standards of care for the staff.

Nurses and nurse managers carry the accountability for the supervision of others, who are often unlicensed assistive personnel. Supervision includes monitoring the tasks performed, ensuring that functions are performed in an appropriate fashion, and ensuring that assigned tasks and functions do not exceed competency or require a license to perform.

Nurse managers use their autonomy to make decisions about practice situations. They are accountable for carrying out supervisory responsibilities; proper notification; assessing the competency of staff; training, orientation, and evaluation of staff; reasonable staffing decisions; and monitoring and maintenance of professional treatment relationships with clients, called *nonabandonment* (Aiken, 2004; Guido, 2010).

DEFINITIONS

In addition to law included in the federal and state constitutions, United States law is composed of **statutory law** (law enacted by the U.S. Congress, state legislatures, and local government bodies), **administrative law** (regulations promulgated and adopted by federal or state agencies to implement statutory law adopted by Congress or state legislatures), and **common law** (decisions of courts setting precedents to be followed, at least in that court's jurisdiction, until overturned

by a higher court). The law recognizes two classes of wrongful acts that may cause harm. These are **criminal acts** (conduct that is offensive or harmful to society as a whole) and **civil acts** (wrongs that violate the rights of individuals by tort or by breach of contract). Persons found guilty of crimes are generally fined, jailed, or both, whereas persons who commit civil wrongs are usually required to pay monetary damages to those who are wronged.

Nurses, nurse managers, and health care facilities are all subject to being found **legally liable** (i.e., legally responsible) for harm caused to others by civil wrongs. More specifically, liability is created when the law imposes a civil obligation on a wrongdoer to compensate an injured party for the consequences of a wrongful act. As shown in Figure 6-1, there are two sources of legal liability—torts and contracts.

The most common source of legal liability for nurses and nurse managers is a *tort*—that is, a wrongful act (other than breach of contract) committed against another person or organization or their property that causes harm and can be remedied by a civil (rather than criminal) lawsuit. Although torts most commonly give rise to *personal* (or *direct*) liability for the person committing the wrongful act, in some cases another person or organization may also be held *vicariously* liable for the same wrongful act they did not commit. For example, when a nurse commits a tort, the nurse may be found to be directly liable and the nurse's employer also may be found to be vicariously liable for the nurse's wrongful action.

As indicated in Figure 6-1, determination of legal liability as a result of a tort depends on more than just the various technical elements of the tort that must be proved by the injured party (plaintiff), the presentation of various available defenses by the defendant, and the formal rules of the judicial system regarding the litigation process. In the case of torts, the legal outcomes are often influenced also by what may be termed *judicial risk*—various aspects of the litigation process that can introduce further uncertainty and additional cost into the determination of legal liability. Judicial risk can result in findings with respect to legal liability that are not based solely on the merits of the case nor on the rules of law applicable to the case.

There are three categories of torts: negligence, intentional torts, and strict liability torts. **Negligence** is the failure to exercise the proper degree of care

LEGAL LIABILITY
A civil obligation imposed by law on a wrongdoer requiring compensation of an injured party through money damages or some other legal remedy for the consequences of a wrongful act

"JUDICIAL RISK" FILTER
Various aspects of the litigation process that can introduce further uncertainty and additional cost into the determination of legal liability
- Witnesses' perceptions of the facts can change over time
- Courtroom conditions can influence the jury

TORTS
Tort—a wrongful act (other than a breach of contract) committed by one person that causes harm to another by invading a legally protected right
- **Personal (Direct) Liability**—liability imposed on the person who committed the wrongful act
- **Vicarious Liability**—a person or organization that has not behaved wrongfully can be held legally liable for torts committed by others

CONTRACTS
- **Breach of Contract**—if a party to a contract does not perform as promised, the other party can sue for money damages or seek the remedy of specific performance
- **Hold Harmless or Indemnity Agreements**—one party assumes the liability of another party for damage in situations in which the first party would not otherwise be liable

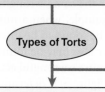

Types of Torts

Negligence
- An unintentional tort
- Negligence—failure of a person to exercise the degree of care that an ordinary prudent person would have exercised under similar circumstances
- Malpractice—failure of a professional person to act as other prudent professionals with the same knowledge and education would have acted under similar circumstances

Intentional Torts
- A wrongful act that was intended to cause harm

- Examples
  - Assault and battery
  - False imprisonment
  - Defamation—libel and slander
  - Invasion of right of privacy
  - Fraud
  - Intentional torts against property (trespass, conversion)

Strict Liability Torts
- Tort liability imposed when the defendant acted neither negligently nor with intent to cause harm

- May be applied in cases involving dangerously defective products—medical devices, use of unlicensed medicines

FIGURE 6-1 Sources of legal liability.

required by the circumstances. In general, the standard of care is defined as that which a reasonably prudent person would exercise under the circumstances to avoid harming others. Malpractice is a special type of negligence that applies only to professionals and employs a higher standard of care than ordinary negligence (Weld & Bibb, 2009). **Malpractice** is the failure of a professional person to act as other prudent professionals with the same knowledge and education would act under similar circumstances. Depending on the nature of the situation involved, nurses and nurse leaders may be subject to either ordinary negligence or malpractice. An example of ordinary negligence would be a situation in which a nurse saw that food had been spilled on a client's floor but failed to have it cleaned up, and as a result, the client slipped and broke her hip. Because this is an act not requiring the exercise of professional judgment, the standard of care in determining negligence would be the degree of care that an ordinary prudent person would exercise under the circumstances. However, if the client had fallen and broken her hip because a nurse had failed to raise the side rails on the client's bed, the standard of care in determining malpractice would be the degree of care other prudent professionals with the same knowledge and education could be expected to exercise under similar circumstances.

Although negligence involves unintentional wrongful acts that harm another person or his or her property, *intentional torts* are voluntary and willful acts intended to cause harm by interfering with another person's rights. Common intentional torts occurring in the health care field include, among others, assault and battery, medical battery (surgical procedures performed without patient consent), false imprisonment, trespass to land, conversion of property, and intentional infliction of emotional distress.

In some cases, tort liability can be imposed without the defendant acting either negligently or with intent to cause harm. *Strict liability* requires that the responsibility for some accidents automatically rests with the defendant. With strict liability, anyone who engages in an activity known to endanger others assumes responsibility for any resulting damages. In general society, situations requiring strict liability include such activities as blasting, keeping dangerous animals, and selling dangerously defective products. In the health care field, the concept of strict liability has been applied in some cases involving harm caused by, among other things, the use of unlicensed medicines, defectively designed medical devices, tainted or contaminated drugs, and the prescription of dangerous combinations of drugs without obtaining a sufficient medical history to ensure that problems do not occur.

As shown in Figure 6-1, contracts are also a source of legal liability. In most states, employment of nurses generally follows the employment-at-will doctrine in which there is no written contract specifying the term of employment. However, in some cases, nurse managers, especially those at higher levels in an organization, negotiate written employment contracts. In addition, a few courts have ruled that contracts existed on the basis of language used in advertisements and statements made during the interviewing process. Courts also have held that contracts may arise after employment based on statements made in employee manuals and handbooks. With an increasing number of nurses negotiating various types of consulting arrangements with facilities, working as independent contractors and operating their own privately owned businesses, contracts are playing an even greater role in nursing.

Legal liability based on contracts can arise in two ways: breach of contract, or an agreement to assume another party's liability. The most common is *breach of contract,* in which one party to the contract fails to perform as promised in the contract. For example, if a nurse has an employment contract stating that he or she can be discharged only for incompetence but then is discharged for another reason, the nurse can bring a suit for wrongful discharge under contract law due to breach of contract. Less likely to be encountered by nurses is legal liability arising from *an agreement to assume another party's liability.* For example, in signing a lease for property needed to carry on his or her privately owned business, the nurse likely would be agreeing to assume responsibility for all injuries occurring on the premises, including any caused by the owner of the property.

LAW AND THE NURSE MANAGER

The managers of any health care organization are responsible to the policy-making body of the organization. The managers also hold an obligation to comply with the laws of society at local, state, and national levels. Managers are responsible for ensuring that laws are adhered to in the actions of management itself and also in the actions of those employees who assist the managers in carrying out the mission of the organization. Concern for the law involves three general areas: personal negligence in clinical practice, liability for delegation and supervision, and liability of health care organizations.

Personal Negligence in Clinical Practice

Activities of clinical client care involve corresponding legal accountability and risk. Errors do happen. Some lead to injury to a client. At minimum, nurses have an ethical obligation to nonmaleficence, or to do no harm to clients. This duty is discharged in part by remaining competent in knowledge and skills and the standards of practice. Nursing negligence/malpractice occurs when the nurse's actions are unreasonable given the circumstances or fail to meet the standard of care or when the nurse fails to act and causes harm. In nursing, harm related to clinical practice commonly arises from negligent acts or omissions (unintentional torts) and a variety of intentional acts (intentional torts) such as invasion of privacy or assault and battery (Aiken, 2004).

To establish legal liability on the grounds of malpractice (professional negligence), the injured client (plaintiff) must prove the following four elements:

1. A duty of care was owed to the injured party.
2. There was a breach of that duty.
3. The breach of the duty caused the injury (causation).
4. Actual harm or damages were suffered by the plaintiff.

Critical in determining liability for malpractice (professional negligence) is the definition of the duty (standard) of care owed by the nursing professional to the client. The standard of care, the minimum requirements that define an acceptable level of care, is "the average degree of skill, care, and diligence exercised by members of the same profession under the same or similar circumstances" (Aiken, 2004, p. 39). Standards of care can be found in the state nurse practice act, standards published by the American Nurses Association, other professional organizations and specialty practice groups, federal agency guidelines and regulations, and the facility's policy and procedure manuals. In malpractice cases, the standard of care owed to the injured client is commonly introduced into evidence by expert witnesses and the impact of that evidence is ultimately determined by the jury after receiving instructions from the judge on the law applicable to its use.

Common clinical practice areas that give rise to allegations of malpractice include the general areas of treatment, communication, medication, and the broad category of monitoring/observing/supervising/surveillance. Examples of common negligence allegations in nursing malpractice suits include patient falls, use of restraints, medication errors, burns, equipment injuries, retained foreign objects, failure to monitor, failure to ensure safety, failure to take appropriate nursing action, failure to confirm accuracy of physicians' orders, improper technique or performance of treatments, failure to respond to a patient, failure to follow hospital procedure, and failure to supervise treatment (Aiken, 2004; Weld & Bibb, 2009).

Because intentional torts differ in nature from negligence (unintentional torts), establishing legal liability for these intentionally harmful acts is based on elements different from those used in proving malpractice. To establish liability on the grounds of an intentional tort, the injured client (plaintiff) must prove that a voluntary and willful act by the nursing professional (defendant) was intended to interfere with the plaintiff's rights and was a substantial factor in doing so. Unlike negligence, intent is necessary in proving intentional torts. However, proof of actual injury or damage is not required, because intentional torts interfere with another person's rights. Also, there is no need to determine duty or standards of care in proving intentional torts.

Liability for Delegation and Supervision

Over and above personal liability for clinical practice, nurses and nurse managers have accountability and liability for their acts of delegation and supervision. Both nurses and nurse managers are obligated to report incompetent practice that occurs at any point in the care delivery process. Nurse managers have a duty to train, orient, and evaluate the ability of nursing staff to perform specific functions and tasks. Health care organizations have a duty to monitor the competence and ability of nursing and medical professionals and to inquire about their credentials (Aiken, 2004).

Both nurses and nurse managers have a duty to follow policies and procedures when reasonable. Nurse managers are advised to review policies and procedures carefully, including the language used, in order to adhere to legal and ethical parameters more closely. Clearly, management in nursing practice means that nurses must fulfill obligations and duties both to clients and to the organization. This means using knowledge, skill, and decision-making abilities to reduce the incidence of negligence and malpractice by employees as a way to reduce harm to clients and legal risk to the organization. As the primary coordinators of care, nurses need to manage the environment of care delivery. Ensuring staff competence and reporting incompetent practice are key activities. For example, in nursing, legal and ethical issues arise when a nurse is impaired by substance abuse. The overall consideration is protecting the client from harm. Confronting suspected abuse must be done carefully. However, when an incident occurs, the nurse manager has a responsibility to intervene.

Liability of Health Care Organizations

In addition to the liability faced by nurses and nurse managers arising out of malpractice in clinical practice and negligence in the process of delegating and supervising, health care facilities face extensive exposure to legal liability from several sources. These sources include negligence of their employees, negligence of independent contractors, corporate negligence arising out of the facility's responsibilities to hire qualified employees and monitor and supervise their activities, and failure to comply with numerous laws and regulations, especially those related to employment issues. Nurse managers have important roles to play in helping their organizations control facility liability arising from each of these sources.

Under the doctrine of *respondeat superior* (meaning "let the master answer"), an employer may be held vicariously liable for the negligent act or omission of an employee. For the employer to be found vicariously liable, the employee's act or omission must occur both during the course of employment and while the employee was acting within the scope of employment. For example, if a nurse negligently injured a client during the course of and within the scope of employment, not only would the nurse be directly liable for damages but also the health care organization would

be vicariously liable. Because of their "deep pockets" (their ability to pay larger settlements or judgments) and the concept of vicarious liability, health care facilities are almost always named as defendants in malpractice suits. Nurse managers can play a key role in assisting facilities to avoid payments for vicarious liability by ensuring that the nurses they supervise deliver competent care to clients while following facility policies and procedures (Guido, 2010).

Under the doctrine of ostensible authority (or apparent agency), facilities may also become liable for the negligence of an independent contractor if it would appear to a reasonable client that the independent contractor is a facility employee. For example, a hospital might be held liable for the negligence of an agency nurse who appeared to a client to be a nurse employed by the hospital. Guido (2010) recommends that when dealing with agency or temporary personnel, nurse managers should, among other things, do the following:

- Consider their skills, competencies, and knowledge when delegating tasks and supervising their actions.
- Ensure that they are made aware of facility policies and procedures, resource materials, and documentation procedures.
- Assign a resource person to each temporary staff member to serve in the role of mentor and help prevent potential problems from occurring because of a lack of familiarity with institution routine or where to turn for assistance.

Under the doctrine of corporate liability, health care organizations themselves are held legally responsible for "ensuring that competent and qualified practitioners deliver quality health care to consumers" (Guido, 2010, p. 307). Under this doctrine, facilities can be held liable for a variety of activities that are beyond the control of any single employee, including the following (Aiken, 2004):

- Failure to check references, educational credentials, license status, disciplinary actions, and criminal record for applicants
- Failure to protect the clients from health care providers who can cause harm
- Failure to monitor the quality of care provided by all medical and nursing personnel within the facility
- Failure to periodically review staff competency
- Failure to terminate an employee who has harmed a client and then injures another client

Nurse managers can help the facility avoid corporate liability by, among other things, ensuring that those who report to them remain competent and qualified and have current licensure. Nurse managers should also report to appropriate managers dangerously low staffing levels or incorrect mixes of staff for effectively meeting the health care needs of clients, as well as report incompetent, illegal, or unethical practices to appropriate authorities (Guido, 2010).

In addition to facility liability arising from vicarious liability, the doctrine of ostensible authority, and the doctrine of corporate liability, health care organizations are constrained by specific laws related to employment issues. Although the various health care providers and their employing organizations have specific legal and ethical obligations to clients, such as executing informed consent and following the Patient Self-Determination Act of 1990, organizations carry specific legal and ethical obligations toward employees. The employer has an obligation to provide a safe and secure care delivery environment (Aiken, 2004).

Management policies and procedures must be in compliance in the areas of hiring, performance appraisal, management of employees with problems, and termination (Aiken, 2004). Lawsuits also have formed the basis for the standards to be met for the termination of employees. Discharges may occur for lack of adherence to employer-established policies or standards, "good cause" per institutional policy, illegal activity, assault, insubordination, or excessive absenteeism. Written notice and the reasons for termination avoid misunderstandings and show justice through due-process procedures. Careful documentation is important. If the employee is a member of a protected group, the employer may be required to submit formal justification for the termination (Aiken, 2004).

The various legal and ethical considerations of nursing management span client, provider, and employer rights and obligations. Nurses and their employing organizations are responsible for knowing and following the various applicable laws and regulations. In-service education can increase knowledge and awareness. Nurse managers will need to manage the environment of nursing care to ensure client safety, provider justice and safety, and organizational compliance with the law.

LEADERSHIP AND MANAGEMENT IMPLICATIONS

Clearly, nurses, nurse managers, and the facilities that employ them face legal liability from a wide array of sources. Although it is not possible to avoid legal liability in all cases, nurse managers can take a number of steps to protect themselves, staff nurses reporting to them, and their facilities where possible. The first step is summed up in a statement often attributed to football coach Vince Lombardi: *The best defense is a good offense.* Nurse managers can do a number of things in applying this strategy of using a good offense to defend against problems leading to legal liability. First, because problems generally can be dealt with more effectively if anticipated, nurse managers should see that both they and the staff nurses who report to them are knowledgeable concerning the most common problem areas related to malpractice and the other sources of legal liability, especially new ones that have not yet been experienced within the unit. Likewise, nurse managers should ensure that both they and their staff nurses are aware of the many prevention activities that can aid them in avoiding these legal liability problems. Providing this information to staff nurses and using examples will probably improve both recognition and retention. In addition to the previous brief discussion of the sources of legal liability faced by nurses and nurse managers and the activities for preventing them, extensive information, including examples, is available from numerous sources. These include books (e.g., Aiken, 2004; Brothers, 2005; Guido, 2010), articles in nursing journals (e.g., Austin, 2011; Frank-Stromborg & Christensen, 2001a, b; Miller & Glusko, 2003), and a variety of websites that present articles and continuing education materials about recommendations for avoiding malpractice (e.g., Croke, 2003; Nurses Service Organization [NSO], 2012; Wetter, 2007).

Many, if not most, of the lawsuits seeking to determine legal liability involve the alleged failure of nurses to meet appropriate standards of care, especially those reflected in the policies and procedures of their facility. Therefore nurse managers must not only ensure that they and their staff nurses know the standards of care that apply to them and are competent to satisfy them but also actively participate in facility committees as well as those at the state, national, and even international level that make decisions as to the standards of care to which nurses will be held.

Although the first step in defending against problems of legal liability involves taking positive action in an effort to prevent them from arising, it is not possible for nurses, nurse managers, and health care facilities to avoid legal liability in all cases. This is so, if for no other reason than the existence of what might be termed *judicial risk*.

RESEARCH NOTE

Source

Reising, D.L. & Allen, P.N. (2007). Protecting yourself from malpractice claims. *American Nurse Today, 2*(2), 39-43.

Purpose

Malpractice is a form of negligence for which nurses have been sued. The purpose of this article is to prepare nurses to respond effectively to the increased legal risk that accompanies greater nursing autonomy.

Discussion

After defining malpractice and briefly describing the elements of a malpractice suit, including the standards of care applied to nursing practice, the author discusses the six most common malpractice claims made against nurses for failure to exercise reasonable care in their own practice as well as a nurse's liability exposure arising from delegation to others. Suggestions are provided for preventing malpractice claims and dealing with the challenges that arise in the event of a lawsuit. Additional useful suggestions are presented in display boxes entitled "Avoiding Communication Breakdowns" and "Keeping Your Cool in the Courtroom."

Application to Practice

A negligent professional act that causes injury is known as *malpractice*. For a successful lawsuit, the injured party must prove that the nurse's conduct lacked due care. Knowledge of the most common problem areas, the use of examples, and the display of prevention tips aid the nurse in avoiding problems.

Judicial risk can result in findings with respect to legal liability that are not based solely on the merits of the case or on the rules of law applicable to the case. In the case of torts, aside from all the lists of elements that must be proved by injured plaintiffs, all the legal defenses available for attempting to block their arguments for damages, and the formal rules of the judicial system regarding the litigation process,

legal outcomes also are often influenced by judicial risk—that is, various aspects of the litigation process that can introduce further uncertainty and additional cost into the determination of legal liability. The following are some examples:

- Any client can sue a staff nurse, nurse manager, and/or health care facility for a tort, and if no response is filed within the legal time frame, the court will enter a default judgment against the defendant. Thus, at a minimum, regardless of the apparent validity of the grounds for the lawsuit, the defendant must incur defense costs or lose.

- Given the typical lengthy period between the defendant's act or omission and the introduction of evidence into the trial, many things can happen that will alter the perception of the facts. Witnesses, for example, may be questioned repeatedly, coached, or simply forget exactly what they witnessed.

- Conditions in the courtroom can also influence the jury. Some jury members may be influenced by the dress or behavior of the defendant's attorney and form subsequent opinions despite the facts (e.g., a high-priced lawyer with an arrogant attitude may elicit feelings such as "We'll show him"). Or the appearance of the plaintiff may influence jurors (e.g., "How could a little old man like that be partly responsible for his own injuries, and besides, who cares anyway since the defendant has liability insurance?").

- Often more than one principle of law applies to a case, and the outcome may be influenced by which one the judge uses in giving his or her instructions to the jury.

- In suits such as those alleging malpractice in providing or failing to provide proper end-of-life care, juries and even judges can be sufficiently influenced by their emotions so as to rationalize a finding of legal liability against the defendant, especially when, as is generally the case, liability insurance is available to pay the judgment. In fact, in some cases, a jury can actually change the law of a jurisdiction in making its decision. (See Case Study.)

In some cases, the elements of judicial risk make impossible even one's best efforts to prevent legal liability from being imposed on them and/or their facility. Thus all nurses, whether staff or managers, should carry adequate professional liability insurance to protect themselves against defense costs and liability judgments (or settlements). Although nurses are often covered as employees under a facility's professional liability policy, a number of reasons exist why they should also carry their own individual professional liability insurance. An employer can sue a nurse found guilty of malpractice for reimbursement (indemnification) of any damages the facility was required to pay as a result of vicarious liability. In addition, because a facility's professional liability insurance protects a nurse only while acting within the scope of employment or the nurse practice act, individual liability coverage would be required by private-duty nurses and off-duty nurses providing volunteer services. Although a facility's policy may provide only a single attorney to represent the different interests of the facility and the nurse, an individual policy will provide an attorney to specifically represent the nurse's interests. An individual policy will also provide funds to cover a nurse's defense costs and a portion of the judgment (or settlement) in the event that the total judgment exceeds the limits of liability of the facility's coverage. Individual policies generally provide coverage for personal injuries such as libel, slander, assault, battery, and violation of privacy, which may not be covered for employees in facility policies. Despite the large size of potential judgments and thus the high limits of liability required to adequately protect against them, many nurses can obtain individual coverage with limits of $1 million per claim and $6 million aggregate for an annual tax-deductible premium of approximately $100 (less than $70 if within 12 months of graduation).

ETHICAL ISSUES

In addition to potential legal concerns, nurses and nurse managers are often faced with ethical dilemmas in connection with decision making. Ethical dilemmas require that decisions be made about what is right and wrong in situations in which an individual has to make a choice between equally unfavorable alternatives. Traditionally, nurses, like other health care professionals, have faced ethical dilemmas arising primarily out of clinical practice. These dilemmas have involved conflicts among principles and/or rules attributable to common morality (socially approved norms of human conduct), standards articulated in professional codes of ethics, public policies

promulgated by government agencies, and in some cases, the personal values of the health care professionals themselves (Beauchamp & Childress, 2001). More recently, ethical dilemmas faced by nurses and nurse managers have increasingly involved clashes between the principles, rules, values, and standards of clinical/professional ethics and those of organizational/business ethics (Austin, 2007; Johnson, 2005).

Although the domain of clinical ethics is the care of clients, the domain of organizational ethics is a facility's business-related activities, including, among others, marketing, admissions, transfer, discharge, billing, and the relationship of the facility and its staff members to other health care providers, educational institutions, and payers, activities that also directly affect the care of patients. Organizational ethics reflect a health care facility's basic values that serve as guides for proper and acceptable behavior in decision making. According to Nelson (2011) "Basic ethics principles that make up our common morality, including respect for patients, acting in patients' best interest, avoiding bringing harm to patients and treating patients in a fair and equitable manner, serve as the foundation for healthcare values" (p. 46). The Joint Commission further supports these basic ethical principles as guides to a hospital's business practices in Standard LD. 04.02.03, where the standard is that care, treatment, and services are provided based on patient needs (Schyve, 2009).

Together, clinical and organizational ethics reflect a health care facility's concern that, whether related to the continuum of care or the continuum of services related to that care, ethical dilemmas should be resolved based on values-centered principles that center on doing the right thing and taking the right action.

ETHICAL DECISION MAKING IN CLINICAL HEALTH CARE

Many of the decisions nurses and nurse managers make on a daily basis have an ethical component and may involve conflicts among ethical responsibilities. These conflicts may involve clashes between the following:

- Two ethical duties to the client (e.g., duty to respect autonomy and duty to benefit the client)
- The client's rights and benefits (e.g., withholding or withdrawing treatment in respect for a client's right to die by forgoing treatment at any

time and treating or continuing treatment that is expected to produce more good for the client)

- Duties to self and duties to the client (e.g., a nurse's desire to remain on the same shift because of parental responsibilities and the need to advocate for better treatment of the clients by some health care practitioners on that shift)
- Professional ethical provisions and religious ones (e.g., a professional code requiring the recognition of the client's right to self-determination and a nurse's religious beliefs prohibiting abortion)

When ethical dilemmas are encountered in dealing with clinical matters, health care professionals commonly refer to various principles, rules, and standards for guidance in making moral decisions. Principles and rules are normative generalizations that provide guidance in ethical decision making. Although rules are more specific in content and restricted in scope than principles, neither can fully guide action but, rather, must be complemented by judgment for a decision to be made (Beauchamp & Childress, 2001; O'Neill, 2001).

Definitions

Like other health care practitioners, nurses apply four fundamental morality principles and a number of related rules in dealing with ethical dilemmas encountered in clinical practice on a daily basis. The four principles that form the cornerstone of biomedical ethical decision making are (1) autonomy, (2) beneficence, (3) nonmaleficence, and (4) justice. **Autonomy** refers to the client's right of self-determination and freedom of decision making. **Beneficence** means doing good for clients and providing benefit balanced against risk. **Nonmaleficence** means doing no harm to clients. **Justice** is the norm of being fair to all and giving equal treatment, including distributing benefits, risks, and costs equally (Aiken, 2004; Beauchamp & Childress, 2001; Guido, 2010).

Biomedical ethics also recognizes a number of rules that are related to the four fundamental principles and, likewise, provide guidance in dealing with ethical dilemmas (Beauchamp & Childress, 2001). Examples of commonly applied rules are fidelity, veracity, confidentiality, and privacy. **Fidelity** means being loyal and faithful to commitments and accountable for responsibilities. **Veracity** is the norm of telling the truth and not intentionally deceiving or misleading clients. **Confidentiality** prohibits some disclosures of

some information gained in certain relationships to some third parties without the consent of the original source of the information. **Privacy** is a right of limited physical or informational inaccessibility (Aiken, 2004; Beauchamp & Childress, 2001; Guido, 2010).

Code of Ethics

In addition to these basic moral principles and rules of biomedical ethics, nurses are also provided standards of conduct by professional codes of ethics. For example, the ANA's *Code of Ethics for Nurses: With Interpretive Statements* (2001) provides nonnegotiable standards as to the ethical obligations and duties of those who enter the nursing profession. The ANA (2001) indicated that the Code "provides a framework for nurses to use in ethical analysis and decision-making" (p. 3).

As with the principles and rules just discussed, the Code's provisions and accompanying interpretive statements, for the most part, do not focus on giving precise answers to specific ethical problems but, rather, provide general guidance as to how to act when faced with ethical dilemmas. The Code does, however, identify and provide somewhat more specific advice related to several currently unresolved ethical problems such as those involving the following:

- Practitioner decisions surrounding a client's right to die
- The introduction of incentive systems to decrease spending
- Responding to questionable and impaired practice
- Handling situations in which a client's needs are beyond a nurse's qualifications and competencies
- The existence of organizational barriers to ethical practice

Decision-Making Model

Although a number of decision-making models and processes have been proposed for use in resolving ethical dilemmas encountered in clinical practice (Aiken, 2004; Guido, 2010), they are all essentially modified versions of the six-step problem-solving model traditionally used in business, as follows:

1. Define the problem.
2. Develop alternative courses of action.
3. Evaluate each alternative course of action.
4. Select the best course of action.
5. Implement the selected course of action.
6. Monitor the results.

Because an ethical dilemma is merely a type of problem, specifically one that involves conflict, the six-step problem-solving model provides a process for making a decision when a moral dilemma arises in clinical practice. The ethical principles, rules, and standards just discussed are moral resources that can be used along with practitioner judgment to evaluate the alternative courses of action in step 3 of the problem-solving process to provide a basis for selecting the most appropriate course of action for resolving the dilemma.

THE CLASH BETWEEN CLINICAL AND ORGANIZATIONAL ETHICS

In today's rapidly changing health care environment, the traditional clinical ethical principles of autonomy, beneficence, nonmaleficence, and justice are being severely tested as they compete with demands for financial performance and demonstration of value. External financial pressures arise out of the reliance by health care facilities on market competition as a vehicle for cost control as derived from social policy (American Medical Association [AMA], 2000). By the very nature of their work, nurse managers play two different and often conflicting, roles: a professional caregiving role and an organizational role involving responsibilities associated with the management of nursing care or other aspects of a health care facility.

Dilemmas arising from the clash between clinical/professional ethics and organizational/business ethics are experienced daily by nurses and nurse managers (Austin, 2007; Johnson, 2005). Unfortunately, despite the passage of time, they continue to present major challenges to the delivery of professional nursing care in many, if not most, health care facilities (Cooper et al., 2002; Cooper et al., 2004; Miller, 2006). Specific examples of nurses' ethical dilemmas include the practice of pulling or floating nurses to areas in which they are not cross-trained, an action that also increases the client-to-nurse ratio to greater limits. Nurse managers may be asked to reduce expenditures by leaving specialty areas, such as labor and delivery, uncovered when no clients are present. Despite the evidence from studies by Aiken and colleagues (2002) about reduced mortality in ICUs with more RNs and the Magnet Recognition Program's® rigorous evidence about the structural and staffing factors

associated with quality of care, workload and staffing continue to be major nursing concerns. Nurses are known to use unauthorized "workarounds," especially in the area of medication administration. Such practices have huge business and risk implications. Along with their ethical concerns, most, if not all, of these dilemmas also have the potential to give rise to unfavorable legal consequences if resolved improperly.

Perceptions of Staff Nurses and Nurse Managers

Studies conducted by Cooper and colleagues provide some evidence as to the perceptions of staff nurses (Cooper et al., 2004) and nurse managers (Cooper et al., 2002) regarding the importance of the clash between clinical ethics and organizational ethics and the key effects on the delivery of quality health care. In each study, randomly selected participants were presented with a list of ethics-related statements that were referred to as *ethical issues* for simplicity (33 issues for staff nurses and 40 for nurse managers). Participants were asked to rate each issue on a 5-point scale, with "5" meaning that the issue was a major ethical problem for health care organizations and "1" meaning that it is not a problem. The high positive correlation coefficient for the group means of staff nurses and nurse managers for the 32 ethical issues common to both studies was 0.9023, which suggests that the order of the 32 issues in terms of the extent to which they present problems for health care facilities is quite similar.

Another area of similarity is reflected in 4 of the 8 ethical issues rated in the top 10 by both staff nurses and nurse managers. Both the 325 responding staff nurses and 295 responding nurse managers identified failure to provide service of the highest quality (defined by both groups of respondents as service that is inconsistent with both the standards of the nursing profession and the ANA Code of Ethics) as a major problem facing health care facilities. Moreover, the respondents to both studies indicated that this disappointment with the quality of service was felt not only by those in the nursing profession and the clients for whom they care but also by other health care providers employed by the organization.

Three other ethical issues rated in the top 10 by both the staff nurses and the nurse managers suggest a potential cause of this purported widespread disappointment with the quality of service provided by health care facilities in general. In both studies, the ethics-related statement rated first in terms of the extent to which it causes problems for health care organizations was the failure to provide service of the highest quality because of economic constraints determined by the organization (Gaudine et al., 2011). This issue is a direct reflection of the conflict between clinical ethics, with its primary focus on the delivery of high-quality client care, and organizational ethics, which has been heavily influenced by cost constraints imposed by the market (Johnson, 2005; Miller, 2006). Both the staff nurses and nurse managers also rated quite high an ethics-related statement pointing even more directly at the ongoing ethics clash, that of conflict between organizational and professional philosophy and standards (Cooper et al., 2002; Cooper et al., 2004). Finally, in rating department closings and layoffs among the top 10 issues in both studies, staff nurses and nurse managers identified an important problem stemming directly from the conflict between clinical ethics, with its focus almost exclusively on health care needs of individual clients, and organizational ethics, with its focus on the responsibility of facilities to provide health care to patient populations by responding to market pressures to remain competitive through cost control (AMA, 2000). These findings appear to suggest that the yet unbridled conflict between clinical and organizational ethics may be a major if not the key cause contributing to the perceived failure of many health care facilities to provide service of the highest quality as anticipated by the standards and codes of ethics of professional nursing.

LEADERSHIP AND MANAGEMENT IMPLICATIONS

Nurse managers have a responsibility to prepare themselves and those reporting to them to deal effectively not only with the yet unresolved issues of clinical ethics, such as full disclosure and end-of-life care, but also with the many unresolved dilemmas arising from the ongoing conflict between clinical and organizational ethics (Andrews, 2004). A study of nurse managers (Cooper et al., 2003) provided suggestions of where the emphasis should be placed to be most productive. The study found that, after their own personal moral values and standards, nurse managers tended to find several aspects of their organizational

environment to be more helpful in dealing with ethical dilemmas than resources related to the professional environment. Resources related to the professional environment include the current ANA Code of Ethics (which was rated least helpful among 17 personal, organizational, and professional resources), professional publications/resources on ethics, literature on ethics/professionalism, and professional meetings in which ethical issues can be discussed.

Within the organizational resources, informal factors related to organizational climate were viewed as being more helpful in dealing with ethical dilemmas than formal organizational resources such as a facility's statement on ethics, the organization's policy for identifying and resolving ethical issues, a contact person within the organization to which unethical activity can be reported, and ethics training provided by the organization (which was rated next to last out of 17 possible resources). Involving merely the *absence* of pressure to compromise one's own ethical standards, the two top-rated factors—the fact that your boss does not pressure you into compromising your ethical standards and an organizational environment/culture that does not encourage you to compromise your ethical values to achieve organizational goals—suggest that an important way health care facilities and their managers can assist nursing professionals in resolving ethical dilemmas effectively is by neither explicitly nor implicitly pressuring them to go against their own ethical values (Cooper et al., 2003). Other informal organizational factors rated as being more helpful in dealing with ethical dilemmas than the formal resources provided by one's facility included the organization's culture and management philosophy, management's clear communication of appropriate ethical behavior, and the ability to go beyond one's boss, if necessary, for information and advice on ethical issues. These are all factors that, despite any personal risk involved, nurse managers at all organizational levels can and must continually work to improve and maintain if a culture that encourages and supports ethical behavior is to exist within their facility. In even a broader sense, Miller (2006) pointed out, "Creating a positive culture in which nurses can flourish is the responsibility of leaders in the profession who model the behaviors that support good work in nursing" (p. 482). Shirey (2005) presented a list of strategies for consideration by nurse leaders working to create a positive ethical climate for nursing practice within health care organizations. The increasing commonality of organizational ethics committees and consultant resources is a positive step toward building an organizational culture of support for nurses and all employees as they work through ethical issues.

In addition to the need for nurse managers to prepare staff nurses and others working for them to identify and otherwise deal effectively with ethical issues encountered in their health care facilities (Porter-O'Grady, 2003; Zuzelo, 2007), in recent years, the nursing ethics literature has called on nurse managers to encourage participation by staff nurses, as well as increase participation themselves, on facility ethics committees, especially those dealing with issues of organizational ethics and conflicts between clinical and organizational ethics (ANA, 2001; Guido, 2010; Zuzelo, 2007). Even more directly, the ANA's *Code of Ethics for Nurses: With Interpretive Statements* stated, "Nurse administrators must ensure that nurses have access to and inclusion on institutional ethics committees" (2001, p. 7). The ANA Code continues, "Nurses must bring forward difficult issues related to patient care and/or institutional constraints upon ethical practice for discussion and review" (2001, p. 7). In their role of responsible representation, nurse managers should also ensure that "the clinical and ethical concerns of nurses are heard at the highest levels of organizational decision making" (Curtin, 2000, p. 12).

The logic and critical importance of nurses and nurse administrators having access to and inclusion on the health care organization's ethics committee is clear in view of the membership commonly found and functions generally performed by this body now formed at nearly all U.S. hospitals. Composed of members with diverse professional backgrounds, the typical hospital ethics committee (HEC) deals with ethical issues related to patient care through case consultations producing recommendations for best handling ethical conflicts encountered in the course of treatment, development and review of the organization's ethics policies, and preparation and delivery of ongoing committee and staff ethics education (Cotter & Vaszar, 2008; Lachman, 2010a). Given their fundamental role, responsibilities and experiences associated with patient care, nursing professionals are ideal members of a committee of diverse professionals whose mission is dealing with clinical ethical issues

and policies. By serving on the HEC, nurses and nurse administrators have an opportunity to express their points of view and voice concerns regarding ethical decisions and policies that will affect their practice and leadership efforts (Bailey & Aulisio, 2011). Nurse access to the HEC is critical to enable them to seek consultations when encountering ethical dilemmas and conflicts. In contrast to an ethical dilemma which exists when a nurse must choose between two or more ethically justifiable actions, an ethical conflict involves a situation in which a nurse knows the ethically appropriate action to take but is constrained from taking it by conflicting opinions or policies of physicians, other health care providers, patients, family members, surrogates, administrators and others involved in a particular case (Epstein & Delgado, 2010).

Although many incidents encountered in nursing practice have been identified as giving rise to ethical conflicts leading to negative emotions commonly referred to as moral distress (Pavlish et al., 2011a), the two most frequent causes relate to unsuccessful advocacy in attempts to protect patients' rights, patient autonomy, and informed consent to treatment (Ulrich et al., 2010). Left unaddressed by ethical consultations or other strategies (Epstein & Delgado, 2010), repeated episodes of moral distress are found to have a variety of negative impacts on nurses and nurse leaders, including, among others, a variety of physical and emotional symptoms (Schluter et al., 2008), becoming morally numbed to ethically challenging situations (Epstein & Hamrick, 2009), feeling powerless (Ulrich et al., 2010), reduction in job satisfaction, and burnout. Clearly it is essential for nurse managers to take the lead in identifying, advocating and implementing both specific actions (Pavlish et al., 2011b) and strategies (Bell & Breslin, 2008; Epstein & Delgado, 2010) that enable both nurses and themselves to recognize (Pavlish et al., 2011a) and respond effectively to ethical dilemmas and conflicts arising in practice.

Although increased and improved training would undoubtedly contribute to better preparing staff nurses and nurse managers to identify and deal with ethical issues (Zuzelo, 2007), the key factor for success is an organizational culture that encourages, supports, and rewards ethical behavior (Lachman, 2002; Upenieks, 2003). In this context, organizational culture can be defined as a set of shared core values that members of an organization have reflected on, articulated, and accepted as normative (Silverman, 2000). As principles of right action, these shared core values serve as guides for proper and acceptable behavior in making decisions within the organization. Creating an organizational culture that will serve as a resilient base for a successful organizational ethics initiative requires that the core values not only be identified and effectively communicated to the organization's members but also be championed and demonstrated by the organization's top managers (Douglas, 2007; Shirey, 2005).

In reality, the organizational cultures of health care facilities are arrayed along a continuum ranging from those based on letter-of-the-law compliance with regulatory and accrediting requirements to those that encourage, support, and reward ethical behavior. Therefore nurses and nurse managers will face varying types and degrees of challenge in their efforts to carry out the activities related to improving education and training, increasing participation, and implementing strategies that permit more effective response to ethical dilemmas and conflicts arising in the organization. In many cases, it will take pressure from nurse managers to encourage senior management to recognize the need and provide their support for these activities of staff nurses and nurse managers. In facing this challenge, nurse managers should remember that, among other things, leaders are expected to have courage and to take risks in constantly challenging the status quo. Nurse managers should also encourage risk taking among the nurses reporting to them by defending and supporting them when they do (Porter-O'Grady, 2003). The current spotlight shining on patient safety and quality of care can be a powerful motivator for change.

In view of the significant degrees of change and uncertainty associated with the legal and ethical aspects impacting decision making in nursing care management, there is certainly no shortage of current issues and trends in this area. A major current issue, of course, is the nursing shortage, which for a number of reasons is expected to continue in the foreseeable future despite recent growth in the number of young RNs entering the profession (Auerbach et al., 2011). This issue gives rise to a number of legal and ethical challenges for nurse managers and staff nurses. Resulting largely from increases in cost-cutting measures and other financial constraints, as well from deterioration of working conditions (American Hospital Association [AHA], 2002; Gordon, 2005; O'Neil & Seago, 2002),

the nursing shortage has resulted in a major problem called *short staffing*. This refers to the use of an insufficient nursing staff on a unit or in a facility for the number of patients requiring care at various acuity levels (Aiken, 2004; Guido, 2010). Consequences commonly associated with short staffing (Cooper et al., 2004) include the following:

- Deterioration of patient outcomes in terms of increased mortality and failure-to-rescue rates (Needleman et al., 2011)
- A general decline in the quality of patient care (Buerhaus et al., 2005, 2006, 2007; Hassmiller & Cozine, 2006)
- Deterioration of nurse outcomes resulting from increased burnout and greater job dissatisfaction (Agency for Healthcare Research and Quality [AHRQ], 2004; Aiken et al., 2002)
- Increases in organizational costs resulting from increased turnover (AHA, 2002; Hassmiller & Cozine, 2006; PWC, 2007)
- Legal liability

In an effort to deal with short staffing, nurse managers are often required to do the following: float nurses to areas in which they are not cross-trained, an action that also increases the client-to-nurse ratio closer to staffing requirements; use agency (temporary) personnel; and use unlicensed personnel. Staff nurses, nurse managers, and health care facilities all face numerous possibilities of legal liability, as well as dilemmas involving conflicts between clinical and organizational ethics, as a result of short staffing and actions taken in an effort to temporarily solve this problem.

Potential legal and ethical problems are encountered also in connection with the predominant issues of unnecessary patient suffering and patient autonomy, especially at end of life (Pavlish et al., 2011a, b), as well as unresolved issues of clinical practice such as decisions about withholding or withdrawing life-support systems. Just as the AMA's *Code of Medical Ethics* (AMA, 2012-2013) provides physicians with guidance in dealing with issues related to the withholding or withdrawing of life-sustaining medical treatment, the ANA's Code of Ethics (2001) provides guidance for nurses regarding the responsibilities they may face in dealing with key issues associated with end-of-life care. For example, the ANA Code addresses (1) respecting the client's right of self-determination, which is consistent with the ethical principle of autonomy; (2) ensuring that the client is fully informed and understands his or her options; (3) enlisting the use of a surrogate if the client's comprehension is questionable; and (4) handling conflicts between the moral standards of the profession and the nurse's own moral values.

Despite this guidance and the best efforts to apply it to end-of-life care, claims of legal liability against a nurse, nurse manager, and/or the facility that employs him or her (not to mention the physician) can arise from a variety of alleged torts related to the withholding or withdrawal of life support. For example, economic, non-economic (emotional distress), and/or punitive damages might be claimed for negligence (including malpractice) arising out of the following:

- Failure to adequately inform the client in a manner that facilitates an informed judgment
- Failure to obtain proper consent for an organ donation
- Provision of life-prolonging treatment against the client's wishes
- Failure to provide life-sustaining treatment when it is requested by the client
- Failure to recognize that the client's standardized advance directive document did not deal with CPR even though the client was a candidate for a DNR order
- Failure to properly interpret the client's advance directive document because of its unreadable legal language
- Denial of proper medical care
- Failure of a nurse to make timely arrangements for another nursing practitioner to take over a particular client's care when the nurse's own moral values conflict with those of the profession

Damages might also be sought on the grounds of intentional torts such as medical battery for tissue burns, broken bones, or other harm arising out of resuscitation, or intentional infliction of emotional distress. A nurse may also be named in a lawsuit filed primarily as a result of a physician's alleged malpractice or intentional tort. Being named in this lawsuit would at least give rise to costs associated with the nurse's defense. Finally, even when the basic rules to avoid negligence or intentional tort have been closely followed, a nurse, nurse manager, and/or facility may still be found legally liable for payment of damages as

a result of judicial risk. As mentioned earlier, in some cases, juries and even judges can be sufficiently influenced by their emotions so as to rationalize a finding of legal liability against the defendant, especially when, as is generally the case, liability insurance is available to pay the judgment.

Nurses need to focus on their use of expert judgment in practicing the highest legal and ethical standards in the quest for high-quality care and services. In some instances, they may also be called upon to demonstrate moral courage—the courage to honor ethical core values in the face of personal risk (Lachman, 2007a, b). The literature presents a number of strategies that are available to the nurse leader for promoting moral courage in the organization (Edmonson, 2010; Lachman, 2010b; LaSala & Bjarnason, 2010). Chief among these is the use of multidisciplinary teams that can provide an expert group approach to addressing moral and ethical issues.

- As members of a profession, nurses and nurse managers are guided by both legal and ethical considerations in making decisions. Most commonly, nurses and nurse managers are subject to legal liability arising from malpractice and intentional torts they personally commit in clinical practice, from negligence in their acts of delegation and supervision, from failure to follow policies and procedures when reasonable, and from breach of contract. Critical to the determination of legal liability for malpractice (professional negligence), standards of care can be found in the state nurse practice act, standards published by the American Nurses Association, other professional organizations and specialty practice groups, federal agency guidelines and regulations, and the facility's policy and procedure manuals.
- Health care facilities can be held legally liable for malpractice or intentional torts committed by nurses and nurse managers they employ under the doctrine of respondeat superior, for malpractice and intentional torts committed by independent contractors (e.g., agency personnel) under the doctrine of ostensible authority, and for failing to ensure that competent and qualified practitioners are hired and that they deliver quality health care to clients under the doctrine of corporate liability. Judicial risk can result in

findings with respect to legal liability that are not based solely on the merits of the case or on the rules of law applicable to the case.

- The four principles of autonomy, beneficence, nonmaleficence, and justice; several closely related rules of biomedical ethics; and standards of conduct provided by professional codes of ethics provide guidance to nurses and nurse managers when faced with ethical dilemmas arising in the course of clinical practice. Many ethical dilemmas encountered in today's health care environment involve a conflict between clinical ethics with its primary focus on the delivery of high-quality client care and organizational ethics reflecting a number of other human and financial considerations, including the reliance of health care facilities on market competition as a vehicle for cost control. In preparing themselves and those reporting to them to deal effectively with yet unresolved dilemmas of either clinical ethics or the conflict between clinical and organizational ethics, nurse managers should work toward the establishment of an organizational culture that encourages, supports, and rewards ethical behavior in both their own area of responsibility and the entire health care facility.

CASE STUDY

An example of judicial risk is seen in a situation that occurred when the author served as foreman on a jury in a contributory negligence state. The jury was instructed by the judge that if the plaintiff (a very elderly man who would be spending the rest of his life in some type of health care facility as a result of injuries caused by an auto accident) was even partially at fault for his own injuries, the jury had to find in favor of the defendant and the plaintiff would be awarded no damages. During 6 hours of deliberation, feeling sympathy for the plaintiff, all jury members except the foreman repeatedly ignored the fact that the testimony of witnesses had indicated that the elderly man was completely at fault and voted continually to find that the plaintiff's injuries were completely the fault of the defendant (a trucking company and its driver) who had insurance and thus could afford to pay. Because the foreman was concerned that the viewpoint of the other jurors was not consistent with the judge's instructions regarding the state's law and thus not faithful to legal instructions, he held out until the issue essentially became one of whether the jury should return and continue deliberations the next day. In the next round of voting, the entire jury properly applied the state's contributory negligence law and found for the defendant. This case illustrates two aspects of judicial risk. First, the radical change in the jury members' votes was clearly not based solely on the merits of the case but, rather, on their desire to not have to return the next day for further deliberations. Second, if, instead, the jury foreman had changed his vote to provide a unanimous verdict for the plaintiff, the jury would have essentially changed the state's law in reaching its verdict by not applying the contributory negligence doctrine to the facts of the case.

CRITICAL THINKING EXERCISE

Ms. Anna vanDahm, one of the wealthiest and most influential people in town, was placed in the hospital's intensive care unit (ICU) after undergoing kidney replacement surgery. Because of the inability to deliver high-quality care as a result of financial constraints and a high turnover rate related to nurse discontentment with the dictatorial leadership styles of ICU nurse managers, the ICU was regularly short of qualified staff nurses. As a solution to this problem of short staffing, nurses from other units with lower levels of client acuity were routinely floated to the ICU, often without regard to whether they were cross-trained to take on ICU responsibilities.

Abigail Friendly, an RN without prior training or experience in caring for ICU clients, was floated to the ICU, where she was assigned to provide care for Ms. vanDahm, who had responded very poorly to her surgery and was put on a life-support system by a physician just before Nurse Friendly's arrival. While Nurse Friendly was caring for her, Ms. vanDahm communicated, in the presence of her oldest son, that she did not want to be resuscitated in the event of cardiopulmonary arrest.

When her shift ended a few minutes later, Nurse Friendly, exhausted and overwhelmed by what she had just experienced, left for home. Shortly thereafter, Ms. vanDahm sustained a cardiopulmonary arrest; however, in the absence of proper documentation and notification, she was resuscitated. Subsequently, the son, angry that his mother's request had not been followed, consulted an attorney, who promptly contacted the hospital's CEO. The next day, Nurse Friendly, who had always received highly positive performance evaluations over the 5 years she was employed by the facility and also was subject to protection under the provisions of an antidiscrimination statute, was told by the manager of her unit that she was being fired effective immediately.

1. Nurse Friendly
   a. On what grounds could Nurse Friendly be found legally liable for malpractice?
   b. What actions should have been taken by Nurse Friendly to prevent malpractice in this type of situation?
   c. What ethical dilemma(s) did Nurse Friendly face in this situation?
   d. What factors should have been considered by Nurse Friendly in dealing with the ethical dilemma(s) encountered in this situation?

2. Manager of Nurse Friendly's unit
   a. On what grounds could the nurse manager be found legally liable?
   b. What actions should have been taken by the nurse manager to prevent legal liability in this type of situation?
   c. What ethical dilemma(s) did the nurse manager face in this situation?
   d. What factors should have been considered by the nurse manager in dealing with the ethical dilemma(s) encountered in this situation?

3. Nurse manager of the ICU
   a. On what grounds could the nurse manager be found legally liable?
   b. What actions should have been taken by the nurse manager to prevent legal liability in this type of situation?
   c. What ethical dilemma(s) did the nurse manager face in this situation?
   d. What factors should have been considered by the nurse manager in dealing with the ethical dilemma(s) encountered in this situation?

4. Hospital
   a. On what grounds could the hospital be found legally liable?
   b. What actions should have been taken by the hospital to prevent legal liability in this type of situation?

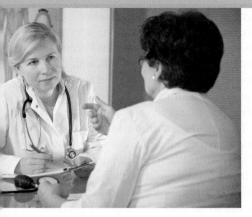

Communication Leadership

Diane L. Huber

evolve WEBSITE

http://evolve.elsevier.com/Huber/leadership/

Communication is a process in which information, perception, and understanding are transmitted from person to person. As an integral part of any relationship, communication is important to nurses. Nurse leaders and managers can view communication as a tool to accomplish work and meet goals. The significance of communication revolves around its effectiveness and the climate in which communication occurs. Effective communication is enhanced by clear, direct, straightforward, and frequent message transmission. Trust, respect, and empathy are the three ingredients needed to create and foster effective communication.

For leaders, communication is a key element of the role. Leaders are in charge of vision, and the vision needs to be communicated as a compelling image. Such a compelling image is thought to induce enthusiasm and commitment in others. Thus a major part of the leader's role is to communicate a vision. Leaders shape values and norms in a way that binds and bonds individuals and groups. Communication is key to this effort. Visions are communicated by means of managing meaning and creating understanding, commitment, and ownership of a vision. Leaders

Photo used with permission from Photos.com.

use communication as a tool for building trust. Trust is the glue that holds leaders and followers together.

DEFINITIONS

Communication is based on mutual understanding. Clarity of meaning is derived from a clear definition of terms related to communication. Relevant definitions are as follows:

- **Humanizing Nursing Communication Theory:** A nursing theory describing the manner of communicating that acknowledges the unique characteristics of the holistic human being. The communication patterns of interaction (communing, asserting, confronting, conflicting, and separating) are conveyed with an attitude that can be identified on the humanizing-dehumanizing continuum (Battey, 2006, 2007; Duldt, 2008; Duldt & Giffin, 1985). Humanizing Nursing Communication Theory (HNCT) is based on "normal" as opposed to "therapeutic" and includes not only professional-client but also inter- and intra-professional communication.
- **Interpersonal communication:** Communication between two or more individuals involving face-to-face interaction while all parties are aware of the others on an ongoing basis. Each person sends and

111

receives information while continually adapting to the other actors.

- **Nonverbal communication:** Unspoken, this communication is composed of affective or expressive behavior.
- **Persuasion, negotiation, and bargaining:** Persuasion is the conscious intent by one individual to modify the thoughts or behaviors of others (Bettinghaus, 1968). Negotiation is a dialogical discussion between two or more parties to arrive at an agreement about some issue. To bargain is to make a series of offers and counteroffers about what each party will do, give, receive, and so on, until an agreement is reached to the satisfaction of all. All three of these involve communication. Persuasion uses argumentation and appeals to logic, whereas negotiation and bargaining may involve some sense of compensation and perhaps coercion, such as bullying or condescending behaviors.
- **Spiritual assessment:** Information needed by nurses resides within each patient, and the professional nurse seeks to use the patient's own definition in developing individualized plans of care. This information may be obtained through informal conversation or a formal assessment interview.
- **Spiritual care:** Interpersonal communication. It exists in the relationship between the caregiver and the care recipient. Whether the spiritual care exists at all is determined by the perceptions of the one receiving the care. The implication of this definition is that nurses need specific communing skills to establish and maintain the relationship.
- **Spirituality:** A dimension of all human beings that is relational in nature, with a higher being and/or with other human beings; may include spiritual and religious practices, perhaps within an organized faith community.
- **Verbal communication:** Includes both written and spoken communication.

BACKGROUND

Communication is a basic and essential skill for leaders and managers. Communicating, along with diagnosing and adapting, is one of the three basic competencies of influencing and leadership (Hersey et al., 2013). It is a critical and important tool for effectiveness in engaging and motivating people and in getting work done

through others. Structuring messages so that people understand them clearly and avoiding emotion-laden triggers enhance the communication effectiveness of a manager. For example, the communication of accurate (correct, truthful, precise), adequate (sufficient, consistent, repetitious), and applied (useful and appropriate to the nurse's individual needs) information was necessary for directing managed care changes (Apker & Fox, 2002). These communication techniques can foster stronger organizational affiliation while maintaining nurses' strong identification with nursing.

Acquiring interpersonal relationship skills, including the ability to communicate, is as essential to a leader's personal set of leadership skills as psychomotor skills are for a clinical nurse. Leadership and management ability is predicated on a facility for communication. In nursing leadership and management, skillful communication is essential for effective implementation of the change process. It is an intervention that leaders and managers in nursing use to accomplish their goals. Communication also is a key component of case management practice.

Language is used by leaders to give meaning to work. Communication problems may be a source of dissatisfaction. Research has indicated that a positive communication atmosphere, positive communication between staff nurses and immediate superiors, and personal feedback on job performance are related to nurse job satisfaction (Pincus, 1986). Farley (1989) identified six areas of organizational communication that can be assessed for communication problems (Box 7-1).

Leaders and managers always communicate in basic ways, whether they want to or not—they always communicate their attitude and their goals and expectations. Trust or distrust is communicated. Leaders

---

BOX 7-1   **COMMUNICATION ASSESSMENT**

- Accessibility of information
- Communication channels
- Clarity of messages
- Span of control
- Flow control/communication load
- The individual communicators

Data from Farley, M. (1989). Assessing communication in organizations. *Journal of Nursing Administration, 19*(12), 27-31.

communicate a vision, subtly or directly, and a sense of where they are going and what they expect from their followers.

One technique used for interpersonal effectiveness in groups, collaborative teams, and interdisciplinary work situations is *persuasion*. The tactics of persuasion are useful when an authoritarian leadership style is not appropriate and the nurse has to convince colleagues to work together.

Harvey (1990) suggested that skillful, positive questioning can persuade people to accept change. People are more willing to commit themselves when they see personal benefits. Positive questioning capitalizes on this fact to establish hopeful, affirmative attitudes. Inviting agreement, commitment, and realization of benefits facilitates necessary changes. Setting a positive and cooperative tone within a work group is each member's responsibility. Nurses frequently may be in situations in which they need to persuade others to cooperate. Therefore they will need to use strategies of persuasion and *negotiation*.

The work of successful nurses and managers depends on the ability to negotiate. Nurses need to be able to articulate needs, positions, and justification for resources. The different techniques of conflict resolution and influencing in nursing include bargaining and negotiation as one method of gaining power and persuading others to grant autonomy by using individual and collective action. The use of collective action at both the work group and the larger profession levels can make a difference in terms of autonomy in professional practice, job satisfaction, and a general positive feeling about the profession of nursing.

Human interaction issues are the general arena in which leaders and managers spend most of their time. Power and conflict become important focal points of human interaction in organizations that may need management or resolution through persuasion or negotiations. Both conflict resolution and negotiation techniques can and should be used to manage change. As nurses are confronted with the impact of mergers, downsizing, restructuring and reengineering, and alterations in skill mix, negotiation skills are needed. These skills can help improve relationships and aid managers to function in their designated roles.

Negotiation is used to educate clients and other professionals about nurses' roles and contributions, to get a fairer exchange in decision-making autonomy, to interact with vendors, to deal with client complaints, to interact with integrated health systems and group health care purchasers, to deal with unionized employees, to respond to the media, and to negotiate with medical staff and managed care groups to consolidate contracts (Sherer, 1994).

COMMUNICATION LEADERSHIP

Nurses work in a complex and highly interpersonal relationship-based work environment. It is known that inter- and intra-professional relationships can be problematic (Duddle & Boughton, 2007). Conflict, poor colleague relationships, decreased job satisfaction, reduced productivity, and quality/safety concerns result. Leaders can help nurses gain insight into their own behavior, how it affects others and the work environment, and how to use strategies to cope, become resilient, and advocate for workplace communication improvements at all levels.

Management Approaches

There is a great need in the health care professions to provide holistic care (body, mind, and spirit) to all clients, regardless of religious, ethnic, or cultural characteristics, in a humane (nonjudgmental and compassionate) manner. Yet today's American health care system emphasizes certain business and management concepts such as efficiency, accuracy, and economy. This is expected in the use of sophisticated medical terminology and highly skilled specialists who operate modern equipment, but the technical and disease-oriented language that is used is often ineffective in aiding some patients to understand their health conditions.

Health care organizations are complex and exist in uncertain environments. Nurse leaders and managers play a crucial role in the management of information and communication for the purpose of effective care coordination and the avoidance of unsafe and error-prone care situations. Medical errors and patient safety in hospitals have been a focus of the Institute of Medicine (IOM). Clearly, providers need high-quality information and effective communication. Nurse administrators are responsible for developing care delivery systems with adequate structure and an effective communication system that enhances care coordination. These systems of communications need to enable patient rescue and safety by coordinating care, preventing information loss, and improving methods of surveillance (Anthony & Preuss, 2002). Interventions have been initiated to augment nurse and physician collaboration in intensive care units (Boyle & Kochinda, 2004) and to capture communication patterns in OR nurses to facilitate automation to reduce adverse events (Moss & Xiao, 2004).

A related concern for the management of information and communication is how to prevent breaches of patient confidentiality. The Health Insurance Portability and Accountability Act (HIPAA) provisions have heightened awareness about and presented strategies to protect patients' privacy and data security in health care transactions. For example, fax transmissions need to be secure and security measures need to be taken to protect computerized databases and electronic transmissions. End-user encryption is commonly used for data security. In a series of interviews with 51 patients, Brann and Mattson (2004) identified both internal and external confidentiality breaches, which were categorized into a typology table. Health care providers' actions that disseminate confidential information can harm patients. Systems, processes, and structures can be altered to prevent many of these situations.

A couple of examples from nursing leadership and management are worth considering. Delivering unpleasant news is one example. In hospital nursing, situations occur in which nurses are sent (*pulling, floating,* and *farming* are the terms used) from the unit in which they normally work to another unit. The person who has to deliver the often unpleasant news determines whether to call the unit and leave a brief note on the assignment sheet or go to the nurse to talk directly about the change. Some might offer to take the nurse to the other unit, introduce the person to the charge nurse, and smooth out the transition. There are different ways to structure and deliver the message to be effective in difficult situations.

One leadership situation occurs when a nurse presents a proposal to a committee who must be convinced to release the money for a project that is vital to the care of clients. Strategic planning and a written business plan are used to determine how to maximize the message delivery. This may include knowing how to structure the communication, nonverbally as well as verbally, so that a positive impression is created to set the stage for a full and impartial hearing. The use of the evidence base and expertise can be leveraged for effect.

Communication effectiveness becomes crucial in times of disaster. In fact, often one of the key outcomes of disaster drills is to identify breaks in the communication system so they can be fixed before a real-time event occurs. Argenti (2002) found that in times of extreme crisis, the internal communication to employees took precedence. It was most important for the leader to effectively rebuild the morale of employees so that they could then serve customers. The five strategies he recommended are as follows:

1. Get on the scene to lead, decide, and show compassion.
2. Choose your channels carefully because normal flows often are disrupted because phone and power lines have been destroyed.
3. Stay focused on the business.
4. Have a contingency and disaster plan in place.
5. Improvise, but from a strong foundation of values, preparation, and training.

Spiritual Care and Holistic Communication

Implementing spiritual care in clinical practice within an agency is an example of communication leadership. Spirituality is in itself complex, unique, and difficult. As a leader, nurses are responsible for their area of knowledge, power, and influence. Nurses cannot expect to change other professions and disciplines but can set realistic goals about major issues within the scope of nursing leadership influence and make a difference in patient care. A plan to address the spiritual dimension of holistic care is offered based on theories, supporting research, and the study of spirituality in healing (Battey, 2006, 2007). This is *not* to be considered *the* final answer but merely an initial way to provide one perspective in developing a plan most appropriate to situational leadership needs.

One issue for leaders in nursing is to implement holistic care—the spiritual dimension of this paradigm in particular. Some may just add the word *holistic* to the mission statement and continue business as usual. This is not enough. The holistic paradigm is becoming the desired mode of health care delivery and needs to be reflected in communication and practice.

In the 2005 manual for hospitals, The Joint Commission (TJC) included requirements about spirituality care (TJC, 2008). Nurses are now charged to define and record social, *spiritual,* and cultural variables influencing the patient's health in their initial assessment. Many facilities have pastoral care departments to provide spiritual care.

The proposed definition of spirituality useful for nurses is that spirituality lies within each patient, and the professional nurse seeks to use the patient's own definition in developing individualized plans of care. Ethically, as nurses strive to deliver just holistic care, they need to keep their own spiritual/religious beliefs to themselves and avoid proselytizing. Although definitions of spirituality are endless, *nurses need be responsible for only five dimensions:* **b**eliefs, **v**alues, **m**eanings, **g**oals, and **r**elationships (BVMGR). The BVMGR rubric is proposed as the most appropriate guide or assessment tool for nurses. Nurses can be alert to the BVMGR topics during routine care of patients.

The core of spiritual care is supporting the following position: **the definition of spirituality that is relevant to a particular patient/client can be found only within that person.** Therefore it should not matter whether the nurse is a Buddhist or whether the hospital is owned by Jews or Catholics or Adventists or whether this happens to be a public hospital in the middle of the Christian "Bible Belt" of the southern United States. What is relevant to the health care decisions to be made for a particular patient is what he or she Believes, Values, finds Meaningful in life, maintains as life Goals, or has as special interpersonal Relationships. For nursing assessment, it is the rubric of BVMGR—the dimensions of a patient's spirituality—that forms the basis for spirituality care.

The following definition is drawn from religious rather than health care scholars and offered as a benchmark for nursing. According to Kraus and Holmes (2007), spiritual care is not technique, technology, maps, guidelines, drugs, or directives that make the impact; rather, *spiritual care is defined as interpersonal communication.* Spiritual care occurs within the relationship between the caregiver and the care recipient. Whether the spiritual care exists at all is determined by the perceptions of the one receiving the care (Kraus & Holmes, 2007). The implication of this definition is that nurses need to develop specific communing skills. Two theories, *Humanizing Nursing Communication Theory* and *Communication Ethics Theory,* offer solid direction to nurses for interacting in a compassionate manner with spiritually distressed clients (Battey, 2006, 2007).

Spiritual Care of Nurses

If spirituality is defined as relational, and if spiritual care is interpersonal communication, then the spiritual care of the nurses also is important. Extensive documentation in the literature exists regarding the disruptive and distracting communication interactions that occur not only between nurses and between nurses and professional colleagues (e.g., physicians, pharmacists, administrators) but also between nurses and patients. The research, the literature, and common knowledge from reading the daily papers indicate that nursing personnel experience high turnover rates, job dissatisfaction, and burnout; many RNs are leaving the profession. The shortage of nursing personnel in most areas of the United States has had a negative effective on retention of nurses and recruitment of students to nursing (Buerhaus et al., 2005; Buerhaus et al., 2007). The work environment is described as hostile to nurses, and patient outcomes of increased severity of illness and mortality have been directly related to poor communication skills of the staff (Kramer & Schmalenberg, 2003). The clinical ambiance and interpersonal communication received by nurses need to change. Leaders can set realistic goals within the scope of their leadership influence and make a difference where nurses live and work.

Are Leaders Prepared to Deliver Outcomes?

The challenge of this issue of leadership and communication, persuasion, and negotiation revolves around *who* is to change *what, when, how, with whom,* and *with what outcome?* How can the leaders (the "who") who are to implement holistic care—especially spiritual care (the "what")—throughout the nursing organization somehow (the "how") involve all nursing professionals (the "with whom") so that nurses will be able to provide spiritual care to patients (the "with what outcome")?

Leaders, to a significant degree, are alumni of an educational system that historically did not teach these concepts. If they did, nursing education about spirituality was likely to be an hour's lecture by a chaplain or minister. In fact, the current literature reveals a wide range of perspectives, including the position that spiritual care is not to be provided by nurses. Fortunately, most nurses are creative, "renaissance" people who are talented in examining, learning, reviving, and adapting to meet new challenges.

Humanizing Nursing Communication Theory (HNCT)

For most of the past century, concern for the manner by which human beings are treated has increased, not only on an international and national level but also in business and industry. The need for humane behavior toward people, especially in communication behavior, is particularly important as health care evolves into a larger and more complex industry. In a conference report (Troupin, 2001) from the Durban South Africa meeting of the World Organization of Family Doctors, David Satcher, the former U.S. Surgeon General, reviewed the history of health care for the past 100 years. His message to family physicians was to take an active role in improving the overall quality of health through focused efforts. He noted that health resources can be more equitably distributed if leadership is directed to improving and humanizing problems in the health care system.

It is proposed that if health care personnel, especially nurses, are regarded in a manner that acknowledges all characteristics of human beings, then these personnel will tend to regard the patients, clients, peers, and professional colleagues in a similar manner. Because registered nurses constitute the largest health care occupation in the United States, with 2.7 million jobs of the approximately 4.8 million people employed in hospitals in the United States (U.S. Department of Labor, Bureau of Labor Statistics, 2012), humanizing efforts become important to the fabric of health care.

Numerous theories of communication have been developed for nursing practice, usually in clinical psychiatric and mental health contexts. Attitudes are an important factor. Nurse leaders can become intellectually aware of and sensitive to the wide range of humanizing and dehumanizing attitudes (Box 7-2) that can be used with different patterns of communication interaction (Figures 7-1, 7-2, and 7-3). The list of attitudes was developed by searching the literature for concepts commonly used in promoting relationships and in counseling; then the antonyms were identified using a thesaurus. The patterns of interactions were identified from the discipline of communication studies and are known to be commonly used in everyday communication.

At the core of the patterns of interaction model is the most humanizing communication, **"communing,"** that involves four necessary elements: **trust, self-disclosure, feedback,** and **listening** (see Figure 7-2). For example, the patient (or follower) needs to trust the nurse (or leader) enough to self-disclose personal concerns often not revealed to anyone else. The nurse (or leader) needs to respond by providing feedback that is informative yet

BOX 7-2	HUMANIZING-DEHUMANIZING CONTINUUM OF ATTITUDES
HUMANIZING	**DEHUMANIZING**
Dialogue	Monologue
Individual	Categories
Holistic	Parts
Choice	Directives
Equality	Degradation
Positive Regard	Disregard
Acceptance	Judgment
Empathy	Tolerance
Authenticity	Role-playing
Caring	Careless
Irreplaceable	Expendable
Intimacy	Isolation
Coping	Helpless
Power	Powerless

supportive to the patient (or follower). Both need to listen with intentionality to what is being said (Figure 7-4). This is communing, and by the definitions offered earlier, this is dialogue, and this also is spiritual care.

As one moves outward on the model of patterns of interaction (see Figure 7-2) to assertiveness, confrontation, and conflict, perceptions increasingly differ, ultimately ending the relationship in separation, if dehumanizing attitudes are consistently used. However, to the degree that humanizing attitudes are used at any level, the relationship can return to the communing level (Box 7-3). Agendas, such as **s**ituation, **b**ackground, **a**ssessment, and **r**ecommendation (SBAR), de Shazer's (1985) solution-focused brief therapy (SFBT), and many "crucial conversation tools" as suggested by Patterson and colleagues (2002) may be used within the patterns of interaction and attitudes continuum. The *Nursing Communication Observation Tool Instruction Manual* (Duldt, 2008) may be helpful in research and in teaching HNCT.

In group process as described in Situational Leadership®, the communing or dialogue of HNCT can be chosen by design for a high probability of positive outcomes in a group as it moves through the forming, storming, norming, and performing sequence of group process.

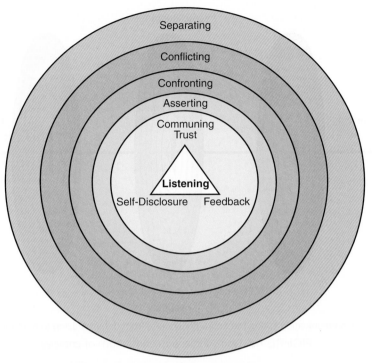

FIGURE 7-1 Communication interaction patterns.

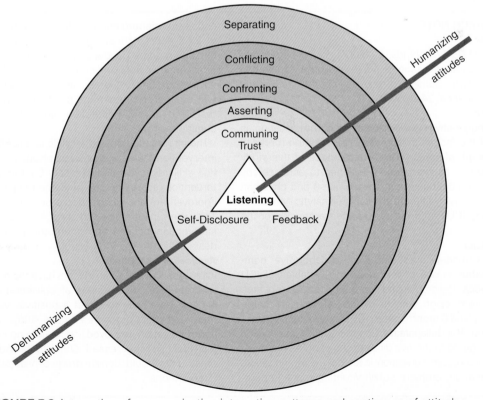

FIGURE 7-2 Interaction of communication interaction patterns and continuum of attitudes.

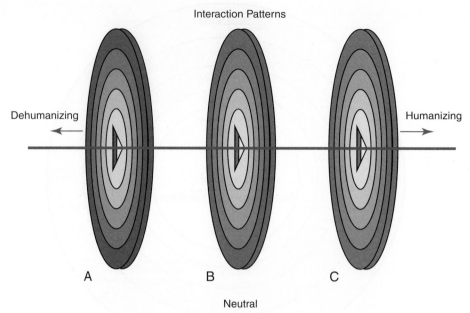

Interaction Patterns

Dehumanizing

Humanizing

A   B   C

Neutral

Communication spans the entire continuum, from dehumanizing to humanizing

FIGURE 7-3 Communication continuum of choices.

RESEARCH NOTE

Source

Boyle, D.K., & Kochinda, C. (2004). Enhancing collaborative communication of nurse and physician leadership in two intensive care units. *Journal of Nursing Administration*, *34*(2), 60-70.

Purpose

Poor nurse-physician collaborative communication is one of the factors in increased risk-adjusted mortality and length of stay in ICUs. The purpose of this study was to test an intervention designed to enhance collaborative communication among nurse and physician leaders in two different ICUs. The Analytic Model for Studying ICU Performance was the framework for the study.

Discussion

In this model, nurse-physician collaborative communication is one of four predictor variables of ICU outcomes. The study used a pretest-posttest, repeated measures design with follow-ups at baseline, intervention, and 6 months after. ICUs in two hospitals participated. The Collaborative Communication Intervention was targeted to the five dimensions of nurse-physician collaborative communication: leadership, communication, coordination, problem solving/conflict management,

and team-oriented culture. The intervention consisted of 23.5 hours of training using six standardized curriculum models: leadership, core skills for communication, guiding conflict resolution, helping others adapt to change, teams, and trust. Evaluation data were gathered pretest and posttest, using a vignette test and a self-perception and staff-perceptions questionnaire.

The intervention proved feasible and useful. After the intervention, nurse and physician leaders' communication skills significantly increased. Six months after intervention, scores on unit outcome measures showed improvement, including a decrease in personal stress. This was a pilot study and small in scope, but it was intervention-focused and attempted an experimental design.

Application to Practice

ICU nurse and physician leaders have the responsibility to create an environment of collaborative communication as a way to effect a positive work environment and affect outcomes. In this study, collaborative communication improved after a training intervention. Individual skills increased. Other ICUs and potentially other units could benefit from similar skills training interventions.

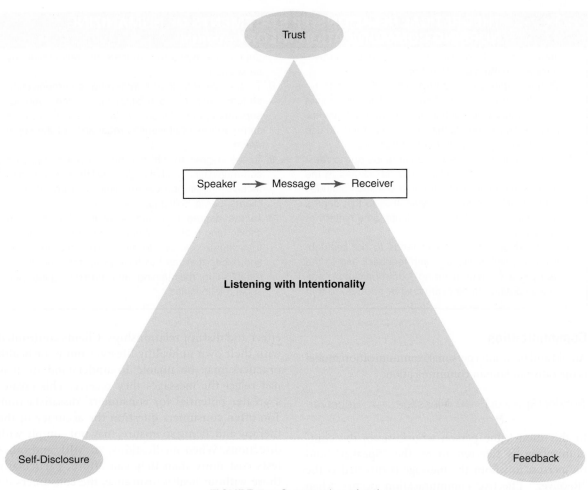

Trust

Speaker → Message → Receiver

Listening with Intentionality

Self-Disclosure

Feedback

FIGURE 7-4 Communing tripod.

BOX 7-3 THEORETICAL RELATIONSHIP STATEMENTS OF HUMANIZING NURSING COMMUNICATION THEORY

1. To the degree to which one receives humanizing communication from others, to that degree one will tend to feel recognized and accepted as a human being.
   a. While applying the nursing process, to the degree to which a nurse is able to use humanizing communication, to that degree will the client, peer, or colleague tend to feel recognized and accepted as a human being.
   b. In a given environment, if a critical life situation develops for a client, to the degree the nurse uses humanizing communication attitudes and patterns while applying the nursing process, to a similar

   degree will the health of the client tend to move in a positive direction.
2. To the degree that listening, trust, self-disclosure, and feedback occur, to that degree humanizing communication or communing also occurs.
3. In the event one tends to experience dehumanizing communication (e.g., monological rather than dialogical communication, categorical rather than individualistic), then one tends to move outward (on the model) to the next pattern of interaction.
4. In an interpersonal relationship of trust, self-disclosure, and feedback, to the degree that dehumanizing communication attitudes are expressed by

Continued

BOX 7-3   THEORETICAL RELATIONSHIP STATEMENTS OF HUMANIZING NURSING COMMUNICATION THEORY—cont'd

another, to that degree one tends to use assertiveness as a pattern of interaction.

5. To the degree that assertiveness tends not to reestablish trust, self-disclosure, and feedback and to the degree that dehumanizing attitudes are expressed by another, to that degree one tends to use assertiveness as a pattern of interaction.

6. To the degree that confrontation tends not to reestablish trust, self-disclosure, or feedback and to the degree that dehumanizing communication attitudes continue to be expressed by another, to that degree one tends to use conflict resolution as a pattern of interaction.

7. To the degree that conflict tends to not reestablish trust, self-disclosure, and feedback and to the degree that dehumanizing communication attitudes continue to be expressed by another, to that

degree one tends to terminate the relationship by separation.

8. To the degree that humanizing communication attitudes occur in a relationship, in the event of separation, the relationship can be resumed to the same degree of closeness regardless of the separation.

9. To the degree to which a nurse uses humanizing communication, to that degree will the nurse tend to receive humanizing communication from others—clients, peers, colleagues, and leaders.

10. To the degree that one is aware of one's own choice (and motives) about interaction patterns, to that degree one can develop communication skills and habits that tend to have predictable results in establishing, maintaining, and terminating interpersonal relationships.

Communication

An old and basic interpersonal communication model is operative in human communication:

Sender(Speaker)   →   Message   →   Receiver

In this model, the person who initiates the communication is referred to as the "Speaker" and the person to whom the message is directed is the "Receiver." Effective communication occurs when the receiver interprets the speaker's message in the same way the speaker intended it (Patton & Giffin, 1977). Box 7-4 displays the ten characteristics of interpersonal communication.

In the nursing context, the model looks like this when the message is negative:

Nurse/other	→	Message	→	Patient/
healthcare		(Bad		Client
providers		News)		

By the very nature of being a nurse or other health care provider, messages to patients or clients may contain negative information and be characterized as "bad news." The messages may be about delayed meals, unpleasant and even painful procedures, and distressing revelations about illness. The age-old pattern of "blaming the messenger" may be in

effect and disrupt relationships. Clients confronted with their own unhealthy lifestyle and poor health practices may be unable to understand or may just reject the messages they receive. This creates a greater potential for consumers' dissatisfaction. Too often consumers question the accuracy of the therapy and, being so unsure, may not comply with directions. When medications, an MRI, and other tests cost more than they can afford, particularly those without health insurance, the consumers do not know where to turn.

Health care providers in general, and nursing as a discipline and practice profession in particular, are basically humanitarian—that is, concerned with and focused on the well-being of people. Yet an unfortunate trend, reported by both health care consumers and providers, appears to be a growing lack of concern for one another. People frequently describe unpleasant encounters that leave them confused, insulted, irritated, and indignant when they seek care. Why this happens and is tolerated is not clear.

Regretfully, there appears to be a trend for people to interact in a dehumanizing manner in the health care system, and this trend can be expected to continue. Too often it is unpleasant for the consumer as well as the professional care provider. In the twenty-first century, U.S. society is moving toward a nationwide shift in the financing and availability of health care resources, increased

BOX 7-4 TEN CHARACTERISTICS OF INTERPERSONAL COMMUNICATION

The following characteristics are presented to stimulate discussion and help identify the dimension of interpersonal communication as opposed to other dimensions such as small group, organizational, and mass communication (Patton & Giffin, 1981, pp. 12-20):

1. Communication is unavoidable and inevitable when people are aware of one another.
2. In interpersonal communication, both the sender and the receiver of "meaning"* must be present.
3. Each person assumes roles as both sender and receiver of messages in interpersonal communication.
4. The choices that a person makes reflect the degree of that person's interpersonal communication competencies.
5. In interpersonal communication, the sender and the receiver are interdependent.
6. Successful interpersonal communications involve mutual needs to communicate.
7. Interpersonal communication establishes and defines the nature of the relationship between the people involved.
8. Interpersonal communication is the means by which we confirm and validate self.
9. Because interpersonal communication relies on behaviors, we must be satisfied with degrees of mutual understanding.
10. Interpersonal communication is irreversible and unrepeatable and almost always functions in a context of change.

***NOTE:** "Meaning" is what a word, sign, or symbol means or what the sender or senders want to convey. It refers to the implications of the content of the message. The receiver needs to understand what the sender intends to convey by the message or what he means in order to avoid misunderstandings.

humanize means to recognize the individual's human characteristics and to address the presented health care issues with dignity and respect. To implement the spiritual aspect of holistic health care, concerted effort is needed by health care leaders in both education and practice to guide people in a careful exploration of interpersonal communication processes that are known to promote humanizing relationships not only between the nurse and client but also between and among health care colleagues.

LEADERSHIP AND MANAGEMENT IMPLICATIONS

Communication, persuasion, and negotiation are core skills in leadership. The long tradition of research has shown that the most important variable in leadership is the communication that occurs between the leader and the follower(s) (Sanford, 1950).

Situational Leadership® focuses on three competencies deemed necessary for a leader's success. These are summarized as follows (Hersey et al., 2013):

- *Diagnosing is a cognitive—or cerebral—competency*. It is the understanding of what the situation is now and knowing what it can reasonably be expected to be in the future. The discrepancy between the two is the problem to be solved. This discrepancy is what the other competencies are aimed at resolving.
- *Adapting is a behavioral competency*. It involves adapting behavior and other resources in a way that helps close the gap between the current situation and what the leader wishes to achieve.
- *Communicating is a process competency*. Leaders need to communicate effectively. If leaders cannot communicate in a way that people can understand and accept, they will be unlikely to meet their goals.

Overview of Groups

Hersey and colleagues' (2013, p. 234) definition of a group is "two or more individuals interacting, in which the existence of the group is necessary for the individual group members' needs to be satisfied." It is important to note that individual group members have differing needs to be satisfied by being a part of the group. As a principle, the degree to which individual need satisfaction is achieved differentiates

numbers of clients, increasing complexity of care, and the lack of personnel in nursing and other health care professions (Johnson, 2000). Health care providers, especially nurses, are experiencing reality shock, anger dismay, job dissatisfaction, and burnout. They frequently choose to resign, resulting in high annual turnover and high inactivity rates among practitioners.

Dehumanizing processes can be counteracted by effective interpersonal communication, the key to humanizing relationships between people. To effective from ineffective groups; the greater the individual's satisfaction, the higher the probability of group effectiveness (Hersey et al., 2013). According to workplace specialists, job satisfaction has been found to include much more than salary increases, decreased overtime, and tangible rewards. Appreciation, trust, and respect do not have direct costs. These, as well as support for individual growth and a sense of purpose, have been identified as important factors in job satisfaction. Job satisfaction means having a leader who is fair and honest, listens to concerns, and helps the followers in developing knowledge, attitudes, and skills to advance their careers. Some have suggested that nurses probably do not leave agencies; they leave dehumanizing nursing leaders (Gardner, 2008). Nurse leaders need to be in touch with the degree to which nursing staff are satisfied. Job satisfaction remains an important issue in the workplace environment, given nurse shortages (Aiken et al., 2001; Buerhaus et al., 2007).

Members assume a variety of roles within the process of a group. Most are constructive in nature, contributing to the discussion, solving the problem, and achieving the group goal. These roles may be questioning, suggesting possibilities, taking notes, and summarizing the group's progress. However, some roles are not helpful. The most disruptive periods in group process are probably in Readiness 1, "forming" with uncertainty and chaos; and Readiness 2, "storming" with intergroup dissonance and competition. It is at these levels that members may behave in roles that hinder group effectiveness, such as criticizing, attacking, or name calling. The leader needs to intervene as appropriate with discussions of goals, standards, and feedback on behavior and progress for individuals or the group, depending on the situation. The degree to which roles are not helpful probably influences member satisfaction, and certainly interferes with communication and collaboration (Hersey et al., 2013).

Situational Leadership® for Groups

Research in small task group process has also revealed movement from an initial organization through a period of disorganization or chaos to reorganization at a level that achieves a goal. A group is defined as two or more people, and it exists to meet the needs of each individual in the group so that each will be satisfied. The leader's four major styles of communication used with task groups are similar to those for individual followers (telling, selling, participating, and delegating). The process includes moving from defining, clarifying, and involving to empowering according to the leader's diagnosis of the maturity level (readiness) of the group (Hersey et al., 2013).

Group readiness levels include four stages: forming, storming, norming, and performing. At the forming readiness level, the group needs direction in defining task goals and objectives as opposed to personal goals. The members are uncertain and insecure about their role in the group. This initial period is chaotic. During the storming period, there is more willingness to accept the group goals and objectives, but there are still differences of opinion, competition for recognition, and attempts to influence the group. During the norming period, there is greater agreement on the task goals as the group develops cohesiveness and adjusts to the group and task. Finally, during the performing period, the members are thinking as one and willingly performing the task. There is camaraderie and team spirit as the group becomes self-managing (Hersey et al., 2013).

When combining the leadership style and the group readiness levels, the descriptions may be summarized as follows (Hersey et al., 2013):

- *Level 1: Group Readiness:* The group is described as uncertain and in chaos, without a common goal. The leader's Style 1, monological communication of "defining," concentrates on setting goals and providing descriptions of roles and responsibilities.
- *Level 2: Group Readiness:* The group members compete for recognition and influence during this storming phase as they begin to bring their personal goals into agreement with the group goal. The leader's Style 2, "clarifying," fine-tunes details of the group's responsibility. The leader's position is central within the circle of the group members.
- *Level 3: Group Readiness:* Group members begin to come together, "norming," as the individuals accept the group goal; they emerge toward cohesiveness. The leader's Style 3, "involving," is dialogical and located within the circle of members of the group. The leader becomes more involved with goal setting and serves as an active member.

- *Level 4: Group Readiness:* The group members begin to function together, "performing" in synergy with one another toward goal attainment. The leader's Style 4, "empowering," lets the team become self-managing. The leader steps outside the group circle to serve as the conduit of communication between the group and the organization and/or its other groups.

Communication Within the Group

Classic research by Bavelas (1953) revealed the best way to communicate within a group for effectiveness in task performance, as well as for group morale. The communication patterns he tested were (1) the autocratic, hub, or star pattern; and (2) the democratic, circle pattern.

Five members were in each experimental group. In the star pattern, members wrote messages only to the leader at the center or hub of the group—a one-way communication pattern. This pattern proved to be fastest but could have negative effects on morale. All the messages went from one member to the leader; the members could not send messages to one another. With each experimental trial, the members developed a low opinion of themselves (except for the leader), and they became dissatisfied. Some sabotaged the task by writing messages in foreign languages or just tearing up messages. The leader at the hub of the group was happy getting all of the messages and participated effectively. However, when confronted with an emergency, the members tended to avoid responsibility and to look to the leader to solve the problem; the group did not perform well. Still, overall, this group proved to solve the problem faster and accomplished more than the circle group.

In contrast, in the democratic circle group, members could send messages to one another—the two-way communication or dialogical pattern. The progress was described as slow and inaccurate, but the members were happy. No one wrote messages in foreign languages and the like, but they seemed to like the task even though they were critical of their own work. No one leader emerged. Because more messages were sent, the circle group had the advantage of check-backs and opportunities to find and correct errors. In the event

of an emergency, the members became cohesive and were able to solve the problem, coping with the situation much better than those in the star pattern.

These experiments show how communication can affect how people feel about their own and the group's job performance, participation, satisfaction, and responsibility. Although experienced nursing leaders may feel comfortable using the circle pattern, leaders with less experience may feel more comfortable with the star pattern. It may be appropriate to use both patterns, depending on the situational variables within the organization as a whole. It is suggested that the circle pattern would be most appropriate in introducing a change in order to develop commitment and involvement of the members. Using the star communication pattern may tend to result in resentment and opposition, and it is to be avoided if a democratic circle pattern of communication is currently in place. Before implementing change, the nurse leader is well advised to first analyze the communication pattern currently in place (Hersey et al., 2013). The nurse leader will probably find a careful study of Situational Leadership® helpful. The relationship styles, defining, clarifying, involving, and empowering describe the highest probability of success for the manner in which the leader relates to the group.

Health care organizations are moving away from bureaucratic and hierarchical organizational structures to facilitate communication effectiveness, innovation, and problem-solving, learning environments. The transition is toward network structures because these allow for communication both vertically through the chain of command as well as horizontally across providers, units, or departments (Clancy, 2007). Network structures may be matrix designs or be as simple as the clustering of patient care into care areas with similar patients, such as under true patient-and-family-centered care models. The strategy is to increase communication links, move information around the organization, and improve information flow to advantage the collective enterprise. Optimal designs are those that capitalize on computerized information systems to enhance communication, use social networks and wikis for group problem solving, and have robust mechanisms for care coordination and integration. These are radical changes but essential as the care delivery paradigm reconfigures to be primary care–based under reforms triggered by the Affordable Care Act.

CURRENT ISSUES AND TRENDS

There is support on a national level to promote effective communication and collaboration. It is important that positive interdisciplinary relationships are active in the organizational culture. The workplace does not have to be hostile. Nurse leaders have a responsibility to communicate zero tolerance for bullying and a hostile environment.

The Hostile Workplace

Registered nurses are often overlooked in the power and decision-making arenas. Nurses represent the largest licensed professional health care provider group in America. The professional nurse traditionally has had the closest and longest interpersonal contact with patients compared with most other health care providers. In this same health care system, technology rules in a labor-intense service industry, as seen in all the buildings, equipment, and sophisticated monitoring machines that need to be operated by human beings. Yet nursing colleagues, as well as other health care professionals, overlook the need to communicate with one another in a holistic and humanizing way. Ulrich (2004) urged nursing leaders to limit the "fear factor" in nursing practice for the welfare of the patients as well as the staff. The Institute for Safe Medication Practices (ISMP) (*www.ismp.org*) reported a survey indicating the role that intimidation plays in the safe administration of medications (Smetzer & Cohen, 2005).

Childers (2004) described the hostile work environments in which professional colleagues behave as "bullies." Lindeke and Sieckert (2005) focused on the nurse-physician collaborative communication and noted that the intentional sharing of knowledge of patients leads to improved patient outcomes as well as increased workplace satisfaction among staff. Namie and Namie (2008), social psychologists and founders of the Workplace Bullying and Trauma Institute (*http://www.workplacebullying.org/*) said that although many good nurses have been driven out by toxic environments, many other nurses have just accepted those environments. The Namie and Namie (2008) studies indicated that 70% of the people targeted by a bully have to quit either because of health (33%) or because they are victims of manipulated negative performance reviews (37%). Keefe (2007) noted that the age-old problem of nurses "eating their young" is bullying, and new graduates do not need to go through a trial by fire when beginning a new job. Plans for changing the culture are outlined by the Institute for Safe Medication Practices (2004). The plans involve long, expensive administrative processes to establish a zero-tolerance policy, a reporting system, conflict resolution, and educational programs. However, polices are limited in changing the way people feel about one another and how they interact. Toxic workplaces are expensive and need to be addressed for nurses and other health care providers.

Spirituality in Practice

The literature reveals there are many questions about the ways in which spirituality assessments are conducted and whether one assessment tool can prove adequate in measuring the significance of spirituality in the lives of individuals, all of whom may interpret its meaning differently. Power (2006) indicated it is unlikely that tools can be developed that are widely applicable for identifying and assessing spirituality. A research report by Baldacchino (2006) identified main competencies of nurses for spiritual care: (1) delivery of spiritual care by the nursing process, (2) nurses' communication with patients, (3) interdisciplinary team and clinical/educational organizations, and (4) safeguarding ethical issues in care. New standards reflect the importance of chaplaincy service, yet inadequate spiritual assessment, unsupportive organizational structure and climate, and lack of understanding of chaplains' role can prevent these services from being fully utilized. Nurses need to recognize when to make referrals to chaplains and how to help develop the organizational infrastructure to support processes of spiritual care (McClung et al., 2006).

Teaching Communication

There are many approaches to teaching communication skills to nursing students. Most approaches are based on procedures, techniques, and/or rubrics that provide an agenda of topics for specific case situations. Communication seems to be such a broad topic that it is unclear what to include. In addition, teaching communication skills is particularly challenging under conditions of cultural diversity.

What is needed is a general communication theory specifically for nursing that will provide a framework from which to teach communication skills to nursing students. The HNCT perspective of communication is believed to be useful in all situations in nursing practice, and thus it can serve as a benchmark theory. This theory aids the nurse in coping with the wide range of messages containing *facts* and *feelings* as well as *patterns of interaction* and *attitudes* experienced in the practice of nursing. This nursing theory can be used with other nursing theories to provide a unique perspective of the communication dimension of interpersonal interactions. The HNCT is realistic in that it recognizes the humanizing as well as dehumanizing attitudes of communication with nurses, clients, and others. This theory is an "is" rather than a "should be" theory. It provides the nurse with options to choose along a continuum of humanizing to dehumanizing attitudes, and nurses can intervene by design so that there can be an escape from negative patterns of communication. It provides direction to change relationships into humanizing interaction patterns and attitudes. Although this theory is easily understandable for clinical nurses, it is not widely used and warrants further research.

There is a need to determine a theoretically based and research evidence–supported approach to teaching communication. It is important that this approach be most effective in developing interpersonal communication skills in nursing students to ensure that they have the highest probability of responding in a humanizing manner with patients in critical life situations. The criterion for determining the degree of humanizing or dehumanizing that has occurred is what is experienced by the receiver of the speaker's message, which is the response of the receiver. This is analogous to the recipient of the sexual harasser's message determining the meaning of the message regardless of the speaker's intent. The dehumanizing message is perceived as unattractive; the receiver's body language indicates defensiveness and distancing

from the speaker, and posture and facial expression changes.

Documentation in the literature is extensive regarding disruptive and distracting communication interactions not only between nurses and between nurses and professional colleagues (e.g., physicians, pharmacists, administrators) but also between nurses and patients. The research indicates that nursing personnel experience high turnover rates, job dissatisfaction, and burnout; many RNs are leaving the profession. The work environment is described as hostile to nurses, and patient outcomes of increased severity of illness and mortality have been directly related to poor communication skills of the staff. There is some evidence that this is an issue in many parts of the world, not just in the United States. The clinical ambiance needs to change. Research by DeMarco and colleagues (2007) on the concept "self-silencing" reveals that women are socialized to value relationships to the degree that they choose not to reveal their needs or feelings to avoid disagreements and potential loss of the relationship. Findings indicate this is a gender issue and may limit the degree to which RNs can be independent and in control of their professional practice. It is suggested that research is needed about the use of assertiveness, confrontation, and conflict as HNCT patterns of interaction.

There is a need for research to determine the distribution of nursing students and staff communication on the humanizing and dehumanizing continuum. One way to do this is to use the Nursing Communication Observation Tool (NCOT), which is designed for use in data collection within the framework of HNCT (Duldt, 1989). Data can be obtained by having groups or subjects view a video, such as "Wit" or "The Doctor," and then identify patterns of interaction and attitudes on the NCOT. Analysis may show a range of sensitivity that would provide direction for educational interventions. How can nurses (and others) be "inoculated" to increase their resilience to a hostile workplace? How can nurses be instructed in the everyday communication skills necessary in clinical practice and not just in specialized communication as is taught in psychiatric nursing? HNCT is designed to suggest directions for educational interventions, but more research is needed.

CASE STUDY

As director of the nursing education department in a large hospital, Evelyn Sullivan is responsible for providing the educational component for nursing staff. The current educational program for the entire nursing staff is spiritual assessment and care. The staff is composed of nurses of a wide variety of Christian religious affiliations. One concern about the content of the workshops Evelyn is planning is conveying convincingly the ethical standards to be maintained (i.e., autonomy, beneficence, confidentiality). Of particular concern is the issue of respecting the patients' beliefs and avoiding proselytizing or trying to convert patients to the nurses' own religion. Nurses are to listen for what patients believe as it is relevant to their health care and try to work within these beliefs. Evelyn devised the following plan.

A group of 30 nurses would be attending the first workshop on spirituality and spiritual care. In an introductory lecture, the purpose of the spiritual assessment is to learn the following:

1. How spirituality/religion influence health care
2. How beliefs help patients cope with illness and stress
3. What spiritual needs can be identified and addressed
4. What referrals are needed to the chaplain, priest, or religious official
5. What the scope of the patients' support systems is
   Evelyn's plan was to ask nurses to write on the provided index card how they defined spirituality and spiritual care. After about 5 minutes, Evelyn would then ask the nurses to meet in small groups to share their ideas and briefly discuss their definitions.

Rather than following the usual method, Evelyn decided to not have the small groups report about their discussions or definitions. Rather, she would ask them to keep this information to themselves by putting the index card in their pocket. That card contains what they personally believe, and they could use this as a reminder about spiritual care principles. In considering spirituality, the nurses were to listen carefully for the **b**eliefs, **v**alues, **m**eanings, **g**oals, and **r**elationships, the BVMGR, to what the patient says comprises spirituality. Although the patient may profess being a member of a certain religious organization, the patient may not believe exactly what is commonly known about that religion or accept all the tenets of that religion.

On the basis of this information, a "designer" spiritual care plan can be developed to provide spiritual comfort to the patient. The focus is to be on the patient's definitions of spirituality, not the nurse's. The rationale for this is based on the ethical principles of autonomy, beneficence, and confidentiality.

Evelyn followed this plan in the presentation of the first workshop. The nurses had no difficulty writing their beliefs and briefly discussing them with one another. Everyone followed her instructions and put the index cards in their pockets. In the remainder of the workshop, the five "*R*'s" role of the nurse and the role of chaplains and community church leaders were discussed at length as spiritual care plans were developed for case situations. Evelyn was relieved to note that the nurses did not discuss their own beliefs but did, in fact, think about how patients they had known thought about and practiced spirituality.

CRITICAL THINKING EXERCISE

Nurse Olivia Witte is in charge of an interdisciplinary team at Sunrise Hospital. The nurses at Sunrise have identified a need to develop a critical pathway for ventilator-dependent patients who are about to be discharged to home with home health care. Nurse Witte knows that these patients have multiple complex care needs. It is urgent that information flow be specific and detailed to make "seamless" the care transfer between the hospital and home care, wherever

this may be. First, Nurse Witte had to manage a few physicians who flatly stated that they would not follow a "cookbook" concocted by nurses. Then the dietary representative presented the team with dietary's protocols and suggested that nurses integrate these because nurses were in charge of the pathway maintenance. Next, Nurse Witte discovered why the local home health care representative was not returning phone calls and could not come to team meetings for quite a while: the group was planning a move in 1 month and was just notified of that The Joint Commission (TJC) would be visiting in 3 months.

1. What is the problem?
2. Whose problem is it?
3. What should Nurse Witte do?
4. What mode of communication should Nurse Witte use?
5. How can Nurse Witte structure a clear message?
6. To whom should Nurse Witte communicate first? Who else needs to be involved in the communication flow?
7. What leadership and management strategies should Nurse Witte use?

8

Team Building and Working with Effective Groups

Jo Manion, Diane L. Huber

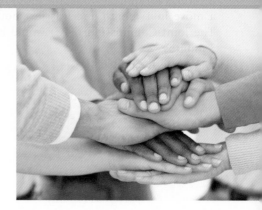

℮volve WEBSITE

http://evolve.elsevier.com/Huber/leadership/

Nurse leaders in today's health care organizations must be skilled group facilitators with an exquisite ability to manage and lead the collective work of people. A significant percentage of work completed in organizations today is done through collective efforts, either in work groups, committees, or teams. Understanding the characteristics of each of these entities and basic principles for attaining successful outcomes increases the leader's effectiveness.

In years past, many health care organizations attempted to convert their traditional hierarchical, bureaucratic structures to a team-based structure, with varying degrees of success. Many of these efforts were less than successful at the broad organizational level; yet the factors driving these changes still exist. There is vastly increased complexity of both today's workplace and the work of patient care. Teamwork has become the imperative for leaders today because the level of knowledge required to meet the demands of both patients and systems of care requires collective pooling of thinking styles, diversity of professional backgrounds, and the collaboration of many. Rapidly changing structures of care delivery and reimbursement protocols, increasing governmental regulations,

increasing complexity, technology advances, rapid information dissemination at the worker level, and the shift to a knowledge worker–based service society are some of the social and economic forces operative in health care. These forces converge to create tumultuous change in health care delivery.

Employees who work in a collaborative manner with others and who are able to work effectively within a team context can provide the strength, structure, and resiliency to deal with work complexities and changes. Today's health care organizations are considered *knowledge organizations,* and there is a renewed emphasis on the role of teams. Although interdisciplinary teams have always played an important role in home care, hospice, and other community settings, hospitals and large health care organizations are placing more emphasis on teams as a part of their core structure and the general way of doing business.

"Knowledge has become so complex and specialized that virtually no single individual can be effective alone" is still true today (Sorrells-Jones & Weaver, 1999, p. 15). Because knowledge workers are specialists, the only way for them to be adequately productive is to work in groups or teams. Thus as the focus shifts to building knowledge work teams, today's leaders must be able to help these teams be more effective and productive.

Photo used with permission from Photos.com.

Developing effective teams of professionals from different disciplines is challenging. However, effective knowledge work teams can create a form of synergism in which the outcome is greater than the sum of individual efforts. Such synergism confers a competitive edge and boosts productivity under conditions of constrained resources. Teams are a way to enlist employee participation and capitalize on possibilities for improved patient safety, increased productivity, better decisions, and process innovation. Team building is a strategy for designing, implementing, developing, and nurturing work teams in organizations. These work teams are a specialized subset of the many types of groups that form or are formed in organizations.

In nursing, group process theory relates to both how to be therapeutic with clients and how to work as an employee within an organization that is often large and complex. Nursing has at its core both a caring and a coordinative function. The nurse's coordinative role is at the hub of all client care information. For example, nurses collect, process, and integrate the initial assessment and laboratory data; handle the tracking of all therapeutic interventions for the client; are at the bedside in hospitals for surveillance of minute-by-minute changes; and are the major point of contact for clinical care delivery in many settings and sites. For example, if narcotics are given in a hospital, nurses track whether that intervention has worked, whether alternative pain strategies might be needed, and what psychological reaction the client might have. Even hospitalists who may see a patient multiple times in a day may not recognize the fine distinctions of change in a client's condition. Nurses predominate in actual client care in home health, long-term care, hospice, and many other settings. The nurse is involved more intimately and more proximately than any of the other health care providers in managing the total health care of the client. Therefore understanding and developing skill in group process and group dynamics is essential within the context of leadership and management in nursing because of the group functioning and coordinative aspects of nursing practice. Nurses need strong group process and interaction skills to communicate clearly and collaborate effectively with a variety of colleagues.

DEFINITIONS

A **group** is defined as any collection of interconnected individuals working together for some purpose. Groups are important in organizations not only because of informal network dynamics but also because of the multitude of formal committees and teams in the contemporary organization.

A **committee** is a relatively stable and formally composed group. Committees are a specific type of group in that they are stable, meet periodically, and have an identified purpose that is part of the organizational structure. There is a mechanism for maintaining and selecting members. Typically, committees have official status and sanction within an organization. For example, there is a policy and procedure committee or a patient safety committee.

Team building is defined as the process of deliberately creating and unifying a group into a functioning team.

A **team** was defined by Katzenbach and Smith (1993) as "a small number of people with complementary skills who are committed to a common purpose, performance goals, and approach for which they hold themselves mutually accountable" (p. 45). Manion and colleagues (1996) modified this definition slightly for health care by noting that the members need to be consistent. This was in reaction to confusion in terminology for many people in health care who had prior knowledge of team nursing, in which whoever was present on a given shift was on the team. In this type of team nursing model, members could vary from shift to shift and from day to day, reducing the overall performance outcomes of the team. Team nursing was an assignment pattern and work allocation methodology rather than a true team model as seen in business and industry.

The distinction between a work group and a true team is crucial. Health care leaders may mistakenly assume that simply calling a group a *team* actually makes it a team. As Katzenbach and Smith (1993) emphasized, the group becomes a true team only by doing its collective work. The team goes through a developmental process that takes time and the investment of energy to materialize. Many collective entities in today's organizations are called a *team* yet clearly function more as a work group than a true team.

A **work group** is a collection of individuals who are led by a strong, clearly focused leader. They come together to share information and ideas, and they may even mutually make some decisions. However, the members of the work group have individual work products for which they are responsible, and these consume their major focus and effort. For example, in a patient care unit, the unit secretary has certain responsibilities as does the charge nurse, patient care nurse, and nurse manager. The boundaries remain fairly clearly separated when the collective entity is a work group. Each person may feel individual accountability, but there is little to no collective accountability.

This is in contrast with a true team, which is a collective entity in which the leadership rotates and is shared by various members of the team, depending on appropriateness and fit of skills and abilities. In a true team, there are collective work products—for example, the provision of quality patient care to all of the patients housed in the department. There is group as well as individual accountability. If one member of the team is having a problem, it is not just that person's problem but, rather, is the problem of and for the whole team to resolve. An example of team thinking is "No one sits down until we can all sit down" or "No one goes home until we all go home." If quality outcomes are difficult for one team member, all team members are affected by this and become engaged in helping the affected team member meet expectations. In the management book *The Goal* (Goldratt & Cox, 2004), the author tells a parable about taking a Boy Scout troop on a hike. When it was discovered that Scout Herbie was slowing the whole group down, the weight in his backpack was redistributed and the troop sped up. This is how a high-performing team works.

Another collective entity apparent in many organizations is a **pseudoteam.** This is a group of people who believe they are already a team, although clearly they fall short of the definition of a true team. Characteristics of a pseudoteam include confusion over their purpose, unhealthy or toxic interpersonal issues and communication patterns, members who put individual needs and ambition above the needs of the team, the presence of hierarchical rituals that preclude full participation of all members, unclear goals, and a lack of evaluation criteria. The true danger of

pseudoteams is that members think they are already a team and thus see no need for improvement. As a result, they do not grow and develop but, rather, just become more and more dysfunctional with the passage of time.

BACKGROUND

Group interactions are a pervasive element of the health care environment in which nurses work. A basic understanding of groups helps nurses function more effectively. These principles apply to any group, whether an actual team, a committee, or an informal group effort. Group interactions are composed of the following elements (Book & Galvin, 1975) (Figure 8-1):

- The *process* that the group undergoes to reach outcomes: This relates to the unique way the group interrelates and begins to work together. The leader can assess group process through observation. What is the process that occurs while accomplishing its task?
- The *standards* that regulate the group's behavior: This relates to the specific values and norms that are chosen for group processing. Which ones are chosen and which are discarded?
- The process of *problem solving* or *decision making* that the group adopts: Does the group solve problems? How are decisions made? Are they group decisions made by consensus, or are they individual decisions made with group input (as occurs when the group participates but the decision is made by a leader or manager)?
- The *communication* that occurs among group members: What are the internal patterns and styles of communication used by group members? To whom does the group communicate? Do they report as a subcommittee to a full committee? If a team, does the team have frequent communication with external team leaders? What are the internal and external modes of communication for group input and output?
- The *roles* played by each member: Members will adopt a variety of group roles within the group, but roles are fluid. Members may take on different roles in different situations. It is important to remember when assessing group interactions that roles in the group may be formal roles, clearly established by the

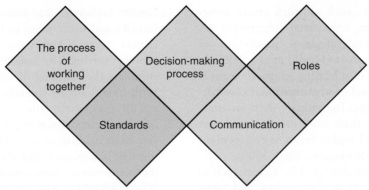

FIGURE 8-1 Group process elements. (Data from Book, C., & Galvin, K. [1975]. *Instruction in and about small group discussion*. Falls Church, VA: Speech Communication Association.)

leader or the group. However, there are additionally roles that each group member moves in and out of that best suit him or her (such as clarifier, harmonizer, devil's advocate, etc.). Clarity in the more formal roles such as team leader, facilitator, recorder, and timekeeper is important to avoid confusion and unnecessary conflict.

Groups tend to go through a series of stages in their work and development. Farley and Stoner (1989) originally identified these as (1) orientation, (2) adaptation, (3) emergence, and (4) working. The first stage, *orientation*, occurs when the group first forms and the members begin to relate to one another and the task. The group needs to develop trust and define boundaries in order to establish involvement and identification. The second stage, *adaptation*, occurs as the group begins to develop a collective identity and differentiate roles. The group needs a facilitative structure and climate to maximize its processing and to work through the establishment of roles, rules, norms, and a common language. The third stage, *emergence*, occurs as control issues arise. Disputes, disagreements, confrontations, alliances, and power struggles mark this stage of determining control over the group in order to emerge with a more consolidated identity. The final stage, *working*, occurs when conflict and dissension dissipate and the group achieves greater cohesion through negotiation. The group is now focused primarily on decision making and productivity. The stages may overlap and are not necessarily sequential. The group leader pays attention to the stage of the group as a way of monitoring the

group's development and progress. For example, in the orientation stage, the leader may need to be more alert to the need to intervene personally than would be the case in the working stage when the group has achieved a higher level of maturity.

WHY GROUPS ARE FORMED

In nursing, the formation of groups occurs primarily for one of two reasons: (1) to provide a personal or professional socialization and exchange forum, or (2) to provide a mechanism for interdependent work accomplishment. Groups can be social, professional, or organizational in purpose. The following are some reasons why groups would be established in organizations:

- Group activities can create a sense of status and esteem.
- Groups allow an individual to test and establish reality.
- Groups function as a mechanism for getting a job done.
- The work to be accomplished requires the complexity of knowledge and skill possible only in a group configuration.

"The ebb and flow of work done by groups is a major part of the working environment of hospital nurses" (Leppa, 1996, p. 23). The work group provides an institutional and professional identity for an individual nurse, and work groups become a focus for interpersonal relationships, support, and social integration. Interpersonal relationship elements such as work group cohesion, communication, and social integration remain consistent moderate-level predictors of nursing job satisfaction (DiMeglio et al., 2005). In addition, being part of a healthy group or team is also related to the level of organizational commitment by the employee. Individuals with an emotional connection to their work group have lower levels of turnover and higher levels of engagement (DiMeglio et al., 2005; Manion, 2004, 2009).

Work groups can be disrupted by factors such as downsizing, reorganization, absenteeism, and turnover. Work group disruption has been shown to be linked to negative outcomes (Leppa, 1996; Kalisch & Begeny, 2005; Kalisch et al., 2008; Kalisch & Lee, 2010). In a study of four hospitals, interpersonal relations were found to be an important part of nurses' job satisfaction. There was a relationship between work group disruption and interpersonal relations (Leppa, 1996). Things get done because of relationships among people; nurses need to build successful collaborative relationships among multiple levels of colleagues, key people, organizations, and clients (Laramee, 1999). The level of nursing teamwork has been found to be directly linked to missed nursing care (Kalisch & Lee, 2010).

Furthermore, informal work group norms exert a strong influence on nurses' behavior and can contribute to forms of nursing deviance. Work group relationships can reinforce behaviors and rationalization, thus leading to deviant behaviors becoming passively or actively accepted. For example, in one study of nurses in practice, nurses used work group norms to neutralize opposition to drug theft and use (Dabney, 1995). Clearly, there is a strong relationship between work groups, interpersonal relationships, and outcomes such as nurses' behaviors and perceptions. Work group relationships are a powerful mechanism influencing both good and bad outcomes in nursing practice.

ADVANTAGES OF GROUPS

There are advantages to group work. For example, groups are one vehicle for solving problems. Veninga (1982) identified the following five major advantages of group problem solving over individual problem solving:

1. *Greater knowledge and information:* Obtaining a broader and wider range of knowledge and experiences creates a higher-quality input into group problem solving. The insights of one member can stimulate the thinking of other group members. With today's highly specialized health care workers, this is especially true.

2. *Increased acceptance of solutions:* If there is a decision to be made in an organization, people can get together in a group to talk about it so that the people themselves are more committed to the decision. When individuals who are going to be affected by a decision are part of the decision-making process, they do not have to be convinced of the rightness of the decision and are more likely to be committed to implementing it.

3. *More approaches to a problem:* Complex problems typically are more manageable when a number of perspectives are mixed together to address the problem. The advantages include blending and complementing individual learning and problem-solving styles to capitalize on strength through diversity.

4. *Individual expression:* Groups allow for individual expression, and in organizations specifically, there may be few mechanisms for expression of individual perspectives. Sharing information and getting input are done best in groups (Veninga, 1982). Sometimes groups allow people to express themselves—for example, if they are anxious about a change or if morale is low.

5. *Lower costs:* If the group is functioning in a positive and constructive manner, the use of a group can be less expensive than the use of individual effort to accomplish a task. Group decision making is cost-effective if it saves time. For example, when a group meets for one session as opposed to the leader meeting multiple times with multiple individuals, the leader and possibly the group members save time.

It is imperative that the purpose of the group be established, especially when the group is part of a larger organization. Ideally this is an early conversation for the group and is determined with the input of all members. The stated purpose should be evaluated periodically. Is it a functional? Is it accomplishing the task to which it was assigned or committed? If not, should the group be disbanded? When the work output of any group is analyzed, meetings can be financially costly endeavors. For example, when the number of hours spent by all committee members is multiplied by their individual hourly salary and fringe benefit cost and added together to compute a committee total, the sum of costs for the group may be astounding. This is one reason for paying attention to how well the group is functioning. Just as important is the increased cynicism found in organizations where groups are ineffective, when people cease to be interested in participating because nothing really changes as a result of their efforts.

A well-tuned and functioning group is positive for an organization. Often such a group is less expensive and time-consuming in terms of solving complex problems. Participation and involvement in a group decision typically results in individuals being more committed to a decision, even if there is disagreement.

DISADVANTAGES OF GROUPS

Group decision making can be derailed at a number of points in the process. The three disadvantages commonly noted about group decision making are the potential for premature decisions, individual domination, and disruptive conflicts (Veninga, 1982).

Premature Decisions

Sometimes decisions result from pressure. Once a majority vote is taken, the minority experience an element of pressure because of psychological dynamics related to subtle pressure for group acceptance and conformity. This is often referred to as groupthink. It may be difficult to be a devil's advocate or to adopt the role of bringing alternative critique points to the group for consideration because of a concern about not being personally socially accepted or fear of retaliation. For example, derision and humiliation can occur if members react with strong negative opinions. This response stifles further input.

Individual Domination

The emergence of dominating or argumentative members who obstruct the group process is a disadvantage. These members not only make it an unpleasant experience for all involved, they sabotage the work of the group. It becomes costly and time-consuming for the group to divert its energy and productivity

to working out interpersonal dynamics rather than moving forward on the group's task.

Disruptive Conflicts

If people perceive an adverse effect on a group member or members or if they feel threatened, conflicts usually emerge. Conflicts can accelerate in a competitive environment when members vest in their own position. Conflicts that are about substantive issues actually help the group become more effective in their decision making. However, when conflicts occur over differences in personality or opinion, or clashes of values, these conflicts can become destructive. Although it may seem contradictory, conflicts can serve as a control mechanism in a group and may actually result in far superior outcomes. When group members are comfortable respectfully disagreeing with each other, a premature acceptance of decisions can be avoided because opposing viewpoints are considered. However, group members and leaders need to become skilled and comfortable in handling interpersonal dynamics.

GROUP DECISION MAKING

Group work can be, and typically is, a slow process. It takes more time for a group to arrive at a decision than for one person to make the decision.

In addition, a continuum of decision-making power may be vested in a group (Figure 8-2). A group or committee has certain powers, tasks, and functions, as well as certain parameters or latitude in terms of how far to go in making a decision. Decision power is a matter of degree, with four distinct points on the continuum of authority for decision making: autocratic, consultative, joint, and delegated.

On one end of the continuum is an *autocratic decision procedure* in which the leader makes all of the decisions. In this process there is input, perhaps, but not necessarily a vote. For example, in certain legislative committees the chairperson may or may not be able to put forth legislation or block a bill. It may be the case that an autocratic leader controls the power and the committee exists mainly for the sake of appearance. This type of committee is set up for reasons other than making participative decisions. It is hoped that very few of these structures are found in human service organizations because they can generate increased cynicism and employee disengagement.

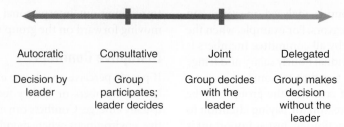

FIGURE 8-2 Range of decision powers.

A *consultative decision procedure* occurs when decisions involve employee participation but the leader still makes the final decision alone. Group members may make certain recommendations, but these must then go to the leader, chairperson, or head of the group, who makes the final decision. There is more participation with this type of procedure, but the ultimate decision is not under the control of the group members.

Some decision procedures result in *joint decision making*. In this approach, the entire group decides, whether by a two-thirds vote, simple majority, consensus, or some other process. In a joint decision procedure, the employees have as much influence as the leader. The leader has one voice, one vote. The leader can use persuasion, but when it comes to the final vote, the leader's vote is equivalent to that of any other member of the group. This is fundamentally different from the leader making the decision with group input. This is the type of decision making used in a multidisciplinary team. Every voice is heard and valued equally.

Finally, at the other end of the decision continuum is the *delegated decision procedure*. This occurs when the committee chair or leader allows participants to make the final decision. For example, in true self-scheduling, the leader may set up the basic parameters, but the staff members (usually through the work of a smaller, designated team) actually decide what schedule they work. The true test of a delegation decision procedure is whether the leader overrides the followers' decision. Technically, the leader would not have the authority to veto or override. If it is truly a delegation situation, the leader would go forward with the approach that the decision is the choice of the group. The group then becomes accountable for the outcome and is responsible for fixing any resulting issues. Hersey and colleagues (2008) labeled these same four procedures as *authoritative, consultative, facilitative,* and *delegative* decision-making styles.

It is advisable for the followers in any group to determine who has the authority to make decisions. Knowledge about what type of group it is and what delegation or decision procedures can be anticipated is critical to participation. A leadership or conflict moment may occur when a group assumes that the decision procedure rule in effect is delegation and the decision is *its* to make but the leader has a different idea. Clarity before beginning work on an issue prevents unnecessary conflict and augments productivity.

WORKING WITH TEAMS

In health care, interdisciplinary care teams are necessary for survival. High-performance teams are essential to an organization's efficiency and effectiveness because high-quality work outcomes and cost control are impossible without collaboration and teamwork.

Nurse leaders need to learn how to create, lead, and manage teams; all nurses must know how to be effective team players. The formation of a well-functioning group or team is never the work of just the leader. Members give input, participate in decision making, share responsibility, and hold themselves accountable for the outcomes of the group. A highly skilled and effective professional is not necessarily a highly skilled and effective group member. There are distinct skill sets involved, and all are needed by nurses today. Leaders and staff members alike must be able to function both independently and interdependently with others. And they must have the judgment to know when which form of functioning is more appropriate.

Types of Teams

Three types of teams found in health care are (1) primary work teams, (2) leadership teams, and (3) ad hoc teams (Manion, 2011). Primary work teams include all forms of client care teams such as an emergency department trauma team. In the operating room, teams are often based on the specialty (e.g., a cardiovascular or an orthopedic team). The senior executive team is an example of an executive or management leadership team. At the hospital department level there may be a leadership team that is composed of the nurse manager, charge nurses, and perhaps an educator. Continuous quality improvement teams, project teams, and problem-solving teams are examples of ad hoc teams found across settings and sites. Specific problem-solving teams in departments are other examples of ad hoc teams. The chief characteristic of these teams is that they are created to perform a very specific piece of work. When that work is completed, the team dissolves. Designing, building, and implementing effective work teams requires a specific methodology and process. A primary work team fails if it behaves like a collection of individuals operating from narrowly defined jobs; if it is composed of the wrong mix of members, size, structure, responsibility, or expertise; or if it cannot fluidly shift activities and adapt to changes. Teams should be designed based on the work responsibilities of the team. After the team design is determined, the next step is to build the team by incorporating the essential elements needed to function. These include a common purpose; agreed-on performance goals or results-driven structure; competent members; a common approach for the work; complementary skills; a collaborative relationships; mutual accountability; standards of excellence; external support; and principled leadership (Manion et al., 1996).

The complementary skills that are needed, in the right mix, to do the team's task fall into at least three categories: technical or functional expertise, problem-solving and decision-making skills, and interpersonal skills (Box 8-1).

BOX 8-1   TEAM PERFORMANCE CHECKLIST

- Small in number, consistent members
- Complementary skills
- Meaningful purpose
- Specific goal(s)
- Clear working approach
- Sense of mutual accountability

Data from Katzenbach, J., & Smith, D. (1993). *The wisdom of teams: Creating the high-performance organization.* New York: Harper Collins.

Managing this development process is a key leadership function. This means that the leader guides the team in the development of its purpose. The team members are more likely to coalesce into a strong team if they have been given the time and opportunity to carefully reflect on their purpose and agree on what they do and for whom they do it. This leads to a unified commitment. The team becomes a true team by doing its work. Specific performance goals give it direction and also provide evaluative criteria by which the team's success can be measured. Although it is simplistic to say that the team has common working approaches, unnecessary conflict occurs in this area if the leader and team members have not established these key processes. Agreement is needed about how things are going to be done and by whom. This ranges from the establishment of team behavioral norms to agreement on procedural issues. This step usually requires a significant amount of time and will continue to be addressed throughout the lifetime of the team. By laying a foundation carefully, effective teams can emerge (Manion, 2011).

Team Dynamics

The dynamics of interdisciplinary teams create some unique issues. Regrouping people into multidisciplinary groups increases the diversity of the team and can result in increased conflict. A lack of common vocabulary and understanding about other disciplines' practices may surface. Many highly skilled, committed professionals are used to functioning very independently and simply do not know how to work together in teams (Sorrells-Jones, 1997). Lencioni (2006) promoted the idea that to overcome the common turf battles and the tendency team members have to function in their own narrow scope (silo thinking), the team needs to have a pressing, time-constricted goal upon which to focus.

Other perils and pitfalls occur when teams are assigned, not designed, including the following (Manion et al., 1996):

- Confusion about the team's work.
- The team lacks real authority.
- Structural team building is not done.
- Dysfunctional behavior occurs and team members don't know how to deal with it constructively.
- Team-based outcome measures and coaching are lacking.

Trust and communication are critical elements of building effective work teams. It is not enough to simply structure the team. Team members need to learn to work collaboratively and interdependently. Team performance and effectiveness are important managerial concerns. Dysfunctional team behaviors can occur. Lencioni (2002) identified five key dysfunctions of a team as absence of trust, fear of conflict, lack of commitment, avoidance of accountability, and inattention to results.

Teams form, grow through stages, and mature. Team dynamics change throughout this process. Teams benefit from team building and developmental training. Articulating and negotiating expectations for healthy interpersonal behavior benefits team development. A key characteristic of an emotionally intelligent team is one that has established norms that guide team member behaviors (Cherniss & Goleman, 2001).

Team norms are best established when the team initially forms. They are continually revisited, modified, and expanded throughout the life span of the team. The process for developing norms is usually leader-initiated and begins with a conversation within the team about how members expect each other to behave and contribute. The norms are usually developed during a group meeting in which ideas are shared, refined, and finally negotiated with all team members. Appropriate topics for behavioral norms include, but are not limited to, expectations around the following:

- Communication, both at the individual and group levels
- How team members treat each other
- How support is to be demonstrated
- Decision-making process
- How conflict is to be handled

For example, one team developed the following expectations of each other:

I expect you to:

- Communicate in an open, honest, and direct manner with me
- Give me feedback when my behavior creates a difficult or uncomfortable situation for you
- Persist and work with me on difficult issues until we reach a mutually agreeable resolution
- Pitch in gladly, provide help when asked, and look for ways to help each other out
- Respect confidences and not share sensitive information we discuss with others without my knowledge or permission
- Be trustworthy as evidenced by honoring and meeting commitments made, by being loyal to absent team members, and by presenting me in the best light to others

Often these norms are referred to as the *team operating agreement,* the *code of conduct,* or *articulated expectations.* In many teams, once they are identified, team members sign them, indicating agreement, and they often are posted in sight in the workplace. These norms are more than just a paper exercise. They signify that the team member agrees to live by the expectations and address other team members who do not.

The greater the performance of a team, the greater is the advantage to the group members, their customers, and the organization. Productivity is impacted, but more importantly team members are likely to experience a higher degree of engagement in their work and commitment to the organization (Manion, 2009).

COMMITTEES

An essential part of any nurse's role is to be involved in committee and group work. Work is accomplished through people, and the quality of care is furthered through committee actions. It also is important to nurses' job satisfaction and autonomy to have an avenue of involvement and participation in which to actively solve problems and retain autonomy over nursing care. Shared governance models incorporate staff nurse participation in groups and committees as a core element of how work gets accomplished.

Some people react negatively to committees because they dislike the time involved and because they are frustrated with the psychodynamics of group process and decision making. However, committees are a mainstay of organizations and can be an important way to make changes in clinical practice. Lencioni (2004) believed there is no substitute for a good meeting—one in which there is passionate, dynamic, and focused engagement—to gather the collective wisdom of the group. Understanding committee workings facilitates the process of being a more effective nurse.

Committee structures are preferable in the following two kinds of situations:

1. *Situations in which each member's input is needed to attain a certain goal.* For example, a committee may be set up to implement self-scheduling or to start a new program to benefit clients. If the work cannot be done alone or if there is a need to have everyone's agreement, then a committee is probably appropriate.

2. *Situations in which diverse representation facilitates implementation of proposed activities.* To have a diverse group of people provide input in order to get the job done, a committee should be created. For example, a multidisciplinary products committee could be established to develop a process in which products would be reviewed before large purchases are made. This approach prevents the nurses at the care delivery site from using products that are potentially unsafe or unusable, and thus costly. And it can prevent a product being purchased because it works well for the way care is delivered in one department, but not for those using the product in another department.

Types of Committees

Several types of committees are found in organizations. One kind is the *standing* committee, which, as the name implies, is a constant, ongoing part of the organizational mission, performing critical and essential functions. For example, policy committees are standing committees because there always are policies to write and review. The same is true for quality assurance/improvement committees or a patient safety committee because these functions and activities are ongoing and continuous.

Contrasted to a standing committee is the task force, also called a *project team* or *ad hoc committee.* This is a committee that is developed in response to some emergent or immediate need. A need arises, and a group is formed. A task force is not part of the organizational core mission. It is formed in response to a specific circumstance that arises or to study a specific problem. The committee is expected to disband when the issue is resolved. Examples are a search committee to replace an advanced practice nurse or a problem-solving group dealing with, for example, patient flow issues or bed space availability in the emergency department, which subsequently affects the entire hospital.

Some groups or committees are structured to gather together members *based on organizational position or job position.* For example, all the nurse managers may belong to a group of nurse managers or staff nurses may belong to a staff nurse council. By holding the position of nurse manager, the person belongs to that committee. This provides an opportunity for peer interaction, support, and problem solving.

There are multidisciplinary interdivisional committees. A *multidisciplinary* committee includes participants from several divisions or specialties. The participants may all be from within the institution or from both inside and outside the organization. These committees often are used to coordinate and eliminate boundary conflicts. Some examples are a products committee, a risk management committee, or a medical liaison committee in which nurses and physicians work together to improve patient care and reduce interprofessional conflicts. In some cases, multidisciplinary teams are formed using a committee structure (e.g., to develop a critical pathway). Other committees may be cross-functional (e.g., nurses meeting with members from the information technology or facilities management department to discuss and resolve issues).

Within organizations, committees perform a central role in the implementation of the strategic plan. A committee is a group that can assume responsibility and be held accountable for planning, implementing, and evaluating the outcomes of a strategic goal translated to the operational level. Committees accomplish some departmental activities and provide a mechanism for increasing staff participation in decision making. In an environment characterized by complex work, committees become a major vehicle for resolving issues related to the organization's mission. Two elements promote efficient and effective committee decision making: appropriate representation (by including people affected by changes) and delegation of an appropriate level of authority to the committee (Manion, 2011).

Committees evolve over time. To remain vital, committees need to be evaluated regularly for congruence with organizational mission and contribution to outcomes. The committee's goals and outcomes should be reviewed annually, with membership reevaluated and changed as necessary. If asked to be on a committee as a unit representative, it is advisable for the nurse to explore the nature and characteristics of the committee.

The nurse needs to determine the authority level delegated to this particular committee, remembering that this delegation may be formal or informal. Another factor involves assessing the personal level of interest in the work of the committee. Other factors include whether the people on the committee are highly motivated, whether they are task- or relationship-oriented people, and what committee politics exist. The feedback mechanisms and the committee's productivity are key characteristics. The track record of the committee is reflected in its output. These characteristics are important for the nurse to understand before deciding to participate. Preparation for followership enhances both personal and committee productivity. It is also helpful to clarify any expectations for the committee role being considered. For example, is the nurse there to share individual opinions or to represent others in the department? This role requires more active solicitation of colleagues' opinions and ideas.

EFFECTIVE MEETINGS

Meetings are common occurrences in health care organizations. Whether a meeting involves a group, a committee, or a team, the leader's role is to maximize the benefits of the meeting. Structuring a meeting for effectiveness requires preparation and effort. To manage effective meetings, the leader should consider the purpose for which they are organized. There are many purposes for meetings and Lencioni believed that some of the most common reasons meetings are ineffective are that the purpose of the meeting is not clear or there are too many competing issues on the agenda for a single meeting (Lencioni, 2004). For example, a brief team huddle would become ineffective if it turned into a decision-making group about a key department issue.

Probably the most common type of meeting is held for *information dissemination or sharing*. For example, the designated leadership person calls the group together to let the members know that direction has come down to cut the budget by 10% because of fiscal retrenchment. A meeting is called to disseminate information about what is happening and to provide time for questions and answers. Perhaps there has been an organizational change, such as the decision that one unit is going to be consolidating with another unit or that a new building, department relocation, or merger is being planned.

One familiar form of *information sharing* is the end-of-shift report. Pertinent, important information about patients is passed from staff members on one shift to those on another. A very common form of this type of meeting seen in many organizations today is the team huddle. This is a very short meeting at the beginning of the shift with all team members to review the upcoming shift or any short topics that need to be communicated.

Second, there are meetings held for the purpose of *opinion seeking*. The goal of these meetings is open dialogue to solicit group and individual opinions and ideas on specific topics or issues. This purpose does not imply that decision making is the prerogative of the group. Seeking opinions is an input strategy and may be used only for gathering data or testing group reactions. For example, an opinion-seeking meeting may be called to invite input on equipment purchases for budget requests.

The third type of meeting is held for the purpose of *problem solving and/or decision making*. The meeting is structured to solicit help in clarifying, analyzing, and solving a specific problem. This type of meeting is more action-oriented. Group participation in decision making is encouraged. For example, group problem solving or unit meetings may be called to discuss ways to solve problems related to disruptive or manipulative clients or family members. Meetings for the purpose of problem solving must follow a methodical structure; otherwise, they are likely either to deteriorate into a complaint session or to result in ineffective or unacceptable recommendations. Effectively leading these groups requires strong facilitation skills and knowledge in problem-solving techniques.

Yet another type of meeting is a *strategy* meeting. These meetings are less frequent, perhaps quarterly or annually, and focus on forging a vision for the department or work group, developing future goals and strategies, or tackling one issue in great depth, such as implementing a shared governance model or a new model of care delivery.

Preparing for Meetings

In the most effective groups, all members are clear about the purpose of the meeting they are attending and help the group stay focused on the purpose. When the group becomes distracted by other issues (for example, getting side-tracked by operational issues during a strategy meeting), focus is lost and the meeting time is wasted.

In many nursing departments, meetings become unmanageable. This is a sign that the entire meeting structure needs to be evaluated. One way to approach committee evaluation is to form a committee to conduct a comprehensive strategic evaluation. A questionnaire is developed to gather information about current committees, including membership, purpose, meeting frequency, and effectiveness. Recommendations are made, including the elimination of some committees, consolidation of others, streamlining of membership, and suggested expectations for committee participation. Committee responsibilities can be realigned to increase effectiveness of nursing employees.

In preparing for a meeting, a leader needs to make certain that the committee's process stays true to the purpose of the meeting. In other words, there should not be a mix of items in the same meeting. For example, basic information dissemination is not appropriate at a quarterly strategic meeting. This does not mean that any of these items are less important, but introducing them in the wrong venue or with the wrong timing will reduce the effectiveness of the meeting.

In the past, using a timed agenda became popular and was recommended as a way to facilitate the group's process. This involved identifying on the agenda, next to each item, the anticipated amount of time allotted for discussion. It was meant to serve as a guideline rather than a rigid parameter. However, in too many cases it was a substitute for good judgment, prematurely cutting off debate or forcing a decision when a particular discussion was productive but took longer than anticipated. Lencioni (2004) believed that, especially for information dissemination or coordinative meetings such as a team huddle or daily operations meetings for leaders, information should be shared and the agenda flow from what members of the group are dealing with at the time. In other words, in the most effective of these meetings, the agenda is not prepared ahead of time. Obviously this does not hold true for problem-solving, decision-making, or strategic meetings and some routine operations meetings. It is most appropriate for brainstorming and shared governance. In addition, meetings can rapidly become disorganized without a prepared agenda.

Leader Duties

The leader of the group can facilitate meeting effectiveness by preparing and dealing with both the task

and the people involved. The leader needs to listen carefully, process the interactions, control the flow, and keep the meeting directed toward accomplishing the objectives. The ideal size of a group depends on the work to be accomplished. If group interaction and getting everyone's input is important, the size of the ideal group is small, perhaps 4 to 7 people, with 12 being the upper limit. Members should be carefully selected for best input, being representative, and potential contribution to the work.

The leader needs to start on time and be alert to seating positions. The leader can facilitate effectiveness by controlling compulsive talkers, drawing out silent members, protecting junior members, encouraging the clash of ideas, discouraging the clash of personalities, preventing the squashing of creative ideas, and closing on a note of achievement (Jay, 1982). The leader also needs to attend to careful meeting wrap-up. Summarizing after the meeting the group's accomplishments and verifying task assignments going forward are important leader responsibilities. Box 8-2 presents a checklist for leading effective meetings.

BOX 8-2 EFFECTIVE MEETINGS CHECKLIST FOR LEADERS

- Identify the purpose of the meeting:
  - Information dissemination
  - Opinion seeking
  - Problem solving
- Prepare an agenda and related materials
- Identify the category of each agenda item:
  - For information
  - For development
  - For implementation
  - For change in the system
- Set the size at four to seven people
- Carefully select members (based on skill and expertise)
- Distribute agenda (if needed) well in advance of meeting
- Start on time
- Listen carefully
- Process the interactions
- Control the flow of interactions
- Keep the meeting directed toward accomplishing objectives

Data from Jay, A. (1982). How to run a meeting. *Journal of Nursing Administration, 12*(1), 22-28.

Without thought and preparation, people go into a meeting focused on their own issues, biases, and perspectives; they may not be tuned into how to be productive within the meeting. However, even in a negative situation, individuals may choose to participate in a way that assists or enhances the process by making constructive suggestions about how things could be done better. This is an ideal situation—one to be encouraged, structured, and facilitated by the leader.

The duties of the chairperson include preparation of the physical environment. Comfort and convenience engineering is part of the leader's responsibility in terms of preparing an environment that is conducive to people being satisfied, productive, positive, and working together. The worst-case situation occurs when members have to sit in an uncomfortable chair in a room that is too cold, too hot, or too noisy because of construction; when members cannot hear or talk to other people; or when the technology does not work. Consider how to facilitate group work through hosting functions related to breaks, food, and beverages. It is human nature for members to be more relaxed and productive in comfortable surroundings.

As all nurses are pressured to do more with less under severe time and travel constraints, conducting meetings assisted by technology has become a major strategy. The prevalence and ease of technology such as Skype, internet-based meeting technology, real-time (synchronous) discussion boards, and related audio or video technology strategies are commonly employed. These become useful ways to save time by eliminating travel to an in-person site. However, specific problems may occur such as technology incompatibility, speed of transmission, connection failures, or other delays in transmission that result in people talking over one another or hesitancy in speaking, a lack of interpersonal modulation due to absence of body language, or a tendency to forget about people who are not actually in the room. Despite these known issues, nurses in the future will increasingly experience meetings assisted by technology.

Positive meeting dynamics are a shared responsibility between the leader and group members. A leader has a responsibility to prepare in advance for the meetings and provide participants support in their preparation. The participants' responsibility is to read and be prepared, show up on time, participate openly and positively, share responsibility for managing the group's dynamics, and attend to the task at hand. If needed for the meeting, the leader needs to prepare an agenda with handouts and background materials and distribute them to the members, giving the members time to read them. The better-prepared members are, the more they can participate, positively impact the quality of decisions, and feel gratified by their participation.

If the leader's preparation activities include generating an agenda or reviewing the status of agenda topics, questions to ask include the following:

- Where are we?
- What else needs to be done?
- What supporting materials might help the committee members?
- Who should be invited? Are there other experts or people from other departments that can contribute to this committee's process?

A leader who comes to the meeting and distributes a handout for a quick look before discussion, input, or a vote violates the participants' ability to think through what is being presented. This may be done as a tactic to avoid thorough deliberation by pressuring for the immediacy of a decision, but more often this behavior results from disorganization or lack of attention to leader responsibilities. It simply wastes everyone's time and increases participants' cynical view of meetings.

CONSTRUCTIVE GROUP MEMBERS

Savvy group leaders and members understand that people in groups assume a variety of roles. In a now classic work, Lancaster (1981) identified both group building roles and group maintenance roles as being a part of group interactions. Group building roles include *initiator, encourager, opinion giver, clarifier, listener,* and *summarizer.* Group maintenance roles include *tension reliever, compromiser, gatekeeper,* and *harmonizer.* The group building roles concentrate more on relationship functions than on task functions; the group maintenance roles focus more on task functions than on relationship functions.

Beyond the more general group roles are specific, structured roles that can help increase the effectiveness of the group. For example, one positive way to handle meetings is to identify a facilitator. Often this is the formal group leader or individual in a position of authority, but it does not have to be. If this is a true team, the role of facilitator may rotate among team members. In a committee, the facilitator is probably the committee chairperson. A facilitator conducts the meeting, ensuring that everyone has the opportunity to speak, maintains the focus of the meeting, and ensures that group dynamics remain positive.

Also needed is a group recorder. The task of taking minutes or summarizing discussion and decisions may need to be delegated to a clerical support person (if possible) if group members are averse to taking on the task of recording outcomes. However, a recorder who is a group member technically can do far more than just take minutes. This person should be in tune with the group processing and with the inputs and roles of group members and help keep the group on time. The recorder can provide feedback to the facilitator in terms of how to improve the process. One key tip is to construct a standardized meeting record (or minutes) form to facilitate the process and flow documentation. It is helpful to decide in advance the level of detail required in the minutes to avoid lengthy minutes and potentially unnecessary effort. One useful way to expedite group work is to use a laptop computer to directly enter draft minutes.

Finally, group members are needed. In this instance, *group members* means active participants, each with equal status in the meeting. The three components of facilitator, recorder, and group members contribute to the design of a positive working group. All can share in the basic group role functions as identified by Lancaster (1981).

DISRUPTIVE GROUP MEMBERS

Another role that the group leader assumes is that of process facilitator. The leader must observe group member actions and be prepared to control or redirect disruptive behaviors. Following are common types of disruptive group members that are encountered (Jacobs & Rosenthal, 1984), with strategies for the leader to use in managing dysfunctional members. In a mature team or highly effective group, although the leader has a responsibility to deal with these nonproductive behaviors, it is also a responsibility of other group members. If the issue is not addressed by a fellow group member, then the leader needs to be prepared to address this dysfunctional behavior.

However, it is very hierarchical thinking to leave this responsibility solely to the leader and doing so reinforces the formal hierarchy in the group.

Compulsive Talkers

A common disruptive behavior is seen in the individuals who are compulsive talker. Often their behavior can be modified. One suggestion is to thank them for their input and then ask to hear from others on that same topic before they are given the opportunity to speak again, as a way of guiding and opening up the meeting to be more effective. If this behavior continues to impact the group negatively and the individual is not receptive to this subtle feedback, meeting with the person after the group work and giving direct, constructive feedback about the negative impact of his or her behavior may be necessary. In a mature team, it would be expected that this issue would be brought up and dealt with by any team member.

Nontalkers

The nontalkers are the quiet ones. They can be asked to write down and submit their ideas or directly asked to share their thoughts on the matter at hand. Anyone in the group can specifically ask them questions to draw them out and thereby open up a broader range of group input. Preparing members in advance by posting the agenda or letting them know where their input will be crucial is also a way to include the nontalkers. Sometimes these people need time to think through their thoughts before they engage in a conversation, unlike their more spontaneous and verbal peers.

Interrupters

The interrupter must be addressed because this person is demonstrating a lack of self-control. The interrupter can be a problem in groups because the person who is interrupted feels violated and wonders why he or she is not given the courtesy of finishing a thought and having his or her full input considered. Any one in the group can halt the interruption, control, and redirect the interrupter. This can easily be accomplished by saying "Let's let Joan finish what she was saying."

Squashers

Squashers try to squash an idea before it is even developed. Suggestions about processes or procedures that have not been proven or even tried are much easier to criticize than are facts or opinions. Persons who are averse to change may have a litany of reasons why a potential solution would never work or why this proposed project simply cannot or should not happen. Often these are people who do not want to take a personal risk or undergo the personal effort of making a change, so it is easier to squash everything and maintain the status quo. Especially during brainstorming sessions, the leader must be alert to and have a method for containing the squasher. An easy way to influence this is to set the expectation at the beginning of the session by saying, for example, "For this exercise, please do not engage in analyzing or saying anything negative about the ideas thrown out until we have them all identified." There will be time later that allows dissecting and critiquing a new idea. Negative remarks adversely affect the level of creativity in any group.

Busybodies

Busybodies really are not committed to the group's work. They frequently arrive late, leave early, take personal messages on personal digital devices or cell phone calls during the meeting, spend the meeting time checking their e-mail or texting, rarely read the agenda, may be passive-aggressive, and simply want to show up for a few minutes for the purpose of appearances but do not contribute any effort. They are meeting their needs by showing up, but they are not contributing to the ongoing group work or the task at hand; nor are they invested in the group's goals. The leader needs to find creative mechanisms to engage the busybodies, perhaps by giving them a concrete assignment with accountability. If this does not work, they may need to be released from the group or placed in an advisory role.

MANAGING DISRUPTIVE BEHAVIOR IN GROUPS

The most useful way to affect these negative behaviors is to lead the group through the clarification of their working expectations. When group members have clearly identified what they need from each other to work together productively in a group setting, they have established the norms for acceptable and non-acceptable behavior.

The nurse leader can take an active role in structuring group work for positive processing and effective outcomes. It is important to control the flow to modulate disruptive group members without humiliating them. Another way is to structure positive and constructive group roles among members. Peer pressure is a powerful group behavior modification tactic only for group members for whom approval of the rest of the group is important. The leader's vision, enthusiasm, interpersonal relationship skills, and empowerment of followers all facilitate group effectiveness.

LEADERSHIP AND MANAGEMENT IMPLICATIONS

The leadership and management role in groups, teams, and committees includes strategically considering the work to be accomplished, determining the structure most suited to doing the work, putting the structure in place, and facilitating the work process. This requires a leader who understands the basic differences among work groups and teams, committees, and informal groups. The leader also must be able to think carefully about the work to be accomplished and determine whether it is primarily collective or individual work.

The leader's role includes inspiring members to participate, preparing critical questions, developing agendas and background materials, continually coaching the group for effective functioning, and guiding the long-range strategy. This is a planning, coordinative, and tracking function. Leaders and managers address questions such as the following: What is the task? What is the best way for this task to be accomplished? Is collective work involved? Do we need a team, or will a good work group or committee suffice? How many meetings will it take? How much effort is required? How can the tasks be divided? How can they be delegated?

In planning for meetings, a good leader puts in the time and effort to provide preliminary information and documents so that all members are prepared when they come to the meeting, they know what the issues are and they are familiar with the background of the task to be accomplished. The leader facilitates the group coming to some agreement about norms for decision making, length of discussion, when to vote or use consensus, and the process through which the task is completed efficiently and effectively. This is done as a deliberate agenda item that the leader initiates, opens for discussion, and brings to closure. Sometimes an off-site retreat is used to employ high-relationship and group-forming mechanisms. Nurses may find that the group leader role challenges them to plan, organize, coordinate, and evaluate the work of the group.

An effective leader understands that a process is involved in creating effective work teams, highly functioning groups, and committees. The process requires facilitation and a significant amount of coaching from the leader. The leader's style must fit the development stage of the group, with the leader providing more extensive structure and direction in early stages and minimal structure and direction in later stages. Coaching involves the transfer of responsibility to the team or the group. Skill, capability, and readiness of the group must be assessed.

CURRENT ISSUES AND TRENDS

Creating Healthy Workplaces

In recent years the creation of positive and healthy work environments has become a key issue throughout health care. Organizations continue to struggle with attracting and retaining highly qualified nurses, and today are concerned with finding employees who experience a high level of engagement in their work. Unless the workplace environment is positive and affirming, new practitioners may leave all too quickly (Manion, 2009).

A key aspect of a healthy work environment is the relationships one has with colleagues and co-workers. Groups and teams with healthy interpersonal relationships help foster a strong sense of connection and community among people (Manion, 2004; Manion & Bartholomew, 2003; Manion, 2009). Another aspect of a positive workplace related to groups is people's need to see problems solved and difficult aspects of work resolved so that conditions improve over time. Effective problem-solving groups are a crucial aspect of making this happen (Manion, 2009).

Collective Leadership Teams

Collective leadership teams are receiving renewed attention as the need for increased leadership capacity in our organizations reaches a crisis. The scope of the nurse manager's role is expanding to include responsibilities for multiple departments and increased strategic leadership demands. Collective leadership is an alternative that increases the capacity of an individual nurse manager struggling to effectively juggle multiple responsibilities. Sharing leadership responsibility is also a way to increase leadership capacity organizationally because it facilitates leadership ability developing at every level in the organization.

TeamSTEPPS

In the early 2000s, the Agency for Healthcare Research and Quality in partnership with the Department of Defense began working on a patient safety initiative that was directed at improving teamwork in health care settings. TeamSTEPPS was the result. The acronym stands for Team Strategies and Tools to Enhance Performance and Patient Safety. Launched in 2006, over 1500 organizations and 12,000 professionals have taken part in this initiative. The premise is quite simple—anyone who touches a patient (nurse, physician, pharmacist, technician) must work together to ensure the delivery of safe and high-quality care. It is aimed at helping health care professionals work together more effectively as a team. TeamSTEPPS teaches professionals to understand each other's roles and collaborate together to improve the quality and safety of the care they deliver.

This program is much like a boot camp in teamwork and interdependent relationships. It offers a host of innovations such as team huddles, patient handoff briefings, time-outs prior to commencement of a surgical procedure, the SBAR technique and so on. The website, *www.teamstepps.ahrq.gov*, offers an impressive number of resources.

Using Groups for Innovation

Groups and committees are used as vehicles to promote innovation and change in organizations. One example in nursing is the institution of research-based nursing practice by using a planned change process and a research utilization committee to facilitate the process of incorporating evidence-based practice in nursing. Groups that are skilled in creativity

RESEARCH NOTE

Source

Kalisch, B., Begeny, S., & Anderson, C. (2008). The effect of consistent nursing shifts on teamwork and continuity of care. *Journal of Nursing Administration, 38*(3), 132-137.

Purpose

To evaluate the effect of using a mixture of 4-, 6-, 8-, and 12-hour shifts on the nurses' teamwork and the continuity of care in a department.

Discussion

The authors designed a process that included the participation of staff on each department in a 210-bed community hospital. The staff members participated in role-specific focus groups where they felt free to share reasons for barriers to teamwork, engagement, and the quality of care without fear of repercussion. Using data from the focus groups, the researchers conducted a comprehensive root-cause analysis examining the barriers to teamwork and quality care. It was concluded that both teamwork and the quality of care for patients were being impacted by the multitude of shifts being used to staff the departments.

Working with the staff members, the research team shared the results and together they developed an intervention which required all nurses to work the 12-hour shifts. Postintervention results revealed that almost all of the nurses (98%) and assistive personnel (96%) stated that they felt teamwork and continuity of care were enhanced by working the same shifts. They

stated that the change had resulted in safer care and better team relationships.

A scheduling data analysis showed that 59 staff worked during a 1-week period before the change, whereas only 49 worked in the week following the intervention. The total number of work contacts (number of people working together on a shift) was reduced from 1319 in a week to 941 following the intervention. After the intervention (of all staff working 12-hour shifts) the number of reporting contacts dropped from 243 in a week to 187. After the intervention, the average number of individuals whom each staff member worked with was reduced by approximately 3 people.

Application to Practice

The findings of this project and research shed important light on a practical aspect of teamwork. Stability of the team is important. Continuity and quality of care are more likely to occur when there is stability of team members and straight shifts are one form of stability. Other research (Adams & Bond, 2003) found that nurses perceive their working relationships to be affected by instability. Team stability affects both the quality of care and the personal relationships and feelings of cohesion within the team.

The major premise behind the consistent scheduling that was examined in this study is that it is essential for high-quality teamwork. Perhaps it is no surprise that although initially there were staff members who resisted changing to the 12-hour shifts, with the benefits experienced, only one reported wanting to return to the previous mix of shifts.

techniques and understand the process of innovation can be very effective in disseminating and implementing evidence-based practice changes.

Other examples of innovation groups and committees are total quality management (TQM) initiatives, continuous quality improvement (CQI) methods such as TQM, and business techniques such as Lean, Six Sigma, and rapid-response teams. These techniques are used as ways of addressing problems related to cost and quality. Total quality management is a concept that comes from the work of Deming (Aguayo, 1990; Darr, 1989), who emphasized moving decision making to the worker level. The worker who is closest to actually producing the work is the one with the greatest knowledge and the greatest potential for solving production problems. Deming further recommended work group problem-solving teams.

Problems, in Deming's methodology, were defined as systems problems. By contrast, a common way of thinking about problems is to look for an individual to blame. The result of systems thinking is to capture the energy of teams to tackle systems problems.

Following the Institute of Medicine's report *To Err Is Human: Building a Safer Health System* (Kohn et al., 2000), the entire health care delivery system has been challenged to focus on systems problems and review and improve processes and procedures. This work is often done in groups and committees. The overall focus on quality has led to adoption of business management concepts such as Lean and Six Sigma. These are customer-focused and data-driven approaches to deriving best practices. The focus is on reducing process variation and then on improving process capability. Lean focuses on process speed; Six Sigma focuses on process quality.

Multidisciplinary Teams

Whether CQI, TQM, Lean, Six Sigma, or some related program, staff nurses are expected to participate more actively in multidisciplinary teams. In an organization that looks at problems as systems problems, the next step is to acknowledge that anyone involved in that part of the system needs to be engaged in solving the problem. Therefore coordinating client care and solving problems through interdisciplinary committees and groups with people of equal status is the strategy best suited to solving systems problems.

The basic strategy behind each of these systems-based approaches is to bring together interdisciplinary collaborative groups. This means that if there is a problem in client care, the physicians, nurses, ancillary staff, and any other direct caregivers are involved. They get together and collaborate about problems with the client care delivery system and discuss how these problems can be fixed. The facilitator does not have to be a content expert or the person with the most expertise in that problem area. In fact, having the most expertise in a problem area can actually be problematic when functioning as a facilitator because it becomes too tempting to take over the process. The individual's facilitation skills are crucially important.

Establishing equality among peers regardless of status and using expertise and responsibility result in a different way of looking at work, which has implications in terms of how nursing practice may change. It also means nurses are going to continue to be involved more substantially in groups, committees, and teams. Multidisciplinary teams are not just for problem solving and process improvement. The current pace and complexity of the world today also demands that research approaches be redefined and new multiple disciplinary partnerships formed (Weaver, 2008). In the research arena, "unidisciplinary research can become stale or predictable and suffer a crisis of ideas, viewing a problem from multiple disciplines" can prevent this (Weaver, 2008, p. 108). Although the principles of

CASE STUDY

A Patient Services Leadership Team

In one midsize community hospital a patient services leadership team was created. The members were the directors of the various nursing divisions, the clinical laboratory, medical imaging, respiratory therapy, pharmacy, and perioperative services. This team established their purpose statement, identified their values and developed a Code of Conduct that outlined their behavioral expectations of each other. Although these people had long worked together, this approach with a shared leadership responsibility for the clinical services was new to them.

Ellen, the director of the laboratory agreed to be the team's first formal leader. One of the biggest challenges facing the team was the need to dramatically and quickly improve the patient satisfaction scores throughout the organization. This was the underlying primary reason for the formation of this team. In the past, this would have been identified as a responsibility of the individual directors and managers, and primarily those in nursing. However, there was serious concern about the quality of care that these low patient satisfaction scores represented and as a result this team was assigned the leadership responsibility for intervening in a positive way to raise the scores. Although the work of the team is only briefly presented here, their approach demonstrates the concept of collective leadership and joint or mutual accountability.

One of the strategies these leaders developed was related to mentoring the inpatient care units where the scores were most problematic. They decided that each team member would accept responsibility for mentoring the staff of a specific in-patient area. Ellen, as the director of the laboratory, for example, agreed to mentor one particularly challenging patient care unit that had recently lost their manager. Patient satisfaction scores had plummeted along with the morale of the staff. Ellen began making rounds in the department, helping the nursing staff troubleshoot patient and family issues, and coaching them in service recovery when there were problems. The results were surprisingly impressive. Not only did the patient satisfaction scores rise, but so did employee morale.

Ellen benefited as well. Her leadership capacity deepened significantly, and she became recognized and sought after for attributes that had not been apparent in her work as laboratory director. It was quite remarkable to see the results when these team members accepted joint accountability for something that in the past had been the accountability of individuals. It was also striking that Ellen was so well accepted by the nursing staff when previously a silo mentality would have prevented the formation of this type of coaching relationship between members of two different disciplines.

team building already discussed are applicable to these multiple discipline research groups, there are some additional challenges. These teams bring together people with different conceptual frameworks, language, methodologies and research interests. It takes skilled team leadership and followership to capitalize on team strengths to create an effective, efficient and highly productive team that endures over time.

Involving members in change and solving shared problems helps both members and management. Members benefit because they are involved in what affects their work. Management benefits because involvement tends to reduce resistance and increase ownership of the change or solution. The health care delivery system benefits as high-performing teams tackle and solve systems problems and improve patient safety.

CRITICAL THINKING EXERCISE

Organize into a small group; then select a leader. Take a few minutes to do this, and then select or appoint a process recorder. Here is your assignment:

The leader is a nurse manager at Our Lady of Great Hope Community Hospital. She has been asked to lead a task force to evaluate the effectiveness of the nursing department committee structure. The task force has been asked to create a methodology for conducting the evaluation and then making recommendations for streamlining the current structure, consolidating committees that overlap, and improving the effectiveness of the committees. The leader must now lead your group to develop a plan while preserving a sense of teamwork. The process recorder is to prepare a summary of the group's work and report as requested.

1. Observe the process the group uses to select its own leader. Did anyone try to avoid selection? Was someone an enthusiastic volunteer? How long did the process take? Were the selection criteria discussed? What were the selection criteria?
2. What method was used to select/appoint a process recorder? What power strategy was used to make this decision?
3. What is the problem identified in the task?
4. What did the group leader do to handle the situation?
5. What should the group leader do to handle the situation?
6. How did group members respond to the task?
7. What leadership and management strategies might be effective?
8. What could the leader and followers consider changing in the situation?
9. How did group members feel about what happened?

Follow up this exercise with one that tackles a similar problem: this time the leader has just been informed of a serious morale issue in the department. A few very vocal, negative staff members are intimidating and using bullying tactics to coerce their co-workers in uncomfortable ways. No one wants to speak up and everyone thinks it's the manager's responsibility to fix the problem. This group of charge nurses and the nurse manager need to work together to develop a plan for dealing with this negative behavior.

Delegation

Diane L. Huber

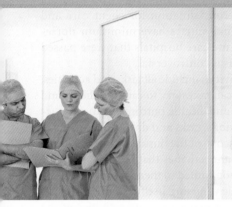

evolve WEBSITE

http://evolve.elsevier.com/Huber/leadership/

Delegation is a fundamental aspect of every nurse's job. The effective delegation of work to others is essential in every type of health care setting and organization. Effective delegation skills also are important for managers whose function is to get work done through the efforts of others. For most nursing jobs, the zone of responsibility exceeds one person's ability to complete all the tasks (Figure 9-1). This is especially true for the care coordination aspects of nursing care management. Nurses need to delegate parts of nursing care delivery to others because, at some point, it becomes impossible to do it all alone.

In the 1800's, delegation was defined by Florence Nightingale (1859) as a critical skill: "But then again to look at all these things yourself does not mean to do them yourself... But can you not insure that it is done when not done by yourself?" (p. 17). Nurses delegate to nurses and paraprofessionals in the health care environment, whether to students, licensed practical nurses/licensed vocational nurses (LPNs/LVNs), orderlies or technicians, corpsmen, medication assistants-certified, nursing assistants, or some other form of nurse extender.

Photo used with permission from Photos.com.

Weydt (2010) noted that nurses have to understand what patients and families need, then engage the right caregivers in the plan of care to achieve outcomes. Meeting the public's increasing demand for quality health care that is both accessible and affordable has created a demand for health care providers and maximized the stress on every health care worker. As a result, the identification of which tasks are appropriate to nursing, which of these tasks can be delegated, and to whom they can be delegated is imperative. Delegation issues have become connected to issues of work overload, safety and quality of care, mix of staff, job security and turf, and nurses' job satisfaction. It has been proposed that delegation of non-nursing tasks also helps reduce health care costs by making more efficient use of nursing time and the facility's resources (Fisher, 2000). Delegation is at the fulcrum of quality and cost concerns.

DEFINITIONS

The American Nurses Association (ANA) and the National Council of State Boards of Nursing (NCSBN) in their *Joint Statement on Delegation* (NCSBN, 2006)

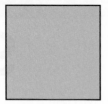

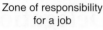

Zone of responsibility
for a job

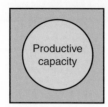

Zone of responsibility
encompassing a less-
than-equal "capacity"

FIGURE 9-1 Zones of responsibility.

defined **delegation in nursing** as "the process for a nurse to direct another person to perform nursing tasks and activities" (p. 1). The ANA described this as the nurse transferring responsibility, whereas the NCSBN called this the transferring of authority. The goal of delegation is workload distribution. It relies on trust. The **delegator** is the person—the RN or LPN/LVN—making the delegation. The **delegate** is the person receiving the delegation. **Supervision** is defined as the provision of guidance or oversight of a delegated nursing task. The availability of the supervising nurse occurs through various means of written and verbal communication. **Assignment** is "the distribution of work that each staff member is responsible for during a given work period" (NCSBN, 2006, p. 1).

The ANA (2005) defined **unlicensed assistive personnel** (UAP) as individuals who are trained to function in an assistive role to the registered professional nurse in the provision of patient/client care activities as delegated by and under the supervision of the nurse. In the past, a nurse extender meant a nursing assistant or a corpsman. A nurse extender is an ancillary person trained to perform some basic client care tasks who may have been given a client assignment or related tasks. The current term is nursing assistive personnel (NAP).

By definition, assistive personnel work under RN/LPN/LVN supervision. The danger is that organizations may deploy them instead of staffing an adequate number of RNs for the care needs and the extra duties of personnel supervision.

A basic distinction is whether the nurse extender performs direct client care. The definition of what assistive personnel can and cannot do is not exclusive and varies by state because of state-specific licensure laws. Alterations in the skill-mix percentage of RNs to assistive personnel occur over time. Nurses

argue that inadequate staffing ratios can create a potentially dangerous situation for client care and safety. In California, nurses have minimum nurse-client ratios in acute care hospitals that were passed in legislation. This is controversial.

Client care activities include all tasks and activities, mental and physical, necessary to care for clients and produce nursing and health outcomes. Nursing activities involve actions, tasks and direct client contact, as well as the full scope of the nursing process. The act of delegating certain activities that are performed by nurses—but are not limited to them—does not create a situation in which nursing itself and the responsibility for it are delegated away. Core activities of the nursing process require specialized knowledge and judgment that only the nurse has.

BACKGROUND

Delegation of care originated from physician responsibilities being delegated to nurses. Nurses began to assume more and more tasks deemed as nursing care up to the point that they could not complete them all in the limited time frame. Thus phlebotomists, respiratory therapists, physical therapists, and NAP emerged to help provide more comprehensive care. The establishment of the health care team formed around these specialists needing to coordinate work. With this work structure, the need to delegate work arose.

The NCSBN has developed a number of tools relating to delegation and the roles of licensed nurses and assistive personnel which have been collected into the document *Working with Others: A Position Paper* (NCSBN, 2005). Key concepts are presented. The NCSBN's position is presented. The delegation decision making process is presented. There are two helpful decision trees (visual flow charts): delegation to nursing assistive personnel (pp. 11-12) and accepting assignment to supervise unlicensed assistive personnel (pp. 16-17). There is a state-by-state review of statutes and rules, a summary of multiple organizations' position statements, definitions, and a literature/case law review.

PROCESS OF DELEGATION

Delegation is a decision-making process that requires skillful nurse judgment. The decision to delegate should incorporate critical thinking and sound

Date _____

Task outcome _____

Task steps _____

Task location _____

Delegator _____

Delegate _____

Time frame _____

Decision responsibility/authority _____

Next communication _____

Other _____

FIGURE 9-2 Delegation tracking form.

clinical decision making. The process outlined by the NCSBN (2005) starts with a preparation phase and then has a 4-step process phase. The steps are (1) assess and plan, (2) communication, (3) surveillance and supervision, and (4) evaluation and feedback.

In most cases, it is recommended that the nurse delegator and the delegate agree on the task, circumstances, and time frame and then arrange for feedback in which the delegate reports or the delegator evaluates progress toward completion of the task. One way to make certain that both delegator and delegate understand what the task is and how to complete it effectively is to follow up a verbal directive with written instructions so that each person can refer to them later. Figure 9-2 displays a sample delegation tracking form that can be generated by NAP to give to the nurse. As a vehicle for clear communication and verification of expectations and consensus, this form can be modified to be specific to each unit. The task should specify a time frame in which the entire task is to be completed. The decision to delegate needs to be consistent with the nursing process. Thus the nurse needs to ensure appropriate assessment, nursing diagnosis, planning, implementation, and evaluation in a continuous process.

Decisions to delegate need to be carefully and thoroughly evaluated. A reasonable first decision rule is to be able to delegate the care of clients whose care requirements are routine and standard. Because care is complex and variable, the competency of the delegate is critical. Once it is assessed that the person to be delegated to has the minimum competencies required for safe care and if the outcomes of care are relatively predictable, delegation is considered safe. If the client's reaction to illness and hospitalization is not threatening to his or her mental health or sense of self, it also is relatively safe to assume that this care can be delegated to NAP. For example, a client experiencing an acute episode of hypertension would require the RN as opposed to NAP to monitor the vital signs.

In making a decision to delegate nursing tasks, the following five factors can be assessed (American Association of Critical Care Nurses [AACN], 2004):

1. *Potential for Harm:* The nurse must determine how much risk the activity carries for an individual patient.

2. *Complexity of the Task:* The more complex the activity, the less desirable it is to delegate. Only an RN should perform activities requiring complex psychomotor skills and expert nursing assessment and judgment.

3. *Amount of Problem Solving and Innovation Required:* If an uncomplicated activity requires special attention, adaptation, or an innovative approach for a particular patient, it should not be delegated.

4. *Unpredictability of Outcome:* When a patient's response to the activity is unknown or unpredictable (depending on how stable the patient is), it is not advisable to delegate that activity.

5. *Level of Patient Interaction:* Will delegation of a particular activity increase or decrease the amount of time the RN can spend with the patient and patient's family? Every time a nursing activity is delegated or one or more additional caregivers become involved, a patient's stress level may increase and the nurse's opportunity to develop a trusting relationship is diminished.

The over-arching determinant for the decision to delegate is the legal scope of delegation as set forth in the state's nurse practice act. With the qualifications of both the delegator and the delegate as a baseline in place, the licensed nurse enters the continuous process of delegation decision making. The situation is assessed, and a plan for specific task delegation is established, considering patient needs, available resources, and patient safety. The nurse needs to ensure accountability for the acts and process of delegation. This includes supervision of the performance of the entire task, any necessary intervention, and evaluation of the task performance and the delegation itself.

The joint ANA and NCSBN (2006) statement identified nine principles of delegation specific to the RN, including the following:

- The RN may delegate elements of care but does not delegate the nursing process itself.
- The RN has the duty to answer for personal actions relating to the nursing process.
- The RN takes into account the knowledge and skill of any individual to whom the RN may delegate elements of care.

The decision of whether to delegate or assign is based on the RN's judgment concerning the condition of the patient, the competence of all members of the nursing team, and the degree of supervision that will be required of the RN if an element of care is delegated.

The RN uses critical thinking and professional judgment when following The Five Rights of Delegation promulgated by the NCSBN (1995) as follows:

1. Right Task (element of care)
2. Right Circumstance
3. Right Person
4. Right Direction/Communication
5. Right Supervision and Evaluation

When determining the *right task* (element of care) to delegate, the nurse determines whether the element of care falls within the guidelines of established agency policies and procedures, the ANA Code of Ethics, and legal regulations for practice. The nurse then must consider whether the element of care can be delegated to any other staff members.

The *right circumstance* to perform the element of care indicates the delegate has the available resources, equipment, safe environment, and supervision to complete the task correctly.

The *right person* has the education and competency to perform the element of care. The right delegate, then, is legally acceptable to complete the element of care.

The *right direction/communication* of delegated elements of care will be a clear, concise description of the task, including its objective, limits, and expectations. The nurse allows for clarification without the fear of repercussions.

The *right supervision* of an element of care includes appropriate monitoring, intervention, evaluation, and feedback as deemed necessary. A process should be in place for the delegate to report to the RN both that the task was completed and the client's response.

In addition to the five rights, the following three organizational principles are to be considered:

1. The RN acknowledges that there is a relational aspect to delegation and that communication is culturally appropriate and the person receiving the communication is treated respectfully.
2. Chief nursing officers are accountable for establishing systems to assess, monitor, verify, and communicate ongoing competence requirements in areas related to delegation, for both RNs and delegates.
3. RNs monitor organizational policies, procedures, and position descriptions to ensure that the nurse practice act is not violated, working with the state board of nursing if necessary.

The five rights can quickly help analyze whether a delegation decision will most likely result in a safe outcome. To facilitate the delegation process in a way that will ensure the client's personal health needs are addressed and the nurse's professional goals are achieved, effective communication techniques must be used (Marthaler, 2003). Box 9-1 outlines a personal checklist for the delegator to use for self-evaluation.

Delegation Facets

True delegation is real to the delegate. Delegators let delegates go on their own but only after instilling in them the highest standards of performance and

BOX 9-1   DELEGATOR'S CHECKLIST

- Develop a good attitude.
- Decide what to delegate.
- Select the right person.
- Communicate responsibilities.
- Grant authority.
- Provide support.
- Monitor the delegation.
- Evaluate.

Data from Nelson, R. (1994). *Empowering employees through delegation*. Burr Ridge, IL: Richard D. Irwin.

adherence to a shared vision. The delegate then functions within the standards set by the delegator, who has given authority to do the job, make independent decisions, and be responsible for seeing that the job is done well. True delegation trust is earned over time. Effective delegation requires that the delegate have the authority to accompany the responsibility. The delegator monitors the element of care completion and is alert for variances or other problems.

The essence of the element of care being delegated is often overlooked. Recognition of the potential vulnerability of the client, and thus the presence of an inherently moral element to health care practice, has raised concerns in relation to proper moral regard and respect for clients (Niven & Scott, 2003). This means that nursing judgment about which elements of care are to be delegated requires consideration of the client's unique individual needs at that point in time. For example, obtaining vital signs on a client who is dying may be a reasonable delegation to NAP. However, because a nurse has spent much time explaining the process of the "do-not-resuscitate" status to the family, a trusting relationship has been established. The client's or family members' preferences for treatment/care need to be considered in delegating care activities.

Safety is a major facet of delegation, addressed over the years by The Joint Commission's (TJC) Hospital National Patient Safety Goals. For example, The Joint Commission's 2007 Patient Safety Goal Requirement 2E, *Implement a standardized approach to "hand-off" communications* (TJC, 2007), is applicable to delegation. Its provisions include the opportunity to ask and respond to questions. This assists in determining whether delegation can safely occur when a responsible delegator is not physically present.

The Joint Commission's (2013) National Patient Safety Goal to maintain and communicate accurate patient medication information (NPSG.03.06.01) is an example of an effort to collect, reconcile, and communicate medication use to enhance patient safety. It speaks to the complexity and fluidity of care and how discrepancies in communication affect safety, especially in the context of multidisciplinary and team-based care systems where gaps can occur.

Communication is a major factor in missed care results of delegation. Research has shown no relationship between leadership style and delegation confidence, although there is an interaction between educational preparation and clinical nursing experience (Saccomano & Pinto-Zipp, 2011). There is, however, a bundle of best practices for delegation and supervision skills that includes planning assignments, including NAPs in shift handoffs and rounding, check-in points, evaluation of organizational practices about delegation and supervision, and coaching and mentoring (Gravlin & Bittner, 2010; Hansten & Jackson, 2009).

Delegation to unlicensed staff is common in long-term care (LTC) and assisted living settings. Thus delegation is a major strategy for care delivery. UAPs can be certified nursing assistants, personal care workers, or other types of unlicensed personnel. Lightfoot (2011) outlined the following eight principles for RN delegation:

1. Delegate tasks only within the RN's scope of practice, expertise and knowledge
2. Assess the patient's condition and stability
3. Only delegate tasks that the UAP is competent to perform and within his/her educational preparation/ability
4. Provide direction and assistance
5. Do not delegate tasks requiring complex nursing skill/judgment
6. Supervise, observe, and monitor UAPs
7. Evaluate the effectiveness of the delegated task
8. Document the delegation.

DELEGATION PITFALLS AND SOLUTIONS

Although it is in everyone's best interest to delegate, the process may be undermined from within the health care setting. Delegation suggests that work is being moved from one member of the primary health care team to another in a downward direction (Richards et al., 2000). As a result, the nurse most commonly delegates to NAP. The RN and NAP will naturally have psychological responses to delegation. The NAP sometimes resent the nurse delegating elements of care that could be completed by the nurse. On the other hand, the nurse may find it difficult to let go of control. When elements of care are delegated, strong feelings and reactions occur, including the nurse's desire to keep control. At times, the nurse reclaims some of the delegated responsibility. Nothing is more demoralizing for delegates than to discover that the delegator has undercut their responsibility. Nurses who are novice or insecure or need to feel indispensable are most likely to resist delegation or to "renege" on it later. Their motto is "If you want a job done right, you have to do it yourself." Box 9-2 displays reasons for reluctance to delegate.

When called on to delegate something important, nurses may suddenly discover that, for some reason, they do not trust their co-workers quite as much as they thought they did. How can work be delegated to people if they are not trusted? On the other hand, how can NAP earn the trust of the nurse who does not delegate to them? This is a real dilemma, facing both delegator and delegate. The absence of trust by the delegator is based on one of the most powerful of all feelings: fear. This fear is very real for the nurse, especially when it involves a loss of control and their license.

An emotional reality surrounds delegation. Delegation inevitably involves risk. Ignorance of the competencies or the scope of practice of health care team members can cause detrimental outcomes. Likewise, over-delegating elements of care also involves risk but, more important, is dangerous (e.g., allowing a nursing assistant in nursing school to start an intravenous line or asking an LPN/LVN to give discharge instructions because you are good friends and are pressed for time). Delegating an element of care that is completed incorrectly translates into potentially harming a patient and possibly incurring a lawsuit.

Conversely, successful delegation of an element of care may be threatening to a nurse's self-esteem or seen as a nurse's failure to personally accomplish work. This is a natural emotion (e.g., the fear that a delegate might surpass the nurse in ability or prestige or mess up and reflect poorly on the delegator), especially for individuals in a new role or job such as a new nurse manager or graduate nurse. The ability to delegate appropriately should be viewed as an achievement and be rewarded, not observed as a weakness or laziness.

In nursing, conventional wisdom and anecdotal experiences indicate how difficult it can be for nurses to delegate effectively. In fact, some nurses may find themselves unable to delegate. Historically, the RN was responsible for providing most of the direct client care, and total patient care delivery models are still in use. Nurses in critical care areas continue to care for patients in this manner. Nurses can become used to providing care themselves and may not learn how to delegate. Graduate nurses typically have had limited experience delegating in nursing school, and they have been delivering direct client care the majority of their time in the clinical arena. Schools of nursing provide theory in delegation and management of patients but may not have requirements for application of these to vital competencies of patient care.

Under-delegation can be the result of a lack of motivation to delegate. Some nurses may find that they need to delegate, direct, and supervise others, yet they have no power over the rewards and disciplinary action that motivate cooperation. The new graduate nurse may have a tendency to under-delegate to seek recognition from co-workers that all of his or her tasks were completed by his or her own personal effort. Unfortunately, the new graduate may then be reprimanded for excessive overtime. Nurses may be reluctant to delegate because they feel that they need to complete the tasks themselves, lack the ability to

---

BOX 9-2   DELEGATION RELUCTANCE

- The "I can do it better myself" fallacy trap
- Lack of ability to direct
- Lack of confidence in subordinates
- Lack of confidence in self
- Aversion to taking a risk
- Need to feel indispensable and difficulty letting go
- Fear of losing authority or personal satisfaction

Data from *Delegating* (videotape). (1981). Del Mar, CA: McGraw-Hill; and Poteet, G. (1989). Nursing administrators and delegation. *Nursing Administration Quarterly, 13*(3), 23-32.

direct, lack confidence in subordinates and self, have an aversion to taking a risk, have a fear of letting go, and have a fear of losing authority or personal job satisfaction (Poteet, 1989).

At times, delegates attempt to avoid delegation by fostering a myth that delegators are so indispensable that they need to do the work themselves. The delegates can actively foster the illusion of the delegator's indispensability. Sometimes this belief is genuine, but it may instead be a way for delegates to avoid being delegated to or accepting more responsibility. Delegates may fear criticism regarding mistakes because they lack confidence in their own abilities. Delegates' most common complaint is that they already have more work than they can handle, when in fact, the delegated elements of care are not extra work but a part of their job description. In addition, they may not have confidence in their own abilities. This can be a matter of reminding delegates that they do have the necessary skills and abilities, especially if they would push themselves a little. The delegator may feel that the delegates do have the job maturity, knowledge, and ability to handle the task, but the delegates may feel that positive incentives are not present. From the NAP's perspective, why should they take on something extra or put in more effort if they perceive that they are not going to be rewarded? Box 9-3 outlines reasons why delegates avoid delegation responsibilities.

At times a nurse delegator can, in effect, never relinquish authority by hovering after an element of care has been delegated. Hovering, or "breathing down somebody's neck," usually conveys a feeling of distrust. This is sometimes called micromanaging when the delegator keeps stepping in and taking over. This behavior may lead to the delegate feeling that he or she really *does* lack ability. Delegation is not meant to intimidate or isolate the delegator or delegate. Having both individuals regard the goal of delegating as being to provide client-centered care in the most efficient way is the optimal delegation approach. Delegating appropriate tasks to the right person, who can complete the task in an established time frame, will allow care to be completed in a timely manner. Useful strategies are to rotate duties to prevent burnout and capitalize on special expertise (e.g., when a nurse is "good" at starting IVs or caring for disoriented patients). Equally important, delegation can stimulate interest in a nursing career, maintain competencies, spark new interests, and prevent monotony.

Solutions to pitfalls of delegation are straightforward. When individuals are shown respect, they experience a sense of worthiness, of being seen and heard (Rushton, 2007). Licensed nurses and NAPs experience an event as positive when they receive feedback and encouragement after delegation (Anthony et al., 2000). Recognizing the importance of the process of supervision and its implications for educational opportunities that focus on delegation competencies is essential for RNs. Peer staff and nurse managers can be consulted regarding delegating nursing activities to ensure accuracy. Detailed and specific activities need to be communicated to the delegate. By observing good performance, the RN will gain trust and confidence in NAP's abilities. In short, delegation gains empowerment over the care provided to clients. Ultimately, the chief nursing officer is accountable for delegation standard compliance.

LEGAL ASPECTS OF DELEGATION AND SUPERVISION

Nurses are accountable for following their state nurse practice act, standards of professional practice, policies of the health care organization, and ethical-legal models of behavior (Marthaler, 2003). Each state's governmental agency is the state board of nursing, the majority of whose governing board members are licensed practical/vocational and registered nurses who are empowered to license and/or regulate nursing practice (NCSBN, 2012). When this body interprets the law, the formal interpretations become

---

BOX 9-3	WHY DELEGATES AVOID RESPONSIBILITIES

- Fear criticism for mistakes
- Lack necessary information and resources to do a good job
- Overwhelming workload
- Lack self-confidence regarding ability to successfully delegate
- Positive incentives may not be sufficient motivators
- Delegator's personality and preferences may interfere with the delegation process
- Easier to seek answers from the nurse than to decide on their own how to deal with problems

administrative rules that have the force of law. State nurse practice acts and their official interpretations constitute a body of rules, codified within the legal regulatory system, that govern nursing practice and provide direction about delegation and supervision. The American Nurses Association (ANA) and each state's nurses association are the bodies that speak for the profession of nursing to define and guide the professional practice of nursing through definitions, standards of practice, and statements about delegation and supervision. Most state nurse practice acts contain language that allows registered nurses to delegate. The bottom line is that patients vary in needs, and those needs can be met by various providers of care. Ensuring that needs match the competency of the provider can ensure proper delegation and good patient care.

Standards of care are used to determine whether the minimum level of care has been delivered. When a nurse deviates from the internal standards of care of an organization, the nurse can be liable for malpractice or negligence.

Accountability is being obligated to answer for one's acts, including the act of supervision. The RN is expected to recognize and understand the legal implications of accountability by knowing what accountability is and what it means in terms of nursing practice. Accountability includes acts of supervision, among other things. In a legal sense, *supervision* means personally observing a function or activity, providing leadership in the process of nursing care, delegating functions or activities while retaining the accountability, and evaluating or determining that nursing care being provided is adequate and delivered appropriately.

Delegation is considered to be part of the nurse's role. Nurses delegate, and they are delegated to. The nurse delegator is accountable to assess the situation and accountable for the decision to delegate. When a nurse delegates, the task must be performed in accordance with established standards of practice, policies, and procedures (NCSBN, 2005). The nurse is ultimately accountable for the appropriateness and supervision of the delegated tasks. Thus the nurse delegator may incur liability if found negligent in the process of delegating and supervising. The delegate is accountable for accepting the delegation and for the actions in carrying out the delegated tasks (Box 9-4). Therefore

---

BOX 9-4   WHO HAS ACCOUNTABILITY?

Delegator
- Own acts
- Acts of delegation
- Acts of supervision
- Assessment of the situation
- Follow-up
- Intervention
- Corrective action

Delegate
- Own acts
- Accepting the delegation
- Appropriate notification and reporting
- Accomplishing the task

---

both the delegator and delegate share accountability. The nurse is accountable for supervision, follow-up, intervention, and corrective action in the event of an error. Assessment, evaluation, and nursing judgment should not be delegated; tasks and procedures may be delegated. Although others may suggest which acts to delegate, the individual nurse ultimately decides the appropriateness of delegation in a specific situation (NCSBN, 2005).

Delegating requires skillful written and verbal communication to avoid liability. If an activity is not documented, it is considered that it was not done. Clear documentation of assignments and additional clarification of the delegated tasks for each health care team member are required when delegating. The nurse's responsibility is to keep current with updates in the literature and guideline changes in the standards of care of delegation. The institution is responsible for informing nurses of all changes in policy through e-mail, memos, in-services, or staff meetings.

LEADERSHIP AND MANAGEMENT IMPLICATIONS

The nurse has an obligation or duty to act in the event of a breakdown in client care wherever in the chain that breakdown occurs. This means that the nurse is never permitted under law to passively observe substandard care. Delegation and supervision are key areas in which such issues may arise. The most common situation is of a fellow nurse or other health care provider demonstrably or clearly failing to provide the appropriate care to clients. Substandard care also may come about when a health care agency fails to exercise its corporate duty in providing sufficient numbers of RNs with appropriate delegation and supervision skills to ensure quality care. In the event the health care agency is compromising care, the nurse will initiate an assessment of how much client safety is being compromised. If there is clear actual or potential harm, the nurse must act directly. If the situation is ambiguous, such as an ethical issue, then the nurse must take some action appropriate to the circumstance. For example, this may be reported to the immediate superior, or the nurse may refuse to participate if that is appropriate. Ethical concerns may be referred to the Ethics Committee.

Legal and ethical issues surround the tensions and trade-offs between quality and cost. For example, what constitutes an "unsafe" level of nurse staffing is not clear. Nurses face uncomfortable situations when deciding between labor budget pressures and staffing for clients' care needs. At what point does the nurse take action to report "unsafe" staffing levels? What action strategies are effective? Are there whistleblower protections? It is not uncommon for the nurse to find conflicts between an employer's expectations and the nursing standards of care, resulting in problems such as having insufficient time or staffing to adhere to the standards taught in nursing school or receiving poor evaluations for taking too long to render care (Martin & Cain, 2003).

Clearly, client safety and the obligation to do no harm are fundamental starting points. The nurse can analyze the situation and decide on a strategy. A framework for ethical analysis can be chosen to help clarify values and ethical choices. A legal analysis can be done to assess whether the elements of a malpractice claim appear to be in evidence: duty, breach of duty, proximate cause, and damages. Other assessments can be done by consulting organizational policies and standards, the state's nurse practice act and administrative rulings from the board of nursing, ANA's code of ethics and standards of practice, and standards and guidelines of specialty organizations. A clear legal duty to act is more urgent than is a question of ethics. Through reasoned investigation and analysis of the situation, the nurse then decides whether to act immediately, investigate further, document, report, or

analyze the situation for future decision making. The standards of "reasonable," "prudent," and "good faith" form the foundations for legal and ethical decision-making strategies. Ultimately, the chief nursing officer is accountable for ensuring patient safety standards are met (NCSBN and ANA Joint Statement, 2006).

Nurses at all levels should be clear regarding their legal accountability when delegating. Questions regarding situations that may occur include these: What is my responsibility if a student errs or is negligent in caring for my client? What are the legal parameters of delegating to one of the UAP who has had only 2 weeks of training? What can I delegate and to whom?

Managers and administrators know the quality of care delivered to clients can be affected by the type of working relationships that exist between RNs and NAP (Potter & Grant, 2004). Delegation is a critical yet very difficult leadership and management skill. All nurses need to build a competency in delegation.

Leader behaviors for delegation and supervision include being around, being available, and helping the delegate through the task actions and decisions. Coaching actions of delegation are expected. Providing guidance and leadership in the development of the nurse's ability to delegate is an important aspect of RN skill building. Delegation is a managerial technique that helps people build skills and confidence. It is hard work and may not come naturally. Mentored guidance and leadership in building the skills related to delegation enhance individuals and build high-performing teams. This makes the facility accountable for delegation through the allocation of resources to allow for adequate staffing so registered nurses can delegate effectively.

Nursing practice in community health or home health care settings may include supervision and delegation of tasks off-site. The importance of the skills involved in assessing the competencies of UAP cannot be overestimated (McIntosh, 2003). Careful assessment, regular visits, and complete documentation are used when delegating in these settings (Barter & Furmidge, 1994). Boards of Nursing are concerned with which activities can be delegated to UAP under licensing laws (Zolnierek, 2011).

Certain aspects of managerial work should never be delegated. These are discipline, praise, recognition, and morale issues. Sending others to do the manager's corrective directing is a counterproductive approach to a problem requiring attention. When a problem needs to be addressed in a direct, calm, unemotional, and fact-finding/clarifying approach, the manager is the best person to handle the situation. In addition, the manager should handle the discipline of employees. The direct managerial intervention of discipline maintains a climate within the work group, communicates a message, and shows discharge of duty. For example, if there is an area in which client care is not bringing about quality results or if there is some problem with regard to the delivery of client care, the manager needs to be directly active in the resolution of the problem. At the same time, praise and recognition are powerful motivators if given by managers and supervisors.

As delegation and assigning nursing care evolves, potential problems can be assessed. The Institute for Healthcare Improvement (2008) recommended health care facilities use Failure Modes and Effects Analysis (FMEA). FMEA is a systematic, proactive method for evaluating a process to identify where and how care delivery might fail and to assess the relative impact of different failures so that the parts of the process that are most in need of change can be identified. FMEA includes review of the following:

- Steps in the process
- Failure modes (What could go wrong?)
- Failure causes (Why would the failure happen?)
- Failure effects (What would be the consequences of each failure?)

Teams use FMEA to evaluate processes for possible failures and to prevent them by correcting the processes proactively rather than reacting to adverse events after failures have occurred. This emphasis on prevention may reduce risk of harm to both patients and staff. FMEA is particularly useful in evaluating a new process before implementation and in assessing the impact of a proposed change to an existing process. It is a formal strategy useful for continual improvements of care delegation processes.

CURRENT ISSUES AND TRENDS

Delegation of care continues to evolve within health care teams from professional to professional and from the nurse to NAP. All jobs in the health care team have been expanded. At the same time, financial pressures related to reimbursement have hampered health care facilities' ability to generate sufficient funds to offset costs related to staffing patterns. Is delegation the result of expanded roles? Or was the expanded role the result of delegation?

Increasing demands for nursing care and not having enough nurses to meet the demand have created troubled times and add constraints to the number of patients a nurse can care for (Hudspeth, 2007). The ANA's *Joint Statement on Maintaining Professional and Legal Standards During a Shortage of Nursing Personnel* (ANA, 1992) noted that during a time of RN shortage, there is a predictable trend to deregulate, remove, or reduce barriers to entry into the marketplace and substitute less-prepared persons for expediency purposes. Such shifts create serious allied issues related to delegation and supervision for RNs as they attempt to work in environments of fewer RNs and more non-RN personnel.

The end of the 1990s saw economic forces and health care costs come to an intersection. Changes in the health care system led to changes in the numbers and types of personnel who deliver direct care to clients (Potter & Grant, 2004). A decrease in the number of licensed caregivers and an increase in the number of UAP occurred. Hospitals had restructured, redesigned, and downsized RNs without paying attention to evidence-based practice changes or known effects on delegation, supervision, and client safety. Although economic and efficiency concerns may prompt providers to utilize unlicensed assistive personnel, the American Nephrology Nurses' Association (ANNA) (2010) believed that the overall accountability and responsibility for nursing care rendered to patients and the coordination of patient care activities, including the provision of dialysis-related assessments and many specific interventions, rest with and are best accomplished by RNs who have been educated in the specialty of nephrology nursing. This "de-skilling" became visible in the 1996 settlement of a lawsuit in Ohio over the 1994 death of a client who underwent a hysterectomy and died because her caregivers were client care technicians, not RNs. The technicians missed the signs and symptoms of infection and shock (American Journal of Nursing [AJN], 1996a). Such reports sparked a round of legislative hearings and debate about regulating UAP by boards of nursing. The issues became contentious as nurses reported low morale, high workload stress, and a shifting of blame for unsafe care onto nurses who were labeled inflexible and not aware of how to delegate. Nurses insisted that mandated nurse-to-patient staffing ratios be enacted in laws. Hospital officials contended that these reports were exaggerated; nursing administrators opposed mandated staffing ratios (AJN, 1996b). These issues of the past set a precedent for future rounds of organizational cost-containment initiatives and need to be taken into account when using evidence to address nurse staffing policy issues.

The escalating shortage of nurses, greater acuity of patient illnesses, technological advances, and increased complexity of therapies contribute to today's current chaotic and multifaceted health care according to the NCSBN and ANA's *Joint Statement on Nursing Delegation* (2006). Delegation and supervision always will be intertwined with issues surrounding the use of nurse extenders and NAP. Concerns about declining quality of care and nurse staffing shortages led to legislation mandating minimum nurse-to-patient ratios in the state of California (Hodge et al., 2004). The nursing profession is challenged to find ways to balance the tension between professional judgment about care needs and the fiscal pressures of the organization.

RESEARCH NOTE

Source

Gravlin, G., & Bittner, N.P. (2010). Nurses' and nursing assistants' reports of missed care and delegation. *Journal of Nursing Administration, 40*(7/8), 329-335.

Purpose

The purpose of the study was to measure RNs', NAs', and nurse managers' reports of missed nursing care, both frequency and reasons for the missed care, and to identify factors related to successful delegation.

Discussion

The RN-NA care delivery model relies on competent delegation and complex delegation decisions. In previous studies RN-NA direction/communication or RN supervision were factors associated with negative outcomes, often related to tasks such as toileting, feeding, or skin care. In this study the MISSCARE Survey 2 and a delegation questionnaire were given to RNs and NAs on 16 med-surg units in 3 acute care hospitals in the northeast. A unit characteristics questionnaire was given to nurse managers. There were 241 (42.4% of 568 total) RNs, 99 (42.6% of 232 total) NAs, and 16 nurse managers (100%) who responded. Nurses (82%) reported being comfortable with the delegation process, and 83% reported delegating to an average of 2 NAs per shift. However, NAs (65%) reported being assigned more than 10 patients per shift and delegated to by 3 to 4 nurses per shift. The most frequently reported missed care items were ambulation, turning, feeding, attending the care confer-

ence, and mouth care. The reasons for missed care included unexpected increases in patient volume/acuity, inadequate number of assistive personnel, heavy admissions/discharges, level of staffing, urgent patient situations, and NAs not communicating that care was not done. Both RNs and NAs (50%) reported tension or communication breakdowns as reasons for missed care. Reports of missed care by both groups were widespread across the three institutions, mostly involving activities of daily living that are routinely delegated to NAs. Nurse managers (88%) said these had been reported to them, and 67% reported frequent occurrences.

Application to Practice

Personnel resources, the ability to manage patient flow, and rapidly changing patient or unit needs create situations of missed care. Tension and communication breakdowns also contribute. Patient safety, the impact on nurse-sensitive outcomes, financial impact, and RN turnover are related consequences of ineffective delegation and care omissions. These serious concerns need to be addressed in the care environment structure and processes. Delegation competency can be addressed through education and training. RN-NA communication and relationships can be improved through team building and structural changes. A best-practice bundle of delegation and supervision skills for bedside care can be implemented through coaching and supervision, resulting in performance improvement.

CASE STUDY

The beginning of the day shift when patients are to go for scheduled invasive procedures can be viewed as a very hectic time. The night nurse had just finished admitting a patient who was scheduled for surgery within the hour. The consent had not been signed because the patient's daughter was her power of attorney. The patient going for surgery needed cefazolin (Ancef) 1 gram, administered IV piggyback 30 minutes before surgery, as a preoperative medication. The surgery department had called to say "pre-op the patient."

Earlier in the week James and one of the NAP discussed how James would let the NAP "do stuff" since she was in nursing school. She was thrilled with the anticipated experiences. Once surgery had called to pre-op the patient, James asked the NAP to hang the piggyback as a big favor, since he still did not have the required paperwork completed for the patient to go to surgery. She hung the piggyback, and a few minutes later the patient put on the call light complaining of shortness of breath. The nurse went into the patient's room to find the patient in respiratory arrest. James notices that the piggyback was not hung on the correct patient, and the patient was allergic to the medication that was hung.

How could this happen when the student had been taught the 5 rights of medication administration? What should the nurse do?

CRITICAL THINKING EXERCISE

The staff on the oncology unit for the day shift (7 AM to 3:30 PM) for nine patients includes Sherry Trader, the charge nurse; James Fair, a recently hired staff nurse; and Julie Coggeshall, one of the NAP, who is in nursing school.

A 78-year-old woman admitted with the diagnosis of breast cancer is scheduled for a radical mastectomy at 8:30 AM. The patient is nonverbal to James, the nurse assigned to the patient. James tells the charge nurse that he has never prepared a patient who was to go to surgery for a mastectomy. The charge nurse indicates to James that the forms are no different from those for any other surgery.

1. What are the key issues to consider about when to delegate and assign care to this patient?
2. What are the problems presented in this case?
3. What are the possible solutions?
4. To whom and what tasks should be delegated to facilitate the patient's progression to surgery?

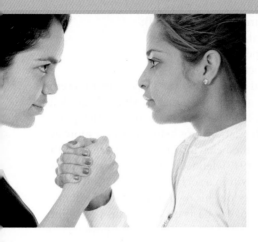

Power and Conflict

Kathleen B. Cox

e**volve** WEBSITE

http://evolve.elsevier.com/Huber/leadership/

POWER

For many nurses, power has had a negative connotation. With major issues and challenges facing the health care delivery system in the United States and the nature of work in today's complex health care organizations, it is imperative that nurses accept the reality and legitimacy of power. Although the United States has one of the most sophisticated health care systems in the world, there are major issues related to costs, access, and quality. The United States spends more on health care than any other industrialized country.

In 2009, national health expenditures grew 4.0% to $2.5 trillion, or $8086 per person, and accounted for 17.6% of gross domestic product (GDP) (Centers for Medicare & Medicaid Services [CMS], 2011). Further, the number of Americans without health insurance coverage rose to 49.9 million in 2010 from 49 million in 2009 (U.S. Department of Health and Human Services [USDHHS], 2011. Despite the abundance of government and private sector safety initiatives,

Photo used with permission from Photos.com.

health care errors persist at alarming rates. Adverse events occurred in approximately 33% of hospital admissions (Classen et al., 2011). According to the Centers for Disease Control and Prevention's CDC Health Disparities and Inequalities Report (CHDIR, 2011), health care quality and access are suboptimal, especially for minority and low-income groups; and although quality is improving, access and disparities are not improving.

President Barack Obama signed the Patient Protection and Affordable Care Act into law on March 23, 2010. Although the Supreme Court deemed the law constitutional on June 28, 2012, much controversy and uncertainty related to the implementation of the law remains. Nursing stands to be at the center of massive changes in health care delivery. In October of 2010, the Robert Wood Johnson Foundation (RWJF) and the Institute of Medicine (IOM) launched an initiative to respond to the need to assess and transform the nursing profession (IOM, 2011). The IOM appointed the Committee on the RWJF Initiative on the Future of Nursing with the purpose of producing a report that would make recommendations for the future of nursing. Through its deliberations, the committee developed four key recommendations:

- Nurses should practice to the full extent of their education and training.
- Nurses should achieve higher levels of education and training through an improved education system that promotes seamless academic progression.
- Nurses should be full partners, with physicians and other health care professionals, in redesigning health care in the United States.
- Effective workforce planning and policy making require better data collection and information infrastructure (IOM, 2010).

The enactment of the health care reform law and issuance of the IOM report on the future of nursing provide unlimited opportunities for the profession to establish a power base and become a force in the U.S. health care system. Manojlovich (2007) noted that power is necessary to influence patients, physicians, and other health care professionals, as well as each other. Increasingly, nurse leaders recognize that understanding and acknowledging power and learning to seek and wield it appropriately are critical if nurses' efforts to shape their own practice and the broader health care environment are to be successful (Schira, 2004). Powerless nurses are ineffective nurses, and the consequences of nurses' lack of power have recently come to light (Manojlovich, 2007). Powerless nurses are less satisfied with their jobs and more susceptible to burnout and depersonalization. Lack of nursing power may also contribute to poorer patient outcomes (Manojlovich, 2007). As the largest health care profession, nursing must use power and influence as a legitimate tool to facilitate change in health care organizations and the health care system.

DEFINITIONS

Although power connotes strength and ability, the term *power* has different meanings. It can mean the ability to compel obedience, control, or dominate; or it can be a delegated right or privilege as occurs in the power to enact the staff nurse role. **Power** can be defined as the capability of acting or producing some sort of an effect, usually associated with the ability to influence the allocation of scarce resources. Other definitions identify power as the potential capacity to exert influence, characteristically backed by a means to coerce compliance. A key element of power is its aspect of being potential as well as actual.

The following are the three formal dimensions of power (Bacharach & Lawler, 1980):
1. The relational aspect
2. The dependence aspect
3. The sanctioning aspect

The **relational aspect of power** suggests that power is a property of a social relationship. Many classic definitions (Blau, 1964; Kaplan, 1964) indicate that power has to do with relationships between two or more actors in which the behavior of one is affected by the other. Weber (1947) defined power as "the probability that one actor within a social relationship will be in a position to carry out his own will, despite resistance, and regardless of the basis on which this probability rests" (p. 52). Dahl (1957) also defined power as an interactive process and stated that "A has power over B to the extent that he can get B to do something B would not otherwise do" (pp. 202-203).

The second formal aspect, the **dependency aspect of power,** was addressed by Emerson (1957), who suggested that power resides implicitly in the other's dependency. Dependency is particularly evident in organizations that require interdependence of personnel and subunits. Daft (2013) defined *interdependence* as the extent to which departments depend on each other for resources or materials to accomplish their task. The highest level of interdependence is reciprocal interdependence. Reciprocal interdependence exists when the output of operation A is the input to operation B, and the output of operation B is the input back again to operation A. Daft noted that hospitals are excellent examples of reciprocal interdependence because they provide coordinated services to patients.

The third formal aspect, the **sanctioning aspect of power,** is the active component of the power relationship, referring to the direct manipulations of the other's outcomes. Sanctions can consist of manipulations of rewards, punishments, or both. Sanctions are a significant part of the process through which parties actually affect one another. In summary, power is a property of a social relationship between two or more actors, in which one is dependent on the other. Sanctions are applied in the form of rewards, punishments, or both.

Empowerment

Empowerment is a corollary concept to power in groups and organizations. **Empowerment** is defined as giving individuals the authority, responsibility, and freedom to act on what they know and instilling in them belief and confidence in their own ability to achieve and succeed (Kramer & Schmalenberg, 1990). Thus empowerment has two meanings: the transfer of actual power and the inspiring of self-confidence. Both aspects enable others to act. Empowerment is a key leadership component.

Empowerment for nurses may consist of three components: a workplace that has the requisite structures to promote empowerment, a psychological belief in one's ability to be empowered, and acknowledgment that there is power in the relationships and caring that nurses provide. A more thorough understanding of these three components may help nurses become empowered and use their power for better patient care (Manojlovich, 2007).

Psychological empowerment is a psychological response to empowered work environments and consists of four components: meaning, competence, self-determination, and impact (Spreitzer, 1995). Psychologically empowered employees feel that the requirements of the job are congruent with their own beliefs and values, which gives the job greater meaning. They are confident in their ability to perform the job, have control over their work, and have an impact on important organizational outcomes. Employees with low levels of psychological empowerment have less capacity to cope with organizational stressors and are more likely to respond passively. Laschinger and colleagues (2007) found that higher levels of structural empowerment were predictive of greater psychological empowerment, which in turn resulted in lower levels of emotional exhaustion and higher job satisfaction. Creating conditions that foster a sense of empowerment in managers is thus important to their well-being and retention.

Employee empowerment became a popular topic in the 1990s, especially in the business literature. With an emphasis on customer service and improving the bottom line through capitalizing on the creative and innovative energy of employees, businesses sought a strategic advantage. Empowerment programs were developed to improve productivity, lower costs, or raise customer satisfaction. However, growing evidence suggests that these empowerment programs fail to meet either managers' or employees' expectations, possibly because although empowerment programs promise employees power, they may not deliver on the promise (Hardy & Leiba-O'Sullivan, 1998).

Empowerment initiatives take two forms. First is the relational approach. The aim here is to improve performance by decentralizing power by delegating power, authority, and decision making. In theory, this reduces organizational barriers to getting the job done. Self-managing teams are one example (Hardy & Leiba-O'Sullivan, 1998).

The second empowerment strategy is the motivational approach. With this approach, there is less delegation of power and more emphasis on open communication and inspirational goal setting. The affective domain is emphasized, with feelings of ownership, responsibility, capability, commitment, and involvement. The goal is to improve employees' self-efficacy, ability to cope with adversity, and willingness to act independently and responsibly. Increasing self-efficacy and decreasing feelings of powerlessness have been linked to effective performance. Examples are training programs for group dynamics and group problem solving.

AUTHORITY AND INFLUENCE

Authority and influence are two major content dimensions of power (Bacharach & Lawler, 1980). There have been three conceptualizations of authority and influence: (1) some authors equate these terms; (2) others tend to equate power with influence and assert that authority is a special case of power; (3) still others view authority and influence as distinctly different dimensions of power. Several points of contrast are summarized in Table 10-1.

Influence Tactics

Kipnis and colleagues (1980) were among the first to investigate the influence behavior of managers. Content analysis led to the identification of 370 different forms of influence behavior, which were condensed into 14 categories. Subsequently, factor analysis brought about the following 8 forms of influence behavior:

1. *Assertiveness* means expressing one's own position to another without inhibiting the rights of others.
2. *Ingratiation* means trying to make the other person feel important—giving praise or sympathizing. Ingratiation is attempting to advance oneself by trying to make another person feel important.
3. *Rationality* means using logical and rational arguments, providing pertinent information, presenting reasons, and laying out an idea in a logical, structured way.

TABLE 10-1 AUTHORITY AND INFLUENCE CONTRASTED	
AUTHORITY	**INFLUENCE**
Authority is the static, structural aspect of power in organizations.	Influence is the dynamic, tactical element.
Authority is the formal aspect of power.	Influence is the informal aspect.
Authority refers to the formally sanctioned right to make decisions.	Influence is not sanctioned by the organization and is, therefore, not a matter of organizational rights.
Authority implies involuntary submission by subordinates.	Influence implies voluntary submission and does not necessarily entail a superior-subordinate relationship.
Authority flows downward, and it is unidirectional.	Influence is multidirectional and can flow upward, downward, or horizontally.
The source of authority is solely structural.	The source of influence may be personal characteristics, expertise, or opportunity.
Authority is circumscribed.	The domain, scope, and legitimacy of influence are typically ambiguous.

4. *Sanctions* are threats. Positive sanctions, or rewards, are addressed within motivation mechanisms.
5. *Exchange* means that to persuade, an exchange is offered; this is sometimes called "scratching each other's back."
6. *Upward appeal* means going to a higher authority—the childhood threat of "if you don't play by my rules, I am going to go tell Mom." Upward appeal simply means taking the appeal to a higher authority to arbitrate.
7. *Blocking* means deliberately keeping others from getting their way, threatening to stop working with them, ignoring them, not being friendly, or simply attempting to make sure others cannot accomplish their aims.
8. *Coalitions* are the result of a group of people getting together to speak or negotiate as one voice.

In their three-nation study of managerial influence styles, Kipnis and colleagues (1984) identified the most to least popular strategies (Table 10-2).

Yukl and Falbe (1991) continued the work of Kipnis and colleagues (1980). They developed an instrument, the Influence Behavior Questionnaire (IBQ), to measure the influence behavior of managers. In later studies, the IBQ was developed further, and psychometric tests were performed (Yukl et al., 1992, 1993). The nine tactics cover a wide range of influence behavior relevant for managerial effectiveness or, in a broader sense, for getting things done in an organization. Influence tactics are identified in Table 10-3.

SOURCES OF POWER

Individual Sources of Power

Although multiple mechanisms of power have been identified, the most widely accepted power base classification is French and Raven's (1959) five sources of power. Their original conceptualization identified the following five power sources (Box 10-1): (1) reward, (2) coercive, (3) expert, (4) referent, and (5) legitimate.

When reward power is used, people comply because doing so produces positive benefits. Coercive power depends on fear. An individual reacts to the fear of the negative consequences that might occur for failure to comply. Referent power is based on admiration for a person who has desirable resources or personal traits. Legitimate power represents the power a person receives as a result of his or her position in the formal organizational hierarchy. Expert power results from expertise, special skill, or knowledge. The problem with the French and Raven typology is that the list is not exhaustive, and it ignores organizational sources of power.

Other Sources of Power

Raven and Kruglanski (1975) and Hersey and colleagues (1979) identified two additional sources of power: (1) connection power, and (2) information power. A third type of power also has been identified: (3) group decision-making power (Liberatore et al., 1989). These three other sources of power are related

TABLE 10-2 MOST TO LEAST MANAGERIAL INFLUENCE STRATEGIES USED IN ALL COUNTRIES

STRATEGY'S POPULARITY	MANAGERS INFLUENCING SUPERIORS	MANAGERS INFLUENCING SUBORDINATES
Most popular ↑ ↓ Least popular	Reason Coalition Friendliness Bargaining Assertiveness Higher authority Sanction	Reason Assertiveness Friendliness Evaluation Bargaining Higher authority

Modified from Kipnis, D., Schmidt, S.M., Swaffin-Smith, C., & Wilkinson, I. (1984). Patterns of managerial influence: Shotgun managers, tacticians, and bystanders. *Organizational Dynamics, 12*(3), 58-67.

TABLE 10-3 DEFINITIONS OF INFLUENCE TACTICS

TACTIC	DEFINITION
Rational persuasion	The agent uses logical arguments and factual evidence to persuade the target that a proposal or request is viable and likely to result in the attainment of task objectives.
Inspiration appeals	The agent makes a request or proposal that arouses target enthusiasm by appealing to his or her values, ideals, and aspirations or by increasing target self-confidence.
Consultation	The agent seeks target participation in planning a strategy, activity, or change for which target support and assistance are desired, or the agent is willing to modify a proposal to deal with target concerns and suggestions.
Ingratiation	The agent uses praise, flattery, friendly behavior, or helpful behavior to get the target in a "good mood" or to think favorably of the agent before asking for something.
Personal appeals	The agent appeals to target feelings of loyalty and friendship toward him or her before asking for something.
Exchange	The agent offers an exchange of favors, indicates willingness to reciprocate at a later time, or promises a share of the benefits if the target helps to accomplish a task.
Coalition tactics	The agent seeks the aid of others to persuade the target to do something or uses the support of others as a reason for the target to agree as well.
Legitimating tactics	The agent seeks to establish the legitimacy of a request by claiming the authority or right to make it or by verifying that it is consistent with organizational policies, rules, practices, or traditions.
Pressure	The agent uses demands, threats, frequent checking, or persistent reminders to influence the target to do what the agent wants.

From Yukl, G., Falbe, C., & Joo, Y.Y. (1993). Patterns of influence behavior for managers. *Group and Organization Management, 18*(1), 5-28.

to groups and organizations specifically, as opposed to French and Raven's (1959) original five sources of power, which relate more to an individual.

Within organizations, the power of connections comes from networking or knowing people and from being able to go across lines laterally to gather information. For example, this occurs when a nurse knows a colleague in another facility with whom to exchange information. For a nurse to know what effective nursing interventions are being used by other institutions helps the institution to be competitive and current. *Connection power* is one strategy to get information accurately and reliably. It also may be manifested as power based on having connections with powerful

BOX 10-1   FRENCH AND RAVEN'S FIVE SOURCES OF POWER

1. ***Reward power*** is giving something of value. For example, in nursing, rewards may be a pay raise, praise, a promotion, or a job on the day shift. Reward power is based on the ability to deliver desired rewards.

2. ***Coercive power*** is force against the will. For example, in nursing, coercive power can be the threat of firing, of disciplinary action, or other negative consequences. Coercive power is the power derived from an ability to threaten punishment and deliver penalties. It is a source of power used to apply pressure so that others will meet what is demanded.

3. ***Expert power*** means the use of expertise. It is knowledge, competence, communication, and personal power all combined in a reservoir of knowledge and experience. Expert power is a source of power held by those with some special knowledge, skill, or competence in a particular area. For example, the nurse with the greatest expertise in wound dressings will be sought out by other people in the work environment for this expertise. Expertise is an artful combination of skill and knowledge. It may be founded on depth of knowledge and/or psychomotor skill. In the use of knowledge and skill is power (i.e., because people need you or can benefit from your expertise, power exists). Therefore the use of expertise can be structured to accomplish or influence movement or action toward certain goals.

4. ***Referent power*** is a little more difficult to understand because it is subtle. It is the use of charisma to influence others. The followers of someone with referent power respond positively to the interpersonal communication and image of the charismatic person. In organizations, this translates into an informal leadership based on liking, charisma, or personal power. Referent power comes from the affinity other people have for someone. They admire the personal qualities, the problem-solving ability, the style, or the dedication the person brings to the work. Referent power can be viewed as an inspirational power, because people's admiration for someone allows that person to influence without having to offer rewards or threaten punishments. For example, in the political arena, occasionally there are charismatic political figures or orators. Their influence comes from their followers' liking or identification with them. An example in nursing is Florence Nightingale, who became a symbol of professional nursing. An emotional upsweep is felt by associating with a charismatic person. Referent power is a personal liking and identification experienced by others. Followers attribute referent power to a leader on the basis of the leader's personal characteristics and interpersonal appeal. Physical attractiveness may contribute to referent power.

5. ***Legitimate power*** means positional power. It is the right to command within the organizational structure, based on the hierarchical position held. The President of the United States has power because of holding the position. Legitimate power is the most common source of power. It is what most often is called *authority*. The authority of position gives the person the right to act, order, and direct others. However, leadership and influence need not be confined to those with authority. Every person possesses the ability to tap different sources of power to use in a variety of situations.

Data from French, J., & Raven, B. (1959). The bases of social power. In D. Cartwright (Ed.), *Studies in social power* (pp. 150-167). Ann Arbor, MI: University of Michigan, Institute for Social Research.

others. Connection power is based on another's perception that the influencer has access to powerful persons or groups.

Information is power. If information is given away, its power may be lost. This is especially true in situations that require negotiation. If information is used strategically, its possession can be a strong source of power. *Information power* is a source of power that can stem from any person in the organization. Kanter's (1977) research suggested that control of resources, especially information, is a major organizational power source. Information power is based on another's perception that the influencer either possesses or has access to information valuable to another.

Another source of power is derived from *group decision making*. This means that a creative synergy and force is created when a group comes together, makes decisions, and acts as a united front. For example, some professional groups have formed strong lobbies to influence state and national legislation. With more than 3.1 million licensed registered nurses in the United States (American Nurses Association, 2011), group decision making with resultant unity of action could be a powerful strategy for nurses to use to advance nursing's goals or policy agenda.

Persuasive power is an additional source of power identified by later researchers investigating French and Ravens' (1959) taxonomy. *Persuasive power* refers to skill in making rational appeals (Yukl & Falbe, 1991). Yukl and Falbe (1991) differentiated between position power and personal power. According to these authors, position power consists of legitimate, reward, coercive, and information power. Personal power consists of expert, referent, persuasive power.

In her structural theory of organizational behavior, Kanter (1977) asserted that "those with sufficient power are able to accomplish the tasks required to achieve organizational goals" (p. 166). Conditions in the work environment influence how much productive power is available to employees. According to Kanter, formal and informal systemic structures are the sources of workplace empowerment. Job discretion, recognition, and relevance to organizational goals are important dimensions of formal power. High levels of job discretion ensure that work is non-routinized and permit flexibility, adaptation, and creativity. Recognition reflects visibility of an employee's accomplishments among peers and supervisors. For example, an innovative staff development director or nurse manager whose techniques are reported in a respected nursing journal will enhance his or her influence in the hospital. Finally, relevance of job responsibilities and accomplishments to the organization's strategic plan or current problems is also important. A nurse who publishes will probably not accrue much power when the hospital's census is consistently low and Medicare reimbursement is down. The nurse may not be seen as contributing to the solution of pressing organizational problems. Another key systemic structure is informal power, which comes from the employee's network of interpersonal alliances or relationships within and outside an organization. Relationships with people at higher hierarchical levels confer approval, prestige, and backing, whereas peer networks provide reputation and "grapevine" information (Kanter, 1977).

Kanter's theory has been tested extensively in nursing populations. These populations have been found to be only moderately empowered, with varying levels of access to information, support, opportunity, and resources (Laschinger & Havens, 1997; Laschinger et al., 2001b). Higher levels of structural empowerment have been associated with higher levels of organizational commitment (Laschinger et al., 2000), greater participation in organizational decision making (Laschinger et al., 1997), higher levels of job autonomy (Sabiston & Laschinger 1995), higher levels of job satisfaction (Laschinger & Havens 1997; Laschinger et al., 2001a), greater organizational trust (Laschinger et al., 2000), and a greater likelihood of feeling respected in the workplace (Faulkner & Laschinger, 2008). All these findings lend support to Kanter's theory.

Kotter (1979) maintained that the basic methods for acquiring and maintaining power are gaining control over tangible resources, obtaining information and control of information channels, and establishing favorable relationships. Basically, acquiring and maintaining power is an exercise in developing credibility by getting people to feel obligated in some way, building a good professional reputation through visible achievement, encouraging identification by trying to look and behave in ways that others respect, and finally, creating perceived dependence either for help or security. Control of information and resources and development of support systems are common elements in both Kanter's and Kotter's theories.

THE POWER OF THE SUBUNIT

Subunit or horizontal power pertains to relationships across departments. Daft (2013) noted that although each department makes a unique contribution to organizational success, some contributions are greater than others. Pfeffer (1981) identified the following structural determinants of power within organizations:

- *Power is derived from dependence.* Simply stated, power comes from having something that someone else wants or needs and being in control of the performance or resource so that there are few, if any, alternative sources for obtaining what is desired.
- *Power is derived from providing resources.* Organizations require a continuing provision of resources such as personnel, money, customers, and technology in order to continue to function. Those subunits or individuals within the organization that can provide the most critical and difficult to

obtain resources come to have power in organizations. Their power is derived from their ability to furnish those resources upon which the organization most depends.

- *Power is derived from coping with uncertainty.* Coping with uncertainty is a critical resource in the organization since it ensures organizational survival and adaptation to external constraints.

- *Power is derived from being irreplaceable.* Members must not only provide a critical resource for the organization but also prevent themselves from being readily replaced in that function. The degree of substitutability is not a fixed thing, however, so it might be expected that various strategies will be employed by individuals and subunits who are interested in enhancing their power within the organization. Some of these might involve the availability of documentation, use of specialized language, centralization of knowledge, and maintenance of externally based sources of expertise.

- *Power is derived from the ability to affect the decision process.* Because decisions are made in a sequential process, it is possible for an individual to acquire power because of his or her ability to affect the premises of basic values or objectives used in making any decision. A person can gain power by influencing the information about the alternatives being considered in the decision process.

- *Power is derived if there is a shared consensus within the organizational subunit.* If individuals within a subunit share a common perspective, set of values, or definition of the situation, they are likely to act and speak in a consistent manner and present to the larger organization an easily articulated and understood position and perspective. Such a consensus can serve to enhance the power of the subunit among other organizational members.

The Theory of Group Power within organizations was developed from a synthesis and reformulation of King's (1981) interacting systems framework and the Strategic Contingencies Theory of power (Hickson et al., 1971). Variables within the Strategic Contingencies Theory of power and their relationships were reformulated within King's framework. These variables relate to controlling the effects of environmental forces, position, resources, and role. Sieloff (2003) noted that although nursing groups are proposed to have a power capacity resulting from controlling the effects of environment forces,

position, resources, and role, not all nursing groups have acted powerfully. Therefore four additional concepts were added to the theory as variables that intervened between a nursing group's power capacity and its ability to actualize that power capacity. These concepts are communication competency, goal/outcome competency, nurse leader's power competency, and power perspective. Every nursing group has a power capacity. The group has the potential to achieve its goals and become a more visible contributor to the progress of the organization. The value of the theory is that it provides nurse leaders at all levels with strategies that could be implemented to improve a nursing group's actualized power (Sieloff, 2003).

LEADERSHIP AND MANAGEMENT IMPLICATIONS

According to Robbins and Judge (2011), leadership and power are two different concepts and need to be defined separately. Leadership is focusing on goal achievement in conjunction with followers. Power is used as a way to accomplish the goal, and often followers contribute to accomplishing the goal. Leaders focus on using their leadership downward to influence others to help them achieve their tasks. On the other hand, power is deployed to influence and to gain something upward or laterally.

POWER AND LEADERSHIP

Power and leadership are closely connected and highly intertwined concepts. This is because power is one of the vehicles by which a leader influences followers to take action. Nurses may be inclined to avoid an acknowledgment or analysis of power. However, to lead and manage, nurses need to acquire, possess, and use power. This begins with understanding it.

Hersey and colleagues (2008) described the relationships among concepts of style of leadership, readiness level of followers, and power base use. They indicated that the readiness of the followers dictates which leadership style is likely to be successful and which power base would most successfully influence followers' behavior. Combining these concepts maximizes the leader's probability of success. Thus nurses should be able to use Situational Leadership® theory

RESEARCH NOTE

Source

Ponte, P.R., Glazer, G., Dann, E., McCollum, K., Gross, A., Tyrrell, R., et al. (2007). The power of professional nursing practice: An essential element of patient and family centered care. *The Online Journal of Issues in Nursing, 12*(1). Retrieved October 1, 2012, from *www.nursingworld.org/ MainMenuCategories/ANAMarketplace/ANAPeriodicals/ OJIN/TableofContents/Volume122007/No1Jan07/tpc32_ 316092.aspx.*

Purpose

Ponte and colleagues' (2007) discussions with nurse leaders were guided by two specific aims: (1) to determine the characteristics of professional nursing power that practicing nurses believe are important at the individual level, and (2) to define strategies to help nurses attain power within their practice. Eleven nurse leaders, including a clinical nurse specialist, nurse manager, vice president, program manager, nurse scientist, dean, chief retention officer, and nurse faculty member, participated in the discussion. In the discussions, seven questions were posed, and the nurse leaders were asked to think about power in the broadest sense and to speak about what power means to them and how it is manifested in their practice and organization.

Discussion

Results of the discussions indicated that nurses who have developed a powerful nursing practice do the following:

- Acknowledge their unique role in the provision of patient- and family-centered care
- Commit to continuous learning through education, skill development, and evidence-based practice
- Demonstrate professional comportment and recognize the critical nature of presence
- Value collaboration and partner effectively with colleagues in nursing and other disciplines
- Actively position themselves to influence decisions and resource allocation
- Strive to develop an impeccable character, to be inspirational and compassionate, and to have a credible, sought-after perspective (the antithesis of power as a coercive strategy)
- Recognize that the role of the nurse leader is to pave the way for nurses' voices to be heard and to help novice nurses develop into powerful professionals
- Evaluate the power of nursing and the nursing department in organizations they enter by assessing the organization's mission and values and its commitment to enhancing the power of diverse perspectives

Application to Practice

Although the theoretical underpinnings that helped guide the methodology and analysis of findings were not presented, the results of the discussions provided insight into these nurse leaders' perceptions of power. As the authors noted, the results support existing literature on power and have implications for other group discussions that will assist nurse leaders to clarify what power means to them and to develop behaviors that enhance power. Finally, the report has implications for future qualitative studies in which the theoretical underpinnings are clearly identified.

to assess and predict style choice and power source use based on the situation and readiness of followers.

Readiness is the ability and willingness of individuals or groups to take responsibility for directing their own behavior in a situation. There appears to be a direct relationship between the level of readiness in individuals and groups and the power base type that has a high probability of effectiveness (Figure 10-1). Readiness is a task-specific concept. At the lowest level of readiness, coercive power is most appropriate. As people move to higher readiness levels, connection power, then reward, then legitimate, then referent, then information, and finally, expert power impact the behavior of people. At the highest level, the followers have competence and confidence, and they are most responsive to expert power (Hersey et al., 2008).

If power is the basic energy needed to initiate and sustain action, then power is a quality without which a leader cannot lead. Power is fundamental to leadership, in that leadership may be the wise use of power. This is especially true for transformative leadership (Bennis & Nanus, 1985). Power need is highly desirable in leaders and managers because power is necessary in influencing others. Assertiveness and self-confidence are associated with power and leadership. Leadership may be characterized as power in the service of others (Kouzes & Posner, 1987). For nurses, this may mean that they need to view power as an integral part of their professional roles in care management and client advocacy. Nursing leadership requires a willingness and ability to take on a power role and to expand the use of power bases.

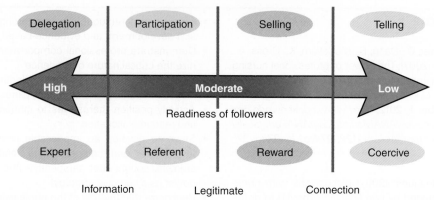

FIGURE 10-1 Power related to leadership. (Data from Hersey, P., Blanchard, K.H., & Johnson, D.E. [1996]. *Management of organizational behavior: Utilizing human resources* [7th ed.]. Upper Saddle River, NJ: Prentice-Hall.)

Centrality and Substitutability

Professional nurses have a high degree of centrality within health care organizations. They are critical to the operation of most health care organizations, and without nurses, many health care facilities would not be able to offer services. Nursing maintains that power by being central to health care services. Strong chief nurse executives with strong formal power are needed to create conditions within the organization and the health care system that address the IOM's call for nurses to practice at the highest level of preparation. Fortunately, research has demonstrated the relationship between RN staffing and important patient outcomes. The Agency for Healthcare Research and Quality (AHRQ) published a systematic review of the literature on workforce characteristics (Kane et al., 2007). The AHRQ review identified 97 observational studies published between 1990 and 2006 and included 94 of these reports in a meta-analysis. This meta-analysis found strong and consistent evidence that higher registered nurse (RN) hours were related to lower patient mortality rates, lower rates of failure to rescue, and lower rates of hospital-acquired pneumonia. Results of the meta-analysis indicated that there was evidence that higher direct-care RN hours were related to shorter lengths of stay. Higher total nursing hours also were found to result in lower hospital mortality and failure-to-rescue rates and in shorter lengths of stay. Based on fewer studies, the review found evidence that the prevalence of baccalaureate-prepared RNs was related to lower hospital mortality rates, that higher RN job satisfaction and satisfaction with workplace autonomy were related to lower hospital mortality rates, and that higher rates of nurse turnover were related to higher rates of patient falls. The conclusion of the meta-analysis was that higher nurse staffing was associated with better patient outcomes but that the association was not necessarily causal. However, this is powerful evidence for nurses' centrality.

CONFLICT

The same turbulent health care environment that demands the use of power also creates the conditions that breed conflict. Health care in the United States has gone through dramatic changes in recent decades. Change increases conflict in organizations. Gerardi (2004) summarized the direct and indirect consequences of conflict in terms of costs, including direct costs such as the following:

- Litigation costs that include attorneys' fees, expert testimony, deposition, lost work time, and document production
- Decreased managerial productivity as a result of time spent on resolving conflict
- Turnover costs
- Disability/stress claims
- Regulatory fines for noncompliance or loss of contracts or provider status with insurers and Medicare/Medicaid
- Costs associated with increased expenditures for patients with preventable, poor or adverse outcomes

- Sabotage, theft, and damage to facilities

Indirect costs include the following:

- Loss of team morale, loss of motivation for organizational change, damaged workplace relationships, and unresolved tensions that lead to future conflicts
- Lost opportunities for pursuing capital purchases, expanding services, enhancing customer satisfaction programs, and developing staff and leaders
- Cost to reputation of an organization and of care professionals; negative publicity/media coverage
- Loss of strategic market positioning because of public disclosure of information regarding the dispute/bad public relations
- Increased incidence of disruptive behavior by staff and medical professionals
- Emotional costs including the turmoil for those involved in conflict.

BULLYING AND DISRUPTIVE BEHAVIOR

There is evidence in the literature that conflict leads to bullying. Leymann (1996) and Einarsen and colleagues (1994) claimed that a bullying case typically is triggered by a work-related conflict. Matthiesen and colleagues (2003) noted that bullying can be described as certain subsets of conflict. When behavior similar to bullying occurs among health care providers from different disciplines, the term disruptive behavior is often used to name the behavior (Dumont et al., 2012). Conflict, as included in definitions of disruptive behaviors, is defined as "any inappropriate behavior, confrontation, or conflict, ranging from verbal abuse to physical and sexual harassment" (Rosenstein, 2002, p. 27). The Joint Commission (2011) acknowledged that unresolved conflict and disruptive behavior can adversely affect safety and quality of care, and they issued leadership standards calling for a stop to disruptive and inappropriate behaviors and a process to manage them. The Joint Commission requires that accredited institutions have a code of conduct that defines acceptable, disruptive, and inappropriate behaviors and that leaders have a process for managing them. In 2011, the elements of performance standards language were changed from "disruptive behavior" to "behavior or behaviors that undermine the culture of safety" (The Joint Commission Online, 2011).

Health care organizations must find ways of managing conflict and developing effective working relationships to create healthy work environments and cultures of safety. The effects of unresolved conflict on clinical outcomes, staff retention, and the financial health of the organization lead to many unnecessary costs that divert resources from clinical care (Gerardi, 2004). In addition, unresolved conflict and behaviors that undermine a culture of safety diminish the nursing profession and limit the profession's power to facilitate change in health care organizations and the health care system. Understanding how to maneuver around and manage conflict situations increases the ability to be more effective in both personal and professional roles.

DEFINITIONS

According to Kelly, a generally accepted definition of conflict does not exist (Kelly, 2006). **Conflict** is defined here as a clash or struggle that occurs when a real or perceived threat or difference exists in the desires, thoughts, attitudes, feelings, or behaviors of two or more parties (Deutsch, 1973). It exists as a tension or struggle arising from mutually exclusive or opposing actions, thoughts, opinions, or feelings. Conflict can be internal or external to an individual or group. It can be positive as well as negative.

Organizational conflict is defined as the struggle for scarce organizational resources (Coser, 1956). Values, goals, roles, or structural elements may be the specific locus of the struggle for scarce organizational resources. For example, two parties may be in opposition because of perceived differences in goals, a struggle over scarce resources, or interference in goal attainment. This opposition prevents cooperation (Deutsch, 1973). **Job conflict** is defined as a perceived opposition or antagonistic process at the individual-organization interface (Gardner, 1992). Conflict levels have an effect on productivity, morale, and teamwork in organizations

A review of the classic literature revealed several definitions of conflict. Social conflict is a struggle between opponents over values and claims to scarce status, power, and resources (Coser, 1956). According to Deutsch (1973), a conflict exists whenever incompatible activities occur or when one party is interfering, disrupting, obstructing, or in some other way making another party's actions less effective. The factors underlying conflict are threefold: (1) interdependence, (2) differences in goals, and (3) differences in perceptions. Conrad (1990) indicated that conflicts are communicative interactions among people who are interdependent and who perceive that their interests are incompatible, inconsistent, or in tension. Conflict is thus the interaction of interdependent people who perceive incompatible goals and interference from each other in achieving those goals (Folger et al., 1997). Walton (1966) defined conflict as opposition processes in any of several forms (e.g., hostility, decreased communication, distrust, sabotage, verbal abuse, coercive tactics). Interpersonal conflict is a dynamic process that occurs between interdependent parties as they experience negative emotional reactions to perceived disagreements and interference with the attainment of their goals (Barki & Hartwick, 2001).

VIEWS OF CONFLICT

Robbins and Judge (2011) described transitions in conflict thought. The traditional view of conflict argued that conflict must be avoided because conflict indicated a malfunctioning within the group. This early approach assumed that all conflict was bad, seen as a dysfunctional outcome resulting from poor communication, a lack of openness and trust between people, and the failure of managers to be responsive to their employees.

The human relations view argues that conflict is a natural and inevitable outcome in any group or organization and that it need not be evil. Rather, it has the potential to be a positive force in determining group performance. Because it is natural and inevitable, conflict should be accepted (Robbins & Judge, 2011).

The interactionist approach proposes that conflict can be a positive force in a group and explicitly argues that some conflict is absolutely necessary for a group to perform effectively. In the interactionist view, conflict is functional if it supports the goals of the group and improves its performance. Dysfunctional conflict, however, hinders group performance (Robbins & Judge, 2011).

Conflict can be competitive or disruptive. **Competitive conflict** is similar to games and sports, in which rules are followed and the goal is to win

---

BOX 10-2   EFFECTS OF CONFLICT

Constructive Effects
- Improves decision quality
- Stimulates creativity
- Encourages interest
- Provides a forum to release tension
- Fosters change

Destructive Effects
- Constricts communication
- Decreases cohesiveness
- Explodes in fighting
- Hinders performance

---

or beat an opponent. A **disruptive conflict** is some activity designed to attack, defeat, or eliminate an opponent. It is not based on rules jointly agreed to, and its objective is not focused on winning but, rather, on disrupting the opponent. The feelings and actions generated by competitive conflict focus on the positive; for disruptive conflict, feelings and actions focus on the negative (Filley, 1975).

Conflict is functional or constructive when it improves the quality of decisions, stimulates creativity and innovation, encourages interest and curiosity, provides a medium through which problems can be aired and tensions released, and fosters an environment of self-evaluation and change (Box 10-2). On the other hand, dysfunctional or destructive outcomes include a degrading of communication, reduction in group cohesiveness, and subordination of group goals to the primacy of infighting among members (Robbins, 2003). Extremely high or low levels of conflict hinder performance. An optimal level is high enough to prevent stagnation and stimulates creativity, releases tension, and initiates change. However, it is not so high as to be disruptive or counterproductive (Brown, 1983) (Figure 10-2).

TYPES OF CONFLICT

Thomas (1992) noted two broad types of conflict. The first refers to incompatible response tendencies within an individual, which Rahim and Bonoma (1979) referred to as *intrapersonal conflict* (Figure 10-3). *Intrapersonal conflict* means discord, tension, or stress inside, or internal to, an individual that results from unmet needs, expectations, or goals. Intrapersonal

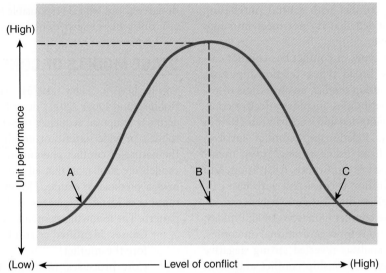

FIGURE 10-2 Conflict and unit performance. (Modified from Brown, L.D. [1983]. *Managing conflict at organizational interfaces.* Reading, MA: Addison-Wesley Publishing.)

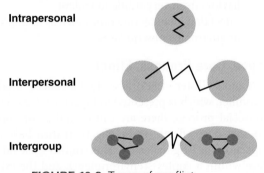

FIGURE 10-3 Types of conflict.

conflict is conflict that generates from within an individual (Rahim, 1983a, b, c). It often is manifested as a conflict over two competing roles. For example, a parent with a sick child who has to go to work faces a conflict: the need to take care of the sick child against the need to make a living. A nursing example occurs when the nurse determines that a client needs teaching or counseling, but the organization's assignment system is set up in a way that does not provide an adequate amount of time. When other priorities compete, an internal or intrapersonal conflict of roles exists.

The second use refers to conflicts that occur between different individuals, groups, organizations, or other social units. Rahim and Bonoma (1979) identified these as interpersonal conflict, a category

that includes intragroup conflict, intergroup conflict, and interorganizational conflict. *Interpersonal* means conflict emerging between two or more people, such as between two nurses, a doctor and a nurse, or a nurse manager and a staff nurse (Rahim & Bonoma, 1979). In this case, two people have a disagreement, conflict, or clash. Either their values or styles do not match, or there is a misunderstanding or miscommunication between them. Interpersonal conflict can be viewed as happening between two individuals or among individuals within a group. When it specifically involves multiple individuals within a group, interpersonal conflict is called *intragroup conflict,* which refers to disagreements or differences among the members of a group or its subgroups with regard to goals, functions, or activities of the group.

Intergroup conflict refers to disagreements or differences between the members of two or more groups or their representatives over authority, territory, and resources. Interorganizational conflict occurs across organizations (Rahim, 1983b; Rahim & Bonoma, 1979). It is conflict occurring between two distinct groups of people. For example, physicians and nurses may disagree about role functions and activities, or lay midwives may seek to perform home deliveries without being prepared as licensed nurse midwives. Sometimes the conflict arises between departments or units as groups. For example, hospital nurses might find themselves in conflict with central purchasing if supplies are provided that do not meet nursing's needs or are defective.

Another view of types of conflict has conflict categorized into three broad types: relationship, task, and process. *Relationship conflict,* an awareness of interpersonal incompatibilities, includes affective components such as feeling tension and friction (Rahim & Bonoma, 1979). Relationship conflict involves personal issues such as dislike among group members and feelings such as annoyance, frustration, and irritation. This definition is consistent with past categorizations of conflict that distinguish between affective and cognitive conflict (Amason, 1996; Pinkley, 1990), with implications for organizational outcomes. Results of a meta-analysis revealed strong negative correlations between relationship conflict and team performance and also strong negative correlations between relationship conflict and team member satisfaction (DeDreu & Weingart, 2003).

Task conflict is an awareness of differences in viewpoints and opinions about a group task. Similar to cognitive conflict, it pertains to conflict about ideas and differences of opinion about the task (Amason & Sapienza, 1997). Task conflicts may coincide with animated discussions and personal excitement but, by definition, are void of the intense interpersonal negative emotions that are more commonly associated with relationship conflict.

Other studies have identified a third unique type of conflict, labeled *process conflict* (Jehn, 1995, 1997; Jehn et al., 1999). It is defined as an awareness of controversies about aspects of how task accomplishment will proceed. More specifically, process conflict pertains to issues of duty and resource delegation, such as who should do what and how much responsibility different people should have. For example, when group members disagree about who is responsible for completing a specific duty, they are experiencing process conflict.

STAGE MODELS OF CONFLICT

Pondy (1967), Filley (1975), Thomas (1976), and Robbins and Judge (2011) described conflict dynamics across a temporal sequence of stages or phases. These models provide significant insight into understanding the nature of conflict phenomena (Table 10-4). These models are similar in that all indicate that conflict follows a predictable course. However, they differ in the number of identifiable stages or elements in a particular pattern. The following elements exist in all the models:

- Causes, identified as conditions, that occur before the conflict
- Core processes, including the perception that conflict exists, followed by some kind of affective state or emotional response
- Conflict behaviors, including a variety of behaviors from very subtle to violent
- Effect that includes outcomes such as resolution or aftermath consequences

Cause, Core Process, Effect

Wall and Callister (1995) described a generic model of conflict, which is presented in Figure 10-4. As with any social process, there are causes and a core process that have effects. These effects in turn have an impact on the original cause. This conflict cycle takes place within a context (environment), and the cycle flows through numerous iterations. Wall and Callister (1995) indicated that the model is a general one that displays how the major pieces in the conflict puzzle fit together. The value of this model is that concepts from all other models may be subsumed under the major concepts of this generic model. In addition, the

TABLE 10-4 COMPARISON OF FOUR PROCESS MODELS OF CONFLICT

PONDY (1967)	FILLEY (1975)	THOMAS (1976)	ROBBINS & JUDGE (2011)
1. Latent (antecedent conditions)	1. Antecedent conditions	1. Frustration	1. Potential opposition
2. Perception and feeling	2. Perceived conflict	2. Conceptualization	2. Cognition and personalization
3. Behavior manifestation (manifest)	3. Felt conflict	3. Behavior	3. Intentions
4. Aftermath	4. Manifest behavior	4. Others' reactions (interaction)	4. Behavior
	5. Resolution or suppression	5. Outcome	5. Functional or dysfunctional outcomes
	6. Conflict aftermath		

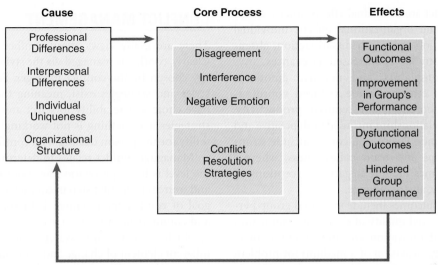

Cause	Core Process	Effects
Professional Differences	Disagreement	Functional Outcomes
Interpersonal Differences	Interference	Improvement in Group's Performance
Individual Uniqueness	Negative Emotion	Dysfunctional Outcomes
Organizational Structure	Conflict Resolution Strategies	Hindered Group Performance

FIGURE 10-4 Conceptual framework for conflict. (Adapted from Wall, J.A., & Callister, R.R. [1995]. Conflict and its management. *Journal of Management, 21,* 515-558.)

simplicity of the model facilitates the discussion of conflict according to cause, core process, and effect.

Causes of Conflict

According to Wall and Callister (1995), conditions that occur before conflict are identified as causes. In a concept analysis of conflict in the work environment, Almost (2005) indicated that antecedents of conflict stem from individual characteristics, interpersonal factors, and organizational factors. Individual characteristics include differing opinions and values; demographic dissimilarity, which includes gender and educational differences; and generational diversity. Interpersonal factors include lack of trust, injustice or disrespect, and inadequate or poor communication. Finally, organizational factors include interdependence and changes due to restructuring.

The Core Process of Conflict

Although conflict has been defined in many different ways, disagreement, interference, and negative emotion are thought to underlie conflict situations (Barki & Hartwick, 2001). Disagreement, interference, and negative emotion can be viewed as reflecting cognitive, behavioral, and affective manifestations of interpersonal conflict. Disagreement is the most commonly discussed and assessed cognition in the literature. Although a number of different behaviors have been associated with and may be typical of conflict, they do not always indicate the existence of conflict. Conflict exists when the behavior of one party interferes with or opposes another party's attainment of its own interests, objectives, or goals. Finally, a number of affective states have been associated with conflict. However, it is the negative emotions such as fear, anger, anxiety, and frustration that have been used to characterize conflict. Barki and Hartwick (2001) proposed that interpersonal conflict exists only when disagreement, interference, and negative emotion are present in the situation.

In 2004, Barki and Hartwick conducted a comprehensive review of the literature in which two dimensions of conflict were identified. The first dimension identifies disagreement, interference, and negative emotion as three properties generally associated with a conflict situation. The second dimension identifies relationship and task content or task process as two targets of interpersonal conflict encountered in organizational settings.

Effects of Conflict

Almost (2005) noted that although conflict includes both positive and negative effects, more empirical evidence for negative outcomes than for positive outcomes was found in the concept analysis. The main effects of conflict are individual effects, interpersonal relationships, and organizational effects. Individual effects include job stress, job dissatisfaction, absenteeism, intent to leave, increased grievances, psychosomatic complaints, and negative emotions. Organizational effects include reduced coordination and collaboration and reduced productivity. Interpersonal relationships included both positive and negative outcomes. Positive outcomes include stronger relationships and team cohesiveness, whereas negative outcomes include negative perceptions of others, hostility, and avoidance.

Functional outcomes include increased group performance, improved quality of decisions, stimulation of creativity and innovation, encouragement of interest and curiosity, provision of a medium for problem solving, and creation of an environment for self-evaluation and changes. On the other hand, dysfunctional outcomes include development of discontent, reduced group effectiveness, disrupted communication, reduced group cohesiveness, and infighting among group members, which then overcomes the focus on group goals (Robbins & Judge, 2011).

CONFLICT SCALES

Three conflict inventories are available to measure conflict. The Rahim Organizational Conflict Inventory-I (Rahim, 1983b, c) is designed to measure three dimensions of conflict: intrapersonal, intragroup, and intergroup. The Perceived Conflict Scale (Gardner, 1992) contains four subscales of conflict: intrapersonal, interpersonal, intergroup/other departments, and intergroup/support services. This scale is designed to measure conflict in nursing. Cox (2004) developed the Intragroup Conflict Scale, which consists of three dimensions: opposition processes and negative emotion, trust and freedom of expression, and views of conflict. The scales can be used for objective measurement not only to determine how much conflict exists but also to determine the causes and effects of conflict and the relationship of conflict to other variables of interest to nursing administrators. Barki and Hartwick's (2004) proposed two dimensions could form the basis for the development of another instrument containing items that reflect these dimensions and expand the ability to comprehensively capture conflict.

CONFLICT MANAGEMENT

There are many views about conflict management. Clearly, conflict is managed via the style and the strategy chosen by the conflict manager. Several conflict styles and strategies exist, meaning that individuals have choices. The ability to select among styles and strategies if something is not working provides flexibility for the person dealing with conflict.

Managing conflict relates to determining whether the level is too high or too low. Assessment of levels and sources is the first step in conflict assessment. The goal of conflict management is to stimulate growth and coping behavior but to avoid reaching the point at which conflict seems overwhelming. Conflict is an inherent element of change and is manifested in resistance to change. This indicates that nurses need to be alert to the predictability of resistance and conflict in any change process.

Personal styles and the interaction of styles contribute to conflict moments. The reality is that most people are more comfortable around people who are similar to them. If people are very different in terms of personality and styles, then how the styles interact contributes to conflict potential. Awareness of one's own style and the recognition of other people's styles contribute to effective management of conflict.

Multiple factors must be considered in conflict management. The important factors can form the basis for conflict management behaviors needed by nurses. These behaviors have been listed in a conflict management checklist (Box 10-3). The checklist can be used as a review or assessment for critically analyzing conflict situations.

BOX 10-3 CONFLICT MANAGEMENT CHECKLIST

- Identify the boundaries of the conflict, the areas of agreement and disagreement, and the extent of each person's aims.
- Understand the factors that limit the possibilities of managing the conflict constructively.
- Be aware of whether more than one issue is involved.
- Be open to the ideas, feelings, and attitudes expressed by the people involved.
- Be willing to accept outside help to mediate the conflict.

Conflict Management Strategies

It is important to take action as soon as a conflict surfaces so that bad feelings will not linger and grow. Conflict in groups adds the complexity of multiple parties to the conflict situation. Usually the best place for a work group to clear the air is in a group meeting. During such meetings, issues can be defined and strategies worked out for managing the points of disagreement. Three overall frameworks or postures for conflict management are the defensive, compromise, and creative problem-solving modes.

The *defensive mode* produces feelings of winning in some and loss in others. Several conflict resolution strategies adopt a defensive mode. Sometimes if creative problem solving and compromise fail, this may be the only way to decrease some of the destructive effects of conflict. A defensive mode may be used initially to gain time to calm down or to think about how to proceed. Following are ways to defensively solve a conflict:

- *Separate the contending parties.* For example, people may be assigned to different shifts or teams or different days off and on.
- *Suppress the conflict.* For example, people may decide not to talk about their differences.
- *Restrict or isolate the conflict.* For example, the parties can agree to disagree about a conflict and move on to items that they do agree about.
- *Smooth it over or finesse it through an organizational change.* For example, sometimes it is possible to solve conflicts by restructuring around the issue.
- *Avoid the conflict to diminish the destructive effects.* For example, people can change the subject whenever the conflict arises or avoid the party or parties involved.

The second mode of conflict management is compromise. With a *compromise mode,* each party wins something and loses something. In the settlement, each side gives up a part of its demands. Thus each side may "go halfway" or "split the difference." A compromise comes about when both sides want harmony or an end to the conflict and are willing to give up something to settle the difference.

The third mode of conflict management is creative problem solving. Use of a *creative problem-solving mode* produces feelings of gain and no feelings of loss for all conflict participants. All parties work together collaboratively to arrive at a solution that satisfies everyone, and all parties feel that they win. Creative problem solving is the most effective mode of conflict management. As part of the creative problem-solving process, the following five steps for conflict management can be identified:

1. Initiate a discussion, timed sensitively and held in an environment conducive to private discussion.
2. Respect individual differences.
3. Be empathic with all involved parties.
4. Have an assertive dialogue that consists of separating facts from feelings, clearly defining the central issue, differentiating viewpoints, making sure that each person clearly states their intentions, framing the main issue based on common principles, and being an attentive listener consciously focused on what the other person is saying.
5. Agree on a solution that balances the power and satisfies all parties, so that a consensus on a win-win solution is reached.

Conflict Handling Intentions

Five conflict-handling intentions can be identified: competing, collaborating, avoiding, accommodating, and compromising.

- Competing occurs when one person seeks to satisfy his or her own interests, regardless of the impact on the other parties to the conflict
- Collaborating ensues when the parties to conflict each desire to fully satisfy the concerns of all parties. The intention is to solve the problem by clarifying differences rather than by accommodating.
- Avoiding emerges when a person recognizes that a conflict exists and wants to withdraw from it or suppress it.
- Accommodating results when one party seeks to appease an opponent; that party is willing to be self-sacrificing.
- Compromising may develop when each party to the conflict seeks to give up something, sharing occurs, resulting in a compromised outcome. There is no clear winner or loser, and the solution provides incomplete satisfaction of both parties' concerns (Robbins & Judge, 2011).

Conflict Resolution Strategies

Conflicts can be a source of chronic frustration, or they can lead to increased effectiveness in organizations and groups. It takes leadership and management to solve them creatively so that people exist more co-operatively with others. Leadership and management for conflict resolution has implications for work group morale and productivity. A fair proportion of a leader's or manager's time is spent on handling conflict.

Conflict management techniques stress the importance of communication, assertive dialogue, and empathy. Thus during conflict situations, the more that individuals look at the total situation and use positive communication techniques, the closer they will come to a successful resolution. Conflict resolution techniques have been identified, described, and categorized in a variety of ways by a variety of authors. Some terms have been used interchangeably, and some terms have similar but slightly different meanings. The following is an overall list of methods or strategies for conflict resolution:

- *Avoiding:* This is the strategy of avoiding conflict at all costs. Some people never acknowledge that a conflict exists. The individual's posture is "If I do not acknowledge there is a problem, then there is no problem." It is sometimes reflected in the phrase "leave well enough alone."
- *Withholding or withdrawing:* In this avoidance strategy, one party opts out of participation and withdraws from the situation. This does not resolve the conflict. However, this strategy does give individuals a chance to calm down or to avoid a confrontation.
- *Smoothing over or reassuring:* This is the strategy of saying "Everything will be OK." By maintaining surface harmony, parties do not withdraw but simply attempt to make everyone feel good. It is similar to "smoothing ruffled feathers." Smoothing over or reassuring strategies use verbal communication to defuse strong emotions.
- *Accommodating:* This strategy is used when there is a large power differential. The more powerful party is accommodated to preserve harmony or build up social credits. This means that the party of lesser power gives up his or her position in deference to the more powerful party. Accommodation may be used when one party has a vested interest that is relatively unimportant to the other party. "Kill the enemy with kindness" is the related phrase.
- *Forcing:* This technique is a dominance move and an arbitrary way to manage conflict. An issue may be forced on the table by issuing orders or by putting it to a majority-rules vote. The hallmark phrase is "Let's vote on it." Forcing is an all-out power strategy to win while the other party loses.
- *Competing:* This is an assertive strategy in which one party's needs are satisfied at the other's expense. Competing is an all-out effort to win at any cost. It is sometimes reflected in the phrase "Might makes right." Competing strategies tend to follow rules and be similar to games and athletic contests. Applying for a job is a form of competition.
- *Compromising:* This strategy is called "splitting the difference." It is useful when goals or values are markedly different. It is a staple of conflict management.
- *Confronting:* This technique is called *assertive problem solving* and is focused on the issues. Individuals speak for themselves but in a way that decreases defensiveness and allows another person to hear the message. It is a staple of conflict management but requires courage. "I" messages are used; "you" messages are avoided.
- *Collaborating:* This is an assertive and cooperative strategy in which the parties work together to find a mutually satisfying solution. It is invoked with the phrase "Two heads are better than one."
- *Bargaining and negotiating:* These strategies are attempts to divide the rewards, power, or benefits so that everyone gets something. They involve both parties in a back-and-forth effort at some level of agreement. The process may be formal or informal.
- *Problem solving:* This strategy's goal is to try to find an acceptable, workable solution for all parties. It is designed to generate feelings of gain by all parties. The problem-solving process is employed to reach a mutually agreeable solution to the conflict.
- *Mediation:* Gerardi (2004) noted that mediation is a useful process to use when the goal of preserving the working relationship is as important as resolving the substantive problems. Although not all conflict situations require mediation, mediation techniques can be used to prevent escalation of conflicts. Effective techniques for improving collaboration and resolving conflicts include listening for understanding, reframing, elevating the definition of the problem, and creating clear agreements. Mediation techniques can be integrated into manager's practice to assist nurses in recognizing issues and addressing the actual needs of co-workers to prevent escalation of conflicts (Gerardi, 2004).

Face Negotiation Theory

Face negotiation is the focus of a theory developed by Ting-Toomey to describe and explain differences in responses to conflict on the basis of cultural backgrounds (Ting-Toomey, 1988; Ting-Toomey & Kurogi, 1998). This theory draws on the idea that *face* is a metaphor for our public identity, or self-image, and is an important element of social situations throughout the world. Specifically, face is "a projected image of one's self in a relational situation" (Ting-Toomey, 1988, p. 215). In the theory, *facework* refers to specific verbal and nonverbal messages that help maintain and restore face loss and uphold and honor face gain. All individuals want others to see them in a certain way, even though they may not be consciously aware of this desire.

Ting-Toomey (1988) originally considered face negotiation theory as a way to explain differences in conflict communication styles stemming from cultural preferences for individualism versus collectivism. She proposed that those in cultures best described as *collectivistic* would be more likely to seek to uphold "other-face," whereas those in *individualistic* cultures would more likely seek to uphold "self-face."

Face negotiation theory builds on the five-style dual-concern framework developed by Rahim (1983a) and is based on the degree to which a person is concerned with self-interest, as well as with the interests of others. The five styles are problem solving (also called *integrating, collaborating,* or *cooperating*), forcing (also called *competing* or *dominating*), avoiding (also called *suppressing* or *withdrawing*), yielding (also called *obliging, accommodating,* or *smoothing*), and compromising (Putnam & Poole, 1987; Rahim, 2001). The theory posits that collectivistic cultures favor the avoiding, yielding, and compromising styles; in contrast, individualistic cultures reputedly favor forcing and problem-solving styles (Ting-Toomey, 1988).

In 1998, the face negotiation theory was revised and the dimension of self-construal (self-image) was discussed in terms of the independent and interdependent self, or the degree to which people conceive of themselves as relatively autonomous from or connected to others (Ting-Toomey & Kurogi, 1998). The revised theory posits that the degree to which people see themselves as autonomous (independent; self-face) or connected to others (interdependent; other-face) is a better predictor of conflict interaction than their cultural or ethnic background. Ting-Toomey and Kurogi (1998) also added the concept of power to the theory to explain communicative differences based on the cultural dimension of power distance. In low-power distance cultures, differences in treatment based on status are less accepted. On the other hand, in high-power distance cultures, differences in treatment based on status are more accepted. The authors proposed that individuals of different status levels in low-power distance cultures are more likely to use the forcing style to resolve conflict, whereas in high-power distance cultures, those in lower-status roles may use styles such as yielding.

Cross-cultural empirical tests of the revised face negotiation theory supported much of the theory (Oetzel & Ting-Toomey, 2003; Oetzel et al., 2001). The 2001 study involved a cross-cultural comparison of four national cultures (Oetzel et al., 2001). In the 2003 study of face-negotiation theory, Oetzel and Ting-Toomey tested the underlying assumption that face mediates the relationship between cultural or individual-level variables and conflict styles. The findings provide supportive evidence of the face-negotiation theory, especially that face concerns provide a mediating link between cultural values and conflict behavior. The authors also suggested that these findings are particularly significant, given the relatively large sample size across four national cultures.

Results of the studies indicated that nursing administrators need to be more attuned to face issues in the conflict dialogue process. The findings of the Oetzel and Ting-Toomey (2003) study demonstrated that display of other-face concern, which is maintaining the poise or pride of the other person and being sensitive to the other person's self-worth, can lead to a collaborative, win-win integrative approach or an avoiding approach. In contrast, individuals who are more concerned with maintaining self-pride or self-image during a conflict episode would devote effort to defending their conflict position to the neglect of other-face validation issue.

Conflict Resolution Outcomes

Whatever the conflict resolution style used, the individual must be aware of the outcome that results from the strategy selected. The outcomes of conflict are what actually happens as a result of the conflict management process. The three ways in which conflicts resolve are (1) win-lose, (2) lose-lose, and (3) win-win (Filley, 1975) (Box 10-4).

Win-Lose
One party exerts dominance.

Lose-Lose
Neither side wins.

Win-Win
An attempt is made to meet the needs of both parties simultaneously.

Data from Filley, A.C. (1975). *Interpersonal conflict resolution.* Glenview, IL: Scott, Foresman; Filley, A., House, R., & Kerr, S. (1976). *Managerial process and organizational behavior.* Glenview, IL: Scott, Foresman.

Filley (1975) described the win-win resolution as the optimum conflict management. Win-lose and lose-lose resolutions also occur, but effective managers should seek win-win resolutions. Win-win strategies focus on problem solving.

Negotiation is a fundamental form of conflict resolution. Negotiation includes bargaining power, distributive bargaining, integrative bargaining, and mediation. *Bargaining power* refers to another person's inducement to agree to terms. *Distributive bargaining* is what either side gains at the expense of the other. In *integrative bargaining,* the focus shifts to problem solving, and negotiators reach a solution that enhances both parties and produces high joint benefits. *Mediation* is a process in which a third party encourages the two parties in conflict to acknowledge that they have injured the other but also are dependent on each other (Hampton et al., 1987).

Integrative bargaining tends to be more cooperative, and distributive bargaining tends to be more competitive. In general, integrative bargaining is superior to distributive bargaining. Fisher and colleagues (1992) proposed an alternative called *principled negotiation.* This approach calls for negotiators to use the following five fundamental principles to negotiate effectively with each other instead of against each other:

1. Separate the people from the problem.
2. Negotiate about interests, not positions.
3. Invent options for mutual gain.
4. Insist on objective decision criteria.
5. Know your best alternative to a negotiated agreement (BATNA).

Although there is no one best method of conflict resolution, competence in managing conflict is essential.

Conflict Resolution Inventories

Several instruments have been developed to measure conflict handling styles. In the Organizational Conflict Inventory-II, Rahim (1983b, c) divided the handling of interpersonal conflict into the two dimensions of concern for self and concern for others, both in high and low degrees, to form a grid. Rahim then adapted Blake and Mouton's (1964) five types of handling interpersonal conflict (forcing, withdrawing, smoothing, compromising, and problem solving) into five styles of handling interpersonal conflict (avoiding, obliging, compromising, integrating, and dominating). The inventory measures the five identified styles.

Thomas and Kilmann (1974) also developed a style assessment and diagnosis inventory, called the *Thomas-Kilmann Conflict Mode Instrument (TKI).* Their grid uses dimensions of assertiveness and cooperativeness on high to low degrees. The five styles are avoiding, accommodating, compromising, competing, and collaborating. This model blends a description of an individual's behavior on assertiveness and cooperativeness dimensions in situations in which the concerns of two people appear to be incompatible. The behaviors of individuals are thought to be a function of both personal predispositions and situational contingencies. Avoiding is low on both assertiveness and cooperativeness; collaborating is high on both aspects. Competing is high on assertiveness and low on cooperativeness; accommodating is low on assertiveness and high on cooperativeness. Compromising is in the middle.

Bartol and colleagues (2001) described the development of a scale designed to determine attitudes toward managing conflict. The authors indicated that the Bartol/McSweeney Conflict Management Scale is simple to use and suitable for nurses working in different settings. They pointed out that knowing one's predisposition toward conflict is the first step in creatively managing conflict.

Studies of Conflict Management in Nursing

Older studies in nursing found that avoiding and compromising were the most frequently used conflict handling intentions in nursing. More recently,

Sportsman and Hamilton (2007) conducted a study to determine prevalent conflict management styles chosen by students in nursing and to contrast these styles with those chosen by students in allied health professions. The associations among the level of professional health care education and the style chosen were also determined. A convenience sample of 126 university students completed the TKI. The difference was not significant between the prevalent conflict management styles chosen by graduate and undergraduate nursing students and those in allied health. Some of the students were already licensed in their discipline; others had not yet taken a licensing examination. Licensure and educational level were not associated with choice of styles. Women and men had similar preferences. The prevalent style for nursing students was compromise, followed by avoidance. The prevalent style for allied health students was avoidance, followed by compromise and accommodation. When compared with the TKI norms, slightly more than one half of all participants chose two or more conflict management styles, commonly avoidance and accommodation at the 75th percentile or above. Only 9.8% of the participants chose collaboration at that level.

LEADERSHIP AND MANAGEMENT IMPLICATIONS

Organizational Conflict

Thomas (1976) identified a "big picture" structural model of conflict that examines four factors that seem to influence the way conflict is handled in organizations: behavioral predispositions of individuals, social pressure in the environment, the organization's incentive structure, and rules and procedures. The different levels of power exist as a result of bureaucratic hierarchy and the resultant position power.

Organizational conflict is a form of interpersonal conflict that is generated from aspects of the institution, such as the style of management, rules, procedures, and communication channels. Conflicts that arise when an individual's needs and goals cannot be met within the system are generally organizational. Conflict may be necessary to groups and organizations. Conflict serves to unify and bind together a group by setting boundaries and strengthening a group's identity. Conflict may help stabilize a group by serving as a test of opposing interests within the group. Conflict may help integrate a group by distributing power. Conflict may be necessary for the growth of a group and its members and serves to stimulate creativity, innovation, and change (Coser, 1956).

Organizational leadership sets a tone for conflict and conflict management (Barton, 1991). This occurs because leaders and managers model behaviors of positive or negative conflict management and choose when and how to intervene in conflict situations. Choice of intervention style and timing of conflict management are functions of the individuals' behavioral predispositions and environmental pressure coupled with the organization's reward structure and coordination and control methods.

Specifically related to organizational conflict and the focus on groups in organizations, Pondy (1967) identified three strategies to use when attempting to resolve organizational conflicts—bargaining; using rules, procedures, and administrative control; and using a systems integrator. Bargaining might be useful when a conflict exists over scarce monetary resources. The administrative control approach might be helpful when clarification of role boundaries is needed. The systems integrator approach might be appropriate in a matrix structure or where there is a need to coordinate personnel in vertical and horizontal organizational structures.

Sources of Conflict in Organizations

The sources of conflict frequently encountered in organizations are power, communication, goals, values, resources, roles, and personalities. Conflict arises from a variety of sources. Power clashes lead to conflict. This happens if one person has more power than another. For example, in organizations, relationships exist between and among individuals with unequal power such as that between physicians and nurses, which can hinder effective teamwork.

Another source of conflict is the misunderstanding or breakdown of communication. Conflicts can be the result of clashes between deep-seated, sincere, but diametrically opposed views. Communication may be used to clarify opposing views. Because values are internalized, they are not easily changed but may be clarified by communication or become a barrier as a result of miscommunication. Conflict situations often arise suddenly with the awareness of conflict existing on an emotional level. Emotional intensity may be the first element communicated. The emotional reaction may include responses such as frustration or wanting to lash out with a strong verbal communication.

The roots or causes of conflict are many and varied. Other general sources of conflict that occur frequently in organizations are different goals, different ways to reach a goal, different values, overlapping or unclear designation of responsibility, lack of information, and personality conflicts. Irresolvable conflicts will need to be carefully managed within any work group to balance conflict levels. For example, nurses may thrive when the conflict level is sufficient to stimulate a clash of ideas that leads to creativity and innovation or growth. However, nurses may expend energy in nonproductive activity if the conflict level is too high or becomes destructive.

Conflict appears to be an inherent part of the work of nursing. Nurses are prime candidates for conflict because of the need to work collaboratively with people of varying social, ethnic, and educational backgrounds. Collaboration implies a distribution of power, yet nurses may be employed in a hierarchical system. When nurses work in groups, they work with a number of different colleagues and a variety of client types and personalities. These are complex interrelationships. Added to the complexity is the fact that multiple providers (e.g., physicians, nurses, nurse managers, ancillary personnel, the client, and the client's family) with differing perspectives require coordination and communication to manage the care for any client.

Within health care, there is interdependence among members. This situation also provides conditions ripe for conflict to arise. Multiple care providers rely on one another to carry out portions of the work. For example, physicians depend on nurses to achieve certain client outcomes, nurses depend on physicians to achieve certain client outcomes, and both nurses and physicians depend on a variety of assistive or allied care workers to deliver the therapies or promote client outcomes. Nurses and physicians also depend on each other's expertise. For example, nurses need the physician to prescribe an analgesic if medication would be the appropriate intervention for pain. When physicians request certain therapies, they rely on nurses to assess and evaluate the client, coordinate the care, get the laboratory results ordered and processed, and see that therapy is delivered. The complexity of the interrelationships and the nature of interdependent work create conflict moments for nurses. This coincides with Kotter's (1979) ideas about dependency, power, and conflict in organizations. He viewed power as a mechanism to resolve conflict.

The source of a conflict can be interpersonal or organizational in nature. Furthermore, these categories often overlap. In some cases the conflict situation grows to involve multiple groups or pairs of groups.

Personal and organizational goals and values may clash over general policies. *General policy* refers to the course of action taken by an institution, department, or unit. Policies are the guidelines developed to handle specific issues. They are designed to give guidance about standardized ways to make decisions in recurring circumstances. However, professionals and other care providers may approach situations with diverse viewpoints about the "best" way to handle a specific problem. Disputes between and among nurses, physicians, and assistive personnel arise over methods and procedures involving specific diagnostic, therapeutic, clerical, or managerial routines. Clashes may result when a nurse's professional judgment as an autonomous professional intersects with standardized policies developed by the institution and designed to produce uniform behavior.

Resource allocation is an issue associated with the definition of organizational conflict. Cost-containment strategies have created conflict over scarce resources in organizations. Nurses often are placed in the center of this conflict. The scarcer the resources, the greater is the potential for conflict.

Power divisions occur across organizational and interpersonal lines to produce role conflicts. Role conflicts often manifest themselves in role overload and role ambiguity. Role overload is a common source of nursing conflict. It occurs when nurses are expected to perform the work of other employees or disciplines in addition to providing nursing care. The result of overload often is burnout. Another facet of role conflict, role ambiguity, occurs when the nurse's responsibility expands faster than is officially recognized. When roles are unclear, conflict can surface.

Another stress point for conflict in nursing occurs when the individual's needs intersect with the organization's needs and goals. Role stress and strain are a reality in the work existence of nurses. For example, other decision makers in the environment may hold one view about what the nurse's role should be, whereas nurses may have an entirely different view, and the two views may conflict. For instance, nurses consider a part of their role to be client advocacy. When an unfavorable outcome occurs, the nurse's client advocacy role may be placed in opposition to the institution's image or legal liability needs. Furthermore, nurses as individuals may need job security, practice autonomy, or pay equity. These needs may conflict with the organization's needs to hold down labor costs or control the practice decisions of its largest category of workers.

Sometimes conflict stems from individuals' attitudes, personalities, and personal behavior. *Personal behavior* refers to style, mannerisms, or work habits. Chronic lateness is an example of a personal behavior that frequently causes conflict. In all cases, it is important for leaders and managers to separate issues related to persons and personalities from issues arising from work-specific problems.

Whatever the cause, when a conflict occurs, an individual can expect that more information will be needed to process the conflict constructively. Similar to problem solving, conflict situations require information gathering and clear problem definition. However, the conflict may be difficult to define, especially if more than one causative factor contributes to the tension. Furthermore, the conflict may involve a covert, less obvious issue than what is presented on the surface. Conflicts often appear larger and more difficult to manage than what actually can be done about them. For example, intense or high levels of emotion are a part of conflict. Both the emotional and issues content of the conflict will need to be managed. By identifying both the areas of agreement and areas of disagreement and then defining the extent of each party's aims, a nurse leader or manager can begin the process of constructively reducing a seemingly overwhelming conflict to a manageable and functional one.

Clearly, if not handled productively, conflicts can be a disruptive rather than a creative force. Conflict involves energy. Within an organization, consistently avoiding or suppressing conflict is usually not effective because conflict can be the first process that occurs in an attempt to create changes or to innovate. If managed appropriately, conflict can motivate people to look at situations and others in new ways. It can lead to increased productivity and harmony. Modes of behavior such as aggressive, hurtful competition maximize the destructive effects of conflict. For nurses, the techniques of problem solving form a useful basis for handling conflict. However, nurses need to cultivate an understanding of conflict and an attitude of self-confidence in constructive conflict management.

Marshall (2006) discussed approaches to prevent and manage conflict.

1. Get education and training in conflict and conflict management. Conflict resolution education and skills training should be part of all health care professional programs and all health care facilities' continuing education programs. In addition, there are numerous publications on conflict resolution skills and techniques that are easily accessible.
2. Improve communication skills. Active listening is especially important in conflict resolution.
3. Recognize that men and women frequently, but not always, have different communication styles and responses to conflict. Women tend to seek each other's company in times of stress and want to discuss and share their experiences. Women turn outward, whereas men tend to turn inward.
4. Adopt an AVID approach to others. Nurses are not alone in being surrounded by stressful, conflict laden situations on a daily basis. In order to deal with the stress of everyday life, suggest using the AVID approach:

A: Assume the positive about others and their behavior. Assume that they are reasonable and are not trying to cause you grief or pain. Assume that if someone is difficult to deal with, they have something problematic going on in their life. Assume it is about them and not about you.

V: If you cannot assume the positive, then you must Validate the situation. Talk to the individual directly and find out what is going on with them.

I: If you are unable to assume the positive and are unable (or unwilling) to validate the situation by talking to the individual, then Ignore it and let it go.

D: If you cannot think positively, cannot or will not validate, and can no longer ignore, then DO something. There are a number of things you can DO:

- Debrief the situation with a trusted friend and get advice.
- Discuss the situation and your response with a therapist.
- Do introduce relaxing activities and techniques into your lifestyle.
- Consider meditation as a way to become more self-aware and positively focused (Marshall, 2006).

The goal of conflict resolution is to create a win-win situation for all. Although it is not realistic to think that every conflict can be resolved in such an ideal fashion, win-win solutions are a worthy goal requiring hard work, creativity, and sound strategy.

CURRENT ISSUES AND TRENDS

The passage of the Patient Protection and Affordable Care Act (PPACA) provided tremendous opportunities for nurses to be at the forefront in the implementation of the health care reform law. Principles of uncertainty, centrality, and unsubstitutability can be applied to increase the power of the nursing profession within the health care system. The following strategies may be used to demonstrate that nurses can cope with uncertainty, become unsubstitutable, and establish centrality in order to establish a power base.

Nurse-Led Innovations

To meet the challenges of health care reform, implementation will require new approaches to health care delivery such as Accountable Care Organizations (ACOs), Patient-Centered Medical Homes (PCMHs), and Nurse Managed Health Centers (NMHCs).

ACOs are a new approach to health care delivery, encompassing a network of doctors/providers and hospitals that share responsibility for providing care to patients. In the new law, an ACO would agree to manage all of the health care needs of a minimum of 5000 Medicare beneficiaries for at least 3 years. During this fixed, 3-year term, the ACO will receive a fixed payment for each Medicare patient enrolled with it. Since the various providers within the ACO are jointly responsible for the patient, they will be expected to share that bundled payment. The payment will be based on the average, expected health care utilization of each patient, but no one knows yet how that payment will be determined or how much

it will be adjusted upward for patients with chronic illnesses. This will replace the fee-for-service model that Medicare currently uses to pay providers. Green (2012) identified the following six attributes that ACOs must have to ensure success:

- Information continuity: Patients' records must be available to providers at the point of care and to patients through electronic health record systems.
- Care coordination and managed transitions: Care coordinators must manage care coordination across all levels of care and all care providers, with an emphasis on managing transitions across care settings.
- System accountability: Clear accountability must exist for the total care of the patient, coupled with shared revenue generation based on population outcomes.
- Peer review and teamwork for high-value care: Providers (including nurses) within and across settings have accountability to one another, review one another's work, and collaborate to reliably deliver high-quality, high-value care.
- Continuous innovation: Innovation and learning are inherent in the system to improve the quality, value, and patients' experiences of health care delivery.
- Easy access to appropriate care: Patients have easy access to appropriate care and information at all hours. Appropriate care includes having access to culturally competent providers who are responsive to patients' needs.

Green (2012) noted that as ACOs emerge across the nation, nurses are expected to play an important role in their success, and leadership positions should abound. The expertise and care services of nurses, as the largest group of care providers, will touch more populations of patients than those of any other group in the future health care system. This will create great challenges and opportunities for the nursing profession.

Medical homes, or health homes, are usually small, community-based primary care practices in which an emphasis is placed on care coordination in order to improve the management and outcomes of chronic illness and reduce the numbers of costly hospitalizations and emergency department visits. Nurses who head up health homes, as occurs in many NMHCs, should consider developing proposals for comparative testing of clinical and financial outcomes of their care coordination and should work with state Medicaid offices to ensure that nurse led practices are included in the state's Medicaid projects (Mason, 2010).

NMHCs could help meet the need for cost-effective quality care and for improving access. Currently over 250 NMHCs operate throughout the United States (National Nursing Centers Consortium, 2012). NMHCs are community-based health clinics that are managed by nurses in partnership with the communities they serve. Most are either independent nonprofits or academically-based clinics affiliated with schools of nursing. NMHCs provide a full range of health services, including primary care, health promotion, and disease prevention, to low-income, underinsured, and uninsured clients. They record over 2.5 million client encounters annually and provide primary care to approximately 250,000 patients around the nation. This care is provided by nurse practitioners, clinical nurse specialists, registered nurses, health educators, community outreach workers, health care students, and collaborating physicians. By providing accessible, high-quality, comprehensive primary care services to populations who have trouble accessing care, NMHCs reduce health disparities.

Esperat and colleagues (2012) described the nurse-managed health center (NMHC) as a model for effective health delivery in providing safety-net care to medically underserved populations. There is mounting evidence that demonstrates that NMHCs provide quality and cost-effective care to their target populations. Esperat and colleagues (2012) noted that although the Division of Nursing of the Health Resources and Services Administration has ample data to support the findings that NMHCs are a significant component of the primary health care system in providing access particularly for medically underserved and vulnerable populations, the financial challenges facing NMHCs are enormous. It will take a great deal of effort from the NMHC movement to give NMHCs a fighting chance to survive within the competitive health care climate. Esperat and colleagues (2012) concluded that policy changes are essential to assure that NMHCs remain an integral part of the primary health care safety net for America's vulnerable populations, and that advance practice nurses are at the forefront of policy initiatives.

Research

Nurse researchers must continue to contribute to the development of nursing knowledge. In addition, the economic value of the profession must be demonstrated through research. Although economic evaluation of nursing practice has increased, it is still a rather small area (Lämås et al., 2009). Comparative effectiveness research (CER), a model by which cost-benefit analyses of different treatments for a given condition are compared, provides an excellent avenue to demonstrate economic value.

Scope of Practice

The health care reform law includes various measures to promote primary care, prevention, chronic care management, transitional care, and care coordination—all services that nurses provide (Mason, 2010). As recommended in the IOM 2010 Report on the Future of Nursing, Advanced Practice Nurses (APNs) must be allowed to practice to the full extent of their education and licensure. With 32 million Americans about to receive health insurance under PPACA, it is crucial that APNs be permitted to provide the primary care they are educated to give (Hassmiller, 2010).

Interprofessional Collaboration

Hassmiller (2010) suggested that teamwork and collaboration are critical to seamless high-quality care. The process begins with understanding the roles and responsibilities of each health care discipline through joint education for nursing and medical students, and students from other health care disciplines. The interprofessional collaboration must continue as a cultural norm in practice settings.

Leadership

With more than 3 million registered nurses in the nation, the nursing profession should be a tremendous force in political and public policy debates. The reality offers the nursing profession a formidable power base that is largely untapped (Abood, 2007). Boswell and colleagues (2005) noted that, more than ever, nurses need to be involved personally and professionally in the political arena. Increasingly, decisions that influence nursing and health care are being made by politicians. All nurses are touched by the impact of policy and politics on health care and nursing practice, research, and education. Thus it is essential that nursing become involved in the political process. Barriers to political activism are thought to include heavy workloads, feelings of powerlessness, time constraints, gender issues, and lack of understanding of a complex political process (Boswell et al., 2005). In a recent article, Abood (2007) offered several strategies for effective action in the legislative arena—entering the legislative arena, understanding steps in the process, understanding the power players, understanding committees, and communicating with legislators. Mullinix (2011) noted the need for nurse legislators and explained that the absence of nurses from leadership positions poses a risk to patients and to the future of health care. When nurse legislators are present, health care delivery decisions are made voices with intimate know of direct patient care are present. Health care organization administrators need to appoint nurse executives to positions that have a voice in strategic decision-making processes. Leadership development must be a feature of every work setting and professional association (McBride, 2011) and nurses should provide leadership at all levels (Hassmiller, 2010). Nurses at the bedside need to be empowered through shared governance models to provide evidence-based, cost-effective care (Barden et al., 2011).

Technology

According to Glaser and Latimer (2011), there is reasonable certainty about the major health information system applications our nation's nurses will encounter in the era ahead. These are (1) an integrated electronic health record that spans inpatient, outpatient and emergency department care; (2) a revenue cycle system that also spans this care continuum and is well integrated with the electronic health record; (3) work flow engines that help to improve the performance of core clinical processes, such as patient discharge, chronic disease management and infection management; (4) rules engines that critique a specific clinician decision, such as checking for drug-drug interactions after the entry of a medication order; (5)

business intelligence and analytics technologies that enable providers to measure the quality, safety, and efficiency of their care, monitor clinical performance, and understand the resulting reimbursement ramifications; (6) interoperability technologies that enable providers to exchange such clinical data as patient allergies, problems, medications, and information on events (e.g., an unplanned emergency room visit) with other providers as they jointly manage the care of the patient; and (7) patient-oriented technologies like the personal health record and online patient communities that assist patients in managing their own care (Glaser & Latimer, 2011). The authors noted that now is the time for nurses to exert their leadership and become intimately familiar with their respective organization's strategic information technology vision, especially the implications it will have on patient care.

Through the challenging years ahead, the nursing profession must demonstrate its ability to cope with uncertainty and establish centrality and unsubstitutability in order to establish the power base to shape practice and the health care environment. As McBride (2011) asserted, nurses need to seize the opportunities handed to them.

As has always been the case, nurses derive their core power from being the health care providers that the public trusts the most. Caring generates power in relationships, and nurses can nurture this as a power source. Individually, nurses can use power concepts to establish a power base and gain power in their work setting. For example, nurses can use information and expertise to construct powerful, persuasive arguments. Nurses can collect and analyze data that can be strategically used or controlled. They can be visible and persistent in goal pursuit. They can be creative and challenge the system to innovate. Nurses can use group power strategies such as networking, connecting, and collaborating to achieve professional goals and contribute to the welfare of patients as well as to the health of the population.

CASE STUDY

Mary Jones, an experienced nurse, accepted a staff nurse position on a medical-surgical unit at the University Hospital a year ago. She was on time every day and completed her assignments in a timely manner. Mary took the initiative to assist others or asked what needed to be done when she had completed her assignment. Because of her previous work experience, she was aware that some of the work processes on the unit were outdated and in need of revision to increase efficiency. She offered suggestions to her peers and the Nurse Manager. Her suggestions for change were met with remarks such as "That's not the way we do it," or "That wouldn't work here." After she had been there for 3 months, Mary began to notice a change in the way some of the staff interacted with her. They would withhold certain information about hospital procedures and equipment and often asked pointed questions designed to "trip" her up. Mary noticed that some of the nurses seemed to do the minimum to get by, were often given lighter assignments, and would take long breaks and socialize together. She began to feel excluded and isolated. After Mary had been employed for 6 months, she was eligible for a pay increase. Performance reviews and pay increases were just issued, and one of the nurses who was not productive received a significant increase, which she bragged about. Mary was perplexed and disappointed because her performance review was just satisfactory, and she did not receive much of an increase.

1. What are the dimensions of power and conflict evident in this case study?
2. How is it possible to turn the situation around?
3. How can a win-win situation be created?
4. What power and conflict resolution strategies might be helpful?
5. Which communication techniques would be most constructive?
6. What are the disagreements, interference, and negative emotions involved in this situation?

CRITICAL THINKING EXERCISE

Although Jessica had been working at the community hospital longer than Danielle, the two had been friends and professional work colleagues on the same unit for many years. Both have completed master's degrees and are considered leaders on their unit. Unexpectedly, the nurse manager of the unit submitted her resignation. The position was advertised and there were many applications for the position. Both Jessica and Danielle applied; and, out of numerous applicants, Danielle was hired for the position. Jessica was clearly upset when she was not selected. She felt that she was more qualified for the position. She became distant and cold, and Danielle knew that Jessica was complaining about her and making comments to others. Tensions arose when Danielle decided to introduce a new policy, which made little sense to the rest of the nurses and is likely to increase their already heavy workload. When presented with the policy at the staff meeting, Jessica angrily voiced her opposition to the policy and pointed out all the flaws, obstacles, and potential problems. Other members of the staff began to side with Jessica.

1. What are the dimensions of power and conflict evident in this case study?
2. How is it possible to turn the situation around?
3. How can a win-win situation be created?
4. What power and conflict resolution strategies might be helpful?
5. Which communication techniques would be most constructive?
6. What are the disagreements, interference, and negative emotions involved in this situation?

11

Workplace Diversity

Diane L. Huber

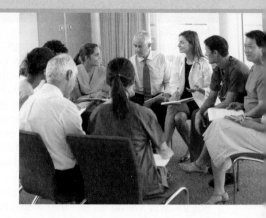

ⓔvolve WEBSITE

http://evolve.elsevier.com/Huber/leadership/

Cultural diversity in the workplace is a growing factor for health care in the United States, both for nurses and the patients and families they care for. More than 80 years ago, following the 1930 census, the U.S. Census Bureau reported that Whites made up **89.8%** of the U.S. population (U.S. Census Bureau, n.d.a). By the time of the 1990 census, the White percentage of the U.S. population declined to **80.3%** (U.S. Census Bureau, n.d.b). Following the 2010 census the U.S. Census Bureau reported Whites made up **75%** of the U.S. population (U.S. Census Bureau, 2011a). Looking into the future, the Census Bureau estimates that "Minorities, now roughly one-third of the U.S. population, are expected to become the majority in 2042, with the nation projected to be 54 percent minority in 2050" (U.S. Census Bureau, 2008, p. 1).

The Affordable Care Act of 2010 (ACA) will increase the diversity of patients seen in health care settings. In an amicus curiae brief filed with the U.S. Supreme Court before that court upheld the constitutionality of the ACA, the NAACP Legal Defense & Educational Fund, Inc., and others noted that "racial minorities are much more likely to be uninsured than

whites… Latinos are the most likely to be uninsured, followed by African Americans" (U.S. Supreme Court, 2012, p. 10). The Kaiser Family Foundation further pointed out that minorities are much more likely to be uninsured than whites. "About one-third of Hispanics and nearly one-quarter of black Americans are uninsured, compared to 14% of non-Hispanic whites" (The Henry J. Kaiser Family Foundation, 2011, p. 11). The Kaiser report provided the following figures for non-elderly Americans lacking insurance coverage in 2010:

White, non-Hispanic=14%
Black, non-Hispanic=22%
Hispanic=32%
Asian=19%
American Indian=30%
Multiracial=15%

The passage of the ACA, with its constitutionality subsequently upheld by the U.S. Supreme Court, results in the provision of insurance coverage to many previously uncovered Americans; and in the process it will also increase the proportion of non-Whites being able to seek and receive health care.

Continuing change in demographics and insurance coverage heightens the importance of dealing with the growing cultural diversity in the workplace. There are two important elements to any workplace effectively

---

Photo used with permission from Photos.com.

dealing positively with the growth of cultural diversity: (1) increasing employee knowledge of other cultures, and (2) taking steps to eradicate ethnocentrism in the workforce. *Ethnocentrism* is defined as being "characterized by or based on the attitude that one's own group is superior" (Merriam-Webster, 2012).

DEFINITIONS

The term **workplace diversity** is a common term today, but it is one that has to be carefully analyzed as its impact on the health care environment and workplaces is considered. An internet search returns many sites containing discussion of actions in pursuit of workplace diversity or multiple applications of or for workplace diversity initiatives. But the question remains as to what is an appropriate definition for **workplace diversity,** especially as it relates to health care.

BACKGROUND

Diversity of Employees and Patients

Nurses deal with diversity in their workplaces every day, and this diversity comes from many perspectives. Some work with patients' families from diverse cultures; some work with co-workers from diverse cultures. The institution has its own culture, as does each nurse or clinician.

In order to make a positive contribution to the effective treatment of patients, it is critical that nurses or clinicians first recognize that they are dealing with this multiplicity of cultures. They include the culture of:

- Each clinician
- The patient/family
- Each co-worker
- The health care institution

From where does culture come? A culture can develop from characteristics such as those enumerated by the U.S. Department of Health and Human Services (USDHHS, 2003, p. 9).

A culture can be defined by characteristics such as the following:

- National origin
- Customs and traditions
- Length of residency in the United States
- Language
- Age
- Generation
- Gender

- Religious beliefs
- Political beliefs
- Sexual orientation
- Perceptions of family and community
- Perceptions of health, well-being, and disability
- Physical ability or limitations
- Socioeconomic status
- Education level
- Geographic location
- Family and household composition

However, when looking at areas from which cultural values are drawn, it is important *not* to assume that the criteria for a certain cultural group are true for every person who belongs to that racial, ethnic, or cultural group. Patients and/or their families, clinicians, and other individuals should not be put into restricted, culturally specific "boxes" nor labeled by virtue of culture and race. Learning cultural values requires moving beyond the group generalization to the individual's specific values. History shows that the differences between the two extremes of any group are usually greater than the differences between the midpoint of two different groups. As President Obama said, "culture matters but that culture is shaped by circumstance" (Obama, 2006, p. 255).

Henry (2012) gives an example about assuming that the criteria for a certain cultural group are true for every person in that group. He tells of the Dalai Lama reflecting on a trip he took to Israel and a discussion he had with one of the chief rabbis. When queried about what doctrine(s) united Jews all around the world, the rabbi responded that there wasn't such a doctrine, and that in fact it was the rituals practiced by Jews that united them. Henry (2012) further noted the non-universality of doctrine in the Roman Catholic Church: "Whatever the few required tenets are that all Catholics must believe, certainly they do not include opposition to birth control, legalized abortion and gay marriage" (p. 1).

There is a large percentage of Roman Catholic women, more than 90% according to some polls, who have practiced some form of birth control. He explained that "This figure is so high because many priests tell women in the confessional to follow their conscience on this issue" (Henry, 2012, p. 1).

Workplace diversity for nurses encompasses not only their nursing colleagues and other health care workers. Just as importantly, it encompasses the patients and families the nurses work with. The U.S. Census (U.S. Census Bureau, 2011b) shows that not only is the nation changing to less and less of a White society, but also it is becoming less identified as a Christian society (Table 11-1). However, race and religion are just two of the things that factor into diversity. What really is diversity?

In the 1990s the U.S. Department of Commerce and the Vice President of the United States created a task force that issued the benchmark study: *Best Practices in Achieving Workforce Diversity*. That task force (U.S. Department of Commerce, 1999, p. 7) verbalized a wide ranging conceptualization of diversity:

A common misconception about diversity is that only certain persons or groups are included under its umbrella, when in fact, exactly the opposite is true. Diversity includes the entire spectrum of primary dimensions of an individual, including Race, Ethnicity, Gender, Age, Religion, Disability, and Sexual orientation. Secondary dimensions commonly include: communication style, work style, organizational role/level, economic status, and geographic origin (e.g., East, Midwest, South). It is a simple fact that each of us possesses unique qualities along each of these dimensions.

HISTORY

In the United States, as elsewhere in the world, social unrest and the evolution of a cultural response to issues of diversity have tended to occur periodically and typically have revolved around one diversity issue at a time. From the ratification of the U.S. Constitution in 1790, it was more than three quarters of a century before the Constitution was amended (13th, 14th, and 15th amendments) in the late 1860s to provide some equality for African Americans. It was still a century later before the 1960s civil rights movement brought about some semblance of equality for African Americans in the United States through the adoption of the Civil Rights Act of 1964, the Fair Housing Act of 1968, and other civil rights laws and related measures. It was 130 years after the adoption of the U.S. Constitution before it was amended to give women the right to vote.

In the mid twentieth century there was significant discussion about religious diversity in the United States. Roman Catholics were frequently denied equal treatment in social and cultural arenas. The election of John F. Kennedy as the first Roman Catholic President of the United States saw a significant reduction in the discrimination experienced by Catholics. The tragic events of September 11, 2001, not only resulted in nearly 3000 deaths but also saw an upswing in Muslim Americans being denied equal treatment in social and cultural arenas. Jews in the United States have experienced their own brand of discrimination, and Mormons and other religious affiliations have experienced theirs. The U.S.

TABLE 11-1	**RELIGIOUS DIVERSITY IN THE U.S.**		
INCREASE IN GROUP POPULATION		**CHANGE IN GROUP'S PERCENTAGE OF TOTAL POPULATIONS**	
	2008	**1990**	**2008**
Total U.S. population	Increased 30.1% over 1990		
Christian	Increased 14.7% over 1990	86.2% of total population	75.9% of total population

Other
  Jewish
  Muslim
  Buddhist
  Unitarian/Universalist
  Hindu
  Native American
  Sikh
  Wiccan
  Pagan
  Spiritualist
	Increased 50.1% over 1990	3.3% of total population	3.9% of total population

No Religion	Increased 138% over 1990	8.2% of total population	14.9% of total population

Source: The 2012 Statistical Abstract, The National Data Book, U.S. Census Bureau, 2011b.

Census Bureau reported that religious diversity in the United States continues to increase (see Table 11-1) (U.S. Census Bureau, 2011b).

In the early years of the twenty-first century, gay marriage became the focal point for denial of equal treatment in social and cultural areas. Many health care and legal matters are impacted by the gay marriage question, including insurance, Medicaid, and hospital visitation.

It is interesting to look at why humans generalize or categorize so much when dealing with the "unique qualities" that the Vice President's workforce diversity task force (1999) said "each of us possesses." Some believe that the human mind generalizes because it cannot deal with a multitude of variables at the same time. Halford and colleagues (2005, p. 70) reported on a study where "the conceptual complexity of problems was manipulated to probe the limits of human information processing capacity… These findings suggest that a structure defined on four variables is at the limit of human processing capacity." This is perhaps an explanation as to why the mind classifies things for us. However, such classification can lead to significant errors when the mind makes inferences about an individual from the group classification it has created. For example, Hilton (2007) provided an in-depth look at the positions of various religions on abortion (Table 11-2), demonstrating diversity and variance.

TABLE 11-2 RELIGIOUS VIEWS OF ABORTION

BUDDHISM	CHRISTIANITY	HINDUISM	ISLAM	JUDAISM
The modern **Buddhist** view on the morality of abortion is more divided. Abortion is permissible when it is necessary for saving the life of the mother, or when it is known that a child would be born with medical conditions that would cause it to suffer.	The **Roman Catholic Church** believes that life begins at conception and thus abortion is considered to be a grave moral offense. Not all Catholics agree with the Vatican line on abortion. Though the **Episcopal Church** recognizes a woman's right to terminate her pregnancy, the church condones abortion only in cases of rape or incest, cases in which a mother's physical or mental health is at risk, or cases involving fetal abnormalities. The official position of the **Evangelical Lutheran Church** in America states that "abortion prior to viability [of a fetus] should not be prohibited by law or by lack of public funding," but that abortion after the point of fetal viability should be prohibited except when the life of a mother is threatened or when fetal abnormalities pose a fatal threat to a newborn.	Nonviolence includes that it is not only wrong to kill living beings, but to kill embryos as well. Abortion is practiced in Hindu culture in India, because the religious ban on abortion is sometimes overruled by the cultural preference for sons.	Muslims regard abortion as wrong, but many accept that it may be permitted in certain cases.	Judaism expects that every case be considered according to its own merits and that the decision to abort only be made after consultation with a rabbi.

Data from Hilton, A. (2007). *The different religions' views on abortion.* Retrieved from *http://www.helium.com/items/716202-the-different-religions-views-on-abortion* and The Pew Forum (2013) retrieved from *http://www.pewforum.org/abortion/religious-groups-official-positions-on-abortion.aspx.*

Although followers of Roman Catholicism, Judaism, Protestant faiths, or Islam may hold given positions on abortion or contraception, many adherents of each faith undoubtedly practice something different than what their faith espouses. Those who generalize about Catholics being pro-life or anti-contraception would many times be wrong when applying those characteristics to individual Catholics. As an example, "nearly 70 percent of Catholic women use sterilization, the birth control pill or an IUD" according to a 2011 report from the Guttmacher Institute, the nonprofit sexual health research organization (Reuters, 2011, p. 1).

At times it seems that most if not all of the "unique qualities" that the Vice President's workforce diversity task force (U.S. Department of Commerce and Vice President Al Gore's National Partnership for Reinventing Government Benchmarking Study, 1999) said "each of us possesses" can become a point of contention both between workers and between workers and those they care for. It is essential for nurses to understand those "unique qualities" of their co-workers and their patients/families as they seek to respond in a holistic way to the needs of those they are responsible for.

The field of health care, and especially nursing practice, must recognize and respond to diversity as much if not more than any other industry in the twenty-first century. That is because workplace diversity in the health care setting includes the following:

- Diversity among employees
- Diversity among patients (customers)
- Diversity as applied by a diverse population of employees to a diverse population of patients
- Application of basic principles of life that are often viewed and valued differently by individuals (both employees and patients) based on individual mores that frequently come from race, ethnicity, religion, and other diverse foundations. But these principles may vary more between individuals within a particular group than they do between groups.

NATIONAL STANDARDS ON CULTURALLY AND LINGUISTICALLY APPROPRIATE SERVICES

The Office of Minority Health (2007) in the U.S. Department of Health and Human Services has established National Standards on Culturally and Linguistically Appropriate Services (CLAS). The CLAS standards are designed to make health care practices culturally and linguistically appropriate. The 14 standards form generally accepted practice standards that nurses need to be familiar with. They are:

Standard 1
Health care organizations should ensure that patients/consumers receive from all staff members effective, understandable, and respectful care that is provided in a manner compatible with their cultural health beliefs and practices and preferred language.

Standard 2
Health care organizations should implement strategies to recruit, retain, and promote at all levels of the organization a diverse staff and leadership that are representative of the demographic characteristics of the service area.

Standard 3
Health care organizations should ensure that staff at all levels and across all disciplines receive ongoing education and training in culturally and linguistically appropriate service delivery.

Standard 4
Health care organizations must offer and provide language assistance services, including bilingual staff and interpreter services, at no cost to each patient/consumer with limited English proficiency at all points of contact, in a timely manner during all hours of operation.

Standard 5
Health care organizations must provide to patients/consumers in their preferred language both verbal offers and written notices informing them of their right to receive language assistance services.

Standard 6
Health care organizations must assure the competence of language assistance provided to limited English proficient patients/consumers by interpreters and bilingual staff. Family and friends should not be used to provide interpretation services (except on request by the patient/consumer).

Standard 7
Health care organizations must make available easily understood patient-related materials and post signage in the languages of the commonly encountered groups and/or groups represented in the service area.

Standard 8

Health care organizations should develop, implement, and promote a written strategic plan that outlines clear goals, policies, operational plans, and management accountability/oversight mechanisms to provide culturally and linguistically appropriate services.

Standard 9

Health care organizations should conduct initial and ongoing organizational self-assessments of CLAS-related activities and are encouraged to integrate cultural and linguistic competence-related measures into their internal audits, performance improvement programs, patient satisfaction assessments, and outcomes-based evaluations.

Standard 10

Health care organizations should ensure that data on the individual patient's/consumer's race, ethnicity, and spoken and written language are collected in health records, integrated into the organization's management information systems, and periodically updated.

Standard 11

Health care organizations should maintain a current demographic, cultural, and epidemiological profile of the community as well as a needs assessment to accurately plan for and implement services that respond to the cultural and linguistic characteristics of the service area.

Standard 12

Health care organizations should develop participatory, collaborative partnerships with communities and utilize a variety of formal and informal mechanisms to facilitate community and patient/consumer involvement in designing and implementing CLAS-related activities.

Standard 13

Health care organizations should ensure that conflict and grievance resolution processes are culturally and linguistically sensitive and capable of identifying, preventing, and resolving cross-cultural conflicts or complaints by patients/consumers.

Standard 14

Health care organizations are encouraged to regularly make available to the public information about their progress and successful innovations in implementing the CLAS standards and to provide public notice in their communities about the availability of this information.

COMMUNICATION

Communication between nurses and the patients/ families they treat is an underlying element with significant impact on the effectiveness of that treatment. Communication failure between the nurse or other health care worker can result from language barriers and/or cultural value differences.

The Council on Graduate Medical Education, Twelfth Report (U.S. Department of Health and Human Services, 1998, p. 4) noted that:

> Although interpreters can assist ... health care professionals should become more involved in the communication process by seeking a greater understanding of cultural differences among their patient populations. The report went on to state: cultural competency includes certain common elements: appropriate communication skills; an ability to identify health beliefs of different groups; and an understanding of biases and barriers that inhibit access to health care. Becoming culturally competent is viewed as a developmental process with five elements: a) valuing diversity; b) making a cultural self-assessment; c) understanding the dynamics when cultures interact; d) incorporating cultural knowledge; and e) adapting practices to the diversity of the population in the setting.

In considering the patent/family's culture, it should be remembered that each individual likely holds varying levels of commitment and/or involvement in his or her culture. This variation will likely result in differences in cultural beliefs and practices among members of the patient's cultural group. It underscores the need for assessment of individual cultural values.

For example, a case presentation routinely includes a racial designation, such as: a 50-year-old Hispanic male presents with chest pain. What meaning does "Hispanic" convey to the clinician? This individual could have been born in Monterrey, Mexico, be a college professor who speaks five languages including English, and lives 6 months each year in the United States and 6 months in Mexico. This patient might also be a monolingual Hispanic man, born in the United States, living alone in a Chicago ghetto, with little education and very low income. Failure to identify such differences not only perpetuates stereotypes evaluations but also can cause the clinician to fail in accurately assessing potential conflicts with the cultural values of this patient or identifying important communication barriers.

Schyve (2007, p. 360) discussed the importance placed on patient communication by The Joint Commission:

Effective communication with patients is critical to the safety and quality of care. Barriers to this communication include differences in language, cultural differences, and low health literacy. Evidence-based practices that reduce these barriers must be integrated into, rather than just added to, health care work processes.

In assessing the individual's own cultural competency for dealing with patients and their families from other cultures, there are numerous tools available, some at no cost and others for a fee, on the internet. Nurses can locate a tool, do a self-assessment, and apply the results. One example is a *Self-Assessment Checklist for Personnel Providing Primary Health Care Services.* This checklist is provided by the National Center for Cultural Competence at Georgetown University *(http://nccc. georgetown.edu/documents/Checklist%20PHC.pdf).* This checklist asks the user to rate themselves on items such as: "I understand and accept that family is defined differently by different cultures; I accept individuals and families as the ultimate decision makers for services and supports impacting their lives; I accept that religion and other beliefs may influence how individuals and families respond to illnesses, disease, and death."

Another example is *Eight Steps to Cultural Competence For Primary Health Care Professionals,* provided by the Nova Scotia Department of Health *(http:// healthteamnovascotia.ca/cultural_competence/Cultural_ Competence:guide_for_Primary_Health_Care_ Professionals.pdf).* Examples of steps are: "Recognize racism and the institutions or behaviors that breed racism; Familiarize yourself with core cultural elements of the communities you serve; Recognize that unique experiences and histories will result in differences in behaviors, values and needs; Learn how different cultures define, name and understand disease and treatment."

LEADERSHIP AND MANAGEMENT IMPLICATIONS

Multicultural Teams

Diversity is a basic component of a strong team. Valuing all team members creates synergistic relationships, which translate into a higher quality of production. Ignoring diversity inhibits full participation and may even disrupt the workings of an effective team. Because much of the diversity of individuals is far below the surface, it may be difficult to recognize that there is a clash of cultures that prevents a team from gelling. In fact, relationships may be significantly damaged before anyone realizes that the conflicts that the team experience are not about what the team members say they are about. Recent research (Brett et al., 2006) has identified the following four categories of challenges that arise from differing styles of communication in multicultural teams and can jeopardize important projects:

- Direct versus indirect communication
- Trouble with accents and fluency
- Differing attitudes toward hierarchy and authority
- Conflicting norms for decision making

Of note are some words of caution. Individuals who cannot articulate their thoughts or feelings may be wrongly judged as less intelligent. Such logic can devalue those team members and subject them to disrespect, ridicule, and ostracism. It is wise to analyze carefully and proceed with caution about approaches to communication style, decision making, and organizational structure. Individuals from Western cultures such as the United States prefer direct forms of communication, such as asking questions, giving opinions freely, and making eye contact; they tend to judge those who do not do so as dishonest and not trustworthy. Westerners also prefer flat instead of hierarchical structures, but colleagues from hierarchal cultures are uncomfortable on flat teams. This is explained by the concept of high context/low context. An approach called *fusion* is getting serious attention from political scientists and government officials. It seems that today, more than ever, multicultural populations want to protect their cultures rather than integrate or assimilate. An awareness of cultural mismatches is the first step in being proactive in the approach to managing multicultural teams or, equally important, being a good team member.

High Context and Low Context

The assumptions of high context and low context are a part of the health care context, which is always dynamic. The context dictates "where one is coming from" and how information or knowledge is communicated in human transactions or relationships, and it is culturally based. From a global perspective, the cultural context of the Western world is "low context." In low-context cultures, the explicit verbal or written message carries the meaning. Low-context cultures require extensive detailed explanations and information because they are making up for what is missing in a situation. In high-context cultures, often found in the non-Western world, that which is written or stated rarely carries the meaning. The meaning of the message is understood by reading between the lines for what is not written or stated. In high-context cultures, most of the meaning is assumed to exist by the nature of the situation (i.e., the context). Most nuclear families are high context, relying on high interpersonal interaction and subtle messages. Leaders from a low-context culture may have the power to define the rules of work and to determine what will be rewarded, who gets promoted, what benefits will be offered, and what values will define the organization. Therefore placing someone from a high-context workplace culture into a setting dominated by leaders from a low-context culture increases the likelihood of perceptions of inequity and workplace conflicts (Hall & Hall, 1990).

Generational Workforce Diversity

A growing challenge in nursing leadership is the management of generational workforce diversity. Sociologists categorize generational groups into *cohorts*. These cohorts are members of a generation who are linked through shared life experiences in their formative years. As each new cohort matures, it is influenced by what sociologists call *generational markers*. Individuals are all products of their environment. Generational markers are events that affect all members of the generation in one way or another. Thus being aware of generational differences is essential for every organization's leadership in managing a multi-age workforce. Each generation possesses unique characteristics and often deems the values and behaviors of another cohort as character flaws instead of cultural differences (Table 11-3).

Baby Boomers

The baby boomers, born between 1946 and 1964, are currently occupying the leadership chairs of many executive suites, including those in health care organizations. Boomers present a striking contrast to members of the previous generation, those born between 1925 and 1945, often referred to as the *Mature Generation* or the *Silent Generation*. Members of the Silent Generation grew up in a period of strong military and political leaders, a time when respect for authority was expected, conformity was the characteristic most treasured and exhibited, and children were to be seen but not heard.

Boomers, historically the second largest generation in the workforce, have dominated U.S. society for many years because of their large number. Beginning in January of 1996 and continuing for the next 18 years (to 2014), a baby boomer will turn 50 every 18 seconds; and their preferences in every facet of American life are affected by their sheer numbers alone (U.S. Census Bureau, 1996). The boomer phenomenon has been known and predicted for many years. As of 2012, the Boomers were turning 65, retiring, and entering the Medicare system. They also were beginning to acquire chronic conditions. The implications for health care delivery and financing are enormous. Efficiency, teamwork, quality, and service have thrived under their leadership. Boomers grew up in a period of unprecedented economic growth during which the United States had virtually no strong economic competitors. They grew up thinking they were special and that they could ignore or break rules and still be successful.

TABLE 11-3	GENERATIONAL CHARACTERISTICS		
MATURES	**BABY BOOMERS**	**GENERATION X**	**MILLENNIALS**
Hard work	Personal fulfillment	Uncertainty	What's next?
Duty	Optimism	Personal focus	On my terms
Sacrifice	Crusading causes	Live for today	Just show up
Thriftiness	Buy now/pay later	Save, save, save	Earn to spend
Work fast	Work efficiently	Eliminate the task	Do exactly what's asked

Data from Wendover, R.W. (2002). *The corrosion of character.* Aurora, CO: The Center for Generational Studies.

They love convenience and brought true meaning to "charge it" when it comes to debt management. Financial security will remain a central issue for many. Consequently, many Boomers will work past the age of retirement. They have questioned traditional authority structures, blurred gender roles, and made vigorous attempts to push systems toward their ideas of perfection. During the Vietnam War, the civil rights confrontations, and Watergate, baby boomers saw clearly the vulnerability of authority; they have been reluctant to accept formal authority since. Their preference is for a more participative and less authoritarian workplace.

Generation X

Support for such a workplace environment comes also from members of Generation X (X'ers), born between 1965 and 1980, who share with boomers an aversion to authority but with a decided preference for a balanced life. X'ers are the first generation of latchkey kids; as such, they found the need to be resourceful at an early age. Their childhood years have been marked with economic uncertainty, and thus they are skeptical of traditional practices and beliefs. In their view, employment contracts are agreements that either side can cancel at will, which means that placing their future in the hands of employers makes them extremely uneasy and is thus highly unlikely to occur. The length of time spent with an organization is less relevant to X'ers than how to protect themselves from the capriciousness of business challenges (Wendover, 2002). Trust imposes its own constraints and has its own rules.

Millennials

Both the youngest group in the workplace and the largest group in U.S. history are the millennial workers, those born between 1981 and 1999. This group is known by several other monikers, including *Generation Y, Generation Why?, Nexters,* and the *Internet Generation.* The common marker of their developmental years is technology. This group is the most demographically diverse generation in this country's history. These workers have astonishing multitasking skills. They also tend to have a positive outlook and a desire to improve the world.

Many believe that millennials are shallow on basic skills; but because they grew up with computers, they can create solutions that other generations could not

have imagined. Technology guides their every move. They are problem solvers who grew up in a flourishing economy. Millennials matured in a world in which shortcuts, manipulation of rules, and situational ethics seem to have reigned. They got the message somehow that the final word is not the final word. They do not live to work; they work to live. Thus they have a different set of expectations about the world of work. Most enjoy the liberty of working on their own in a style that favors their work ethic. Millennials have learned that their presence is in demand. To thrive, they need clear definitions of outcomes, resources to do what needs to be done, and a deadline.

CURRENT ISSUES AND TRENDS

Nurses recognize that cultural diversity, awareness, and unconditional positive regard for people are critical core concepts. Yet somehow, cultural diversity is not seen as a powerful variable in how nurses communicate and interpret behaviors or mediate conflict among themselves. There can be a direct impact on how problems, assessments, diagnoses, and intervention strategies are determined. As global trends in mobility, migration, cultural identity importance, and changing roles increase, the need for awareness is greater. Shifts in the site of care to the community, a rise in moral/ethical issues in health care, and a desire by many, but not all, consumers to control and regulate their own health care—along with a concomitant desire to make it better for others—have created a necessity to know and respect diverse perspectives.

Attracting a Culturally Diverse Workforce

Reaching for cultural competence in the health care workplace requires not only that institutions strive for a greater understanding of the values represented by divergent patients and families, but also that efforts be increased to diversify the makeup of nursing and other health care professions.

Workplace diversity is an issue for both the workforce and the patients/families. The institutions that take the initiative to strive for cultural competence can engender respect for the similarities and differences that both employees and patients/families bring to the health care endeavor. Success with cultural competence concerning employees will improve understanding for culturally diverse patients/families. In turn, success with culturally diverse patients/families will help an institution recruit and maintain a culturally diverse workforce. The inevitable conflicts that can occur when persons with diverse value sets work together will decrease as success is achieved in cultural competence in interpersonal relationships.

Cultural diversity in the workplace has both advantages and challenges. The synergy of diverse viewpoints can improve nursing's knowledge base and care strategies. Yet the differences among people can give rise to communication gaps and conflict. The same issues of communication, interpersonal space, social proscriptions, time sense, and other variations in beliefs and behaviors that are important when interacting with clients need to be balanced and smoothed in work groups and teams. The nurse care manager can employ cultural competence principles in leading and managing work groups. Strategies of respect for differences, exploring beyond the comfort zone, withholding judgment of others, emphasizing the positive, and practicing good communication techniques are strategies for success.

The National Coalition Building Institute (NCBI) is a not-for-profit leadership training organization focusing on diversity training and school violence prevention. NCBI trains local community leaders in effective bridge-building skills to combat intergroup conflicts. Their NCBI Controversial Issue Process is an example of constructive conflict resolution applicable to cultural diversity training for workplace diversity (NCBI, 2012).

Efforts to pursue cultural competence must incorporate the broad base of diversity. The American Association of Colleges of Nursing (AACN) has reiterated the importance of intensifying efforts to increase diversity in programs that educate nurses (AACN, 2011).

Diversity initiatives in the nursing profession will have a marked opportunity in the coming years because the outlook for growth in nursing jobs is bright. The U.S. Bureau of Labor Statistics (U.S. Department of Labor, 2012) projected that the rate of change in employment for the 10-year period between 2010 and 2020 for nurses is 26%, whereas for all occupations it is 14%. Each nurse lives and works within a meld of cultural aspects and values. This includes influences from race, community, ethnicity, lifestyle, and professional and organizational cultures. The nursing leadership and management challenge is to effectively manage diversity for effectiveness.

RESEARCH NOTE

Source

Weech-Maldonado, R., Dreachslin, J.L., Brown, J., Pradhan, R., Rubin, K.L., Schiller, C., & Hays, R.D. (2012). Cultural competency assessment tool for hospitals: Evaluating hospitals' adherence to the culturally and linguistically appropriate services standards. *Health Care Management Review, 37*(1), 54-66.

Purpose

The purpose of this article is to describe and discuss the development and use of the Cultural Competency Assessment Tool for Hospitals (CCATH). This tool was developed for use as an assessment instrument to gauge adherence to the U.S. health care standards for culturally and linguistically appropriate services (CLAS). This focuses attention on developing culturally competent systems of care where cultural competency practices are integrated throughout clinical and management subsystems.

Discussion

The U.S. Department of Health and Human Services' Office of Minority Health (OMH) has identified 14 CLAS standards within three categories of culturally competent care, language access services, and organizational supports for cultural competence. The CCATH was developed as a tool to quantify and then compare hospitals on the extent of adherence to CLAS standards. Comparing the CLAS standards and the National Quality Forum's cultural competency domains, the authors identified six domains for hospital cultural competency. The CCATH was drafted, pilot tested, evaluated via focus groups and interviews, and field tested. The reliability and validity of the CCATH were determined to be acceptable.

Application to Practice

The authors identified using the CCATH as a tool to evaluate hospital performance and for research as being the practice applications. Collecting benchmark data can assist in identifying national and regional norms. Using this reliable and valid tool, cultural competency practices can be assessed and opportunities for improvement evaluated and remediated. The goal is better patient experiences.

CASE STUDY

Maria, a Hispanic woman with three children, presented with a tumor requiring a hysterectomy. Maria did not speak English, and the health care staff had asked her bilingual son to serve as an interpreter in explaining that Maria needed to sign an informed consent form for the surgery. The son explained the procedure to the mother. Staff noted that he appeared to be translating their explanation to the mother and pointed to his mother's abdomen as he translated. Maria willingly signed the consent form. When Maria learned the next day that she would no longer be able to bear children because her uterus had been removed, she became very agitated. Eventually she threatened to sue the hospital. When the health care staff discussed Maria's agitation with her family, they were told that, because it is not appropriate for a Hispanic male to discuss his mother's private parts with her, Maria's son had explained to her that a tumor would be removed from her abdomen and pointed to the general area. Maria's anger about not being able to bear more children was the result of her role in the Hispanic culture where a Hispanic woman's status is derived in large part from the number of children she produces.

CRITICAL THINKING EXERCISE

Mr. Lin was diagnosed with cancer in China before he emigrated to the United States with his wife and their two sons. The older son attends junior college and speaks English well, always accompanying his non–English-speaking father to the clinic. Since his arrival in the United States, Mr. Lin received treatment for locally invasive nasopharyngeal cancer, which progressed to the point of being immediately life-threatening because of the high likelihood of hemorrhage from major blood vessels in his neck. He has been treated with both radiation therapy and chemotherapy and is taking traditional Chinese medicine.

The professionals caring for Mr. Lin began with the assumption that he must be fully informed. However, relying on Mr. Lin's son to translate opens up the possibility of conflicting notions of what constitutes appropriate disclosure. This is because many Chinese are not used to telling their ill family member everything. Ill family members are not used to this either. It is believed that the client cannot tolerate this information and will become more ill if told the worst. In this case Mr. Lin and his son chose to maintain ambiguity and thus hope.

1. What is the problem in this case?
2. Whose problem is it?
3. What should the health professionals do?
4. How can the health professionals be culturally competent in this situation?

Case and Population Health Management

Diane L. Huber

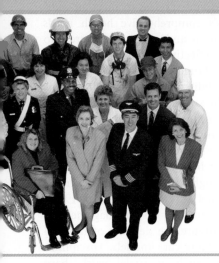

evolve WEBSITE

http://evolve.elsevier.com/Huber/leadership/

It appears that we are in the midst of a care delivery revolution: the radical shift from an acute care–based delivery system to one founded on primary care as the major setting for the delivery of health services. Along with shifts to Patient-Centered Medical Homes (PCMH) and Accountable Care Organizations (ACOs) and reimbursement shifts triggered by the Patient Protection and Affordable Care Act (ACA) of 2010 have come a renewed emphasis on, and reimbursement incentives for, care coordination, integration, and prevention strategies. This is the age of care coordination.

The modern era of case, disease, and population health management began in the early 1990s. The effectiveness of what was called case management (CM) in producing quality and cost containment outcomes began to be noticed anecdotally by providers in the field, but more importantly by health insurance companies who came to believe it worked. However, case management services were rarely paid for outside of rehabilitation and some social services areas, which severely limited the widespread implementation of CM and inhibited care integration. Despite funding restrictions, the belief in the effectiveness of CM

Photo used with permission from Photos.com.

spurred research and the development of the knowledge base and evidence for practice. Major professional, certification, and trade associations also grew over the last 20 to 25 years.

The field first split into CM and disease management (DM) (Huber, 2005a). With the criticism that not all health conditions are "diseases," such as behavioral health, the term *disease management* was dropped in favor of population health management (PHM). Rigorous research and federal government funded demonstration grants continued to solidify the evidence base for practice.

When needed services other than acute care are actually added to/provided for in the mix of health care, it is difficult to demonstrate cost savings. However, CM, DM, and PHM strategies all have proven positive clinical outcomes. What is clear is that **care coordination** is the core element common to all provider interventions in CM, DM, and PHM.

CARE COORDINATION AND INTEGRATION

Central to accomplishing the "triple aim" of better care, better health and lower costs is the strategy called care coordination. **Care coordination** was defined by the Agency for Healthcare Research and Quality (AHRQ, 2007, p. v) as "the deliberate organization of patient care activities between two or more participants (including the patient) involved in a patient's care to facilitate the appropriate delivery of health care services. Organizing care involves the marshalling of personnel and other resources needed to carry out all required patient care activities, and is often managed by the exchange of information among participants responsible for different aspects of care."

According to AHRQ (2007, p. vi), "Care coordination interventions represent a wide range of approaches at the service delivery and systems level. Their effectiveness is most likely dependent upon appropriate matching between intervention and care coordination problems, though more conceptual, empirical and experimental research is required to explore this hypothesis."

Care coordination seeks to meet patient needs and deliver high-quality care (AHRQ, 2011a). Its goal is high-quality transitions and referrals to meet the Institutes of Medicine's (IOM) six aims of safe, effective, efficient, timely, equitable, and patient- and family-centered care (Improving Chronic Illness Care, 2012). According to the IOM's report entitled *Crossing the Quality Chasm: A New Health System for the 21st Century*, the U.S. health care system should use the six criteria to ensure that quality care is provided (IOM, 2001). Transitions of care focus on reducing re-hospitalization rates and enhancing post-discharge care, according to the Centers for Medicare & Medicaid Services (CMS) and the IOM (AHRQ, 2011b). The definition of *transition of care* is "a set of actions designed to ensure the coordination and continuity of health care as patients transfer between different locations or different levels of care within the same location" (AHRQ, 2011b, p. 1). Transitions of care have become more imperative than ever before in current health care reform.

DEFINITIONS

The Case Management Society of America (CMSA) is the professional organization representing case managers in practice. It is a multidisciplinary organization. The CMSA (2012a, p. 1) defines **case management** as "a collaborative process of assessment, planning, facilitation, care coordination, evaluation, and advocacy for options and services to meet an individual's and family's comprehensive health needs through communication and available resources to promote quality, cost-effective outcomes." Thus there is a major professional organization that defines case management as a multidisciplinary provider intervention and promotes the knowledge base for practice.

In nursing, the American Nurses Association (ANA) first defined **nursing case management** as a system of health assessment, planning, service procurement, service delivery, service coordination, and monitoring through which the multiple service needs of clients are met (ANA, 1988; Zander, 1990). Hospital acute care nursing case management is an attempt to reconfigure the delivery of hospital care away from previous care models. Disciplines other than nursing, such as social work, have discipline-specific definitions of case management. In addition, there is a consumer definition of case management, that case managers work with people to get the health care and other community services they need, when they need them, and for the best value, that was promulgated as a communication tool to help explain CM to the public.

CASE MANAGEMENT OVERVIEW

Case management (CM) is an intervention strategy used by multiple health care providers and systems to advocate for clients, coordinate health care delivery, and facilitate outcomes of both cost and quality. Arising out of pressures for cost containment, and later valued for quality control in the midst of alarming medical errors, CM came to be seen by health plans, and later hospitals, as a major solution to serious problems of mission and margin.

Case management as a nursing model of care evolved in the late 1980s. It has been defined as both a process (it is a provider intervention) and a care delivery model. CM has developed as a method to manage care. **Managed care** is care coordination that is organized to achieve specific client outcomes, given fiscal and other resource constraints. Managed care has been described as "the systematic integration and coordination of the financing and delivery of health care" (Grimaldi, 1996, p. 6).

Case management and care coordination have been the care delivery models used for years by public health and community health nurses (Mikulencak, 1993). In these settings, CM has been centered on the needs of the client rather than the shift, unit, or system. Because it is an intervention used by many providers and in multiple settings, as management can occur inside or outside the hospital only, extend across the health care continuum, or be linked to a population focus.

Case management is a system of client care delivery that focuses on the achievement of client outcomes within effective and appropriate time frames and resources. CM has components of health services delivery, coordination, and monitoring, all of which are used to meet the multiple service needs of clients. Hospital-based acute care nursing CM was focused on an entire episode of illness, crossing all settings in which the client receives care. Care is directed by a case manager, who is not always a nurse, and can be unit- or population-focused.

Case management is an interdisciplinary provider intervention that crosses settings and sites of care. Previously used as a strategy in social services, rehabilitation, and public health, by the 1990s CM was a popular way to address coordination of care for the ill and the poor and to manage catastrophic injury or illness. Case managers were deployed to decrease fragmentation, reduce expense by streamlining care, and control costs by linking, advocating, coordinating, negotiating, educating, and monitoring. As CM became more popular, case managers' employment settings shifted to hospitals.

Registered nurses (RNs) have emerged as the large majority of case managers, especially in hospitals, in part because of their specialized expertise for the function of determining medical necessity for health care payment and because of care coordination for complex medical discharge planning needs (Park et al., 2009; Zander, 2002). Zander (2002) called CM "the nursing process applied at a system level" (p. 58). This is because CM services by nurses are designed to produce a balance between the demands of the mission (quality health care) and the operational margin (costs and resources). Case management has grown in conjunction with the experience of risk by payers and providers (Zander, 2002). The American Nurses Association (ANA, 2012) has issued a position statement on care coordination and the RN role to recognize and promote RNs' integral role in the care coordination process.

Case management has garnered considerable attention in health care. It has been suggested that the processes associated with CM have the potential to save money, improve effectiveness, and maintain or improve the quality of care (Lu et al., 2008). However, a diversity of CM approaches exists. For example, "case management may describe a patient care delivery system, a professional practice model, a group of activities that a nurse performs within an organizational setting, or a separate service provided by private practitioners" (Goodwin, 1994, p. 29). The term *case management* can be specific to an institution, refer to services rendered to a population or community, or be a separate service provided by independent case managers or health insurance companies (Goodwin, 1994). Models have been implemented in many settings, including acute care, long-term care, and community health care (Huber, 2005a; Zander, 2002). Case management is a central component of integrating and coordinating care across the health care continuum. It is focused on the individual recipient of services.

Case management is an approach to managing care and service delivery that is designed to coordinate care, decrease costs, and promote access to appropriate and needed services. Case management has a heritage more than a century old, but it gained wide implementation and popularity as systems of managed health care emerged in the 1990s. Managed health care, more simply called *managed care,* has gained momentum and evolved as a response to national concern over rising health care costs and expenditures, increasing care fragmentation, and lack of continuity and access under fee-for-service reimbursement. By the end of the 1990s, health maintenance organizations (HMOs) had become the most predominant form of health care coverage among U.S. businesses with more than 100 employees (Coleman, 1999; Tahan, 1998).

Internal and external pressures on the health care delivery system have been intensifying, including a shortage of RNs and the aging of baby boomers. A convergence of cost, quality, and access demands has created a complex and volatile environment. Complexity arises from the simultaneous balancing of needs for quality, productivity, and flexibility. Health care providers are directed to manage both clinical care outcomes and associated resources by providing cost-efficient and cost-effective health care services and being accountable for the value of services relative to the costs of those services. Specifically, the pressure on nurses is to balance quality of care with client advocacy. Thus nurses need to demonstrate and document the effect of nursing care on client outcomes and on the efficiency and price competitiveness of provided services. The benefits achieved need to exceed the costs incurred. The mounting pressures on the health care delivery system since the mid-1980s have provided an impetus for the explosive growth of case management as both an economically important strategy for controlling costs and an opportunity for health care services improvement during economic hard times.

Like health care, CM as a professional practice role is in transition. For example, the Case Management Society of America (CMSA, 2012b), the organization representing case managers, was founded in 1990. Since then it has grown to an international nonprofit organization dedicated to the support and development of the profession of case management. It has over 75 chapters and more than 11,000 individual members. It has promulgated the following:

- Standards of Practice (CMSA, 2010)
- Statement Regarding Ethical Case Management Practice
- Support of a certification program through the Commission for Case Manager Certification (CCMC), which is an independent separate entity
- State of the Science papers on adherence and patient participation

Case Management

Multiple disciplines lay claim to CM. **Case management** is a term that refers to client-focused strategies concentrating on the coordination and integration of health services for clients with complex or costly health problems. CM has a strong interdisciplinary component. There have been a variety of definitions of CM, often reflecting the perspective of a specific discipline and creating confusion. As the professional organization representing case managers, CMSA's definition is used by convention.

Despite the variety of definitions, the general meaning of CM is any method of linking, managing, or organizing services to meet client needs. Thus CM entails the coordination and sequencing of care. It helps tighten the plan of care and link direct caregivers and services across facility and service boundaries.

Acute care hospital nursing CM is a system in which the accountability for the care management of clients in a specific diagnosis-related group DRG category, disease group, or other population over an entire hospitalization is assigned to an RN. The nurse case manager coordinates care across the continuum of services. Hospital nursing CM usually is targeted at high-risk, high-volume, and/or high-cost populations. Although all clients need to have their care coordinated, CM functions best to coordinate health care services for high-risk populations across community, acute, and long-term care settings (Simpson, 1993). Zander (1991) defined CM as a matrix model at the clinician-provider level in acute care.

Case management in acute care nursing is an attempt to reconfigure the delivery of hospital care into a more integrated system management care modality. CM and care coordination have been the care delivery modalities employed by public health and community health nurses (Mikulencak, 1993). In these settings, CM has been centered on client needs rather than being shift- or unit-centered. CM can occur in the hospital only, extend across the health care continuum, or be linked to a population.

CM is described as a system of client care delivery that focuses on the achievement of client outcomes within effective and appropriate time frames and resources. It is a system of health services delivery, coordination, and monitoring through which multiple service needs of clients are met. CM operates at the intersection of organizational systems and the delivery of clinical care. It is focused on an entire chronic or catastrophic condition or conditions, crossing all settings in which the client receives care. New services across the continuum of health care are incorporated as needed. Care is directed by a case manager, often a nurse, and focuses on an interdisciplinary team effort.

A term related to CM is **disease management**, which is defined as a comprehensive, integrated approach to care and reimbursement based on a disease's natural course. Disease management programs contain a series of clinical processes and services across the health care continuum that rely on informatics to identify and manage a medical or chronic condition in a particular at-risk population to improve care, promote wellness, and manage or reduce costs (Ward & Rieve, 1997). Such disease state CM programs are population-based approaches to the identification and management of chronic conditions. Health status is assessed, plans of care are developed, and data are collected to evaluate the effectiveness of the program (Levitt et al., 1998). These programs are focused on the group level of aggregation and may be community-focused or population health–focused.

Critical Pathways

A *critical pathway* is a written plan that identifies key, critical, or predictable incidents that must occur at set times to achieve client outcomes within an appropriate time frame, such as a length of stay in a hospital setting. A critical pathway has been defined as an "outline or diagram that documents the process of diagnoses or treatment deemed appropriate for a condition based on practice guidelines" (MediLexicon, 2012, p. 1). Critical pathways are tools used to help providers identify, measure, and analyze care processes and desired patient outcomes (Renholm et al., 2002). As a pathway, they are a tracking system for the timing of treatments and interventions, health outcomes, complications, activity, and teaching/learning. They detail essential care steps and describe the expected progress. They include time-dependent functions and organize and integrate provider interventions in a multidisciplinary format and across multiple settings or levels of care (Cesta & Tahan, 2003).

Providing an overview of the whole process, critical pathways are best practice tools that identify and document the standardized, interdisciplinary processes that need to occur for a patient to move toward a desired outcome in a defined period of time. Elements include all providers' assessments and interventions, laboratory and other diagnostic tests, treatments, consultations, activity level, patient and family education, discharge planning, and desired outcomes (Renholm et al., 2002). Critical pathways have been described as protocols of interdisciplinary treatments, based on professional standards of practice and placed in order on a decision tree (Simpson, 1993).

Critical pathways are called by a variety of names, such as critical path, coordinated care path, clinical pathway, clinical protocol, care track, care step, or evidence-based practice protocols. They are case management tools that map out the plan of care and guide and document care within a framework that reflects the research, experience, and consensus priorities of a multidisciplinary group of providers actively engaged in providing care to the target population. Critical pathways are cause-and-effect visual grids or paths to direct care toward goals. They show key incidents and expected behaviors. Critical pathway elements include an index of problems, a timeline, a variance record, and the path or grid. Critical pathways are one form of structured care methodologies (SCMs), or streamlined interdisciplinary tools, used to "identify best practices, facilitate standardization of care, and provide a mechanism for variance tracking, quality enhancement, outcomes measurement, and outcomes research" (Cole & Houston, 1999, p. 53). Examples of SCMs are critical pathways, evidenced-based algorithms, protocols, standards of care, order sets, and clinical practice guidelines. The use of best evidence is considered the gold standard to reduce practice variation in an environment focused on patient outcomes. Critical paths outline time and the sequence of events for an episode-of-care delivery. Resources appropriate in amount and sequence to a specific case type and individual client are managed for length of stay, critical events and timing, and anticipated outcomes. Variances are noted and analyzed. The process of developing and using critical paths encourages both critical thinking and accountability. Critical paths can be used to educate, prepare, and orient care providers and to negotiate expectations and care roles with clients. Critical paths can and should be individualized to each client. They are major tools of outcomes management and coordination of care delivery.

Critical pathways display expected outcomes. A difference between what was expected and what actually occurred is called a *variance*. A variance is a deviation from a standard. Variances can be either positive or negative. Sources of variance include client- and family-related, systems-related, or provider-related factors. A process needs to be in place to document, collect, and analyze variances for trends and opportunities for cost reduction and quality improvement (Cesta & Tahan, 2003). A literature review revealed that the use of critical pathways has a positive impact on patient care outcomes (Renholm et al., 2002).

Benchmarking and evidence-based practice are used in constructing and evaluating critical pathways. Benchmarks form a frame of reference against which an institution can compare itself relative to others. Benchmarking is a useful strategy for helping to understand internal processes and performance levels. Benchmarks help identify performance gaps. Consensus benchmarks can be established by professional societies, health systems, national databases, or texts and manuals (Cesta & Tahan, 2003).

BACKGROUND

Case Management Models

A variety of case management models have arisen; some are nursing models, and others are non-nursing models. The core elements center around a case manager who coordinates and monitors the care given to clients by multiple health care providers and services in an attempt to decrease service fragmentation and improve the quality of care (Rheaume et al., 1994). Weil and Karls (1985) identified eight main service components common to all case management models (Box 12-1).

CM exists in many contexts and settings, including insurance-based programs, employer-based programs, workers' compensation programs, social services programs, independent CM practice, for-profit CM companies, medical practice, nursing practice, public health nursing and home health care agencies, maternal-child settings, and mental health settings.

BOX 12-1 SERVICE COMPONENTS OF MANAGEMENT MODELS

1. Client identification and outreach
2. Individual assessment and diagnosis
3. Service planning and resource identification
4. Linking clients to needed services
5. Service implementation and coordination
6. Monitoring service delivery
7. Advocacy
8. Evaluation

Data from Weil, M., & Karls, J.M. (1985). *Case management in human service practice: A systematic approach to mobilizing resources for clients.* San Francisco: Jossey-Bass.

CM programs incorporate assessment and problem identification; planning; procurement, delivery, and coordination of services; and monitoring to ensure that the multiple services needs of the client are met. These are clinical systems that focus on the achievement of client outcomes, within effective and appropriate time frames and resources, or the entire episode of illness, crossing all settings in which the client receives care. The case manager's role is as a practitioner who actively coordinates the client's care. CM is by definition a *process*. It expands on components of the nursing process to respond to the needs of clients along the care continuum and across multiple settings.

Using patient-focused strategies to coordinate care, CM becomes a system or design for moving a recipient through the health care system. A model of CM will be designed for a large, rather generic target group or population (e.g., hospitalized, long-term care, chronic care, rehabilitation) or for a specified "expanse" on the health care continuum (e.g., an episode in one setting, in one organization, or for the whole continuum). A model of CM will specify the standards for care and resource use, relationships, and responsibilities in a more general sense. The nurse may or may not be a direct care provider.

Several organizing frameworks or methods of classification have been considered in grouping CM models. Because of the variability in how CM programs are set up, classification into model types helps describe and better compare them. The following are common ways of describing CM models:

- Organizational versus practice models
- External versus internal case management models
- Episodic versus continuity models
- Provider versus purchaser models
- Hospital-based CM versus community-based models
- Case management programs that cross the continuum of care

Using these distinctions, CM models can be understood in terms of perspective (e.g., organization or providers), scope (e.g., services inside an organization), and time (e.g., one episode or across time and settings).

In the literature, many types of CM models and labels are found. There are multiple discipline–related models and one generally accepted overarching general model. Two factors are common across all CM models: the core component is coordination of care, and the core principle is advocacy. In addition to coordination of care, advocacy, brokering of services, and resource management, there are fairly common process elements in CM models regardless of the specific discipline. These models are typically tailored to fit unique target groups, vulnerable populations, settings, or other factors found in the discipline.

Nursing and health care models tend to focus on the management of health/illness or disease or the rehabilitation needs of an individual or population. These models are sometimes called *medical models, medical-social models, acute care nursing CM models,* or *disease management models.* In the nursing literature, there has been some confusion about whether CM is a care delivery model or an intervention that entails a process. In both nursing and social work, there is a differentiation between CM designed to *deliver* services and CM designed to *coordinate* the provision of services (Ridgely & Willenbring, 1992).

There are two basic CM models that were identified in the nursing literature: the New England Medical Center model of acute care nursing case management and the community-based model of Carondelet St. Mary's.

The New England Medical Center model is an extension of primary nursing methodology called *nursing CM* and is focused on the acute care hospital episode (Zander, 1990, 1991, 1992, 2002). This model exemplifies organization-specific models; it is hospital-based CM. It is best known for structuring the episode of care. In the mid-1980s, this model was introduced at the New England Medical Center, using principles of planning and concurrent management from engineering and other fields to extend primary nursing into outcomes management. The goal was to balance cost, process, and outcomes. The New England Medical Center model is a client-centered approach instituted during episodes of acute illness. It focuses on outcomes, resource utilization, and nursing accountability (Clark, 1996). Written, standardized documents such as case management plans, timelines, and critical paths were developed and evolved into CareMap® tools that formed the basis for a comprehensive hospital case

management system at the New England Medical Center. The complete CareMap® system includes the following:

- Variance analysis
- Use of an outcome-time focus in all multidisciplinary communication
- Case consultation and health care team meetings for clients at more-than-acceptable variance
- Continuous quality improvement

The New England Medical Center model defined CM as a care delivery model called *nursing CM.*

Carondelet St. Mary's Community Nursing Network, or the Arizona Model (Forbes, 1999), used professional nurse case managers (bachelor's and master's level), organized as a nursing HMO, at the hub of a network to broker services. This model type is known as a *beyond-the-walls, medical-social, across-the-continuum of care model.* It is best known for its innovative work in moving beyond the episode of care and into the continuum. This hospital-to-community model used case managers to follow the movement of high-risk clients from acute care to community to long-term care settings. Case managers are responsible for clients with chronic health problems, and the relationship is long-term (Clark, 1996).

There are four models in social work: brokerage, primary therapist, interdisciplinary team, and comprehensive. Social casework emphasizes the development of new resources, linkages to existing service agencies, coordination of care, advocacy, and teaching. Casework typically includes increasing the individual's self-reliance and independence, as well as coordinating and integrating care (Ridgely & Willenbring, 1992). The emphasis is on vulnerable populations.

The brokerage model emphasizes the case manager's traditional linkage function. Clients are linked to a network of providers and service coverage using assessment and referral and ensuring the availability of service activities (Raiff & Shore, 1993). The brokerage approach is sometimes described as a generalist approach. The case manager is a professional responsible for an individual client or a set of clients. The generalist carries out all CM functions and provides the basic direct service, coordination, and advocacy necessary in all CM programs (Weil & Karls, 1985). The primary goal is to increase the likelihood that clients will receive the right services, in proper sequence, and in a timely fashion. To achieve this, the case manager plans a comprehensive service package and negotiates through barriers that prevent clients from accessing needed services. Cost savings may or may not be an explicit goal, but such savings may be expected because the case manager facilitates better access to cost-effective alternatives, achieves better coordination and less duplication of services across agencies, reduces utilization of more expensive and less effective sites of care or services, and diverts clients from admissions (Ridgely & Willenbring, 1992).

In the primary therapist model, the case manager's relationship to the client is primarily therapeutic, and CM functions are undertaken as a part of, or an extension of, therapeutic intervention. The client has one person to relate to about treatment, service access, and case coordination. However, the therapist may feel that CM is a secondary activity to therapeutic work (Weil & Karls, 1985).

The interdisciplinary team model uses a specialized interdisciplinary team in which each member has a specific responsibility for service activities in his or her area of expertise. In combination, the activities of these specialized case managers constitute a complete CM process. The team might divide responsibilities by activity, such as intake, service linkage, and case monitoring (Weil & Karls, 1985). Team structures vary considerably. In some, all case managers on the team are interchangeable and serve the total group of clients. Other programs consist of multidisciplinary teams in which each professional provides specific services to the clients assigned to the team. In other cases, individual case managers carry individual caseloads but provide backup assistance to each other. Despite being called "teams," the specific configuration actually may be critical to the program's success (Ridgely & Willenbring, 1992).

The comprehensive service center model is used in service centers that provide comprehensive services, including social and emotional support, vocational training, and residential facilities. This type of program is often rehabilitative (Weil & Karls, 1985) and is seen in areas such as developmental disabilities and long-term physical disabilities. A personal strengths model may be used to help clients focus on and achieve goals (Huber, 2005a).

Other models of CM in health care include independent practice or private case management. Private CM covers those services contracted for by individuals or families or those subcontracted for by other groups. This approach arose because of the concern over rising health care costs and the confusion that accompanies the choices consumers must make. The case manager has three main functions: coordination, advocacy, and counseling (Clark, 1996). Some examples include entrepreneurial or small independent case managers and practices in for-profit, large, national CM companies.

Long-term care, rehabilitation, occupational health, workers' compensation, pharmacy, and medical case management models exist. Many medical models fall within disease management programs.

Insurance models include brokerage, gatekeeper, catastrophic, HMO types, and governmental models. The brokerage model within insurance companies includes an emphasis on linkage with no provision of direct services. It is similar to the broker in other social work models except for a strong emphasis on conserving benefits utilization.

Gatekeeper (managed care) models manage access to services and promote the use of cost-effective alternatives to expensive services (Ridgely & Willenbring, 1992). They can produce cost savings by managing care, including substituting less costly, more appropriate services and sometimes simply by not authorizing higher-cost services. Rather than facilitating access, gatekeepers must restrict access to control utilization and, thereby, costs. The ability of these case managers to create savings depends on the availability of appropriate cost-effective alternatives, case manager authority within the care system, and case manager ability to control financing for the care they deem appropriate (Ridgely & Willenbring, 1992). The case manager functions much like a purchasing agent (Clark, 1996).

Focused on catastrophic diseases or events such as acquired immunodeficiency syndrome (AIDS) or brain injuries, catastrophic CM is often used with workers' compensation cases and life-care planning. It is designed to manage and maximize insurance and health care benefits, which may be capped at a lifetime maximum. Early warning strategies are adopted to detect the potential for high-cost cases and to deal with both clients and service providers proactively to optimize and economize the health services used (Cline, 1990).

In HMO (managed care) models, prospective or capitated reimbursement systems put providers at financial risk. This creates pressure on providers to control total costs, provide and promote prevention-oriented services, and substitute lower-cost services, preferably without sacrificing quality. One example of managed care models is integrated health care, defined as a network of organizations that provides or arranges to provide a coordinated continuum of services to a defined population and is held accountable for the population's health status (Shortell et al., 1993). Federal, state, and local government agencies also manage and reimburse care via programs such as Medicare, Medicaid, and workers' compensation.

Few interdisciplinary models exist. The following two were described in the literature:

1. One model for acute care case management for nurses and social workers has been described (Dzyacky, 1998). It is a program designed to integrate utilization management functions with discharge planning and separate the practice of social work from discharge planning activities. Discharge planning tasks were divided into two categories—simple and complex. Case facilitator nurses became responsible for simple discharge planning cases; social workers handled the complex category.

2. One model for nurse–social worker collaboration in managed care also has been presented (Hawkins et al., 1998). Called the Biopsychosocial Individual and Systems Intervention Model, it is derived from a combination of interdisciplinary collaboration models at the organizational and administrative levels and a case management intervention approach for individuals and small systems levels. Nurses and social workers are assumed to collaborate as equal partners in interdisciplinary team case management using a transdisciplinary model.

The one general, overarching model that is becoming widely accepted as the generic case management model is Wagner's Chronic Care Model (Improving Chronic Illness Care, 2012; Wagner et al., 2001). The Chronic Care Model addresses concerns about how to manage chronic illnesses. The six elements of the health care system that encourage quality chronic illness care are the community, the health system, self-management support, delivery system design, decision support, and clinical information systems. The specific concepts related to the six elements are patient safety, cultural competency, care coordination, community policies, and case management. Chronic disease/illness care is

important because almost one half of all Americans (145 million people) live with a chronic condition. For older adults, 43% have three or more illnesses (Improving Chronic Illness Care, 2012). This order of magnitude has generated great interest in strategies to be proactive and focused on keeping people as healthy as possible. Case management is an attractive strategy because it is aimed at care coordination and decreased system-related fragmentation.

History of Case Management

Different disciplines practice case management; thus the history of its development varies according to the perspective of the specific discipline reporting it. The social work perspective is that the roots of CM grow from social work's historical tradition and the work of Mary Richmond in the era of the early settlement houses and charity organization societies (Raiff & Shore, 1993). This was a social casework concept at the turn of the twentieth century. Since the 1970s there has been a resurgence in CM as a result of shifts in the locus and financing of health care and human services and problems with service fragmentation and inaccessibility.

The insurance companies' perspective is that CM arose in insurance companies because of the need to manage catastrophic and high-cost cases. For example, Liberty Mutual is often credited with having pioneered the concept of in-house case management/rehabilitation programs in insurance companies in 1943 as a cost-containment measure for workers' compensation. This concept was expanded in 1966 by the Insurance Company of North America (now CIGNA) when it started an in-house program incorporating vocational rehabilitation and CM that later became the company *Intracorp*. Some view George Welch of CIGNA as the true father of modern CM, as demonstrated in the following perspective (Siefker et al., 1998, p. 3):

> *Case management as part of the insurance industry or other third-party payer systems seems to have had two somewhat separate origins: the worker's compensation system and the accident and health insurance system.*

The history of CM in nursing began with private duty nursing, the oldest care modality in U.S. nursing. With the rise of the early settlement houses, coordination of health care services for immigrants and the poor was a concern. This was the beginning of public and human services in the United States. Both nurses and social workers were key initiators. The Henry Street Settlement was founded in 1895 by two nurses (identified as social workers), Lillian Wald and Mary Brewster. In 1902, Lillian Wald founded the first school of nursing. By 1900, visiting nurse services were established to provide comprehensive community services and case coordination (Tahan, 1998).

Community service coordination, a forerunner of CM, began at the turn of the twentieth century in public health programs. The Visiting Nurse Service was one of the first community health programs. Providing service coordination has always been a focus of public health nursing. Service coordination has since evolved into CM, but case management considerably expands on coordination of community services. The concept of a continuum of care was used after World War II to describe the extended community services needed for mental health clients. The term *case management* first appeared in the early 1970s in social welfare literature, followed by a use in the nursing literature. The 1981 Omnibus Budget Reconciliation Act plus Medicare prospective reimbursement encouraged comprehensive, coordinated services. As a result of changing reimbursement structures, insurers have been focused on programs to contain the rising costs of health care. Case management emerged in the fields of psychiatry and social work in the 1920s, was used by visiting nurses in the 1930s, developed and flourished in acute care in the 1980s, and was found in all settings in the 1990s (Cesta & Tahan, 2003).

In nursing, CM historically has been the care delivery model associated with public health and community health nursing. Thus it was operational in settings outside hospitals and operated without the umbrella of managed care. In these settings, CM focused on accountability of process and outcomes of care delivery. Traditional CM principles also were operational in several care models that evolved over time. CM also was used in social service agencies, community mental health services, rehabilitation settings, and long-term care.

In the 1960s, contemporaneous with government legislation enacting Medicare and Medicaid coverage, the insurance industry began to evolve CM models

(Siefker et al., 1998). This pre-emergence decade set the stage for a series of dramatic evolutionary changes in CM each decade since the 1960s.

Many trace the "rise" of CM models to the 1970s. Certainly the past 35 years or so have brought about an amazing growth and change. The effects have been dramatic. In the 1970s, as the federal government began to analyze actuarial data on health care costs, expenditures, and projections, CM became a useful strategy in health maintenance organizations (HMOs), long-term care demonstration grants, and social work efforts to manage the deinstitutionalization of the chronically mentally ill. The 1970s saw the rise of both solo providers of CM services (independent companies) and large national CM companies. Models of catastrophic CM and workers' compensation predominated, and the certification as certified rehabilitation counselor (CRC) began.

The 1980s saw a decade of rapid spread and wild growth in CM models. With the advent of DRGs and prospective payment mechanisms, CM came to be seen as one answer to cost stabilization and cost predictability. It spread into models of social health maintenance organizations and other insurance settings. Independent CM companies grew and thrived. The certified disability management specialist (CDMS) certification was begun, and the New England Medical Center's nursing CM (acute care) model was developed and disseminated into hospital-based CM.

The decade of the 1990s was a time of integration and knowledge explosion. Interest that had been sparked in the 1980s carried over into the 1990s as health care providers, payers, employers, health plans, and professional organizations struggled to integrate CM practice and identify the knowledge base. Two groups merged to form the professional organization representing CM practice: the Case Management Society of America (CMSA). The Commission for Case Manager Certification (CCMC) was established and offered the certified case manager (CCM) credential. A proliferation of other certifications, usually within provider disciplines, occurred. CMSA developed and published standards of practice (SOP) for CM in 1995 and updated this in 2002 and again in 2010. Both CMSA and CCMC adopted the same consensus definition of CM, although CMSA modified its definition in 2002. The managed care technique of utilization management became more closely aligned with CM. Models of CM also proliferated, usually within hospitals and the acute care sector, but without standardization. Jobs for case managers began to shift into acute care, the insurance industry, and large private companies. Organizational accreditation for CM programs was introduced by the Commission on Accreditation of Rehabilitation Facilities (CARF) and the Utilization Review Accreditation Commission (URAC). Rigorous research results began to emerge to demonstrate the value of CM models. CM models came under scrutiny for their value and cost-effectiveness.

Interest arose in using CM principles and applying them to populations with chronic diseases, which was the pre-emergence phase of disease management. With the multiple reports from the IOM and the passage of the ACA in 2010, care coordination became front and center. There is intense interest and activity now around both strategies of CM for individual patients and PHM for disease and population health management.

THE CASE MANAGEMENT PROCESS

Sometimes called *care management, outcomes management,* or *clinical resource management,* CM has elements related to access, decision support, and outcomes achievement. Other CM functions are access, utilization review and management, discharge planning or transition management, episode tracking and continuous quality improvement, health prevention and disease management, and contracting. These functions may be stand-alone or combined in various ways, especially in hospitals in which the functions of utilization review and discharge planning can be balanced (Birmingham, 2007). The CM process is represented by the activities that case managers perform. CCMC (2012) has identified the eight essential CM activities with direct client contact as: (1) assessment, (2) planning, (3) implementation, (4) coordination, (5) monitoring, (6) evaluation, (7) outcomes, and (8) general activities. The six core components to CM practice, for exam purposes, are: (1) psychosocial aspects, (2) health care reimbursement, (3) rehabilitation, (4) health care management and delivery, (5) principles of practice, and (6) case management concepts.

According to the CMSA's *Standards of Practice for Case Management* (2010), the key functions of a case manager are assessment, planning, facilitation, and advocacy. Collaboration with the client and with those involved in the client's care is essential. Specialized skill and knowledge are needed in positive relationship building; effective communication; negotiation; knowledge of contractual and risk arrangements; ability to affect change, perform evaluation, plan and organize, and promote autonomy; and knowledge about funding sources, health care services, human behavior, health care financing, and clinical standards and outcomes. The process of CM begins with the identification of individuals with high-cost, complex care needs who can benefit from CM services. The case management intervention begins with first contact with the client and/or family and continues as an ongoing relationship until termination.

Assessment

To develop a plan of care, a comprehensive assessment of health needs is done. Tools such as surveys or questionnaires, assessment batteries, telephone assessment strategies, or electronic communication may be used. Interviews of the client and/or family, physician and other providers, and other health care team members are important. Assessment needs to cover health behaviors, cultural influences, and belief and values systems and must include identification of potential barriers, negotiating realistic goals, and searching for alternatives (CMSA, 2010).

Planning

To maximize the client's health status and achieve goals and outcomes, planning is done with the client, family, health care providers, payers, and the community. The plan of care needs to be evidence-based and individualized. The goal of planning is to derive an action plan that is appropriate, fiscally responsible, high-quality, evidence-based, and feasible. Contingency plans need to be in place for variances. Reevaluation should be ongoing (CMSA, 2010).

Facilitation

Facilitation uses strategies of communication and coordination and the involvement of the client and family throughout the CM process. Facilitation also is focused on linking parts of the service delivery system and streamlining care delivery. Coordination and education are key strategies (CMSA, 2010).

Advocacy

Case management advocacy is a function related to client empowerment, autonomy, and self-determination. Advocacy actions are supportive and educative and represent the client's best interests. Representing the client's best interest includes advocating for early referral, necessary funding, appropriate treatment, and timely coordination of services. When conflicts arise, the case manager's role is to advocate for the needs of the client (CMSA, 2010).

CASE MANAGEMENT IMPLEMENTATION

In hospitals, CM has become a popular and effective means to decrease length of stay and secure important outcomes. CM has been identified as a major strategy for cost containment that also folds in quality control. Persuasive arguments exist for implementing CM. For example, close follow-up, continuous reinforcement, and systematic treatment adjustments by nurse case managers helped adult clients with diabetes (Aubert et al., 1998).

Four basic principles guide nursing CM:
1. Coordination and integration of a continuum of holistic care
2. Promotion and preservation of health through periods of transition and risk
3. Conservation and allocation of scarce resources
4. Provision of follow-up care that tracks and guides service delivery over the long term and across episodes and settings

Thus the nurse case manager remains in a relationship with clients over time and across boundaries. The nursing concept of discharge is replaced by accompaniment as the nurse follows the client, acting to connect and coordinate a broad continuum of sites and services (Hinitz-Satterfield et al., 1993). Nurses accompany clients in a cognitive and communication sense. Only in certain models will nurses literally provide care across the continuum.

Coordination and continuity are the keys to managing care over the health care continuum and across organizational boundaries. Thus care must be managed carefully within each area or unit and between health care areas. Case management focuses on provider continuity; managed care focuses on the continuity of the insurance plan. Both must be integrated into the care delivery system using a systems perspective (Falk & Bower, 1994).

The unit or area is the most basic locus at which to begin the coordination of care. In nursing, the care delivery system functions to coordinate care at the unit or population level. Coordination and continuity can be shift-based or unit-based. If the existing care delivery system does not accomplish goals of coordinating care, then a unit-based role with accountability for coordinating care across time will need to be developed (Falk & Bower, 1994).

Despite widespread dissemination of CM as a provider intervention and system strategy, some problem areas remain. These include the confusion over definitions and identification of exactly what CM is. Organizations also have struggled with whether and how to internally combine or separate CM and related functions. With an emphasis on financial viability or "margin," CM programs have been analyzed and challenged to justify the allocation of scarce resources to them.

Controversies exist in the field regarding methods and measurements to assess the value of CM. The two basic outcomes categories to be captured are clinical outcomes and financial outcomes. For clinical outcomes, CMSA (Braden, 2002) identified the following six direct outcomes of CM:
1. Patient knowledge
2. Patient involvement
3. Patient participation in care
4. Patient empowerment
5. Patient adherence
6. Coordination of care

Thus changes (improvement) in a key indicator such as patient knowledge can be a direct measure of the clinical effectiveness of a CM intervention. When the outcome of improved patient knowledge is linked by research evidence about improved patient knowledge reducing chronic relapse or use of health care resources, then the effectiveness of CM is further strengthened.

Proving financial gain has been somewhat more problematic for CM. In some areas such as diabetes, congestive heart failure, and mental health, CM has acknowledged acceptance. In other areas such as substance abuse treatment, financial benefit has been difficult to demonstrate. This is partly because CM is an intensive one-on-one service delivered by expert providers. In adding on a service cost, CM programs do not result in the same dramatic savings as reducing a day of hospital care or eliminating a procedure or treatment. The Centers for Medicare & Medicaid Services (CMS) have noted this dilemma, as follows (CMS, 2003, pp. 9675-9676 retrieved February 24, 2013 from *http://www.cms.gov/Regulations-and-Guidance/ Regulations-and-Policies/QuarterlyProviderUpdates/ Downloads/cms5002n.pdf*):

> *In the past, we have conducted several demonstrations of case management for chronic illnesses, including the national channeling demonstration and the Alzheimer's Disease demonstration. The evaluations of these demonstrations found that none of them showed sufficient savings to cover the additional costs of case management. There are several possible reasons for the lack of positive results. First, the most appropriate individuals were not always targeted and enrolled into the demonstration. In many cases, the sites enrolled patients with less severe, and therefore less costly conditions, making it more difficult to achieve cost savings by avoiding normal utilization patterns of acute or long-term medical care. The disease management demonstration Web site … contains additional information about these demonstrations. We are currently conducting other demonstrations that test either case or disease management. In one demonstration, Lovelace Health Systems in Albuquerque, New Mexico, was chosen to operate demonstrations of intensive case management services for high-risk patients with congestive heart failure and diabetes to improve the clinical outcomes, quality of life, and satisfaction with services. The other is a larger scale demonstration involving 15 sites authorized by the Balanced Budget Act (BBA) of 1997 (Pub. L. 105-33, enacted on August 5, 1997) to evaluate methods such as case management and disease management that improve the quality of care for beneficiaries with a chronic illness. The coordinated care demonstration was designed based on the findings of a review of best practices for coordinating care in the private sector.*

Fortunately, research is beginning to emerge and be identified to substantiate savings from CM interventions. Peer-reviewed research studies on effectiveness include Allen and colleagues (2002), Fitzgerald and colleagues (1994), Goodwin and colleagues (2003), Laramee and colleagues (2003), Norris and colleagues (2002), Riegel and colleagues (2002), Sesperez and colleagues (2001), and Weiman (1995).

DEVELOPMENT OF CASE MANAGEMENT PROGRAMS

Case management programs are structured around roles and functions of case managers. The case manager's role balances the aspects of provider, care coordinator, and financial manager. Frequently identified case manager roles are advocate, facilitator, provider, liaison, coordinator, collaborator, broker, educator, negotiator, evaluator, communicator, risk manager, mentor, consultant, and researcher. Case management functions are often identified as care coordination, facilitation and brokerage, education, advocacy, discharge planning, resource management, and outcomes management.

For provider-based case managers, a CM program can be built based on CMSA's *Standards of Practice for Case Management* (2010). The practice components identified in the standards document can be used as the foundation for establishing a step-by-step process. Following the standards as an outline emphasizes comprehensiveness and professional practice (Birmingham, 1996). Job descriptions also can be revised or composed to reflect the CMSA's *Standards of Practice*.

CM programs are developed using a number of situation-specific elements. Two initial assessments are helpful: assessment of the organization and assessment of client populations. The organizational assessment focuses on identification of resources, whereas the client population assessment focuses on how care is experienced by clients and the characteristics of client populations served by the organizations (Box 12-2 lists related assessment questions). If CM is used for specific client populations, priority would go to clients who demonstrate the following (Falk & Bower, 1994):

- Have a high rate of recidivism or frequent emergency department encounters
- Have unpredictable needs for care

BOX 12-2   CASE MANAGEMENT ASSESSMENT QUESTIONS

Organizational Assessment
- What clinical and support services are needed?
- When in the client experience are services most appropriately provided?
- How should services be provided?
- Where are services best delivered?
- Who are the most appropriate providers?
- Where and by whom are services best managed?

Client Assessment
- What are the major client populations served by the organizations—by volume, diagnosis, cost, payer mix, and high-intensity/resource use outliers?
- What is the service path followed by client populations—by entry point, internal flow, discharge, and recidivism?
- What groups of clients fall into high-risk categories—by volume?
- What clients are at risk for less-than-desired outcomes—by morbidity, mortality, infection rates, falls, and clinical outcomes?

- Have significant complications, comorbidities, or variances in usual care patterns
- Fall into high-risk profiles
- Are high-cost

The general process for the development of a case management program can be synthesized as follows:

1. Assess the organization and the client population served. This assessment provides a baseline for implementation.
2. Identify high-volume or high-risk case types. This assessment will indicate priority areas for care coordination.
3. Determine the usual client care problems, issues, or difficulties related to the high-volume or high-risk case types. Determine desired goals.
4. Form an interdisciplinary care team of the interrelated care providers who will be involved with the case types.
5. Develop and design a multidisciplinary critical pathway for each selected case type. The path should outline and specify measurable clinical outcomes, key professional care processes, and exact corresponding timelines as based on

practice patterns, professional standards of care, and length-of-stay parameters. The input and involvement of the client and each provider group, in relation to achieving client outcomes, should be clearly specified. The pathway would mark the occurrence of routine treatments, tests, consults, client activities, medications, diet, educational interventions, and discharge planning. Variance from the path triggers analysis and intervention.

6. Develop a pilot program or trial site.
7. Evaluate the pilot program and consider system-wide implementation. Review the pilot program's articulation with the existing mode of nursing care delivery.

Tahan (1996) mapped out a 10-step process for developing CM programs: (1) design the format, (2) select the target population, (3) organize the interdisciplinary team, (4) educate the team, (5) examine the current process, (6) review the literature, (7) establish the length of the plan, (8) develop the content, (9) conduct a pilot study, and (10) standardize the plan. This process emphasizes the interdisciplinary team approaches needed and highlights the importance of preparing people and the organization to facilitate success.

LEADERSHIP AND MANAGEMENT IMPLICATIONS

All nursing roles contain a component of management. This may range from basic clinical care management to executive leadership of an organization. McClure (1991) has noted that nurses have two roles: caregiver and care coordinator. Nurses in management positions in an organizational hierarchy are organization managers and coordination specialists who integrate units and systems. Management of client care by nurses makes them clinical managers. The shift to managed care in integrated health systems has highlighted CM as a key strategy for nursing practice management and empowerment of nurses. It also has made multidisciplinary collaboration an imperative.

Future effectiveness is thought to be based on decisions about what types of organizational structures and nursing care delivery systems best enable nurse-managed client care and best support nurses in practice. One related question is, How much management structure does a nurse require to be effective?

One assessment is the extent to which a nurse provides client care or manages the care of clients. Case management is one specific approach to redesigning care delivery for client care improvement. This may mean that some traditional management practices and habits will need to be changed or discarded. Case management has come to be a part of care delivery management that emphasizes the expertise of nurses.

Mark (1992) advocated an approach to determining the organization of practice that starts with clients at the core of care delivery systems. Then the goals, roles, and activities valued by nursing staff, medical staff, critical support services, and other stakeholders can be explored. A new practice model and structure can then be created to be consistent with client characteristics, nursing resources, and available organizational support. Various practice models incorporate dimensions of the following:

- Degree of integration of nursing care given to a client
- Degree of continuity of assignment of nurses to clients
- Type of coordination used to plan and organize care

As nursing care delivery systems evolve, the configuration of these dimensions will need to be addressed and evaluated. Nurse leaders can examine the state of health care management in their organizations and develop strategies to implement coordination of care models to best meet client, organizational, societal, and professional priorities, often referred to as patient-and-family-centered models. Given the interdisciplinary nature of CM, model development and success may require a "buy in" by other health care disciplines and other organizational stakeholders. Physicians and hospital administrators are crucial stakeholders for the success of CM programs.

Another leadership and management implication is the human resources deployment of personnel for CM. Who should be a case manager? What roles and functions should case managers be assigned? How much secretarial/clerical support is needed? How will case managers be organized? What is the best mix of RNs and social workers? Given the decision to implement a CM program, leaders and managers will need to make these personnel and systems decisions. In addition, appropriate credentialing for the job is a consideration. Certification typically is an official credential of an individual granted by a nationally recognized agency based on eligibility and passing a national examination. It affirms an advanced degree of competence and is a peer review process (Cesta & Tahan, 2003). Individual certification, as a mark of professional achievement, is more rigorous than a certificate of attendance or merit and differentiated from accreditation, which is a review of an agency or program. Some accreditation bodies are granting "certification" to programs. This essentially is a certificate of achievement or quality designation.

CURRENT ISSUES AND TRENDS

"Effective and efficient patient management is important in all health care environments because it influences clinical and financial outcomes as well as capacity" (Bower, 2004, p. 39). Case management is a premier strategy to manage patient care within and across settings. This is a major concern in both nursing and health care. Case management operates at the nexus of care coordination of systems and between and among parts of the health care delivery system.

CM as a process and intervention strategy continues to grow and develop. Trends and issues in CM reflect its complexity and centrality to health care delivery systems.

The first decade of the 2000s has included standardization and precision in CM models. Certification and accreditation are becoming imperatives for case managers and their programs. Interdisciplinary team models are becoming the norm. Automated systems are required for documentation and population health management because they efficiently integrate, identify, risk stratify, capture, and report care trends and alert providers to variance in outcomes. Value and return on investment are imperatives for CM models. Because chronic diseases are on the rise and consume a significant segment of financial resources, disease management programs for populations with chronic diseases also are blossoming and becoming more sophisticated.

Top trends in CM include establishing definitions; shifting case management roles, job functions, and employment settings; and demonstrating outcomes and financial return on investment. Patient safety and other consumer issues have resulted in greater consumer communication and education. Chronic care management is gaining momentum and may accelerate the integration of CM and disease management. Outcomes research is growing and needs to expand. Nurses are employed by hospitals as case managers; thus the nurse shortage has had an impact on CM. Education for CM needs to be addressed, as well as the confusion around certificates, certification, and continuing education. Multidisciplinary teams are becoming the norm for CM. Relationships with physicians need to be collaborative and collegial. There is a trend toward increasing legislation and rules and regulations in CM practice. Interest in legal and ethical issues in CM practice continues to grow.

CM is growing as a role and a job for nurses. As organizations struggle with definitions, models, and organizational arrangement choices, nurses will increasingly have opportunities and challenges related to implementing CM roles and functions.

In the shift of nursing care delivery systems toward CM, the balance between nurses' roles may shift. Some of the primary caregiving component may be exchanged for care coordination roles. This is the movement away from service provision and into service coordination as the central component of nurses' practice. The emphasis now is shifting to focus on population segments, either those specifically at risk or entire populations. New technologies for tracking large groups of people have assisted this evolution and will be an important factor of ACOs.

The nurse case manager is pivotal to overseeing critical paths and facilitating interventions and coordination activities; advanced registered nurse practitioners (ARNPs) have been used in some models. There is opportunity in the strategic economic importance of the CM process.

DISEASE MANAGEMENT

Disease management (DM) is presented here because it contains a useful and important background. The term DM is being dropped in favor of PHM. However, DM is an important and effective intervention designed to coordinate care and services delivery for better outcomes and lower costs. It is one of three initiatives that are used in the realm of coordination of care: case management (CM), DM, and population health management (PHM). First is CM, which basically involves an intensive focus on an individual patient in relation to one or more health conditions. Case management is often triggered by complex, high-cost, or high-volume conditions. The second initiative is DM, which moves up a level of aggregation. DM generally involves an intensive focus on a disease or health condition of a population group, which is subsequently applied to individuals. It often is used to address chronic conditions. The third initiative, which moves up yet another level of aggregation, is PHM. PHM is a community-based population strategy, such as devising health strategies for all adolescents in a school system or all elders in a community. DM, then, is a population-based strategy for the management of groups needing specialized health care services. Differentiating DM and PHM may be more useful in acute care. Although some combine DM and PHM under the category of PHM, for this chapter, CM, DM, and PHM are discussed and differentiated.

Two major forces have triggered the rise and proliferation of DM programs: (1) the proliferation of managed care systems as a prevailing form of organized health care delivery (the influence of health plans), and (2) the national attention generated by the Institute of Medicine's (IOM) (2004) health care quality initiative, *Crossing the Quality Chasm: The IOM Health Care Quality Initiative.* Health plans led the charge to address the care coordination and service integration needs of clusters of members who had identifiable health conditions, generally chronic in nature. In 1996, the IOM launched an ongoing effort focused on the assessment and improvement of the United States' quality of health care. The IOM's 2001 document, *Crossing the Quality Chasm: A New Health System for the 21st Century,* highlighted the need for profound changes in the environment of care, including revamping practices that fragment the care system. The report identified the coordination of care across patient conditions, services, and settings over time as a major organizational challenge yet a key dimension of patient-centered care.

Certain diseases manifest in clinical conditions that need careful, extended management to achieve the greatest possible health or quality of life and avoid potentially large costs. Disease management efforts usually target people with chronic conditions for which long-term management, patient education, and close monitoring of symptoms can minimize or prevent complications and acute exacerbations.

Reducing emergency department visits and hospitalizations saves money and is better for the health of people. Thus DM programs aim to help individuals cope with chronic conditions in a way that reduces detrimental clinical and functional effects and the need for and cost of medical care (Johnson, 2003). In an acute care, episodic-based care and reimbursement system, care coordination is too often ignored.

Disease management programs were developed and implemented largely as managed care health plan initiatives. They have evolved into proven and effective strategies to make groups of individuals healthier while saving scarce health care coverage dollars (Lipold, 2002). In the early 2000s, the federal government's Centers for Medicare & Medicaid Services (CMS, 2003) took notice of DM programs, sponsored DM demonstration projects, and encouraged contracting with DM vendors for outsourced medical management programs (Lewis, 2004) because DM has been found to be effective in select populations.

It is widely recognized that health care delivery can and must be improved. Clearly, the pressures to provide access to care, maintain a high level of quality, and control expenditures are converging on a traditionally fragmented and acute care–focused system. Projections are that socio-demographic and economic tidal waves are set to converge into a "perfect storm" of crisis over health care in the near future. These tidal waves include the aging of the U.S. population, the effect of the maturing of the baby boom generation, high pharmaceutical costs, advancing medical technology, dramatic increases in chronic health conditions, and U.S. government budget deficits. The solutions are not easy or obvious. However, DM is one major innovative strategy that is being closely watched, carefully analyzed, and undergoing research testing to determine its potential to improve health outcomes across multiple populations while lowering costs and improving patient satisfaction with care delivery (Huber, 2005b).

The community has become a more viable focus for health care services. Social and economic pressures demand that health care organizations focus on ways to provide cost-effective, population-based care. These pressures and the ACA have spurred rapid shifts in care delivery to community-based primary care settings for the management of health and chronic condition care. Thus viability rests on the ability to respond appropriately to the needs of a specific population group. This requires accurate identification of the population's needs along with subsequent development of essential, relevant, and cost-effective programs that provide planned interventions and create disease and population health stability.

DEFINITIONS

To better understand **disease management (DM)**, the term needs to be defined and differentiated from similar terms. Although there are various definitions of DM, the standardized definition is the one developed by the Care Continuum Alliance (CCA), the professional trade organization of the DM and PHM community. The definition of DM promulgated by CCA (2012a, p. 1) is as follows: "Disease management is a system of coordinated health care interventions and communications for populations with conditions in which patient self-care efforts are significant. Disease management:

- Supports the physician or practitioner/patient relationship and plan of care,
- Emphasizes prevention of exacerbations and complications utilizing evidence-based practice guidelines and patient empowerment strategies, and
- Evaluates clinical, humanistic, and economic outcomes on an on-going basis with the goal of improving overall health."

It is seductive to think of DM as the medical management of a disease. At least two major characteristics that distinguish DM programs would be overlooked by viewing this strategy as the medical management of a disease. First, this would imply that DM fell within the domain of physician practice. CCA (2012b) has stressed the multidisciplinary nature of DM, although medical care is a central component. Clearly, the management effort in DM programs is aimed at a population or group, and it is targeted at health, not just the cure of diseases. Second, this would imply that only biophysiological diseases were of concern. This connotation would leave out behavioral health domains and other conditions such as obesity or high-risk pregnancies. Although discrete and specific diseases are a large segment of DM efforts, it is important to revisit the definitions and note the emphasis on populations and conditions. PHM has become predominant because it is more specific to the breadth of conditions and programs. Zitter (1997) noted that population-based care was based on DM principles. The Chronic Care Model (Improving Chronic Illness Care, 2012; Wagner et al., 2001) best displays a PHM conceptualization of chronic DM.

The following six components of any DM program have been identified by CCA (2012a):

1. Population identification processes
2. Evidence-based practice guidelines
3. Collaborative practice models to include physician and support service providers
4. Patient self-management education (may include primary prevention, behavior modification programs, and compliance/surveillance)
5. Process and outcomes measurement, evaluation, and management

6. Routine reporting/feedback loop (may include communication with patient, physician, health plan and ancillary providers, and practice profiling)

According to CCA (2012a, p. 1), "Full Service Disease Management Programs must include all six components. Programs consisting of fewer components are disease management support services".

These components have been reformulated into a flow schematic model by Wilson and MacDowell (2003) in which population selection and evidence-based guidelines flow to providers and patients, which flow to measures and evaluation, which has a feedback loop to providers and patients. The CCA components have been formulated into an evaluation checklist in Table 12-1.

TABLE 12-1	CHECKLIST TO EVALUATE DISEASE MANAGEMENT PROGRAMS	
COMPONENT	**PRESENT (YES); ABSENT (NO)**	**SPECIFIC METHOD OR METRIC USED**
Population identification and selection		
Risk assessment		
Risk stratification		
Use of evidence-based practice guidelines		
Type of practice model		
Collaborative mechanism		
Single-discipline predominates (identify)		
Patient self-management		
Education		
Primary prevention		
Behavior modification		
Lifestyle change motivation		
Telephone contact		
Health advocates		
Compliance/adherence		
Surveillance		
Process, outcomes management		
Process identification and measurement		
Process evaluation		
Outcomes identification and measurement		
Outcomes evaluation		
Process and outcomes management		
Feedback loop		
Communication to:		
Patient		
Physician		
Health plan		
Ancillary providers		
Practice profiling		

From Coggeshall Press. (2008). *Care for the total population.* Coralville, IA: Author.

Differentiation of Case Management and Disease Management

It is not immediately clear or obvious how CM and DM are the same or different. This has caused some confusion in the field. CM and DM are distinct and separate strategies, but a considerable area of overlap exists because both are interventions designed to co-ordinate care for better outcomes and lowered costs. Thus CM and DM might be thought of as looking at two sides of the same coin. Figure 12-1 displays this visually.

Case management generally involves work with an intensive focus on coordinating the care of the individual client in relationship to one or more diseases or health conditions. Disease management generally involves intensive focus on a disease or health condition in relationship primarily to a population group, with application subsequently to individuals. DM is more population-based than client-centered and more proactive in approach than episodic (Huston, 2001).

Thus CM and DM are two different strategies, employed at two different levels of aggregation. The focus (individual versus group, episode versus continuum) varies. However, both are critical interventions for coordination of care and integration of systems.

Related Definitions

Concepts of the continuum of care and population health are related to understanding DM. These terms are each defined next.

Continuum of Care

A continuum of care is a linkage of health services across health care delivery settings and sites of care. In one view of the continuum of care, Aurora Health Care (2004) listed prevention and early detection, family and community services, primary and specialty care, pharmacies, behavioral health care, emergency care, hospital care, rehabilitation, home care, long-term care, and end-of-life care as components of its continuum of care. From a systems integration perspective, Aikman and colleagues (1998) divided the continuum of care into community care and acute care, with community care on either side of acute care in three overlapping circles. The continuum contained health promotion/illness prevention, public health, primary care, diagnostics/drugs, ambulatory care, acute inpatient, rehabilitative/chronic, long-term care, home services, and palliative care segments.

Both DM and CM programs will vary according to the specific characteristics of the setting of service delivery, the target population, and the scope of the continuum of care. The setting may

Case Management	...two sides of the same coin...	Disease Management
Assessment	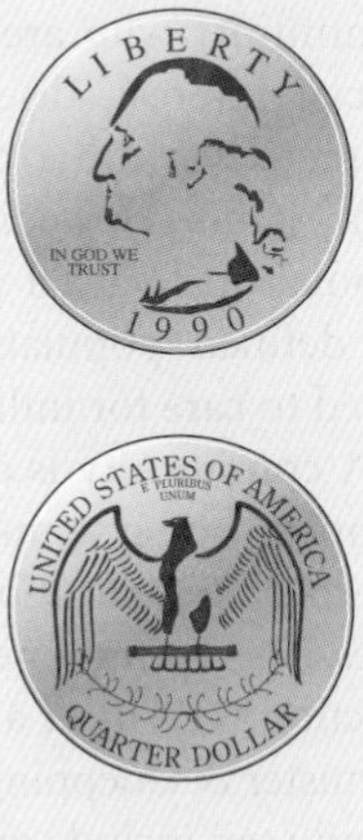	Population identification processes
		Evidence-based practice guidelines
Planning		Collaborative practice models to include physician and support-service providers
		Patient self-management education (may include primary prevention, behavior modification programs, and compliance/surveillance)
Facilitation		Process and outcomes measurement, evaluation, and management
Advocacy		Routine reporting/feedback loop (may include communication with patient, physician, health plan and ancillary providers, and practice profiling)

FIGURE 12-1 Differentiation of case management and disease management. (From Coggeshall Press. [2008]. *Care for the total population.* Coralville, IA: Author.)

be acute care, long-term care, community health, or other settings. The target population may be a specific medical disease, chronic condition, age cohort, insurance group members, catchment area, or other group. The continuum of care may be conceived of as within a facility, across the life span, across specific transitions, or other defined episode or time span. Clarity in the specification of what the continuum of care encompasses is important for understanding and comparing disease and case management programs.

Population Health Management

As the field of DM grew and evolved, it merged with the concept of population health management (PHM). Since 2007, the Care Continuum Alliance (CCA) is the name for the previously named Disease Management Association of America (DMAA). CCA (2012b, p. 1) advocates a Population Health Improvement Model, described as having:

> *"the central care delivery and leadership roles of the primary care physician; the critical importance of patient activation, involvement and personal responsibility; and the patient focus and capacity expansion of care coordination provided through wellness, disease and chronic care management programs. The convergence of these roles, resources and capabilities in the population health improvement model ensures higher levels of quality and satisfaction with care delivery. Further, coordination and integration are important tools to address health care workforce shortages, individual access to coverage and care, and affordability of care."*

The key components of the population health improvement model are (CCA, 2012b, p. 1):

- *Population identification strategies and processes;*
- *Comprehensive needs assessments that assess physical, psychological, economic, and environmental needs;*
- *Proactive health promotion programs that increase awareness of the health risks associated with certain personal behaviors and lifestyles;*
- *Patient-centric health management goals and education which may include primary prevention, behavior modification programs, and support for concordance between the patient and the primary care provider;*
- *Self-management interventions aimed at influencing the targeted population to make behavioral changes;*
- *Routine reporting and feedback loops which may include communications with patient, physicians, health plan and ancillary providers;*
- *Evaluation of clinical, humanistic, and economic outcomes on an ongoing basis with the goal of improving overall population health.*

An important feature of CCA's population health improvement model is its identification of outcomes. The five outcomes are as follows (CCA, 2012b, p. 2):

> *Accountable measurement of progress toward optimized population health should include:*
> - *Various clinical indicators, including process and outcomes measures;*
> - *Assessment of patient satisfaction with health care;*
> - *Functional status and quality of life;*
> - *Economic and health care utilization indicators; and*
> - *Impact on known population health disparities.*

Population-based care management is defined as the integration and coordination of health services to a specified population. Population-based health care is focused on aggregates and communities. The basic definition of a **population** is a "collection of individuals who have in common one or more personal or environmental characteristics" (Williams, 1996, p. 25). Also called an *aggregate,* the members of a community who are defined in terms of geography, special interest, disease state, or another common characteristic are a population. The research-related term is *target population.* In community health, population-focused practice is directed toward care for defined populations or subpopulations as opposed to care for individual clients (Williams, 1996).

A **community** is defined as "a locally-based entity, composed of systems of formal organizations reflecting societal institutions, informal groups, and aggregates. These components are interdependent, and their function is to meet a wide variety of collective needs" (Schuster & Goeppinger, 1996, p. 290). The term *community* can include groups of diverse or similar people living in one geographical location; an interactive link of families, friends, and organizations; or systems or groups bound by shared needs and interests (Carroll,

2004). The concept of community includes dimensions of people, place, and function. The community is considered to be the client when the nursing focus is on the collective or common good rather than on the health of an individual. Thus community-oriented nursing practice is directed toward healthy change for the whole community's benefit. The unit of service may be individuals, families, groups, aggregates, institutions, or communities, but the purpose is to affect the entire community (Schuster & Goeppinger, 1996). Thus the term *community* denotes a local entity, whereas the term *population* refers to an aggregate with any common characteristic (not necessarily tied to a place).

The term *community health* involves meeting the collective needs of a group by identifying problems and managing interactions both within the community and between the community and the larger society. Risk factors, health status indicators, functional ability levels, health promotion, health outcomes, and prevention of identified chronic diseases are the focus of data gathering, program planning, and implementation processes and activities. Community participation and partnership are key concepts because active participation in a decision-making process induces a vested interest in the success of any effort to improve the health of a community. Community partnership is a basic tenet of community-oriented approaches. For nurses, the concept of community as client directs the nursing focus to the collective or common good instead of individual health. Population-based care draws on partnership and community as client concepts. These community health concepts also foster culturally competent health care services (Schuster & Goeppinger, 1996).

BACKGROUND

Chronic health conditions pose a formidable challenge to the health care delivery system. The management of chronic conditions is a particular burden for health care payers and employers. Chronic disease creates two particular difficulties for businesses. First, these conditions in the workforce lead to diminished productivity. Second, these conditions result in a greater portion of the business's revenue being diverted into health care expenditures (Javors et al., 2003). Further effects impact the health care delivery system, society, and individuals' functioning and activities. Of particular concern is the increasing trend of chronic illness in relatively younger people (Javors et al., 2003).

Population and health trends are tracked by governmental agencies such as the U.S. Census Bureau, Centers for Disease Control and Prevention (CDC), Bureau of Labor Statistics (BLS), and Health Resources and Services Administration (HRSA), as well as private foundations and organizations. Clearly, health and health care delivery systems data are continually in flux. However, the available statistics are impressive. Costs are a considerable pressure, because, on average, individuals with chronic conditions cost 3.5 times as much to serve as others and they account for a large proportion of services (80% of all bed days and 69% of hospital admissions) (Nobel & Norman, 2003).

According to the CDC (Centers for Disease Control and Prevention, 2012, p. 1):

> *Chronic diseases—such as heart disease, cancer, and diabetes—are the leading causes of death and disability in the United States. Chronic diseases account for 70% of all deaths in the U.S., which is 1.7 million each year. These diseases also cause major limitations in daily living for almost 1 out of 10 Americans or about 25 million people. Although chronic diseases are among the most common and costly health problems, they are also among the most preventable. Adopting healthy behaviors such as eating nutritious foods, being physically active, and avoiding tobacco use can prevent or control the devastating effects of these diseases.*

The chronic conditions that pose a particular economic burden but can be helped by DM and PHM are characterized by high prevalence, high expense, relatively standardized treatment guidelines, and a significant role played by the member's behavior on the progression of the condition (Cousins & Liu, 2003).

PHM has arisen as a major strategy to address these concerns. It has demonstrated effectiveness in mental health (Ziguras & Stuart, 2000) and Medicare (Martin et al., 2004) populations. Attractive features include effective population management, coordination of care for chronic conditions, consistency of care for at-risk populations, customization of care support, encouragement of adherence to treatment, and proactive interventions.

Disease Management Programs

DM programs offered by health plans can be developed in-house or purchased either from a vendor or another organization such as a hospital. In a stratified random sample of 65 health plans, all of which were members of the American Association of Health Plans (AAHP), 64% of the diabetes DM programs were developed in-house, 27% were purchased from a vendor, and 9% were purchased from other sources (Welch et al., 2002). Employers also contract directly with DM providers.

Proactive outreach is a major strategy of DM and PHM programs. Nursing outreach programs are the core element. Personal communications (usually via telephone) between an expert nurse and the health plan participant build a personal relationship, help identify knowledge deficits and counseling needs, facilitate close monitoring and progress toward goals, enhance treatment adherence, and promote clinical and cost stabilization.

The personal nurse, functioning as a personal health advisor, establishes a single point of contact and coordination of care and service for patients having health problems and promotes a trusting relationship. Whether employed by a health plan or a contracted outside vendor, the PHM provided by nurses functioning as personal health advisors and advocates is central to effective outcomes.

The core of the DM concept is to comprehensively integrate care and reimbursement based on a disease or health condition's natural course. Both clinical and nonclinical interventions are timed to occur where and when they are most likely to have the greatest impact. This sequencing and targeting ideally prevents occurrences or exacerbations, decreases the use of expensive resources, and creates positive health outcomes through the use of prevention and proactive CM strategies. Chronic conditions are the focus, and systematic ways of delivering health care interventions to patients with similar characteristics are the methods used (Zitter, 1997). PHM models focus on the identification, standardization, and coordination of services across the continuum of care and for populations with the same or similar health care needs.

Disease Management Models

Two useful models, one for CM and one for DM, visually illustrate concepts related to PHM across the continuum of care. The CM model (Coggeshall Press, 2008) (Figure 12-2) depicts CM following traditional public health concepts and incorporating concepts of Pareto's Law (2008). The DM translation of the Pareto

Law is that 80% of the CM target population would be able to follow a standardized DM care program but 20% would vary or "fall off the path." Intensive resources would then be targeted to the 20%. This is called managing variance. The pyramid shows a base of strategies applied to all members, with gradual narrowing and focusing of interventions for greater precision and conservation of resources. Applied to DM, the pyramid visual can be drawn simply as wellness, DM, and CM (Figure 12-3). A model integrating

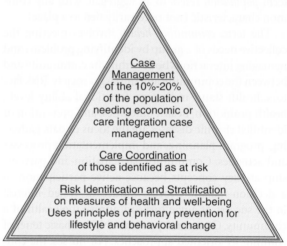

FIGURE 12-2 Case management model. (From Coggeshall Press. [2008]. *Case management model.* Coralville, IA: Author.)

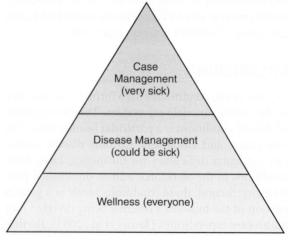

FIGURE 12-3 Levels of intervention. (From Coggeshall Press. [2008]. *Care for the total population.* Coralville, IA: Author.)

both DM and CM is depicted in Figure 12-4. The entire population (base of the triangle) would be targeted for prevention and assessed for risk identification and stratification. Care coordination and DM would be used for those individuals identified as at-risk. Then case management would be applied as an intervention for the 10% to 20% of the population projected to need intensive intervention, surveillance, and follow-up for complex care needs.

The second model was reported in the literature (Ho, 2003) as PacifiCare Health System's approach to DM. Using the same pyramid visual, segments started at the base with preventive health management (e.g., screening, education), followed by acute episode management, DM, special population care, and catastrophic care management of complex cases. Such conceptual models assist with understanding and communicating the array of programs and the level at which each is targeted. The coverage of the continuum of care is evident.

A related model that addresses aspects of chronic care is called the *Chronic Care Model.* This model identifies the essential elements of a health care system and community that encourage high-quality chronic disease care. The six basic elements are (1) the community, (2) the health system, (3) self-management support, (4) delivery system design, (5) decision support, and (6) clinical information systems. Developed by the staff of the MacColl Institute for Healthcare Innovation and supported by the Robert Wood Johnson Foundation, the model can be applied to a variety of chronic illnesses, health care settings, and target populations. The model is being tested by the Improving Chronic Illness Care program. Themes of care coordination and CM fall under the basic elements (Improving Chronic Illness Care, 2012; Wagner et al., 2001).

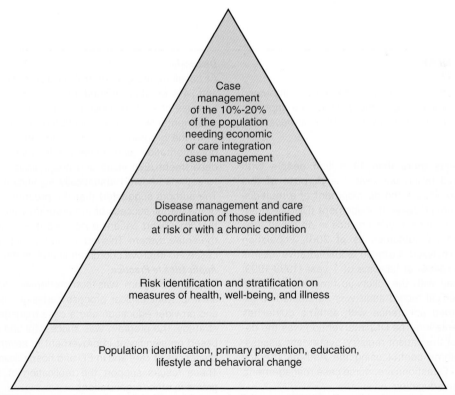

FIGURE 12-4 Integrated model. (From Coggeshall Press. [2008]. *Care for the total population.* Coralville, IA: Author.)

History

The genesis of the rise of DM occurred in the late 1980s and into the 1990s in the U.S. health care delivery system. Nested within the general evolution of CM practice, managed care organizations and health plans began to look closely at DM after initial CM programs had been launched. Further refinements in program quality and cost savings were desired. With some experience in CM to draw upon, the unique challenges of chronic conditions occurring on a large scale needed to be addressed. In pharmaceutical companies, DM emerged as a way to encourage medication adherence.

Todd and Nash (1997) described four generations in the history of DM. This view identified DM as an evolving phenomenon that is progressing in sophistication. The first generation was distinguished by enhanced services. One or more services outside the usual medical care were added to help address illness care. These developments often were prompted by quality report card or accreditation requirements.

The second generation saw the targeting of the sickest patients because they are the highest risk for generating costs. Outreach, education, and proactive, ongoing follow-up to reduce costly acute care episodes are featured.

The third generation saw the true integration of care and a true population-based focus. Risk identification and stratification occur. All important elements of care are addressed for the population using evidence-based protocols. Treatment is centrally coordinated, and health outcomes and costs are tracked.

The fourth generation was projected to contain a true health management model that focuses on optimizing health through wellness and prevention. Lifelong health education and strong incentives for healthy lifestyle behaviors will be featured. Resources will be allocated based on who is most likely to respond and benefit. DM programs are moving into PHM, considered the future fourth generation.

RESEARCH NOTE

Source

Patel, P.H., Welsh, C., & Foggs, M.B. (2004). Improved asthma outcomes using a coordinated care approach in a large medical group. *Disease Management, 7*(2), 102-111.

Purpose

Asthma affects more than 14 million people with costs at $11.3 billion per year. The purpose of this study was to discuss the development of a multidisciplinary asthma disease management (DM) program in one large medical group practice in an urban area and evaluate its outcomes as of 2001. Population data were analyzed from an administrative claims database (n=3486) at baseline of 1 year (1998-1999) and compared with the follow-up time frame (1999-2000). A medical record audit was conducted to examine recorded adherence with asthma guidelines and documentation. The DM intervention was the development of the patient registry, systematic assessment of asthma control using the Asthma Therapy Assessment Questionnaire, nurse case management, and physician education.

Discussion

At baseline, disease control problems were frequent, and 34% of adult respondents reported missing work because of asthma. Documentation needs for written treatment plans were uncovered. Beneficial results from the program included improved medical record documentation and patient education. Emergency department (ED) visits and hospitalization as related to asthma showed statistically significant decreases. The authors suggested that the greatest determinant of the overall success of the program was a realization that improving patient outcomes is a shared goal of the entire system. This led to the redesign of care processes to improve coordination and continuity of care.

Application to Practice

This DM program was comprehensive and involved an important clinical process redesign using patient and provider education and a case management (CM) strategy. The program was successful and sustainable based on significant improvement in several essential processes of care and in ED and hospitalization events. These results support the replication of similar programs in other organizations.

POPULATION-BASED PROGRAM PLANNING

Both DM and PHM tend to occur within organized programs. Nurses need to have skills and knowledge in health care program planning to best showcase their unique contributions.

Health care program planning emerged in the early 1980s. It began as a key aspect of health education and health promotion endeavors. Early models contained operational planning, program development, and strategic planning. In the late 1980s, business plans became more common as tools for both new ventures and health care program development. Now, program planning also needs to address the evidence base for practice and outcomes evaluation criteria. Programs also must be evaluated for their potential and relative worth in terms of cost, quality, and value. A comprehensive program plan enables an assessment of the potential for success before allocating resources, provides a plan to streamline and facilitate implementation, identifies all needed resources, and outlines a way to obtain reliable and valid evaluation data. An integrated population-based program planning model contains the following four components (Hall, 1998):

1. Contextual analysis
2. Implementation plan
3. Budget
4. Evaluation plan

A program outline would discuss the problem, state the need, identify assumptions, and present objectives and standards (Hall, 1998).

Community-focused or population-based care delivery planning follows the nursing process. The six basic steps are as follows (Schuster & Goeppinger, 1996):

1. Establishing the contract partnership
2. Assessing
3. Determining the nursing diagnosis of the problem
4. Planning
5. Implementing interventions
6. Evaluating interventions and outcomes

Assessment involves gathering data, developing a composite database, and interpreting the data. Data gathering usually involves obtaining existing data about the demography of a community. Data such as population characteristic distributions of age, gender, socioeco-nomic status, and race; vital statistics such as morbidity and mortality; disease incidence and prevalence; community institutions and resources distribution; and health care provider characteristics and distribution are gathered (Schuster & Goeppinger, 1996). Because of the influence of managed care reimbursement, the top few employers in the community might also be determined, since the health care needs and policies of the largest groups of insured individuals will have an influence on community health needs and resources.

Population and community health status may be profiled by vital statistics such as births and deaths, the incidence and prevalence of the leading causes of mortality and morbidity, health risk profiles of selected aggregates, and functional ability levels. The structure of community health may be profiled by the number and location of health facilities such as hospitals and nursing homes, the health-related planning groups, health workforce types and numbers, and health resources utilization patterns. Data may be gathered by existing databases, surveys, interviews of key informants, or published reports. The five key methods of collecting data are (1) informant interviews, (2) participant observation, (3) windshield surveys (the drive- by equivalent of simple observation), (4) secondary analysis of existing data, and (5) surveys (Schuster & Goeppinger, 1996).

After data gathering and assessment, a nursing diagnosis of the problem is generated. A modification of the nursing diagnosis format can be used. The three parts are "risk of," "among," and "related to." Each part is filled in to identify the problem clearly. The planning phase is then begun. It consists of problem analysis, problem prioritization, goals and objectives determination, and intervention activity development. Problem analysis may use a matrix or spreadsheet to map and identify direct and indirect precursors and consequences; relationships among problems, precursors, and consequences; and supportive data. Origins and impacts of the problem, points for intervention actions, and parties with an interest in the problem and solution need to be identified (Schuster & Goeppinger, 1996).

The problems identified as part of the assessment need to be ranked to determine relative importance. Priorities are established by using predetermined criteria. The following six criteria are recommended (Schuster & Goeppinger, 1996):

1. Community awareness of the problem
2. Community motivation to resolve it
3. The nurse's ability to influence problem solution
4. Availability of relevant expertise
5. Severity of consequences
6. Speed with which resolution can be achieved

Goals and objectives for high-priority problems need to be established in precise, clear, behaviorally stated, incremental, and measurable terms. A search for the evidence base for any recommended interventions needs to be done. If standardized evidence-based protocols exist, these should be used. Intervention activities also can be mapped on a spreadsheet, along with a probability rating of the likelihood that the activity will foster achievement of the objective and be implemented. Interventions are then implemented and evaluated. Evaluation criteria include successful intervention implementation, meeting of partnership objectives, problem resolution, participant satisfaction, and development of community strengths. Evaluation of both costs and effectiveness is important. The process includes a feedback loop to renegotiate the partnership if needed (Schuster & Goeppinger, 1996).

POPULATION-BASED RISK ASSESSMENT

The aggregate health care costs of chronic conditions increase yearly as individuals grow older. Older individuals tend to have chronic conditions that require complex care. It is estimated that one third to one half of all health care spending is consumed by the elderly. With the shift in demographic trends toward increasing numbers of elderly, there is a shift in the need for preventive care and chronic illness management services (Coleman, 1999). To meet this challenge, managed care organizations have created infrastructures of population-based risk assessment, demand management (self-management and decision support systems such as call centers), DM, and CM.

Illustrating the continuum of care as spanning the well and worried well (self-directed care and primary care), the acutely ill (secondary and tertiary care), and the chronically ill (tertiary care and long-term care), Coleman (1999) identified the corresponding infrastructure. Demand management spans the entire continuum. Case management and DM cover primary care through long-term care and focus on acute and chronic conditions. Case management is identified as valuable for high-volume, high-risk conditions and those who have catastrophic illnesses.

To be effective at individual and population-based care management, both case and DM programs need to identify, assess, and define the populations to be served early in the program planning effort. After the population has been defined, individuals within the population need to be selected and assessed for the appropriateness of case or disease management as an intervention. Profile characteristics may be age, number of chronic illnesses, or number of medications. Extensive surveys, such as a comprehensive health assessment questionnaire, are used to screen the whole population for high-risk indicators.

Population-based risk identification is an innovation that helps determine the best use of staff and clinical resources while also identifying the long-term health needs of groups and populations. Risk identification can be comprehensive when it spans health promotion, wellness, chronic disease, illness, and disability. It can be specific when identifying persons at risk for high-cost, high-intensity, or long-term health care needs. Levels of risk are primary (prevention), secondary (early detection), and tertiary (management of an episode of care) (Burgess, 1999).

A more detailed model of population care management contains these six levels: population needs assessment, identification of health services, targeted health planning, wellness and prevention, care management, and case management (Qudah & Brannon, 1996). Population-based risk identification leads to referring individuals into CM and DM programs. "Disease management is largely an ambulatory care program" (Goldstein, 1998, p. 102) because it is designed to manage chronic conditions rather than addressing an episode of acute illness. Extended CM often is targeted at persons with complex conditions, multiple diagnoses, or extended-term care requirements. Cost-effectively managing populations requires careful risk identification and then the application of population-based principles and care strategies.

Zitter (1997) outlined the following six key success factors for the development and implementation of any DM program:

1. Understanding the course of the disease
2. Targeting patients likely to benefit from the intervention
3. Focusing on prevention and resolution
4. Increasing patient adherence through education
5. Providing full care continuity
6. Establishing integrated data management systems

The selection of a specific DM program for initiation and implementation can be guided by an analysis of the environment and potential target populations. Nobel and Norman (2003) identified the following four modules used by effective DM programs:

1. Candidate identification and stratification
2. Enrollee recruitment
3. The intervention itself
4. Evaluation

Each module contributes an important link in the process, and the four combine to form a process loop. Timely access to critical information is needed in each of the four modules.

Gillespie outlined the following seven criteria useful in the selection of a condition as a candidate for implementing a DM program (Gillespie, 2002, p. 226):

1. *Availability of treatment guidelines with consensus about the appropriateness and effectiveness of care*
2. *Generally recognized problems in therapy that are well documented in the medical literature*
3. *Large practice variation and a variety of drug treatment modalities*
4. *Large number of patients with the disease whose therapy could be improved*
5. *Preventable acute events that are often associated with the chronic disease (e.g., an emergency department or urgent care visit)*
6. *Outcomes that can be defined and measured in standardized and objective ways and that can be modified by application of appropriate therapy (e.g., decreased number of emergency department visits or hospitalizations)*
7. *The potential for cost savings within a short period (less than 2 years)*

In a stratified random sample survey of 65 health plans in 2000, Welch and colleagues (2002) found that virtually all DM programs exhibited the following characteristics:

- Used evidence-based guidelines
- Identified the population with a disease
- Stratified the population by risk
- Matched the intervention with the need
- Educated patients in self-management
- Evaluated the program's process and outcomes

LEADERSHIP AND MANAGEMENT IMPLICATIONS

Managing the Continuum of Care

Nurses need to focus on managing the continuum of care as a basis of nursing practice. Collaboration and communication are essential elements of coordination and integration across a "seamless" continuum of care: "Continuity of patient care involves a series of coordinating linkages across time, settings, providers, and consumers of health care. Communication is a core task in coordinating patient care" (Anderson & Helms, 1998, p. 255). Continuity of care, as a care management strategy, often requires that clients be tracked through multiple organizations or settings of care. The communication of client data and care needs is fundamental to continuity of care. Therefore coordination of care involves communication across boundaries. This need is increased with the multiple and complex elements of chronic illness management and decreased hospital inpatient stays (Anderson & Helms, 1998). As the emphasis on DM and PHM accelerates, nurses have a leadership role and opportunity to use their skills creatively with DM and PHM perspectives. The principles and protocols of CM, DM, and PHM hold value for advanced registered nurse practitioners (ARNPs). These three care management strategies can provide the organization and administration frameworks useful for all nurses as they manage their specialty populations.

One critical application of managing the continuum of care is the facilitation and management of interdisciplinary and interorganizational communication for continuity of care. This is an imperative because information transfer is necessary for planning and planning is necessary for continuity of care.

Information exchange problems and gaps were found in a study of CM and interorganizational referral communication between a hospital and a home health agency within one health care system (Anderson & Helms, 1998; Anderson & Tredway, 1999). The need for barrier reduction in interorganizational communication is an urgent continuity-of-care need. Resources need to be redirected toward reducing obstacles and facilitating data and information transfer to improve the health of individuals and to manage population health care better.

Three major strategies of DM and PHM programs are (1) the use of an interdisciplinary team, (2) outcomes evaluation to measure results, and (3) the application of information management technologies. These three core techniques are used with a population health focus to improve overall health outcomes.

An interdisciplinary team needs to form and collaborate on the total plan of care, with each discipline integrating its expertise. For medical conditions, physicians, nurses, pharmacists, dietitians, social workers, and any other allied health professional with specific expertise need to be incorporated into the team. Communication among team members is the key to a successful program.

CURRENT ISSUES AND TRENDS

A current trend is for the development of integrated population-based programs as care becomes community and primary care centered. Nurses' roles include integrating, coordinating, and advocating for individuals, families, and groups to improve continuity and enhance appropriate service use. The PHM manager's role is to screen for risks, monitor risk factors over time, and initiate both preventive and treatment measures.

Another current trend is the identification of patient adherence as a driver of disease cost and the need for intervention with clients to foster adherence (Aliotta, 1996, 1999). *Adherence* is the extent to which the client continues a negotiated treatment. *Maintenance* is the extent to which a client continues health behavior without supervision. This compliance/adherence engagement is critical because the ultimate benefit of a treatment plan depends on the

extent to which the client implements it. Adherence may directly improve outcomes. For example, poor adherence has been implicated in drug-resistant strains of tuberculosis. Aliotta (1999) stated, "Current best evidence suggests a strong potential for establishing linkages between adherence and better outcomes in the area of chronic illness" (p. 82). Nurses have the skills to deliver adherence interventions.

Information management technologies are critical at every stage of a PHM program. Nobel and Norman (2003) divided the information management arena into information gathering, information integration and analysis, and information deployment. Effective programs need timely access to clinical, administrative, financial, and logistical information flows. Once acquired, these large databases need to be analyzed to identify opportunities for effective interventions to enhance the management of care and services. Deployment of information is reflected in strategies of notification, alerts, reports, and assessment of trends and the impact of interventions. A variety of information management technologies are emerging, such as biometric and handheld devices that can collect and distribute information (Nobel & Norman, 2003).

Technological innovations in informatics have made possible the rapid analysis of large databases. In turn, statistical analyses have become more sophisticated. Currently, claims databases are the primary sources used for data mining and profiling for PHM, although related databases such as pharmacy and nursing care are being linked or merged with claims databases for more robust disease profiling and prediction. An important application of information management technologies in PHM is predictive modeling. Predictive modeling is the use of statistics to calculate expected costs based on variables such as demographics, diagnoses, pharmacy claims, and survey data (Kramer, 2004). Predictive models have been used in other industries, such as credit card companies and retailers, for years. Applied to PHM, predictive models would be able to analyze data to answer questions such as, How much of a cost trend is being driven by age and how much by illness? Which complications and comorbidities drive costs (Kramer, 2004)?

CASE STUDY

The conference room was packed. Tension filled the air. No one wanted to speak up or "tip their hand" by stating a position. The group was gathered to address a serious issue: what to do about the exponential rise in obesity-related health care costs. First, there was the practical matter of illness, disability, and expense associated with the physical and organ-systems damage as a result of nutrition and weight-bearing issues. Then there was the genuine concern for shortened life span or decreased quality of life.

However, the pall hanging over the group was an unspoken concern for being labeled as discriminatory toward overweight people. The challenge for the group

leader was to initiate a balanced dialogue that moved the group into strategy and action.

The group leader began with a review of the data on incidence and prevalence, local population statistics, the evidence base for health effects, cost figures, and recent media attention on this issue. This generated a lively discussion. Many problems and issues were identified. A new evidence-based care protocol was located that could be used for PHM. The next step was to identify a desired action plan. Was it better to implement a CM program for targeted individuals identified as high-risk/high-cost or to implement a disease management program for the entire population?

CRITICAL THINKING EXERCISE

Nurse Gloria Davis just got her dream job as a case manager for diabetes care in a large integrated delivery system. Nurse Davis is deeply committed to high-quality client care. She has structured an excellent teaching program that is administered through the ambulatory clinics. She has instituted population data collection using the SF-36 and Diabetes Quality of Life tools. Nurse Davis has begun to collect trend data on HbA_{1c} values and frequency of blood glucose instability or complications. The next outcome to measure is client satisfaction. Nurse Davis assumes that client satisfaction is related to compliance with treatment. The first step is a small focus group. In the focus group meeting, Nurse Davis discovers that client interactions with a health care provider are becoming more impersonal. The clients have fewer choices

about to whom and where they can go for services, must get complicated authorizations, need to fill out more forms, have to listen to more recorded messages, and are waiting longer for appointments. On clinic days they wait a long time to see their provider only briefly. The process of coming in for care actually makes many of these clients feel worse.

1. What is the problem?
2. Why is it a problem?
3. What are the key issues?
4. What should Nurse Davis do first?
5. How should Nurse Davis handle this situation?
6. What problem-solving style should Nurse Davis use?
7. What leadership and management strategies might be useful?

13

Organizational Structure

Raquel M. Meyer

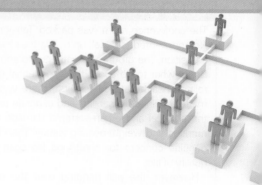

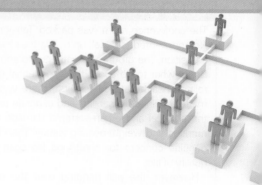

e**volve** WEBSITE

http://evolve.elsevier.com/Huber/leadership/

Structure refers to the arrangement of the parts within a larger whole. *Organizations* are entities that contain groupings which consolidate smaller elements into a larger, systematized whole. When membership in an organization comprises humans, organizations essentially become social structures that rely on human activity. An organization meaningfully coordinates group activity toward a shared goal because collective efforts are often necessary to manage large-scale work processes and outcomes efficiently and effectively. Many types of organizations are necessary to deliver nursing and health care services to diverse populations across sectors and geography. In health care, obvious organizational goals might be safety and quality of care, cost reduction, and increased efficiency. Understanding organizational structure helps nurses be more effective and efficient in their work lives.

DEFINITION

Organizational social structure is defined as the ways in which work is divided and coordinated among members and the resulting network of relationships, roles, and work groups (e.g., units, departments).

Photo used with permission from Photos.com.

The social structure of an organization influences the flow of information, resources, and power among its members. Whether as employees or as independent practitioners, nurses work for, or interact with, organizations. How nurses' roles interface with the structure of the organization influences the accomplishment of organizational goals. Research examples throughout this chapter highlight associations between the organizational structures in which nurses work and clinical, nurse, and organizational outcomes.

ORGANIZATION THEORY

There are many ways to understand organizations, and each understanding reflects different assumptions and tensions regarding the nature and dynamics of organizations. The history of organization theory has been shaped by multiple disciplines, including management, engineering, psychology, sociology, and anthropology. Although this has created a rich and varied understanding of organizations, the field of organization theory contains a variety of approaches to and assumptions about the phenomenon of "organization." Objectivism, subjectivism, and postmodernism reflect three broad perspectives regarding the nature of reality and the nature of knowledge with respect to the concept of "organization" (Hatch & Cunliffe, 2006). These perspectives are reviewed briefly with attention to the meanings of social structure, management, and power.

Objective Perspective

When approached as an objective entity, an organization exists as an external reality, independent of its social actors. Organizations are viewed as logical and predictable objects with identifiable and scientifically measurable characteristics (e.g., size) that can be predicted, observed, or manipulated (Hatch & Cunliffe, 2006). The purpose is to uncover laws that enhance the generalizability of knowledge. Organizational structure is a consequence of the division of and the coordination of labor, which results in a formal set of interrelated and interdependent roles and work groups. Management determines the *formal* relationships and standardizes the behaviors of individuals and groups in order to align organizational functioning with internal demands (e.g., technology) and external demands (e.g., market conditions, regulatory standards) (Reed, 1992). Typically, power is conceptualized as a resource to be allocated among roles and groups. Modernist theories related to bureaucracy and systems, as well as the schools of scientific management and human relations, have focused on improvements to efficiency, motivation, and performance in the achievement of collective goals (Reed, 1992). These theoretical approaches, which focus on the *formal* aspects of organizations, are examined in detail in this chapter.

Subjective Perspective

In contrast to objectivism, a subjective approach to the phenomenon of organization asserts that an organization cannot exist independent of its social actors. The organization is a social reality that can be known only through human experience, relationships, and shared meanings and symbols (Hatch & Cunliffe, 2006). Because knowledge is considered to be relative, open to interpretation, and context dependent, the purpose of inquiries is to uncover collective meanings that resonate with the experiences of those involved (Hatch & Cunliffe, 2006). Social structure therefore arises from and is continuously transformed through social interaction, which is played out against

a backdrop of formal rules and material resources directed by management (Reed, 1992). Power is reflected in the struggle between social actors who proactively and self-consciously shape organizational arrangements and secure scarce resources to serve their interests (Hatch & Cunliffe, 2006; Reed, 1992).

The subjective perspective focuses on the *informal* aspects of organization and on the freedom of individuals to make choices and to influence organizational life. Symbolic-interpretive theorists are interested in "how the everyday practices of organizational members construct the very patterns of organizing that guide their actions" (Hatch & Cunliffe, 2006, p. 126). Examples of daily social practices include routines (e.g., care maps), interactions, and communities of practice. For example, instead of viewing routines as mechanisms to standardize the behavior of individuals (i.e., an objective approach), a subjective approach might examine the changing nature of routines as members selectively modify, adapt, and retain practices in response to varying contexts and conditions (Feldman & Pentland, 2003). In a community of practice, learning occurs through voluntary social interaction whereby clinicians who are committed to a common interest self-organize informally to build ongoing relationships, partake in joint activities, and share resources (Wenger, 2008). An example in nursing would be an informal group of staff nurses who routinely have lunch together and who come to rely on this activity as a source of knowledge related to patient care in terms of problem solving, information exchange, and networking (Wenger, 2008).

Postmodern Perspective

Departing from the polarization between objectivism and subjectivism, the postmodern view challenges the meanings and interpretations associated with the concept of organization. The basic premise is that the world is known through language. Because language is continually reconstructed and context dependent, knowledge is essentially a power play (Hatch & Cunliffe, 2006). Notions of order and structure are the subject of scrutiny. Organizations may be thought of as disorderly entities characterized by conflicts and misunderstandings (Reed, 1992). Managerial practices and structures within organizations are seen to legitimize the interests of those in power (Reed, 1992). Even classic organization theorists such as Weber (1978) cautioned that bureaucracies were essentially domination structures that shape the form and purpose of social action through a system of rational rules and norms. Those who control bureaucracies therefore exert significant power over social action. Thus the postmodern organization is understood both as an arena in which power struggles between dominant and subordinate groups play out and as a text to be rewritten to free its members from exploitative and controlling influences (Hatch & Cunliffe, 2006; Reed, 1992).

Postmodernists challenge the assumption that social structure results from the division and coordination of work among roles and groups. Clegg (1990) suggested that excessive fragmentation of work results in a disjointed and confusing experience for workers who become dependent on more powerful members in the hierarchy to make sense of work flow and goals. To counter this excess control over member actions, he proposed the idea of **differentiation** whereby people self-manage and coordinate their own activities. Other examples of postmodern approaches to organization include feminist critiques of bureaucracies (e.g., Eisenstein, 1995) and anti-administration theory (Farmer, 1997). Each perspective contributes to stretching the thinking about how organizations are structured and function.

KEY THEORIES OF ORGANIZATIONS AS SOCIAL SYSTEMS

In the field of organizational design, the organization is most commonly approached as a social system from the objective perspective. Different theories within this tradition have contributed to understanding organizational social structure (Table 13-1). However, these theories have also been critiqued for rationalizing social action, for favoring efficiency and productivity over other values (e.g., equity, justice), and for adopting an elitist view of management (e.g., O'Connor, 1999).

Bureaucratic Theory

Although often criticized for its oppressive qualities and administrative burden, the concept of bureaucracy may be better understood when placed within a historical context. Theorist Max Weber (1864-1920)

was a German lawyer, professor, and political activist who noted the push of industrialism toward mass production and technical efficiency (Prins, 2000). Weber sought to explain, from a historical perspective, how the bureaucratic structure of large organizations differed from and improved upon other forms of societal functioning (e.g., feudalism). He viewed bureaucracy as a social leveling mechanism founded on impartial and merit-based selection (i.e., legal authority), rather than a social ordering determined by kinship (i.e., traditional authority) or personality (i.e., charismatic authority) (Weber, 1978). However, Weber warned of the potential dehumanizing effects of bureaucracies that emphasized purely economic results (i.e., formal rationality) at the expense of other important social values such as social justice and equality (i.e., substantive rationality) (Weber, 1978). Weber's descriptions of authority and rationality are foundational concepts in the study of organizations. His interpretation of hierarchy and its relevance to health care organizations are explored later in the chapter.

Scientific Management School

Arising from the experiences and ideas of business leaders and engineers in manufacturing industries, the scientific management school sought to determine the single best way to structure an organization (Donaldson, 1996). A well-known theorist in this field is Frederick W. Taylor (1856-1915), an engineer who authored *The Principles of Scientific Management* in 1914 (Prins, 2000). Along with colleagues, Taylor's vision was to improve labor relations and the low industrial standards that plagued the American manufacturing industry by the application of technical solutions (e.g., time and motion studies) (Prins, 2000). He proposed that "THE principal object of management should be to secure the maximum prosperity for the employer, coupled with the maximum prosperity for each employé…for each employé (this) means not only higher wages than are usually received by men of his class, but, of more importance still, it also means the development of each man to…the highest grade of work for which his natural abilities fit him" (Taylor, 2003, p. 235). The goal was to enhance organizational performance in a milieu of improved cooperation between management and labor by matching the work performed with the worker's skills and with economic incentives. However, the experiments and

TABLE 13-1 COMPARISON OF THEORIES OF ORGANIZATION AS SOCIAL SYSTEM

	CONTEXT	VIEW OF ORGANIZATION	GOAL OF MANAGEMENT	VIEW OF MANAGERS	VIEW OF WORKERS	EXEMPLAR THEORY
Bureaucratic Theory	Rise of industrialism	– Closed system – Stable entity – Formalized structure	Enforce legal, rule-bound functioning to achieve technical & economic efficiency	Impartial & qualified decision makers	Obedient & status seeking	Bureaucracy (Weber, 1978)
Scientific Management School	Early 20th century manufacturing industry	– Closed system – Stable & predictable entity – Formalized structure	Apply scientific methods & monetary incentives to plan, control, & evaluate work flow & outputs	Impersonal & goal oriented	Reliable, predictable & economically motivated	Principles of Scientific Management (Taylor, 2003)
Classic Management Theory	Early 20th century manufacturing industry	– Closed system – Stable & predictable entity – Formalized structure	Apply administrative principles to divide & coordinate work activities	Specialists in planning coordination & supervision	Skilled & specialized technicians	Theory of Organization (Gulick, 1937)
Human Relations School	Post World War I—Increasing activism & unionism	– Closed system – Behavioral structure	Enact leadership skills to empower workers & gain their cooperation to improve performance	Democratic leaders & open communicators	Socially & psychologically motivated	Theory of Structural Power (Kanter, 1972)
Open System Theory	Post World War II	– Open & adaptive system dependent on environment – System of interdependent activities – Organization as a process	Integrate system functioning to balance stability, flexibility, growth & survival	Internal & external boundary spanners	Semiautonomous agents	Nursing Services Delivery Theory (Meyer & O'Brien-Pallas, 2010)

Compiled by the author. © 2012 Raquel M. Meyer. Used with permission.

engineering techniques associated with this approach were ultimately criticized for reducing the worker to a mere input in the production process (Prins, 2000). The application of scientific principles to improve the task performance and productivity of workers reflected a bottom-up approach to organizational design (Scott, 1992). In nursing, efforts to redesign nursing jobs or to measure nursing workload often rely on this tradition.

Classical Management Theory

In contrast, classical theorists such as Fayol, Urwick, and Gulick evolved a top-down approach to organizational design. Based on experience as company executives, these practitioners identified principles of administration and management functions that could be applied in the design of organizations. Key concepts such as differentiation, coordination, scalar principle, centralization, formalization, specialization, and span of control became central to the study of organizational structure. These concepts, which describe the *formal* aspects of an organization's social structure and their application to health care organizations, are examined in relation to nursing later in the chapter.

Human Relations School

Theorists in the human relations school emphasized the *informal*, rather than *formal*, aspects of organization social structure. The disciplines of industrial psychology and industrial relations founded this approach, which now persists as the field of organizational behavior (O'Connor, 1999). The social and psychological needs and relationships of workers and groups were thought to be important to work productivity. Improved cooperation between management and workers was proposed to enhance performance and to reduce industrial strife (O'Connor, 1999). The famous Hawthorne experiments were influential in this school of thought. Initial interpretations of the Hawthorne experiments suggested that psychological factors influenced worker motivation because improved worker productivity was observed when researchers gave special attention to workers, regardless of changes to physical surroundings (Scott, 1992). Concepts such as job enlargement and job rotation were promoted to offset the alienation workers experienced because of excessive

formalization and division of work processes (Scott, 1992). Formalization is the extent to which the organization uses explicit rules, procedures, job descriptions, and communications to prescribe roles and role interactions, govern activities, and standardize behaviors (Hatch & Cunliffe, 2006).

Streams of study included leadership behavior, small group dynamics, participative decision making, morale, motivation, and other worker characteristics and behaviors (Scott, 1992). In nursing, this school of thought is reflected in efforts to meet the professional development needs of nurses, to enhance nurse autonomy and empowerment, and to involve nurses in decision-making processes to improve organizational functioning.

Open System Theory

Open system theory emphasizes the dynamic interaction and interdependence of the organization with its external environment and its internal subsystems. Meyer and colleagues (2010) conceptualized the health care organization as an open system characterized by energy transformation, a dynamic steady state, negative entropy, event cycles, negative feedback, differentiation, integration and coordination, and equifinality. Inputs (i.e., characteristics of care recipients, nurses, resources), throughputs (the delivery of nursing services arising from the nature of the work, structures, and work conditions), and outputs (i.e., clinical, human resource, and organizational outcomes) were theorized to interact dynamically to influence the global work demands placed on nursing work groups at the point of care in production subsystems. Contingency theory is a subset of open system theory positing that there is no single right way to structure an organization. Effective organizational performance depends on the fit between structure and multiple contingency factors such as technology, size, and strategy (Donaldson, 1996). Mark and colleagues (1996) applied contingency theory to the evaluation of nursing care delivery system outcomes. The basic premise was that, to perform effectively and produce quality outcomes, an organization must structure and adapt its nursing units to complement the environment and technology.

Technology is a core concept in contingency theory and refers to the work performed. Technology can be examined in terms of task uncertainty (i.e., repetitive nature of the task), diversity (i.e., number of different components), and interdependence (i.e., degree to which work processes are interrelated) (Scott, 1992). Highly repetitive and distinct tasks are amenable to mass production technologies (e.g., manufacturing industry). In contrast, highly uncertain and interdependent tasks require discretion, improvisation, and more intense coordination structures across team-driven networks (Donaldson, 1996; Scott, 1992). The work performed by health care professionals is often considered to be highly uncertain, diverse, interdependent, and reliant on group coordination. For example, in a study of hospital joint replacements, teams with high levels of shared knowledge and goals and mutual respect positively influenced patient-assessed quality of care despite shortened lengths of stay (Gittell, 2004). In this study, task uncertainty was intensified by time constraints (i.e., shorter lengths of stay), task diversity was reflected by the multidisciplinary roles, task interdependence resulted as multidisciplinary work was performed concurrently, and the coordination device was teamwork.

Theories of networks are also applied to organizational structure. Social network analysis, which builds on a systems view of organizations, examines and interprets the structures and patterns of the formal and informal relationships among members of the organization (Tichy et al., 1979). In nursing, for instance, social network analysis has been used to explore the social and geographical ties of senior nurse executives and physicians in the United Kingdom in relation to profession, gender, age, rank, location, and frequency of contact (West & Barron, 2005).

KEY ORGANIZATIONAL DESIGN CONCEPTS

Division and Coordination of Labor

A formal organization that employs people to achieve predetermined goals divides the work among its members by assigning tasks and delegating responsibilities to positions and work units. Structure is a by-product of the basic need to divide the labor into the specific tasks to be performed and a consequent need to coordinate these tasks to accomplish the activity or goal. The structure of an organization can be defined as the "total of the ways in which its labor is divided into distinct tasks and then its coordination is achieved among these tasks" (Mintzberg, 1983, p. 2).

The division (or differentiation) of work by occupation or by function is a form of **specialization.** Specialization is the extent to which work is divided and assigned to positions and divisions (Hatch & Cunliffe, 2006). As occupations and functions multiply in number, an organization increases in complexity and **size** (Katz & Kahn, 1978). Size is a quantitative measure of personnel, physical capacity, volume of inputs or outputs, or discretionary resources of an organization (Kimberly, 1976).

The advantages of specialization include improved work performance and a critical mass of experts (Charnes & Tewksbury, 1993). In health care, specialist roles have emerged to address the increasing complexities of care and technology. For example, occupations such as social work, physiotherapy, occupational therapy, and respiratory therapy represent specialized areas of knowledge that subdivide care with the aim of improving efficiency and outcomes. Within nursing, specialist roles have also evolved to address specific facets of practice. Advanced practice roles such as clinical nurse educators, nurse practitioners, and nurse anesthetists represent specialized areas of nursing knowledge. Organizations may also differentiate work units by function to serve distinct client populations. For instance, rather than a single, general intensive care unit, an organization may establish several intensive care units by medical specialty (e.g., cardiovascular, neurosurgical, neonatal) or grouped into a "service line." At the work group level, nursing care delivery models (e.g., team, primary, or total nursing care models) reflect different ways of dividing and coordinating the work among a team of nurses caring for clients.

Subdividing work creates breaks in work flow. Organizations address this challenge by integrating work processes across roles and subunits using coordination devices (Katz & Kahn, 1978). **Coordination** (or integration) involves bringing together and connecting the smaller elements of an organization to achieve a set of collective tasks (Van de Ven et al., 1976). Coordination is especially necessary when resources must be shared or the work performed by different work groups or roles is interdependent (Charnes & Tewksbury, 1993). Although coordination mechanisms can improve efficiency, performance, and conflict resolution, their misuse can also result in information overload and communication breakdowns (Van de Ven et al., 1976).

At the work group level, coordination involves programming and feedback devices (March & Simon, 1958). In health care, common programming devices used to control work processes are the following:

- Standardization of worker skills coordinates work indirectly by specifying the kind of training or education required to perform the work. In nursing, the standardization of worker skills occurs for advanced practice nurses when a doctor of nursing practice (DNP) degree is required or certification is mandated.
- Standardization of work processes coordinates work by pre-specifying or programming content before the work is undertaken. In nursing, standardization of work processes occurs when nurses use routines such as clinical protocols or evidence-based best practice guidelines.
- Hierarchical referral may occur when exceptions or unanticipated events arise (Galbraith, 1974). In nursing, hierarchical referral happens when a nurse coordinates the resolution of an exceptional or non-routine clinical situation with a nurse specialist or physician.
- Standardization of work outputs coordinates work, before the work is undertaken, through the specification of the results, product, or performance desired or expected. In nursing, work outputs are standardized when care is specified as outcomes objectives or care is managed for outcomes achievement.
- Standardization of communication methods coordinates work by providing a uniform infrastructure of information to facilitate exchange among those involved in common work processes (Venkatraman, 1994). In nursing, standardization of information is achieved through electronic health records and relational databases with alerts which allow nurses and other care providers direct and simultaneous access to client information in a consistent format (Gittell & Weiss, 2004).

In addition, feedback mechanisms entail the transfer of information in an adaptive and reciprocal manner to foster the exchange of information (Gittell, 2002):

- Mutual adjustment coordinates work by using simple informal communication. In nursing, mutual adjustment occurs when one nurse consults another nurse about practice issues, such as how to interpret a policy; or when nurses, physicians, and allied health professionals participate in clinical rounds.
- Direct supervision coordinates work through the use of a supervisor taking responsibility for the instruction and monitoring of the work of others. In nursing, direct supervision takes place when a nurse supervises the work of assistive personnel.
- Boundary spanning roles coordinate work by managing relationships as well as the bidirectional flow of information and materials across functional divisions (Gittell, 2003). In nursing, case managers exemplify a boundary spanning role because these roles manage relationships, exchange information, and negotiate resources with internal and external parties to facilitate care across occupations, services, sectors, funding agencies, and locations.

The types of coordination that are used depend on the degree of stability and predictability of the work situation (March & Simon, 1958) and the size of the work unit (Van de Ven et al., 1976). For example, acute health care settings are typically characterized as highly uncertain and interdependent work situations. Patient health needs, acuity, and care trajectories are often highly variable and unpredictable. To ensure comprehensive care, nurses coordinate patient care activities with the work of others in a reciprocal manner because the work performed is highly interdependent. Traditionally, programming devices are thought to be effective under stable and predictable conditions (March & Simon, 1958) and with larger work units (Van de Ven et al., 1976). However, as conditions become increasingly uncertain and variable, as in health care, coordination by feedback is more likely to be used (March & Simon, 1958). Improved health care team performance has been associated with both programming and feedback devices because standardized routines and care paths may enhance, rather than replace, the interactions among health care providers, particularly in situations of increasing uncertainty (Gittell, 2002).

At the organizational level, the coordination and division of labor influences size and the degree of organizational centralization and formalization.

As organizations grow in size, work units are increasingly subdivided to ensure tasks are accomplished; however, this process slows as organizations become very large, because the gains achieved by subdividing work occur at the expense of the coordination mechanisms necessary to unify system functioning across subunits (Blau, 1970). The need to balance the division of labor with the coordination of subunits and roles eventually constrains organizational size (Blau, 1970). At the organizational level, coordination is often measured by the degree of centralization and formalization. Health care organizations tend to be decentralized and less formalized because professionals are employed to manage highly uncertain work (Scott, 1992). However, as organizations grow and as the work becomes increasingly complex, specialized, and interdependent, there is a pull toward greater centralization and formalization (Scott, 1992).

Organizational Forms

The division and coordination of labor lead to varied organizational forms. As illustrated by the sloping triangles in Figure 13-1, organizational forms reflect a trade-off between differentiation by function and integration by program. *Differentiation by function* refers to the division of work by occupation. **Integration by program** means the coordination of work around the delivery of particular products or services. Five basic organizational forms can be situated along a differentiation-integration continuum (Charnes & Tewksbury, 1993). Functional and program forms represent extreme examples of differentiation and integration.

The matrix form represents the most balanced form. In reality, organizations are not usually found in these pure forms but rather reflect hybrids of the forms described next.

Functional Form

At the extreme left end of the continuum, dividing the work by occupation leads to a functional organization whereby health professions and nonprofessional services are arranged according to the type of work performed. The emphasis is on the human resources inputs to the organization (Figure 13-2). Examples are nursing, respiratory therapy, admitting, and environmental services. Within each functional department, management develops specific structures, policies, procedures, and human resource practices. In this type of organizational form, professionals report directly to a discipline-specific supervisor (e.g., nurses would report to a nurse manager). Members of a functional group (e.g., nursing) are likely to interact more frequently, develop social relationships, receive supervision and evaluations from within the group, and conform to professional standards (Charnes & Tewksbury, 1993).

By dividing personnel according to the type of work performed, organizations can capitalize on the expertise, experience, efficiency, and professional standards that each discipline offers (Charnes & Tewksbury, 1993). Other benefits include cost reduction through shared resources; enhanced monitoring of cost, performance, and quality; and, promotion of professional development, identity, autonomy,

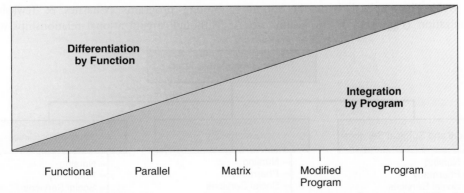

FIGURE 13-1 Continuum of organizational configurations. (Adapted from Charnes, M., &Tewksbury, L. [1993]. *Collaborative management in health care: Implementing the integrative organization* [p. 28, Figure 2.1]. San Francisco: Jossey-Bass. This material is used by permission of John Wiley & Sons.)

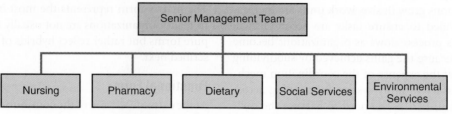

FIGURE 13-2 Simplified functional form.

advocacy, and career advancement (Charnes & Tewksbury, 1993). Disadvantages of the functional form are its potential to overemphasize professional silos, discourage informal relationships across disciplines, and fragment care delivery (Charnes & Tewksbury, 1993). Coordination of activities becomes challenging because group members have functionally based differences in work goals, cognitive patterns, and status (Gittell, 2003). Because the work of nursing is highly interdependent with other professional and nonprofessional work, nurse leaders in functional forms may use coordination mechanisms and leadership behaviors to span the boundaries between disciplines and facilitate the flow and exchange of information, resources, and work activities. Although prevalent in health care in the 1980s, functional forms have gradually been replaced by program or matrix forms to enhance client centeredness.

Program Form

At the extreme right end of the continuum, program organizations emphasize integration of the work by consumer, service, or geography (Charnes & Tewksbury, 1993). The emphasis is on the outputs of the organization (Figure 13-3). In health care,

programs may be managed according to consumer health needs (e.g., diabetes, cancer), consumer age (e.g., elderly, neonates, women), services (e.g., addictions, rehabilitation), medical specialty (e.g., neurosciences, endocrinology), or geography (e.g., catchment areas). Although the corporate structure is shared, each program tends to operate as a semi-autonomous unit with its own management team composed of medical, administrative, and nursing representatives (Charnes & Tewksbury, 1993). Professionals who work in program organizations may not report to a discipline-specific supervisor.

Program designs can optimize service delivery because local experts with accountability for costs, outcomes, and staffing control resources and can make timely operational decisions (Leatt et al., 1994). Patients can access integrated services from an array of health professionals with specific clinical expertise. With the program form, there is a push toward a multidisciplinary team approach (Leatt et al., 1994). However, clients who require access to more than one program may find it difficult to coordinate services among different programs. Integration by program occurs at the expense of decreased coordination among programs (Charnes & Tewksbury, 1993). Although organizational relationships with medical

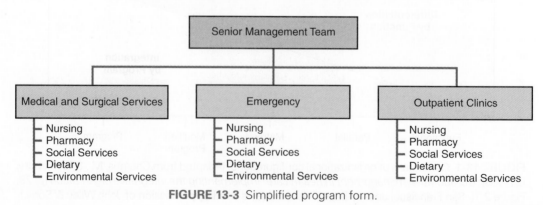

FIGURE 13-3 Simplified program form.

staff are enhanced when programs are grouped by medical specialty (Charnes & Tewksbury, 1993), health care professionals may be isolated from their colleagues in other programs, which has been associated with job dissatisfaction and lack of professional development opportunities (Young et al., 2004). For nursing, the concern is that no organization-wide mechanisms would exist to systematically handle professional nursing issues in terms of standards, resources, or professional advocacy. Because each program operates independently, processes and procedures are likely to be duplicated, and programs may compete for resources or develop goals that diverge from the corporate mission (Leatt et al., 1994).

Parallel Form

To address the challenges of purely functional forms, mechanisms in the parallel form assist in coordinating across functional departments (Charnes & Tewksbury, 1993). These mechanisms can include teams, specialists, task forces, liaison roles, and standing committees. For example, rather than each functional department separately establishing procedures to hire staff, a specialized human resource department may be created to deal with recruitment and employment issues across the organization. Another example is a rapid response team in a hospital that is composed of intensive care physicians and nurses and respiratory therapists. This team assists staff throughout the hospital in detecting and managing imminent patient deterioration and in resuscitating compromised patients. Likewise in home care, nurses with particular expertise such as wound care or palliation might be responsible for referrals across multiple areas. Task forces bring together members from various divisions in an organization to address a concern. For example, developing and implementing critical pathways, evidence-based practices, disease management initiatives, case management projects, or outcomes management efforts generally require an interdisciplinary team of specialists. These types of mechanisms foster collaboration and cross-fertilization of knowledge across divisions and can reinforce consistency in clinical and management practices by standardizing procedures.

Modified Program Form

To offset the fragmentation and isolation of functions in pure program structures, organizations maintain the program structure and develop integrative mechanisms to unify functions and occupations across programs (Charnes & Tewksbury, 1993). For example, a nurse executive could address professional nursing issues related to standards, educational resources, and research activities across the organization. Unlike his or her counterpart in a functional nursing department who has line authority, a nurse executive in a modified program would not directly control operations, finances, or personnel issues (known as *staff authority*). A nurse executive with staff authority must use personal influence and leadership skills to effect change.

Matrix Form

In a pure matrix form, people and work are organized along both functional and program dimensions (Charnes & Tewksbury, 1993). Essentially, the program form overlays the functional form (Figure 13-4). Although some employees may have dual reporting relationships, staff members are evaluated by both supervisors (Charnes & Tewksbury, 1993). The budget and decision making are shared between functional and program divisions. A matrix configuration has the flexibility to adapt to change and to deliver services innovatively and efficiently by drawing on a varied talent pool (Hatch & Cunliffe, 2006). In contrast, innovation in program forms is costly because additional cross-coordination may be required across functional divisions or specialists may need to be hired for each program (Hatch & Cunliffe, 2006). However, true matrix forms are rarely seen and are difficult to maintain because the additional management infrastructure is costly and dual reporting relationships may be ambiguous and lead to conflict (Charnes & Tewksbury, 1993). Success requires well-educated workers who can handle a multifaceted communication and authority web. Nurses in matrix organizations need strong interpersonal and teamwork skills to negotiate these complex environments.

Hierarchy

In bureaucratic and classical management theory, hierarchy is the structure of authority in an organization (e.g., Weber, 1978). Authority is equated with the enforcement of regulations, which brings about a governing order among the formal social

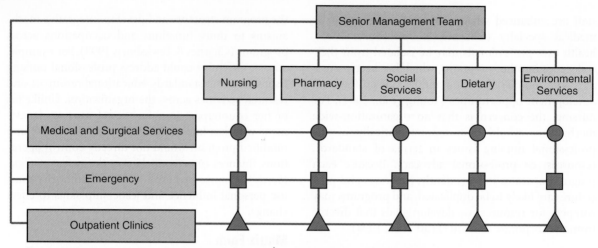

For example, team members for Outpatient Clinics (▲) are drawn from different functions.

FIGURE 13-4 Simplified matrix form.

relationships of organizational members (Weber, 1978). Authority is vested in positions, rather than in persons, and creates an impartial mechanism whereby the supraordinate position directs the actions and the norms expected of subordinate positions (Weber, 1978). Centralization is a multidimensional concept frequently associated with authority and hierarchy. **Centralization** refers to the extent to which decision-making authority is concentrated in the top level of the hierarchy (i.e., centralized) versus spread down through the hierarchy (i.e., decentralized) (Carter & Cullen, 1984). **Hierarchical centralization** can vary according to the decision type (Carter & Cullen, 1984). Hierarchical centralization is the extent to which decision-making authority is vested at the top levels of the hierarchy versus extended down through the hierarchy (Scott, 1992).

Corporate strategy is likely to be decided by top executives, whereas procedural work decisions may be devolved to work units or employees. For instance, a nurse executive could be required to centralize some budgetary decisions, whereas others could be devolved to lower levels in the hierarchy. A specific example would be the need to centralize a component of professional development expenditures required by union contracts (e.g., organization-wide funding for nursing certification) in contrast to decisions at the work unit level to fund nurses to attend ad hoc specialty conferences. Participation is an alternate dimension of centralization that refers to the scope of

involvement and influence of organizational members in decision making (Carter & Cullen, 1984). In a study of Belgian hospitals, nurses who perceived that their work decisions were tightly controlled by a supervisor (i.e., high hierarchical centralization) and that they had little influence on program decisions (i.e., low participative centralization) reported lower job satisfaction (Willem et al., 2007).

In addition, hierarchy creates a reporting structure whereby formal lines of communication, in conjunction with role descriptions, delineate the responsibilities and accountability of each position for work processes and outcomes. Organizational positions are traditionally described in terms of staff and line positions (Gulick, 1937). Staff positions are outside the direct hierarchical authority chain. These positions provide expertise and knowledge to support the line positions in meeting the organization's goals. A nursing example of a staff position is a clinical nurse specialist (CNS) who is hired for knowledge development and expert consultation for selected patient groups. Line positions are in the direct line of hierarchical authority from top to bottom in an organization. These positions are central to controlling or generating the product or service of the organization. Line positions include vice presidents, directors, managers, and frontline nurses because these positions are authorized either to supervise production processes or to produce the organization's output. In nursing, although frontline nurses are commonly referred to as "staff" nurses, these nurses hold line positions that deliver services to care recipients.

Hierarchy also enables organizations to assign responsibilities based on the complexity and skill requirements of the work and to ensure individual accountability (Jaques, 1990). Responsibility is the allocation and acceptance of a task. Responsibility is the obligation to take on and accomplish work and to secure the desired results. A manager assigns or delegates responsibility to a subordinate, and thus responsibility flows down the organizational chain. In accepting the obligation of an assigned task, the staff person is accepting responsibility to accomplish the task. Accountability is the liability for task performance and is determined in a retrospective analysis of what occurred. The assignment of responsibility and the granting of authority create accountability. Accountability flows upward or outward: from staff to manager or from provider to client. Reporting relationships are important to create channels of appeal (Weber, 1978), to ensure employees are held accountable for the work assigned, and to invest managers with the necessary authority to ensure the completion of work (Jaques, 1990). The manager represents the organization at the point of contact with staff, and thus the reporting relationship is also a mechanism by which staff can access organizational resources to identify and solve complex problems (Blau, 1968). Ideally, managers also apply their leadership skills to reporting relationships to release the energy and talents of people in ways that add value to the work performed (Jaques, 1990). Examples of "value added" outcomes include improved employee productivity, organizational commitment, and organizational citizenship behaviors.

ORGANIZATIONAL CHARTS

Hierarchy reflects the *formal* structure of the organization, which can be identified on an organizational chart. An organizational chart is a visual display of the organization's positions and the intentional relationships among positions. The organizational chart reflects the various positions and the formal relationships between and among the positions and, by extension, the people who are a part of the organization. The organizational chart generally presents the line positions, linked together by solid lines to show the flow of authority. Administrative roles are generally shown in vertical and horizontal dimensions. Staff positions or advisory bodies may be depicted on the chart with dotted lines to show consultative relationships. Organizational charts help with administrative control, policy making and planning, and the evaluation of the organization's strengths and weaknesses. They clearly depict who reports to whom. Charts are used to orient personnel because relationships and expected patterns of interaction within the formal organization are made clear. For example, an organizational chart of a matrix structure may show dotted lines for the project or interdisciplinary team relationships. Dotted lines mean that a relationship to the position or the group would form for a project. In the process of applying for a job, obtaining the employer's organizational chart will help understand the relative positioning of individuals within the organization and how the organization is structured—or at least how decision makers believe it is structured.

In addition to a *formal* structure, organizations are characterized by an *informal* structure. The *informal* structure is simply the network or pattern of social relationships and friendship circles that are outside the formal structure. It is an interconnected web of relationships that operate in and around the formally designated lines of communication. The *informal* structure does not appear on the *formal* organizational chart.

ORGANIZATIONAL SHAPES

The shape of an organization structure can be described as relatively tall or flat. Several structural factors influence the shape of an organization. The formal reporting relationships among positions, which ensure the assignment of responsibility, authority, and accountability, result in hierarchical levels. The **span of control** of managers, which is the number of employees reporting directly to a management position, also influences organizational shape (Meyer, 2008). For instance, when managers on average have fewer direct-report staff, the organizational shape is relatively taller. Another structural factor involves decisions about the number of management layers in the hierarchy (i.e., **scalar principle**). Increased layers of management help the organization cope with increasing work complexity and extended time lines (Jaques, 1990). A tall organization structure assumes a pyramidal shape with multiple management layers (Figure 13-5). In contrast, a flat organization structure has minimal management layers (Figure 13-6). Advantages and disadvantages associated with tall and flat organizational shapes are summarized in Table 13-2. However, a narrow focus on the hierarchical structure of an organization without attention to the people and processes within the organization, or the outcomes achieved, can be misleading. For instance, factors that can potentially offset the effects of tall organizations include the competence and leadership of members, the use of merit-based rewards, the effectiveness of reporting relationships, and the sharing of information and authority (Jaques, 1990).

Span of management refers to the number and ordering of management positions and resources relative to other personnel and can be measured at organizational, departmental, managerial, work group, or employee levels (Meyer, 2008). There are many competing theoretical arguments about factors influencing the span of management; and decisions about the amount, type, and distribution of nursing management resources within health care organizations are influenced by a multitude of factors at the consumer, nurse, work group, manager, organizational, and regional levels (Table 13-3) (Meyer, 2008). A key controversy about the span of control of nurse managers relates to supervisory responsibilities. On the one hand, wider spans of control for managers are proposed because nurses and other health care professionals are experts committed to professional codes of ethics and regulated standards, therefore requiring less direct supervision (Meier & Bohte, 2003). On the other hand, narrow spans of control are deemed necessary because (1) nurses require managerial support and access

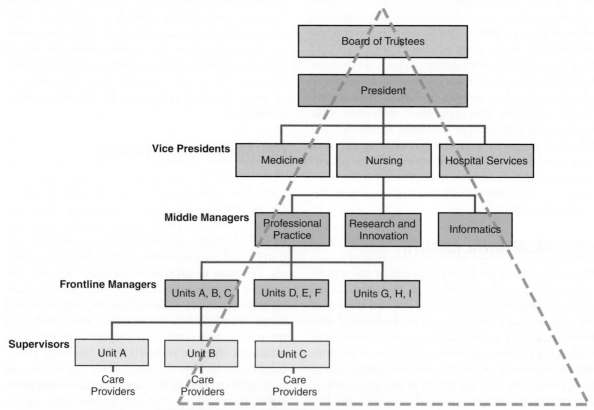

FIGURE 13-5 Simplified tall organizational structure.

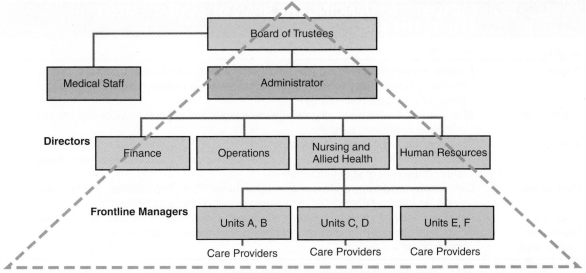

FIGURE 13-6 Simplified flat organizational structure.

TABLE 13-2	**COMPARISON OF FLAT AND TALL ORGANIZATION STRUCTURES**	
	TALL ORGANIZATION	**FLAT ORGANIZATION**
Advantages	• Increased access to managers & organizational resources • Greater supervisory capability • Layers of skill to deal with varying degrees of work complexity • Layers of accountability for work completion • Layers of responsibility to address short, medium & long-term issues & planning	• Fewer divisions facilitate streamlining of goals, problem solving & resource use • Greater hierarchical decentralization; potential for greater staff autonomy through increased delegation • Greater innovation • Enhanced responsiveness to consumers at point of service • Less cross coordination required • Less costly management infrastructure
Disadvantages	• More hierarchical centralization; potential to micromanage staff activities • Slowed vertical decision making & distorted communication • Less innovation • Difficult way-finding for consumers • Greater cross coordination required • Costly management infrastructure	• Decreased access to managers & organizational resources • Decreased supervisory capability • Overextension of managers • Vertical communication delays

Compiled by the author. © 2012 Raquel M. Meyer. Used with permission. Table based on: Alidina & Funke-Furber, 1988; Jaques, 1990; Pabst, 1993.

to organizational resources and information to co-ordinate complex work processes to achieve positive outcomes, and (2) the introduction of unregulated workers into health care settings has required more direct, hands-on supervision to ensure that care standards and organizational expectations are met.

This counterargument suggests that the span of control of frontline nurse managers should factor in the needs of staff for manager support and supervision. In nursing, relationships between the span of control of frontline managers and nurse and clinical outcomes have been investigated (see Research Note).

TABLE 13-3	FACTORS INFLUENCING THE SPAN OF MANAGEMENT IN HEALTH CARE	
LEVEL	**FACTORS**	
Region	Funding and administration models, health care system structures and cultures; degree of reform; cross-border service use; health care worker mobility[e]; population growth; geography; sectors[d]; technology[a]	
Organization	Size; stage of development; degree of decentralization of support services (e.g., human resources, finances)[a]; culture[a,h]	
Manager	Organizational level[e]; scope of responsibilities[a,b,e,h]; mix of assigned areas[b]; profession[b,e]; leadership[c,f]; skills[a,d,e]; education[a,e,h]; experience[a]; budget[b,g]; reporting demands[g]; support roles[a,b,h]; diversity of staff functions[a,g]	
Work group	Care delivery models[a,h,i]; professional and skill mixes[a,g,h]; staffing stability[g]; unit type and size[b,h]; occupancy rates[a,g,h]; task interdependence[a]; distance or location[a,b,h]	
Employee	Profession and need for supervision[a,i]; education[a]; experience[h]; work stability[h]; complexity[a]	
Health care consumers	Acuity; care complexity and duration; immediacy of decisions; degree of coordination[a]	

Reproduced from Meyer, R.M. (2008). Span of management: Concept analysis. *Journal of Advanced Nursing, 63*(1), 104-112. This material is used by permission of Blackwell Publishing.

[a]Alidina & Funke-Furber, 1988.
[b]Altaffer, 1998.
[c]Doran et al., 2004.
[d]Filerman, 2003.
[e]Mahon & Young, 2006.
[f]McCutcheon, 2004.
[g]Morash et al., 2005.
[h]Pabst, 1993.
[i]Redman & Jones, 1998.

POWER

Within the objective perspective, power has been conceptualized as a resource. Kanter's (1977) theory of the structural determinants of behavior in organizations has been investigated in nursing systems (Laschinger, 1996). For Kanter (1977, p. 166), power refers to "the ability to get things done, to mobilize resources". It is not the power to control or dominate others. When power is shared, rather than monopolized, employees are empowered and the organization is more likely to benefit. More activity can be accomplished by organizational members, and the capacity for effective action is increased. Kanter (1977) described three work empowerment structures: opportunity, power, and proportion. The structure of *opportunity* refers to expectations and future prospects (i.e., opportunities for growth, mobility, job enrichment). The structure of *power* stems from access to information, support, and resources. The structure

of *proportion* denotes the social composition of the organization's workforce (e.g., gender, minorities). Empowered work environments are those in which all employees have access to opportunities to learn and grow and to information, support, and resources necessary for the job. Indeed, frontline nurses' job-related empowerment has been positively associated with various nurse outcomes, including organizational commitment (Laschinger & Finegan, 2005; Young-Ritchie et al., 2007); intent to remain in the organization (Nedd, 2006); and interactional justice, respect, trust in management, and job satisfaction (Laschinger & Finegan, 2005). Nurses who occupy positions at higher levels in the nursing hierarchy report increasingly greater degrees of empowerment (Laschinger, 1996). Thus nurses in management positions are likely to perceive greater access to opportunity and power structures than frontline nurses.

In Kanter's (1977) study, effective leaders were seen as both competent and powerful. Sensitivity with

RESEARCH NOTE

Source

Meyer, R.M., O'Brien-Pallas, L., Doran, D., Streiner, D., Ferguson-Paré, M., & Duffield, C. (2011). Frontline managers as boundary spanners: Effects of span and time on nurse supervision satisfaction. *Journal of Nursing Management, 19*(5), 611-622.

Purpose

This article examined the influence of frontline nurse managers' number of direct report staff, time in staff contact, transformational leadership practices and operational hours on nurse supervision satisfaction.

Discussion

This descriptive correlational study collected nurse manager and staff surveys, manager work logs, and administrative human resource data. Managers averaged spans of 86.6 direct report staff (range: 29.0 to 174.3) and spent 3.2 hours daily in staff contact (range: 1.4 to 7.2). Managers usually engaged in transformational leadership practices (mean=7.6; 10-point scale). Hours of operation were extended (n=19) or compressed (n=12). From a convenience sample of 31 managers from 4 acute care teaching hospitals, all were registered nurses and 39% held a master's degree. Of the 558 nurses who rated supervision satisfaction, 88% were registered nurses and 35% held a baccalaureate nursing degree or higher. Nurse supervision satisfaction with the manager's administrative, technical and relational skills averaged 3.8 (5-point scale).

Nurses' supervision satisfaction was higher with more transformational leadership, but was not directly influenced by span, time in staff contact, or hours of operation. A three-way interaction between span, transformational leadership, and hours of operation explained 61% of the variation in supervision satisfaction between managers. When managers were assigned compressed hours of operation, higher leadership enhanced supervision satisfaction when spans were narrow; that is, no matter how highly transformational their leadership style, managers could not overcome wide spans to positively influence supervision satisfaction. When managers were assigned extended hours of operation, higher leadership enhanced supervision satisfaction, and this effect was surprisingly more pronounced under wider spans. Other factors did not predict supervision satisfaction.

Application to Practice

As health care organizations contend with staffing shortages, frontline managers are critical to the retention and supervision of nurses. In this study, the authors surmised that hours of operation are important because the density of staff during the manager's work day and the manager's capacity to be accessible to staff vary relative to operational hours. Hours of operation influenced the number of direct reports on a daily basis. For example, a manager of weekday clinics interfaces with nearly all staff daily and covers all of the compressed hours weekly, whereas a manager of a 24/7 inpatient unit interfaces with ½ of staff daily and covers only ¼ of the extended hours weekly. Moderate daily spans for nurse supervision satisfaction were enabled by narrow spans with compressed operational hours and by wide spans with extended operational hours. Consistent with previous leadership research, this study also recommended investments in transformational leadership training to enhance nurse satisfaction. Further research is needed to understand the conditions under which the job design of frontline management positions influences organizational, human resource and clinical outcomes.

subordinates was secondary to having upward credibility within the organization; leaders to whom others listened, who accessed resources, and who produced results within the broader organization were perceived to be effective. Kanter (1977) proposed that effective leadership evolves from both *formal* and *informal* sources of power in the organization. *Formal* power is derived from work that is relevant to pressing organizational issues and that provides opportunities to perform extraordinary and highly visible activities; *informal* power comes from relationships and alliances with people in the organization.

Kanter (1977) also theorized that "power begets power" (p. 168). Research indicates that nurses who are managed by empowered leaders also are empowered (Laschinger, 1996). For example, frontline nurses in organizations in which chief nurse executives had line authority reported significantly greater global empowerment with respect to resources than their counterparts in organizations in which chief nurse executives had staff authority (Matthews et al., 2006). The authors suggested that the *formal* power accessible to nurse executives with line authority enabled them to secure the staffing resources necessary for frontline nurses to provide high quality of care. Magnet hospitals typically consist of flat organizational structures with nursing councils that empower nurses through decentralized decision making (Kirkley et al., 2004). This structure engages staff nurses in decisions impacting their work, for example, when inter-professional staff work together to redesign workflow. Considered overall, the research suggests that empowerment structures positively impact both nurses and managers and can inform the design of the organizational structures in which nurses work.

LEADERSHIP AND MANAGEMENT IMPLICATIONS

The global and local challenges for nursing within organizations and across systems are numerous. Leaders and managers can influence the structure in which goals are accomplished. In fact, determining the structure is a key responsibility of leaders and managers in planning an organization that is conducive to high-quality nursing care. As environments and technologies evolve, the leadership and management team may need to rethink and redesign the organization and work-group structures to better match the changing conditions and to achieve the desired outcomes. In nursing, determining the structure is a planning and organizing aspect of the management process that can be informed by evidence and theory from the management field. According to the Institute of Medicine (2004), just as clinicians are compelled to seek, evaluate, and apply empirical evidence, so too should managers incorporate evidence-based management practices.

Leaders and managers may be involved in revising or changing organizational structures. *Restructuring* means revising or modifying the structure to reshape it or switch to another structural form. Restructuring efforts have typically been geared toward fixing existing operational processes. Lean, decentralized, self-governing organizations that empower first-line caregivers are the preferred structures. Reengineering is a radical redesign of business processes (Champy, 2010). To begin anew, processes are analyzed from the point of view of the consumer (patient and family), as well as the requirement to achieve greater cost containment, quality, service, and speed. User-friendly processes, efficiency, and economy are key ideas. Job redesign focuses on who does what tasks and on maximizing flexibility, cross-training, and productivity (Curtin, 1994).

Changes to organization structure afford opportunities to empower nurses. Strategies include maximizing nurses' scope of practice, creating autonomous and visible nursing roles relevant to organizational priorities, providing more leadership opportunities for nurses at all levels, and clinical laddering (Registered Nurses' Association of Ontario [RNAO], 2006). Fiscal and material resources can also be deployed to empower nurses by facilitating access to knowledge development opportunities (e.g., courses, conferences) and by providing adequate resources for job completion (e.g., staffing). A decentralized, participative structure can be promoted through coordination mechanisms that involve nurses in shared governance councils and task forces (e.g., related to clinical practice or nurse retention) and in information exchange (e.g., newsletters, open forums, web technologies).

A transparent and participative approach to the development of programming devices to standardize work processes (e.g., care maps, electronic health records) can be used to build shared goals for interdisciplinary teams. Organizations can also deliberately foster informal coordination mechanisms to enhance the relational and functional networks in which work is accomplished (Galbraith et al., 2002). For example, physical co-location, communal space, communities of practice, rotational job assignments, electronic chat groups, and interdisciplinary training programs can foster spontaneous interactions and relationships across functional, professional, and geographical silos, resulting in knowledge sharing, problem solving, and innovation (Galbraith et al., 2002).

Hierarchical reporting relationships can be greatly enhanced by transformational leaders who establish trust with nurses by communicating role and behavior expectations, by giving constructive performance feedback, and by recognizing and rewarding successes (RNAO, 2006). When workers fall outside organizational lines of authority (e.g., outsourced services, nursing agencies), managers and leaders require skill in negotiating standards and performance outcomes, in resolving problems across organizational boundaries, and in building relationships and shared goals to overcome differing alliances (Porter-O'Grady, 2003).

In more highly matrixed organizations, nurse managers and leaders must network with interdisciplinary stakeholders within and across programs and support services. Success for leaders with line authority requires strong relational skills, credibility, an ability to link resource use to outcomes using a business model, and an in-depth understanding of the needs of clients and staff (Lorenz, 2008). The trends toward increased outsourcing, decreased reliance on traditional inpatient services for revenues, and increased specialization of health services require an entrepreneurial skill set and innovative leadership roles to build business partnerships and alliances and to foster change at the point of service delivery (Porter-O'Grady, 2007). In the context of nurse and manager shortages, organizations need to recruit and deploy management resources in line with objectives by reevaluating the number of management layers and the span of control of individual positions, as well as by developing a nursing leadership succession plan. To be supportive of nursing staff, nurse managers need access to the support and information of senior management and peers, professional development and mentorship, an office easily accessible to staff, administrative support, and a strong and shared organizational culture (Kramer et al., 2007).

CURRENT ISSUES AND TRENDS

During the 1990s, health care systems in many developed countries were subjected to restructuring, decentralization, specialization, and performance management, resulting in the de-layering of management structures in an effort to contain costs and achieve outcomes (e.g., Mahon & Young, 2006). Those managers remaining in the system faced expanded roles. Instead of a traditional head nurse position responsible for patient care on a single unit, the role of the nurse manager typically grew to encompass the management of finances, operations, and human resources across multiple clinical areas and services in program management structures with regulated and unregulated multidisciplinary staff (Duffield & Franks, 2001).

The twenty-first century has ushered in significant concerns related to the global community and public safety. These issues are intensified by calls for transparency, accountability, and public reporting in the management of health care services, which in turn, have increased demands on the internal structures and external boundaries of organizations. There is a trend toward planning and coordinating efforts across organizations and jurisdictions, which has been mirrored in the field of organization theory. The focus has shifted from "intra-organizational" to "inter-organizational" phenomena (e.g., clusters, networks, international strategic alliances) (Clegg & Hardy, 1999).

At a global level, increasing shortages of nurses and other health care professionals has engendered a call for developed countries to create self-sufficient and sustainable nursing workforces by increasing domestic supply (Little & Buchan, 2007). This requires jurisdictional planning and coordinated activities and investments across health systems and organizations. At the organizational level, employers need to attract and retain nurses through changes to work conditions and structures (e.g., creating full-time positions, re-dividing work to remove non-nursing tasks, supplying adequate staffing and material resources to accomplish the work) (Little & Buchan, 2007). These strategies are necessary to stabilize the nursing workforce within organizations and to ensure that the knowledge, skills, and competence that nurses possess are retained and appropriately deployed in the organization.

At a societal level, preparedness for disasters, bioterrorism, and pandemics has required health care organizations, communities, and jurisdictions to pool resources and coordinate activities along the external boundaries of organizational structures. In addition, the movement toward clinical integration across settings to provide seamless care and to better manage chronic illness has generated significant boundary and inter-organizational work. Clinical integration is a delivery mechanism whereby hospitals and physicians share responsibility and information about care recipients across settings for a single care episode or longer (Taylor, 2008). However, clinical integration efforts continue to be challenged by significant legal, financial, regulatory, and leadership issues across jurisdictional and organizational boundaries (Taylor, 2008). With the passage and staged implementation of the Affordable Care Act, including the structuring of Accountable Care Organizations (ACOs) and Patient-centered Medical Homes, health care delivery is set to be dramatically restructured to emphasize primary care. Traditional institutional health care services have decreased in intensity and duration and shifted to outpatient or community-based formats (Porter-O'Grady, 2007). An associated consequence has been the compression of nursing care because of shortened lengths of stay and increased patient acuity, as well as the outsourcing of support services (Porter-O'Grady, 2007).

Increased awareness and disclosure about medical errors and preventable adverse events have encouraged organizations to address consumer safety through risk reduction and the development of cultures of safety (e.g., Leape & Berwick, 2005). To address safety, new coordination mechanisms and safety standards are based on the science of human factors engineering, which takes a systems approach to understanding and preventing critical incidents (Hoffman et al., 2006). A systems approach considers how adverse events occur in relation to management, organization, and regulatory factors such as policies and procedures, information technology, staffing practices, and physical structures (Hoffman et al., 2006). Recall that policies, procedures, and information systems are coordination devices. For instance, safety risks may be reduced when nurses standardize care through the use of evidence-based care maps. Organizations are also compelled to collaborate in the development and sharing of safety innovations. The Center for Quality Improvement and Safety in the United States and the Canadian Patient Safety Institute in Canada are examples of how safety innovations can be widely shared and standardized across organizations.

CASE STUDY

Bed Turnaround

Between 11 AM and 8 PM, as many as 17 patients will be discharged and new patients will be admitted on a 34-bed medical-surgical unit. The support associate (SA) is responsible for patient transport and housekeeping duties. The SA is pulled away from cleaning a room four or five times per room to transport patients for discharge or to and from ancillary testing. Meanwhile, new admissions are held in the emergency department or outpatient center, awaiting a clean bed. Often, a centralized housekeeping team is STAT-paged to clean the room.

Further analysis identifies that the lack of trust between departments in this facility often results in sending out a staff to other units to "truly assess" bed status. Lack of teamwork exists between the SAs and housekeeping personnel. The average bed turnaround time from the point of patient discharge to the bed being ready for occupancy is 82 minutes.

As a result, a multidisciplinary team is formed to identify options for reducing bed turnaround time and to evaluate the SA role. Team members consist of an administration representative, the medical-surgical unit manager, three SAs, two housekeeping personnel, a unit clerk, the house-wide bed coordinator, and one registered nurse (RN).

Through this team, the reporting relationship of the unit-based housekeeper responsible for cleaning the common areas (e.g., nurses' station, waiting rooms, and hallways) is changed to a matrix reporting structure in which the housekeeper reports directly to the Director of Environmental Services but also has a dotted-line relationship to the individual department director. In addition, a centralized support associate STAT team is initiated to work from 1 PM to 11:30 PM, Monday through Friday, and 7 AM to 3 PM on Saturdays. Dispatch of the STAT team is delegated to the charge RN via a beeper as opposed to going through the centralized Environmental Services Department. On the off-shift, the STAT SA team reports to and is dispatched by the off-shift supervisor. Finally, one SA per unit is assigned to perform strictly discharge room cleaning, which eliminates transport interruptions. As a result of these structure and role changes, the time from discharge of a patient to the time a bed is ready is decreased 53% to 38 minutes.

Bed Turnaround Process

INDICATOR	BASELINE JULY/AUGUST/ SEPTEMBER 2008	FEBRUARY 2009
Discharge of patient to bed ready	82 minutes	38 minutes

CRITICAL THINKING EXERCISE

Nurse Caitlin Schultz recently transferred from a director role in an inpatient nursing unit to assume the director role of another department. The previous department director had established a council for recruitment and retention. Composed of three RNs and two social workers, this team established a program to fund flowers for any staff member experiencing a family death, wedding, or birth; organized holiday activities at the department level; and assisted the director in recognizing staff members during Nurses' Week.

As part of the annual Nurses' Week celebration, each nursing employee was recognized at the department level with an awards luncheon, attended scheduled events, and received a tote bag with the hospital's logo. Within 1 month of starting the new role, the director attended the first Recruitment and Retention Council meeting, at which the team was preparing for the upcoming week by recognizing one of the nursing specialties practiced in their department.

Staff discussions centered on how to obtain more money from the budget to buy yet another gift for only RN staff members. As the conversation continued, the director became concerned that the team's focus was centered on recognizing only the RNs (as accomplished during Nurses' Week activities) versus focusing on the work and contributions of the entire department as it pertained to that particular specialty.

1. Is there a problem?
2. What is the problem?
3. How can the director's authority, responsibility, and accountability be explained?
4. What elements of organizational structure could be helpful in this situation? Which could be barriers?
5. What options are there to refocus the team?
6. What problems and decisions face the staff nurses?
7. What challenges face the director?

14

Decentralization and Shared Governance

Cheryl Hoying

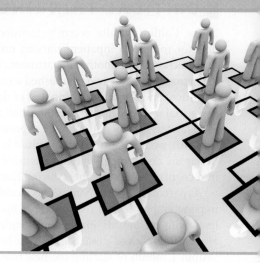

e**volve** WEBSITE

http://evolve.elsevier.com/Huber/leadership/

In early 2012, Google created an online petition to halt two anti-piracy bills that would censor parts of the Internet. Popular websites like Wikipedia blacked out their content in protest, and 4.5 million people sided with the websites and signed the petition. The overwhelming requisition caused 18 U.S. senators—including some of the bill's own co-sponsors—to reverse their positions of support (Kain, 2012; Tassi, 2012).

Social media and other advents in technology like smart phones and Wi-Fi have made it easier for the majority to voice their opinions, but the desire to communicate is nothing new. Plato himself believed the only way to reach the truth was by dialogue (Poe, 2011), yet it took centuries before the voices of the masses were heard. In the nineteenth century, the labor rights movement encouraged workers to address fair treatment and safe work environments. In the 1960s, organizational theorists Herzberg and McGregor championed employees as the most important asset of an organization, and they encouraged companies to invest in their motivation and growth (Anthony, 2004). This paradigm shift caused companies to view employees not as a means to an end, but

as a potential source of innovation and creativity if the environment fostered such ideals.

Luckily these ideas have filtered into health care, and into the field of nursing in particular. Based on these and other management theories, **shared governance** has ascended to become the go-to decentralization structure for hospitals in the twenty-first century. Shared governance is an accountability-based system for professionals that empower individuals within the decision-making system and increases nurses' authority and control over their practice. A model of organizational decision making in which staff nurses are empowered through autonomy and accountability, shared governance will only further legitimize a generation who has grown accustomed to voicing their opinions.

DEFINITIONS

Centralization and Decentralization

Hospitals are organized and their work is structured around a guiding philosophy. The philosophy serves as the institutional framework that shapes the direction of knowledge and skill acquisition. It is the pivotal factor in the long-term development of the institution.

Photo used with permission from Photos.com.

The **mission,** core values, and **vision** are the instruments that give voice to the organization's philosophy. The mission is an aim to be accomplished. It influences the philosophy, goals and objectives of an organization. The vision is a mental image or the power of imagination to see something that is not actually visible. Likewise, the **organizational chart** is a diagram that displays how the parts of an organization are connected. It shows organizational relationships and areas of responsibility (Tomey, 2009). If there are many layers of management with reporting lines cascading down from the top, then the structure is hierarchical. Figure 14-1 illustrates an example. At a glance, the chart permits the trained observer to make a statement about the organizational philosophy of the organization—whether the authority is primarily centralized or decentralized (Straub & Attner, 1994).

Centralization and **decentralization** are organizational philosophies about power distribution that pertain to the hierarchical level of decision-making authority in the institution. **Centralization** means that decisions are made at the top levels. **Decentralization** means that decision making is diffused throughout the organization. The higher the degree of decentralization in an organization, the more decision making is done at lower levels and with less supervision. Institutions organize and structure themselves by defining departmental function and authority to achieve a more coordinated effort. It drives plans and decisions about responsibilities and who reports to whom. Executives may use **selective decentralization,** where power for decision making is concentrated in the functional areas of staffing, purchasing, and operations, for example (Kops, 2011). Alternatively, they may choose to set purchase limits at each level of the organization by dollar amounts.

Centralization and decentralization are relative terms when applied to the operating philosophy of institutions. In institutions where the executive leader retains more decision-making authority, the operation takes on a more centralized philosophy. However, as institutions evolve into more complex global operations—where nurse managers are held accountable for transactional processes such as budgets, productivity, and quality monitoring, on top of their roles as coaches, mentors, and leaders to staff nurses (McGuire & Kennerly, 2006)—it becomes difficult for them to manage the information overload.

An institution with centralized decision making is demonstrated in the first scenario as follows:

Olivia Witte is the nurse manager of 2 Main, a medical nursing unit in General Hospital. As such, Nurse Witte interviews nursing applicants to fill the open nursing positions on 2 Main. At the conclusion of the interviews, the nurse manager is free to contact the applicant and offer the candidate the open position.

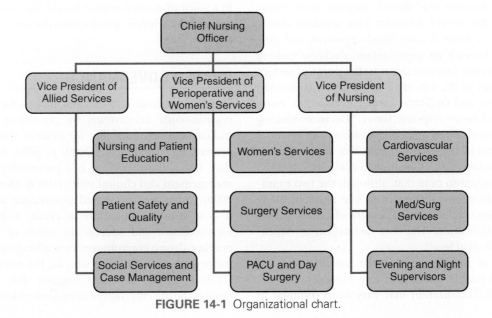

FIGURE 14-1 Organizational chart.

Although this is a somewhat simplistic example, the reader should note that the decision-making authority is vested solely in the nurse manager. That example is compared to the following second scenario:

Steve Smith is the nurse manager of 4 East, a medical nursing unit in City Hospital. With three staff nurse positions vacant, he posts the openings and asks the unit council, made up of nurses and other staff on the unit who have had human resources training on behavioral interviewing, to act as part of the selection committee. Based on the needs of the nursing unit and the availability of nursing applicants who match those criteria, human resource staff screens the files of the applicants. They pass the files of those nurses who meet the requirements for the positions to the selection committee, which then schedules interviews with the applicants. Once the selection committee has interviewed each candidate, it decides on the best candidate for each position. The committee's recommendations, along with the rationale for its choices, are discussed with Nurse Smith. Nurse Smith meets with the candidates and takes into consideration the recommendations by the selection committee, interviews them, and makes the job offers.

The professional staff nurses are involved in making a hiring decision that directly impacts their workplace in the second scenario. This scenario clearly illustrates a more decentralized organizational philosophy. In such an organization, decision-making authority rests in levels closer to the point of service rather than in the executive levels. Decentralization encourages and facilitates greater innovation, more input, and faster response times. "Decision-making that is decentralized and collaborative is an essential component in care environments that support excellence in patient care" (Golanowski et al., 2007, p. 342). It is important to note that, although the two examples would appear distant from one another, many institutions exhibit varying degrees of centralization or decentralization. The core distinction is: decentralized to what level?

Span of management is the number and diversity of people who report to a manager. The degree of decentralization may vary from minimal to maximal. Centralized decision making results in a narrower span of control and more levels of management, whereas decentralized decision making generally means that the **span of management** is larger for each manager (Tomey, 2009). Managers who delegate authority find that they can devote more time to planning and evaluating outcomes. Fewer levels of management will be required because the staff take on great accountability for decisions at the point of service, or operational level.

Staff must be empowered with education, decision-making skills, conflict resolution, and communication techniques to feel comfortable enough to practice autonomously and make effective decisions. Staff members in decentralized organizations are more accountable because fewer people provide functional supervision, quality monitoring, or unit-specific responsibilities that were previously part of the role of the manager. Nurse managers and staff nurses can have differing views on who handles the actual decision making in shared governance (Scherb et al., 2011), so managers must be clear about decision-making domains.

Institutions that employ a decentralized organizational philosophy emphasize planning and evaluation, and communicate clear goals and objectives to their employees. Therefore they are more likely to develop synergy within the institution. **Synergy** results from bringing different perspectives together in a spirit of mutual respect to seek the best solution, because the whole is greater than the sum of its parts (Tomey, 2009).

SHARED GOVERNANCE

Shared governance is "a dynamic process for achieving organizational effectiveness by promoting decision-making and accountability for practice through empowerment" (Bednarski, 2009, p. 585). It is more than just a framework; it is a partnership between management and clinical staff (Frith & Montgomery, 2006). Advocates of shared governance argue that it is a strong foundation to create a framework for excellence and address the needs of a nursing practice-driven environment by reallocating power in the organization to those who do the work (Porter-O'Grady, 2009). Research suggests that registered nurses who are empowered to make decisions through shared governance have higher nurse autonomy and increased confidence in decision making (Newman, 2011, Tourangeau et al., 2006).

History

Kanter's (1993) theory of organizational empowerment provides the theoretical underpinnings for shared governance. Her theory asserts that social structures in the workplace have a larger impact on attitudes and behaviors than do individual personalities. Kanter suggested that avenues of power provide for the sources of structural empowerment in an organization. Avenues of power include access to information, access to resources required to do the job, having the opportunity to learn and grow, and being supported. In addition, she suggested that the informal job factors that influence empowerment are the alliances that workers have with fellow workers at all levels of the organization. Workplaces that are structurally empowering provide many of the opportunities for involvement, commitment and transparency. Empowered workers are more likely to have increased feelings of respect for and trust in management and organizational justice, which relates to one's commitment to an organization (Moore & Hutchison, 2007) and may impact retention, which ultimately affects recruitment.

Decentralization and shared governance were strategies first introduced in the late 1970s to enable nurses to exercise control and make decisions about their practice, as a means to promote relationships and responsibilities between nurses and the organizational leaders, as well as develop equality and parity. Shared governance is touted as a strategy to transform organizations, improve productivity, empower staff nurses, enhance staff nurse autonomy, increase job satisfaction, and reduce nursing turnover (Anderson, 2011). This was seen as a radical departure from the traditional hierarchical hospital management structure in which nurses had little authority, little voice in governance, and low control within the organization (Hess, 1994).

Shared governance is not a theory, a conceptual framework, or an organizational principle. Shared governance is a vehicle for engaging organizations and creating the necessary forums and intersections that assure the decisions and actions remain dynamic and as close to the point of service as possible

(Porter-O'Grady, 2009). It is an accountability-based model through which nurses actively engage in making decisions regarding nursing practice, quality of patient care, education, nursing peer issues, and issues in the work environment. Shared governance promotes involvement, investment, participation, sharing of power, interdependence, cooperation, horizontal relationships, autonomy, and accountability for nursing decisions. Nursing effectiveness is enhanced through the sense of ownership that comes with more active involvement in the leadership of the organization. Professional practice environments, known for their improved patient outcomes, are characterized by institutions in which nurses have a high level of autonomy, strong leadership, support from administration, and control over their practice, all of which are results of shared governance (Tourangeu et al., 2006). Shared governance is seen as a strategy for fostering professional nursing practice through empowerment of nurses.

Empowerment refers to a process whereby nurses recognize that they have legitimate power and authority to make decisions regarding their practice. There is no transfer of power, but merely a change from an external to an internal locus of control. Authority is not given or taken away. Clinicians at the point of service are given the opportunity to be an integral part of the decision making process; but even more important, they act on the opportunity and are responsible for implementing changes to improve patient care quality and the work environment. Empowerment is accomplished through the shared governance journey. Evidence suggests a statistically significant positive relationship between registered nurses' perceptions of shared governance and empowerment (Barden et al., 2011).

Implementation

The degree of nurse participation in decision making varies with shared governance models and may range from minimal, or informal participation, to true sharing of authority and accountability. Porter-O'Grady and colleagues (1997) developed the councilor model as a focus on shared governance. The councilor model structures staff and manages governance through the use of committees or councils of elected representatives. Each council is responsible for certain functions and has clearly defined authority. Councils within nursing may include practice, quality improvement/inquiry, education and management. Figure 14-1 displays the councilor model as it is defined in one large teaching hospital in a metropolitan area.

For successful implementation of the shared governance concept, a supporting structure must be designed to fit the individual operating philosophy of the institution or health system. Regardless of the structure, implementation of shared governance establishes the expectation for staff nurse participation and the acceptance of personal accountability.

At its start, shared governance requires the education and support of organizational executives, managers and point of care staff. All levels of an organization must collaborate on a shared purpose to become innovative and efficient (Adler et al., 2011). The challenge for administrators is not in creating the structure that supports shared governance but, rather, in developing a culture that supports, encourages, and maintains it. More than just the structure needs to be created; the philosophy of accountability must be implemented as well (Anderson, 2011). Perhaps the greater challenge for administrators is justification of the cost in terms of personnel time, effort, and financial commitment. The chief nursing officer needs to build the cost of maintaining shared governance into the operational budget for it to become successful.

Shared governance "is truly a journey, not a destination; a process, not a project" (Frith & Montgomery, 2006, p. 282). It is a dynamic process, one that is constantly changing. It changes as the organization, personnel, and time change. "Because shared governance is a continuum, people need to be met where they are on their journey and coached to progress to the next point" (Moore & Hutchison, 2007, p. 566). Education must be continually available to employees in institutions that practice shared governance. Programs are needed to instruct new employees and newly elected unit representatives, to continually develop leadership behaviors in nursing staff, and to support and guide nurse managers. Educational programs should include consensus building and conflict resolution; planning and conducting effective meetings; successful communication techniques and skills; collecting, aggregating, and displaying meaningful data; and strategies for successful problem solving. Nurse managers are key in determining the degree of shared decision making that will actually occur at the unit level. Those managers willing to relinquish control are likely to find additional time for coaching and mentoring, as well as for planning and strategizing. Evidence also shows shared governance plays a part in developing future nurse leaders (Beglinger et al., 2011), so the nurse manager must foster the development of leadership behaviors in staff nurses.

If governance is restricted to the level of the nursing unit, staff autonomy and participative decision making may increase without affecting the overall organizational structure (Hess, 1994). Thus initial identification of spheres of influence and boundaries associated with shared governance is important to prevent frustration (Ballard, 2010). Accountability must always be located at the place where decisions are most appropriately made for shared governance to work (Porter-O'Grady, 2009, p. 55). If an institution employs a shared governance model in which patient care quality is truly the primary focus and clinical staff members are empowered as decision makers, this will be reflected in both the organizational chart and resource allocations. One example of such an organizational chart is depicted in Figure 14-2.

Challenges

Shared governance remains out of reach to some and an endless process to others because it requires slow, gradual development, role modeling and mentoring by nurse leaders, and continual coaching, nurturing, and education for nursing staff and management.

Case studies suggest that shared governance results in an increase in collaboration, staff recruitment and retention, autonomy, shared values, organizational culture, high morale, quality patient outcomes, versatility, competency, collegial communication, productivity, empowerment and satisfaction (Hess, 2011). Yet questions have been raised as to whether the implementation of shared governance represents a true change in hospital management style or merely serves as a cosmetic Band-Aid. Variations exist in the theoretical underpinnings of shared governance models, so the successful results of individual health organizations must be analyzed on a case-by-case basis (Anthony, 2004). The new Index of Professional Nursing Governance (IPNG), a survey that measures organizational governance, is beginning to systemize the metrics across hospitals and connect the model to favorable outcomes (Hess, 2011).

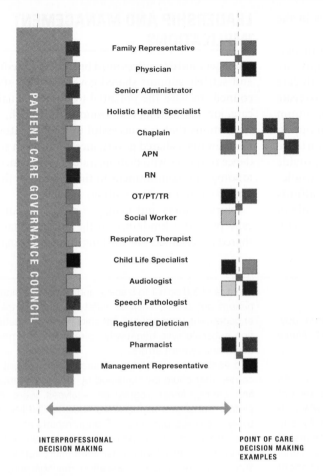

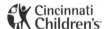

© 2013 Cincinnati Children's Hospital Medical Center

FIGURE 14-2 Model of interprofessional shared governance. (Courtesy Cincinnati Children's Hospital Medical Center, 2013.)

Currently, the direct evidence regarding the financial cost and benefits of its implementation (Brooks, 2004; Hess, 2004) is inadequate.

One challenge to implementation is the various levels of understanding that registered nurses bring to the health care setting regarding shared governance. Traditionally, nurses have worked in strong, hierarchical institutions with centralized decision making and clear authority structures, rigid approval mechanisms, and extensive policies and procedures. This presents an obstacle in that such conditions constrain peer-based, lateral, and collegial dialogue. As a result, nurses may not have depth of experience in attending and conducting committee meetings, setting agendas, developing consensus, and dealing with conflict. Additional barriers to shared governance include inadequate time for education and buy-in by the nursing staff, staff apathy, role confusion, insufficient incentives, and a lack of support and recognition (Ballard, 2010; Golanowski et al., 2007).

With the emergence of multidisciplinary teams and new health care delivery systems, nurses will need to reevaluate models of shared governance to make way for developing partnerships. Additional analyses will be necessary as health care reform and revised payment mechanisms drive changes in the health care delivery systems.

Furthermore, as integrated networks form new organizations, lateral and relational designs are emerging to support community-based health care delivery. These organizations are challenged to create delivery systems that promise a seamless continuum of care. Clinical accountability and personal buy-in by staff nurses become issues of higher importance as partnerships of multidisciplinary players provide service in multi-site care environments. This whole-systems thinking (Porter-O'Grady, 2009) affords nurses the opportunity to take a leadership role in integrated care networks, based on experiences with decentralization and shared governance.

LEADERSHIP AND MANAGEMENT IMPLICATIONS

Managers and executives must be sufficiently educated and actively support shared governance for staff-led councils to have the potential to improve quality of care, job satisfaction, and vision (Brody et al., 2012). Institutions that are successful in implementing and maintaining a shared governance culture can see evidence of nurses who demonstrate empowerment, autonomy, and commitment to the institution through improved staff nurse retention.

Nurse leaders and managers who rule autocratically present a hindrance to the implementation of shared governance. For the long-time nurse manager,

---

RESEARCH NOTE

Source

Rheingans, J.I. (2012). The alchemy of shared governance: Turning steel (and sweat) into gold. *Nurse Leader, 10*(1), 40-42.

Purpose

The purpose of this research was to support or refute that shared governance positively enhances patient outcomes. The author studied a 450-bed Magnet-designated community health care system by surveying the nursing staff about their perceptions of shared governance using the Index of Professional Nursing Governance (IPNG), the Caring Nurse-Patient Interactions Scale (CNPI-Short Scale), the Measure of Job Satisfaction, the Safety Climate Survey, and a demographic form. Data on other variables available at the unit level were collected, including risk management, quality improvement, and patient and staff satisfaction. Over a 2-month period, 140 nurses representing 31 nursing units responded to the survey. The respondents averaged 45.8 years old and had 19.1 years of experience in nursing. Twenty-five percent of RNs had a bachelor's degree in nursing, and 63% had an associate's degree in nursing. Sixty-one percent were members of unit-based practice councils, and 47% were members of a global nursing council.

Results

Staff was found to have knowledge of shared governance, though levels varied significantly between full-time and part-time staff, unit, certification, and participation on councils. Also statistically significant was the correlation between job satisfaction (high, with an average of 3.9 on a 1 to 5 scale) and several nursing and patient outcomes, such as safety climate, employee engagement, and patient satisfaction. A job satisfaction subscale was negatively correlated with medication management errors.

To assess the variability in nursing and patient outcomes that could be explained by shared governance and caring, linear regression analyses were completed. Subscales of the IPNG and the CNPI-S effectively predicted outcomes. Though mostly at the unit level, trends show the potential influence shared governance has on fall rates, fall with injury rates, pressure ulcer incidence, medication management, and patient identification errors. Furthermore, the study validated that integration in professional development activities (council participation and professional certification) improves both adoption of shared governance and job satisfaction.

The relationships between the subgroups of shared governance and caring suggest the need for further investigation, and the relationship of caring and satisfaction suggests the importance in nurses' confidence with clinical care as a driving force for ownership of practice and career advancement.

Application to Practice

The study's findings provide evidence for important linkages between shared governance and nursing and patient outcomes. The results show the importance of studying these impacts across multiple sites in order to legitimize the undocumented, perceived importance of shared governance in driving the quality of patient care and forging the links among structure, process and outcomes.

this radical departure from the traditional autocratic management style presents a whole new paradigm, along with the challenges and uncertainty that accompany it.

In institutions that practice shared governance, the responsibility broadens from the skill and expertise of nurse managers to the skill and innovation of the clinical nursing staff. The responsibility for unit outcomes rests with the whole team, not just with the individual nurse manager. The credibility of the unit's staff nurses impacts the relationships, communications, collegiality, and ability to collaborate with other health care professionals. The nurse manager's role shifts to one of mentoring, coaching, facilitating, enabling, and supporting the staff personnel. Sustainable change can occur at the unit and organizational level if the nurse manager works within the framework of transformational leadership, shared governance, and action processes (Bamford-Wade & Moss, 2010). Further, the institution that espouses a shared governance philosophy needs to continually focus on recruiting leaders who understand and support the concept (Golanowski et al., 2007), while continually supporting leaders, managers, and nursing staff with the education and tools to encourage active participation, accountability, and effective decision making.

In the seminal report, *The Future of Nursing*, the Institute of Medicine (IOM) clamored for nursing transformational leadership, stating, "The nursing profession must produce leaders throughout the health care system, from the bedside to the boardroom, who can serve as full partners with other health professionals and be accountable for their own contributions to delivering high-quality care while working collaboratively with leaders from other health professions." They must do this by being involved in the design, implementation and evaluation of system reform. And while that includes collaboration, there are times when nurses, for the sake of delivering exceptional care, must step into an advocate role with a singular voice (IOM, 2011, pp. 221, 225). Implementation of shared governance is one strategy to create a culture in which individual professional accountability and autonomy are respected and encouraged. Evidence suggests that feelings of accountability and ownership by staff lead to improved patient outcomes (Rheingans, 2012).

Furthermore, shared governance is an important component of the American Nurses Credentialing Center's Magnet Recognition Program®. Organizations are striving for Magnet designation more than ever, as the model has proven to result in improving costs through increases in nursing satisfaction, patient satisfaction, and clinical outcomes (Drenkard, 2010). The recognition as Magnet, now given to 6.1% of U.S. hospitals, honors health care organizations for quality patient care, nursing excellence and innovations in professional nursing practice (American Nurses Credentialing Center, 2012). Magnet hospitals also have significantly better work environments and lower levels of nurse job dissatisfaction and burnout than non-Magnet hospitals (Kelly et al., 2011). To earn the recognition, organizations must demonstrate evidence of formal structures of empowerment and nurses' involvement in governance regarding their practice (Hess, 2011). The traditional organizational structure is no longer adequate to support a professional practice model of nursing because of the increasing numbers of nurses who have pursued advanced nursing education and continued emphasis on this by the IOM.

Shared governance has far-reaching implications for nurse leaders in today's health care environment in which the focus is to provide patient care safely, efficaciously, and efficiently. Organizational benefits include increased commitment of staff to the organization; accountability of the nurse; a new level of professional autonomy; a more efficient model for point-of-service decision making; more expert involvement at the point of service; a more assured, confident patient advocate; and improved financial outcomes. Patients benefit from a more efficient model of health care service, more committed health care professionals, quicker responses at the point of service, and a more assured, confident patient advocate.

Nurse leaders stand to realize numerous organizational gains as professional nurses embrace the quest for empowerment and professional autonomy. However, the journey to shared governance can be both invigorating and tedious, as staff nurses are groomed for opportunities of empowerment and accountability and are taught how to manage these responsibilities. Guiding counsel from the nursing profession's most nurturing leaders is needed to support both staff nurses and nurse managers as they cope with the change from a hierarchical system to one of shared leadership. Mentoring by clinically credible role models will be an important facet of the transformation toward shared governance.

The goal is to transfer leadership wisdom not only to aspiring leaders but also to all employees. The role of today's leaders is to encourage transformation through their own commitment to the journey and to coordinate and facilitate the efforts of others (Porter-O'Grady & Malloch, 2011).

CURRENT ISSUES AND TRENDS

In 2005, the World Health Organization declared the need for the health care workforce to organize care around the patient and collaborate across disciplines, rather than remain in their individual scopes of practice. All professions, including nurses, need to shift from a service-oriented delivery to a patient and family-centered collaborative approach (Orchard, 2010). Nurses are an essential part of this team-based care, as they provide a unique clinical perspective to policy development and strategic planning.

An emphasis on organizational redesign and systems thinking was not introduced until the 1990s, when the vision of a seamless continuity of care that focuses on the welfare of the patient and family was finally recognized as an urgent need. Although bureaucracy and notions of power continued to be seen as areas of conflict, redesign efforts have focused on open communication across disciplines and shared decision making. The traditional view of organizational barriers within hierarchies, caused by the "silo" effect within disciplines, has been replaced by a more contemporary valuing of multidisciplinary delivery of care.

Collaborative leadership in health care has been associated with improved patient outcomes, a reduction in medical errors, and lower staff turnover; it may also reduce the amount of workplace bullying and disruptive behavior. But even with repeated documentation of the benefits of interprofessional health care, the collaboration is frequently not the norm in the field (IOM, 2011). To catalyze this culture shift, nurses at all levels must increase their levels of collaborations among themselves and with physicians and other health care professionals.

The skills developed in a shared governance role can be transferred easily into interprofessional patient and family-centered care. As nurses learn to collaborate in a decentralized structure, they feel empowered to make decisions that affect patients they care for. Models of shared decision making, such as shared governance, make sense in a patient and family-centered care environment in which workers are valued, supported, and respected. Leaders who capitalize on those principles possess the ability to use synergy to transform the workplace by partnering with the staff who function at the point of service. It allows staff to question long-time practices to establish new, more efficient practice models. Such "out of the box" thinking will be beneficial to the entire health care team as they strive to give patients the best care possible.

The future health care team will also require changes in the shared governance structure, allowing for more specialties to sit at the table. As health care moves toward an emphasis on prevention and primary care (IOM, 2011), it is essential that care is coordinated around the patient, not around the professional giving the care. Patient and family-centered care will require all disciplines to unite in collaboration for the common cause of developing evidence-based changes for the health of the patients they serve.

CASE STUDY

The purpose of this case study is to consider one example of implementing change in a large academic teaching hospital in Cincinnati, Ohio, that has had shared governance in place in nursing since 1989. The case study describes the chronological timeline at Cincinnati Children's Hospital Medical Center as related by Patient Services Senior Vice President Cheryl Hoying, PhD, RN, NEA-BC, FACHE, and Assistant Vice President of Education Susan Allen, PhD(c), RN-BC.

Since the following article's publication date, Cincinnati Children's has increased to 577 beds.

Cincinnati Children's Hospital Medical Center is a 577-bed pediatric academic medical center in a large metropolitan area with a main campus in the center of the city and 13 neighborhood locations, a psychiatric hospital, and two pediatric emergency departments. Shared governance had been part of the nursing infrastructure since 1989. After allied health was integrated with the

CASE STUDY—cont'd

division of nursing to create the Department of Patient Services in 1995, a second interprofessional structure for allied health was created in 1999.

1. Based on the information presented thus far, is Cincinnati Children's a centralized or decentralized organization? What factors do you look for when determining whether an institution has a centralized or decentralized organizational structure?
2. Do you think adding a second shared governance model will increase staff empowerment or limit them?

The two shared governance structures operated in parallel for years, with few occasions for collaboration. The silo structures were described as inefficient, burdensome to navigate, and unclear in role and responsibility. Overall governance structure weakened, and training for chairs, mentor accessibility, and new employee orientation to shared governance had diminished.

In 2002, the Medical Center began pursuing perfect patient care, which created an increase in interprofessional activities and collaborations. In 2005, the allied health Interprofessional Coordinating Committee approached the senior vice president and shared concerns that the structure did not have as much authority and autonomy as the nursing structure. Assistant Vice President Susan Allen helped oversee improvements just as Dr. Cheryl Hoying began working at Cincinnati Children's as the new senior vice president/chief nursing officer CNO. As Dr. Hoying familiarized herself by attending meetings, she noted a vast replication of activities in both shared governance structures. She began to consider altering the structure and requested that the nurses and allied health professionals jointly address the changes.

The Interprofessional Coordinating Committee and the Nursing Executive Council began their combined meetings in 2006, uniting to re-strengthen shared governance. After analyzing each structure's strengths and weaknesses, they developed a vision and desired characteristics of the new model, and drafted a shared governance model revision. Additional funding, manager education, and training for effective governance participation were introduced to support shared governance among Patient Services staff. Aligning shared governance with the Patient Services strategic plan in 2008, along with the Medical Center's Magnet journey, helped renew the department's commitment to shared governance. To ensure consistent oversight and direction, the CNO hired two unit-based facilitators—a master's prepared nurse and a master's prepared social worker—to assist in the standardization and implementation of shared governance across disciplines. With their coordinated efforts, the Cincinnati Children's Interprofessional Shared Governance Model was launched in 2008 (see Figure 14-1). Part of the launch included the creation of the Patient Care Governance Council (PCGC), the highest level council in the structure, made up of members from each of the professional disciplines, along with medical staff and patient/family representatives. Using Hess' Index of Professional Nursing Governance tool (IPNG), the shared governance team continually collects data on staff perceptions as the councils work together to unify the department's goals and initiatives across disciplines.

1. Based on the additional information given in the case study, did the two shared governance structures empower or limit the staff? Explain.
2. How might a shared governance committee including allied health, physicians, and families differ from a committee comprised solely of nurses?
3. What key factors in the case study help you determine whether the interprofessional shared governance structure will be successful?
4. What should the council's next steps be?

Data from Hoying, C. & Allen, S. (2011). Enhancing shared governance for interprofessional practice, *Nursing Administration Quarterly, 35*(3), 252-259.

CRITICAL THINKING EXERCISE

Olivia Witte and a number of other nurses on the unit complain upon seeing the new schedule posted in the nurses' lounge. Once again they are scheduled to work on the days that were requested off, and now Nurse Witte has to reschedule her dentist appointment for the second time. Lately nursing staff have been absent from work, and the continuity of patient care is suffering.

1. What are the areas of concern in this scenario?
2. With shared governance in mind, what should Nurse Witte do? What would you do?

CHAPTER

15

Professional Practice Models

Diane L. Huber

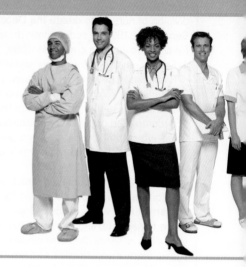

evolve WEBSITE

http://evolve.elsevier.com/Huber/leadership/

The goals of safe and successful patient care delivery include high-quality and low-cost care with the achievement of patient and family outcomes and satisfaction levels. The ability to reach these objectives depends on the organization's approach to the matching of human and material resources with patient characteristics and health care needs via a model of professional practice for care delivery.

Both assignment and delegation are methods used by managers to deliver patient care within the structure of the health care system. The determination of the structure and method by which assignments are made is a managerial responsibility. Although this is part of a process of developing a model of nursing care delivery, pure nursing care delivery models, mainly reflecting the care of the patient by registered nurses on a discrete hospital unit (Minnick et al., 2007), are characteristic of the "siloed" approaches of the industrial age. These approaches are seen as not well matched to organizational effectiveness in an era of primary care–based service delivery such as in Patient-Centered Medical Homes (PCMHs) and Accountable Care Organizations (ACOs).

Nursing leaders are the primary designers and stewards of systems for the provision of client care and the betterment of the organization (Morjikian et al., 2007). Nurses, as the major providers of care, develop and implement patient plans of care in collaboration with the multidisciplinary health care team within the framework of the care delivery model. The model of care delivery has a direct relationship to the allocation of control over decisions about client care. It is the means through which nurse managers delegate effectively and thereby free up and manage time as a scarce resource. The type of care delivery system or care model is seen as determining whether professional practice exists among the nursing staff on a particular unit because delivery systems constrain nursing decision making. This means that autonomy over practice decisions is determined largely by the care model and the resultant nurse decision-making latitude. The type of care delivery system used has implications for job satisfaction, the character of professional practice, and the amount of authority that is actually transferred to the staff.

The determination of a nursing care model or system of care delivery depends on the identification of organizational structures, patient care processes, and

BOX 15-1	DIRECT AND INDIRECT PATIENT CARE FUNCTIONS

Direct Patient Care Functions
- Assessment
- Monitoring
- Prioritizing goals
- Care coordination
- Therapeutic interventions
- Evaluation
- Communication
- Patient education

Indirect Patient Care Functions
- Clinical practice
- Education/research
- Leadership
- Operations
- Personnel management
- Quality improvement
- System coordination
- Other

Data from Fuzard, R.T., Fox, D.H., & Wells, P.J. (1999). Performance of first-line management functions on productivity of hospital unit personnel. *Journal of Nursing Administration, 29*(9), 12-18. Reprinted from Deutschendorf, A.L. (2003). From past paradigms to future frontiers: Unique care delivery models to facilitate nursing work and quality outcomes. *Journal of Nursing Administration, 33*(1), 52-59.

health care provider roles that are necessary to achieve care goals. Examples of structure and process criteria are found in Box 15-1. Trends in the health care environment strongly influence organizational structure.

DEFINITIONS

There is confusion over the differences between the terms *professional practice models* and *models of care delivery* (Wolf & Greenhouse, 2007). These concepts are often used interchangeably, yet their meanings are quite different. **Professional practice models (PPMs)** refer to the conceptual framework and philosophy under which the method of delivery of nursing care is a component. PPMs describe the environment and serve as a framework to align the elements of care delivery. The professional practice model can be thought of as a link between the problems presented by client populations, the purposes of professional occupations,

and the purposes of health care organizations. For any practice model, the degree of integration of the nursing care given to a client, the degree of continuity in assignment of nursing personnel caring for a client, and the type of coordination used to plan and organize the client's care need to be consistent with general client characteristics, available nursing resources, and the organizational support available to nursing (Mark, 1992). The five subsystems of a PPM are: professional values, professional relationships, care delivery model, governance, and professional recognition and rewards (Shirey, 2008).

Examples of professional practice models include Relationship-Based Care (Koloroutis, 2004), the Synergy Model (Hardin & Kaplow, 2005), and Watson's Caring Model (Watson & Foster, 2003). Hoffart and Woods (1996) described five subsystems in a professional nursing practice model:
- Professional values
- Professional relationships
- A care delivery model
- Management or governance
- Professional recognition and rewards

Models of care delivery are the operational mechanisms by which care is actually provided to patients and families (Person, 2004). A **care delivery model** is defined as a method of organizing and delivering care to patients and families to achieve desired outcomes. It organizes the work. The basic elements of any care delivery systems are identified as nurse/patient relationship and clinical decision making, work allocation and patient assignments, interdisciplinary communication, and the leadership or management of the environment of care (Manthey, 1991; Person, 2004). Coordination is a critical component that must be considered to manage task interdependencies upon which process and clinical outcomes rely. Relational coordination (Gittell et al., 2000) is described as the management of the multiple dimensions of communications and relationships between and among health care providers that are necessary to provide quality and efficient care.

Care delivery models must address both *direct patient care functions* (hands-on or delivery of health care services) and *indirect patient care functions* (management of providers and the environment) (Deutschendorf, 2003) (see Box 15-1). Direct patient care functions are facilitated by and depend on management, or indirect functions. For example, the client care assignment system is an aspect of operations included in indirect patient care functions. It is how the work is distributed. Using human resource decisions such as staffing and skill mix, a framework for the deployment of nursing staff and other interdisciplinary providers and their assignment to client care can be determined. Although the nurse manager is ultimately accountable for the achievement of direct and indirect patient care functions, the scope of responsibility necessitates appropriate delegation and assignment to competent unit staff. Delegation and assignment of management functions are vital to developing and maintaining professional nursing practice.

BACKGROUND

Executive leadership is responsible for making decisions about and designing strategies to create a climate and environmental context around the provision of nursing and health care services. Organizational environments exert a strong influence over patient care delivery, either positive or negative. Nursing care delivery can be seen as the dynamic balance between routine resource management and the structure, process, and outcomes of practice. One feature is that the system for distribution of nursing personnel must ensure that staff members of the right skill mix and numbers are promptly deployed so that clients are cared for in an appropriate and timely manner. Studies have demonstrated the impact of skill mix and nurse staffing on patient outcomes (Aiken et al., 2002; Kane et al., 2007; Needleman et al., 2001), further clarifying the need for appropriate role and resource deployment. The four strategic decisions to make are a philosophy of resource utilization, a choice of delivery system, common and individual practice expectations, and a development of the role of the registered nurse (RN) (Manthey, 1991). These four strategic decisions may be made at different levels in any organization. If these decisions are made only by the chief nurse executive, then shared governance and decentralization do not exist.

Professional Practice Models

A PPM is a framework and a structure that glues together elements of the work environment, management and governance, and the needs of patients and families to ultimately achieve outcomes, including care coordination and integration. The nursing practice environment contains those organizational or unit attributes that facilitate/constrain professional nursing practice (Arford & Zone-Smith, 2005). The concept of "magnetism" arising from the Magnet Recognition Program® addresses organizational attributes necessary for attracting and retaining nurses. Nurses want a work environment that allows them to feel productive, have control over work, exhibits respect for employees, and gives feedback on job accomplishment (Arford & Zone-Smith, 2005). The Exemplary Professional Nursing Practice component of the Magnet model measures aspects of the PPM and model of care and their outcomes (Wolf et al., 2008). In one example of a PPM (Erickson & Ditomassi, 2011), the nine components were: (1) vision and values, (2) standards of practice, (3) innovation and entrepreneurial teamwork, (4) clinical recognition and advancement, (5) research, (6) patient care delivery model, (7) collaborative decision making, (8) narrative culture, and (9) professional development. Traditional aspects of the PPM, which are often also incorporated into strategic planning, are organizational mission statements such as mission, vision, values, and philosophy. Organizational structural elements that are the foundation of a PPM are policies and procedures.

Mission Statements

Within an organization there is an established framework for management. For each organization, a characteristic collective of power and authority is vested in the managerial hierarchy. This legitimate authority, given by position, is used with the management process, management skills, and whatever resources are available to meet the organization's goals. The elements of management and the resources available combine to form the basic framework for the management and functioning of an organization. Organizations have a mission—to produce a product or service. This goal will be expressed in mission statements and carried through into policies and procedures, all documents that form the basis for guiding standard operations. These documents are generally gathered into an overall strategic plan.

As a service industry, health care has a product. The basic product of health care is client care service, such as disease treatment or health promotion. Health may be the ultimate outcome to be achieved. An interesting question is whether the product of nursing is the same as the product of health care. Quality care is one ideal product of health care. Kramer and Schmalenberg (1988a, b) said that the product of a hospital is a quality, accessible, cost-effective service called *client care.* In hospitals, 90% of client care is delivered by nurses. If the product is "quality care," valid and reliable measurement is needed to ensure that quality care is delivered and received. The idea has been presented that nursing is not a service composed of tasks but, rather, a business with a product of enhanced client outcomes and contained costs (Zander, 1992). This idea takes Drucker's (1973) conceptualization and merges ideas about a service industry with ideas about traditional for-profit businesses. For nursing, the product is derived from the use of expertise to solve problems for clients. Similarly, the product of nursing administration relates to the use of expertise to solve problems for nurses within systems of care.

Mission, values, and vision are the glue that holds an organization together. They describe what the organization is trying to do, how to go about it, and where it is headed. This helps keep an organization on track and provides yardsticks for measuring present performance. Groups can be brought to crisis by conflicts over basic issues of mission, values, and vision. Without these agreements in place, no organization is truly viable (Adams, 2004).

Mission, vision, and values statements can be mere words on a page, or they can be "living documents" that unify an organization around a purpose. The process of development of these statements needs to begin with bringing members into basic agreement and alignment around the statements.

Using a goals-based strategic planning method, the first step is to develop a mission statement. The mission of any organization is its purpose, function, and reason it exists. Organizations exist to do something such as produce a product or deliver a service. The founders' intentions for what they wanted to achieve by starting this organization need to be reexamined and refreshed periodically to keep the organization dynamic (Adams, 2004). For a health care organization, the mission relates to health care services—for example, client care, teaching, and research. For a

nursing department's purpose, constraints include the organization's purpose, the state nurse practice act and other legal parameters, the context of the local community, and the directives of regulating agencies. The mission statement should be short, concise, and clear. The mission of the nursing department should mesh with the mission of the institution.

In developing a mission statement, factors such as the organization's products, services, markets, values, public image, and activities for survival need to be considered (McNamara, 2008). In addition, the intent of the organization's founders and its history are useful to review. Often employees are unaware of historical background. Because the mission statement needs to describe the overall purpose of the organization, the wording should be carefully crafted. It needs to be derived by a process that respects the organization's culture. The statement needs to have sufficient description to clearly identify the purpose and scope and suggest some order of priorities (McNamara, 2008).

Vision Statements

Vision statements are designed to address the preferred future of the organization. They draw on the mission, beliefs, and environment of the organization and are positive and inspiring. Vision statements are crafted to describe the most desirable state at some future point in time. Often, one step in planning is a gap analysis of the difference between the current state and the vision (Drenkard, 2001). The advantage of vision statements are that they transcend bounded thinking; identify direction; challenge and motivate; promote loyalty, focus, and commitment; and encourage creativity. Vision statements are designed to rise above fatigue, tradition, routine, and complacency. Visioning is setting a high-level direction through turbulent times and creating a compelling picture of a desirable future state. Imagery and stories may be used to sustain the vision. Vision statements need to be vivid enough to keep the organization moving forward.

Values Statements

Core values are strongly held beliefs and priorities that guide organizational decision making. Core values are things that do not change. They are anchors or fundamentals that relate to mission and purpose and hold constant, whereas operations and business strategies change. Values drive how people truly act in organizations. They are the bridge to align how people actually behave with preferred behaviors (McNamara, 2008). Adams (2004, p. 2) stated, "Articulating values provides everyone with guiding lights, ways of choosing among competing priorities, and guidelines about how people will work together."

One way that core values are expressed are through lists or values statements as part of a strategic plan. Another way to express values as statements is to compose a statement of philosophy. Some organizations have philosophy statements, and others use a mix of mission, vision, and values statements as a proxy for their philosophy. Both individuals and organizations can compose a statement of philosophy. For an individual, this would be an expression of personal and professional values, vision, and mission. Although difficult to do, writing a personal professional statement of philosophy is an exercise in clarity and communication.

A statement of **philosophy** is defined as an explanation of the systems of beliefs that determine how a mission or a purpose is to be achieved. An organization's philosophy states the beliefs, concepts, and principles of an organization. It serves as a guide for and an explanation of actions (Poteet & Hill, 1988). The philosophy is abstract: it describes an ideal state and gives direction to achieving the purpose. It may begin with "We believe that…" For example, the system of beliefs, or philosophy, might be stated in any of the following ways:

- We believe that everyone has a right to the highest quality of client care.
- We believe that we have an obligation to render quality client care at a cost-effective price.
- We believe that any person who walks through the door should receive care, regardless of his or her ability to pay.

The philosophy has implications for a nurse's practice role. If an organization's stated mission includes client care, teaching, and research, then all employees will be expected to be involved in all three aspects of the mission. Part of the nurse's job will be to teach students and be involved in research. The nursing department's philosophy should be congruent with the organization's philosophy. The three vital components that form the core of a nursing department

philosophy are the client, the nurse, and nursing practice (Poteet & Hill, 1988).

The organization's philosophy is important to assess as it relates to one's personal philosophy. For example, a potential employee on a job search might compare his or her own philosophy, both of nursing practice and of management, with the philosophy of an organization in which he or she might secure employment. Is there a match? For example, hospitals owned by religious organizations may prefer to hire people who share this same religious faith. If the nurse is not of that religious faith or if he or she has a prejudice or a lack of knowledge about that religious faith, it is advisable to assess personal fit with that particular organization. If some part of the philosophy is personally distasteful, it can have implications for functioning within the practice environment. For example, a specific religious tradition may still be pervasive within the organizational culture, even though the stated philosophy may say that the organization provides care to people of all faiths. That may be bothersome. One example occurs when an organization that is owned and run by a religious group opens each administrative meeting with a prayer. Another example occurs when a nurse believes in providing the total scope of public health services to clients but the organization is run by for-profit principles that dictate the provision of only those services that make a profit. Taking a job in an organization suggests an implicit agreement to cooperate with the organization's values while at work.

Policies and Procedures

Policies and procedures are two functional elements of an organization that are extensions of the mission statements. Both are written rules derived from the mission statement. Together they determine the nursing systems of the work unit and the department of nursing. The purpose of policies and procedures is to provide some order and stability so that the unit functions in a coordinated manner within the larger structure of nursing and the institution. Organizations need to integrate the behaviors of employees to prevent random chaos and maintain some order, function, and structure. These plans are often referred to as *standard operating policies and procedures*. They guide personnel in decision making.

Policies

A **policy** is a guideline that has been formalized. It directs the action for thinking about and solving recurring problems related to the objectives of the organization.

There will be specific times when it is not clear who is supposed to do something, under what circumstances it should be done, or what should be done about unusual circumstances. For example, often there are controversies about the dress code because of disagreements about the definition of what is appropriate. This occurs, for example, when the dress code says, "Nurses will come to work dressed in appropriate attire."

Policies direct decision making and serve as guides to increase the likelihood of consistency in decisions and actions. Policies should be written, understandable, and general in nature to cover all employees. If written, they should be readily available in the same form to all employees. Policies should be reviewed during employee orientation because they indicate the organization's intentions for goal achievement.

After institutional approval, policies need to be collected in a manual or computerized database that is indexed, classified, and easily retrievable. Policies so organized can be easily replaced with revised ones, which often become necessary in light of new environmental circumstances. Policy formulation in any organization is an ongoing core process. Hospitals will have a standing committee for the review of policies as a part of the organizational structure. Policies establish broad limits on and provide direction to decision making; yet they permit some initiative and individuality for unique circumstances.

Policies can be implied, or unwritten, if they are essentially established by patterns of decisions that have been made. In this situation, the informal policies represent an interpretation of observed behavior. For example, the organization may expect caring treatment for all clients. This expectation may not be written as a policy of the organization. However, by the decisions and disciplinary actions that occur, an employee can infer that there is a policy that will be enforced even though it is not written. However, the vast majority of policies are and should be written. Informal and unwritten policies are less desirable because they can lead to systematic bias or unfairness in their application and enforcement (Box 15-2).

BOX 15-2 POLICIES

- Serve as guides
- Help coordinate plans
- Control performance
- Increase consistency of action
- Should be written
- Usually are general in nature
- Refer to all employees

Some general areas in nursing require policy formulation. These are areas in which there is confusion about the locus of responsibility and in which lack of guidance might result in the neglect, malpractice, or "malperformance" of an act necessary to the client's welfare. For example, clear policies need to be in place about medication error reporting and follow-up. In those areas in which it is important that all persons adhere to the same pattern of decision making given a certain circumstance, a policy is necessary so that it can be used as a guideline. Also, areas pertaining to the protection of clients' or families' rights should have written policies. For example, the use of restraints to manage difficult clients came under scrutiny as the Omnibus Budget Reconciliation Act of 1987 (OBRA) pushed restraint-reduction strategies and created policy revisions. Other examples are policies related to "do not resuscitate" and end-of-life care. Areas involving matters of personnel management and welfare, such as vacation leave, should have written policies. In such cases, the lack of a uniform policy would be considered unfair. Many conflicts arise about the scheduling of vacations. How many people can be off at any one time? How long in advance must a vacation request be made? How is the priority for granting requests to be determined (e.g., by seniority or order of request)? The policy is the guideline for determining specific decisions.

Procedures

Procedures are step-by-step directions and methods for actions to follow in common situations. **Procedures** are descriptions of how to carry out an activity. They are usually written in sufficient detail to provide the information required by all persons engaging in the activity. This means that procedures should include a statement of purpose and identify who is to perform the activity. Procedures should include the steps necessary and the list of

BOX 15-3   PROCEDURES

- Provide step-by-step methods
- Are written in detail
- Provide guidelines for commonly occurring events
- Provide a ready reference
- Guide performance of an activity
- Should include the following:
  - A statement of purpose
  - Identification of who performs activity
  - Steps in the procedure
  - A list of supplies and equipment needed

supplies and equipment needed. A procedure is a more specific guide to action than a policy statement. Procedures usually are departmentally or divisionally specific, so they will vary across an institution. They may be very detailed as to how to perform a specific procedure on a specific unit. They help achieve regularity. They are a ready reference for all personnel (Box 15-3).

The similarities between policies and procedures are that both are a means for accomplishing goals and objectives. Both are necessary for the smooth functioning of any work group or organization. The difference between a policy and a procedure is that a policy is a general guideline for decision making about actions, whereas a procedure gives directions for actions. For example, policies about the use of restraints to manage difficult clients would indicate when such restraint use is appropriate. Procedures would cover how to apply specific devices.

A policy is a more general guide for decision making; a procedure is more like a cookbook recipe or a how-to guide giving specific directions about how to perform a certain act or function. There are legal implications to the application of policies and procedures. For example, the nurse may be held liable for failing to follow written policies and procedures. Thus it is important for nurses to be informed about the policies and procedures governing practice in an institution. In addition, both policies and procedures need regular, periodic reviews.

Healthy Work Environment

Nurse leaders and managers can create and maintain an environment that facilitates the practice of the professional nurse. Leadership is required to bring about a good environment. Three elements form the basis for the creation of a positive professional work environment: fun, hope, and trouble. Nurses can use these elements to support each other, stimulate creativity, and work together successfully (McCloskey, 1991). Another aspect of leadership and management in times of change is the creation of a healthy work environment as a nursing core value. Striving for a healthy work environment is a conscious choice. Respect is a hallmark criterion. Elements for constructing such an environment include acknowledgment of the reality of the present environment, clear behavioral expectations and standards, systems and structures to ensure that organizational changes are enduring, and a means to continually assess the health of the work environment. Bylone (2011) noted that nurses still struggle to create a healthy work environment. The six standards of a healthy work environment (American Association of Critical Care Nurses, 2005) are: skilled communication, true collaboration, effective decision making, meaningful recognition, appropriate staffing, and authentic leadership. They have direct relevance to PPMs.

Both older and newer systems and models of patient care delivery are in use. The complexity of the health care environment strongly influences organizational decisions regarding patient care. Fiscal responsibility, accountability to the consumer, and quality and safety outcomes are priorities in an environment of increasing health care costs and health care errors. The development of new models is characterized by changes in the health care climate, including costs, consumer expectations, patient characteristics, and new medical information and technology (Wolf & Greenhouse, 2007). Although all models have their advantages and disadvantages, there is no one right way to structure patient care. The appropriate care delivery model is the one that maximizes existing resources while meeting the objectives of direct and indirect patient care functions (Deutschendorf, 2003). In addition, pieces of older systems often are incorporated into new delivery models as they are developed. Therefore it is important to understand the variety of models available, both old and new. Pure nursing models (effective in less complex times) have yielded to collaborative practice and interdisciplinary approaches with the proliferation of health care provider roles, expedited care processes, and increased severity of illness.

RESEARCH NOTE

Source

Minnick, A.F., Mion, L.C., Johnson, M.E., & Catrambone, C. (2007). How unit level nursing responsibilities are structured in U.S. hospitals. *Journal of Nursing Administration, 37*(10), 452-458.

Purpose

There is a lack of consistent evidenced-based definitions regarding the elements of nursing care models and their influence on outcomes of care. The purpose of this article was to describe the prevalence of standard nursing care models in acute and intensive care units, as well as the assignment of non–unit-based personnel resources. Standard nursing care models included team, functional, primary, total patient care, patient-focused care, and case management. Forty acute care, nonfederal hospitals were selected from six different metropolitan areas, which encompassed 56 intensive care units (ICUs) and 80 adult medical and surgical units. Average daily census for each hospital was at least 99 patients. The selection of hospitals was representative of all U.S. geographical regions and included at least one large academic medical center. Data collection was achieved through staff and leadership structured interviews related to staffing deployment, roles, and care delivery models. Definitions of the elements of each patient care delivery model were identified through a comprehensive literature review.

Discussion

None of the elements of traditional care delivery models were fully implemented on any unit and were inconsistent intra-organizationally as well. Although many nurses reported that they used a primary care model, the defined elements of primary care were not evident. Although the ICUs were more likely to identify a "primary nurse," there was a wide variation in consistent nursing/patient assignments across both ICUs and adult acute care units. Nursing personnel such as nursing assistants and licensed practical nurses/licensed vocational nurses (LPNs/LVNs) might be assigned to patients rather than tasks. Non-unit supportive personnel were not designated to specific units and were not considered to be part of unit staffing. Case management was inconsistently implemented across units in the same organization.

Application to Practice

Although nursing care models are well-defined in the literature, implementation of these models including their defined elements is varied and incomplete. Nursing administrators need to understand how the sporadic use of nursing personnel, such as case managers or LPNs/LVNs on one unit but not another will impact the work of the RN who may have to assume additional responsibilities. This study revealed the prevalence of inconsistent practices of patient care assignments, roles, and responsibilities intra-institutionally as well as inter-institutionally. Future research focused on the understanding of how nursing and non-unit providers are deployed will be key in developing patient care delivery models that will result in positive clinical outcomes.

TRADITIONAL NURSING CARE DELIVERY MODELS

Historians mark the emergence of modern nursing from the time of Florence Nightingale's work in the Crimea. Nightingale believed that nursing care of patients included spiritual well-being as well as the environment. The evolution of nursing models of care has resulted from the impact of economic, social, and political agendas over the past century (Tiedeman & Lookinland, 2004). There are five traditional nursing models of care: (1) private duty, (2) functional, (3) team, (4) primary, and (5) case management. Of these, functional, team, primary, and case management were and are currently associated with hospital nursing practice. Private duty and case management were associated with public health, home health care, and community health but have been adapted to the inpatient setting. Private duty, later called *case* or *case management*, was the original way nursing care was delivered; it later became the foundation for public health nursing and community service delivery.

Private Duty Nursing

Private duty nursing, sometimes called *case nursing,* is the oldest care model in the United States. Private duty nursing is defined as one nurse caring for one client. In this model, complete and total care is provided by one nurse, but the nurse carries only one client assignment. Originally, when the nurse went into the home, the nurse did the cooking, cleaning, bathing of wounds, and organizing of the household functions, basically functioning as a home manager. In American nursing practice, private duty was the original way that graduate nurses found employment, although some had administrative positions in hospitals and some worked in public health (Reverby, 1987). A form of hospital case nursing evolved between 1900 and the 1930s. When the Great Depression hit, most families were too poor to afford private duty nurses and so nurses were without jobs. Hospitals then began to employ graduate nurses.

Reverby (1987) noted that during the depression years, a great transformation from private duty to hospital staffing took place in nursing. As the graduate nurses who had been doing private duty moved into the hospital, they wanted to retain the type of care model to which they had become accustomed. Private duty, the idea that one nurse does the total care of one client, was transplanted into hospital settings for as long as nurses were paid by clients. When nurses became employees of hospitals, the kind of client care that private duty allowed was not possible within the organizational structure of hospital staff nursing. The organization of work in hospitals was task-focused, not client-focused (Reverby, 1987).

The advantage of private duty nursing was that the nurse's focus was entirely on one client's needs. This fostered closeness in the nurse-client relationship and increased RN and client satisfaction with care delivery. The disadvantage was that private duty is a costly model because of its low efficiency. Furthermore, job security was tenuous and irregular (Lee, 1993; Reverby, 1987). Other disadvantages were that nurses had little job mobility and were relatively isolated from colleagues.

Two main variations to the basic pattern of private duty nursing developed: group nursing and total patient care. Group nursing was an early alternative model that combined private duty concepts with hospital staff nursing. Total patient care was a hospital care model characterized by 8-hour shift accountability.

Group nursing was a care model proposed in the 1930s by Janet Geister, then the executive director of the American Nurses Association (ANA). Defined as nursing group practice, the idea of group nursing in hospitals was similar to divisional private duty in which several clients shared a private nurse. The plan was to reorganize private duty from individual to group practice, both inside and outside the hospital. Thus the registry of private duty nurses would be transformed into a group practice and linked to a community's public health nursing service. Facing political pressure, the plan died. Hospitals also experimented with a group nursing care modality, described as being halfway between a private duty arrangement and graduate nurse hospital staff nursing. Under this plan, clients were grouped together in a special unit in which several clients shared a private nurse. Thus three nurses could do 8-hour shifts for two clients instead of four nurses being needed for 12-hour shifts. The hospital paid the nurses' wages but charged the clients directly as a surcharge on the hospital bill. The advantages included shorter hours for nurses, order and regularity in hospital staffing, steady employment for nurses, slightly cheaper rates for clients, and responsibility for the total care of several clients for the nurse. Nurses obtained the autonomy and care delivery method of private duty without its isolation and uncertainty. Nurses were members of the hospital's staff, yet their time was specifically allocated only to a set number of clients who paid for this service directly. However, economic and political pressures for more efficiency, productivity, and service cut off the adoption of this system in hospitals (Reverby, 1987). It is interesting to note the parallels between group nursing and what eventually came to be the way physicians organized themselves.

Total patient care has been defined as a case method for organizing nursing care in which nurses are responsible for total care of a client for the hours in which that specific nurse is present (Glandon et al., 1989). Examples initially occurred in intensive care, hospice care, and home health care. The term *total patient care* has come to mean the assignment of each client to a nurse who plans and delivers care during a work shift (McCloskey et al., 1991; Minnick et al., 2007). Total patient care reemerged in the mid-1990s as a prevalent care delivery system after reengineering and restructuring occurred. The term has become confused with team or primary nursing care delivery systems. Total patient care has been described as a "form of primary nursing" (Reverby, 1987); however, the accountability for patient care coordination throughout the acute episode does not happen. The advantages are the intensity of focus with shift-only responsibility. Significant disadvantages are lack of communication and continuity of care for the client over time. Models of total patient care have contributed to task- and shift-based care that diverts attention from achievement of future patient goals (Bower, 2004). Total patient care has been called the oldest model of nursing care delivery (Shirey, 2008).

Functional Nursing

Functional nursing emerged as a care model in the 1940s. In this model, the division of labor is assigned according to specific tasks and technical aspects of the job. It has been defined as work allocation by functions or tasks, such as passing medicine, changing dressings, giving baths, or taking vital signs (McCloskey et al., 1991). Under functional nursing, the nurse identifies the tasks to be done for a shift. The work is divided and assigned to personnel, who focus on completing the assigned task. Tasks are divided based on the complexity of judgment and technical knowledge and a variety of workers other than RNs to complete the assignment. Functional nursing has the advantage of being efficient for taking care of the tasks related to handling a large number of clients and using workers with varying skill levels (Tiedeman & Lookinland, 2004). Because the division of labor is clearly delineated, administrative efficiency is maximized.

Functional nursing was the norm in U.S. hospitals from the late 1800s through the end of World War II. Factors such as increases in client acuity, greater complexity of care delivery, and expansion of the number of paying clients increased demand for hospital nursing services. As hospitals searched for ways to improve efficiency and service yet control labor costs, the functional division of tasks was instituted to get the work done. Cyclical shortages of nursing labor, exacerbated during times of war, accelerated staffing shortages and the demands of work. This organization of work, combined with frequent understaffing, forced nurses to be task oriented rather than client oriented. It was a major reason why graduate nurses disliked staff nursing as compared with private duty (Reverby, 1987).

In the early 1900s, business and industry concepts of "scientific management" emphasized efficiency. The efficiency was gained by breaking down a work process into its component task steps and then analyzing and timing the steps, establishing standards, and determining the best way to perform each task. Thus managerial control over the planning and execution of work could be established. Assembly lines in factories were one result. Functional nursing was

developed as a result of this concern for task analysis and proper division of the nursing workload. Under this model, there might be a "temperature nurse," a "medication nurse," a nurse for the right side of the hall, and a nurse for the left side of the hall (Reverby, 1987). Functional nursing was not oriented to individualized and holistic client care but, rather, facilitated a fragmented approach to patient care. One advantage was that there was little confusion about roles and duties. When applied to nursing, this method was efficient and inexpensive but nurses and clients hated it. Client satisfaction dropped under this kind of care delivery system. Clients felt that they could not identify who was their nurse caregiver.

Team Nursing

Team nursing is a care model that uses a group of people led by a knowledgeable nurse. It is a delivery approach that provides care to a group of clients by coordinating a team of RNs, licensed practical nurses/licensed vocational nurses (LPNs/LVNs), and aides under the supervision of one nurse, called the *team leader* (Glandon et al., 1989). Team nursing has been defined as the assignment of a group of clients to a small group of workers under the direction of a team leader. Each team member provides most of the care to his or her assigned clients, although some tasks (e.g., medications) may be assigned separately (McCloskey et al., 1991).

Team nursing is designed to make use of each member's capabilities to meet the nursing needs of his or her group of clients. It is a delegation of care to a designated team of staff members. The staff members have various levels of expertise, but they are formed into a team. The nurse leader takes into account the level of expertise and then divides the assignments accordingly so that the clients who are assigned to a team of caregivers have their needs appropriately met. Team nursing developed in the early 1950s in response to a shortage of RNs and in reaction to the dissatisfaction with functional nursing.

The advantages of team nursing are that each member's particular capabilities can be used to the maximum. This model supports group productivity and the growth of team members. Communication is vital. A sense of contribution via the team can be fostered. Oversight for novice nurses and temporary personnel can be facilitated. However, it takes a skilled RN to be a team leader. Furthermore, an RN team member may not be functioning up to his or her full potential because of being assigned an ancillary role, which creates some underutilization of the RN personnel.

One variation of team nursing is **modular nursing.** Modular nursing is based on the existence of specific facilities and on actual structural and spatial changes to enable hospital nurses to stay near the bedside. Structural modules based on client acuity are clustered in larger districts based on geography. Nurses are stationed near their clients, and a wider range of responsibility is delegated to them. Open design and convenient access architecture provide for decentralization of care delivery based on the spatial arrangement of the unit and enhanced communication (Magargal, 1987). The development of an innovative new care delivery system needs to be in synchrony with the philosophy of care (Guild et al., 1994). The essential features of modular nursing are as follows (Anderson & Hughes, 1993):

- A module consists of a group of nurses and a group of clients.
- Clients are grouped by spatial or floor-plan clustering.
- Nurse/client assignment is standardized.
- Modular care-planning rounds occur regularly.
- A unit-based modular committee is established.

In one facility, decentralizing nursing activity to three modular substations for a 50-bed unit allowed for a reduction in RN skill mix from 63% to 46% (Abts et al., 1994).

Functional nursing was a precursor of team nursing. Both models emphasized efficiency and care delivery with a limited number of RNs. However, team nursing corrected some deficiencies in care fragmentation and regimentation that were a problem with functional nursing.

Primary Nursing

Primary nursing began in the 1970s as a way to overcome the discontent with functional and team nursing's emphasis on tasks and discrete functions that directed nurses' attention away from holistic care of the client. This matched a societal trend toward accountability, as well as nursing's rising level of professionalism. Primary nursing is an approach in which a nurse has responsibility and accountability for the continuous guidance of specific clients from hospital admission through discharge. Thus the primary nurse provides for the total nursing process for the client during a period of hospitalization (Glandon et al., 1989). Primary nursing has been defined as the assignment in a hospital of each client to a primary nurse who plans, delivers, and monitors care under a 24-hour responsibility from admission to discharge (McCloskey et al., 1991). The hallmark of the primary nursing concept is the 24-hour accountability element. Autonomy, authority, and accountability in the primary nurse's role are basic to primary nursing. When the nurse is not actually taking care of clients, an associate delivers the care. However, the primary nurse makes the care and treatment coordination decisions, supervising the entire stay, 24 hours per day, for the length of the hospital stay. This increases continuity of care and consistency in assignments. Primary nursing does not mean that the primary nurse takes care of clients 24 hours a day. Rather, the 24-hour accountability is for the supervision and delegation of client care. Primary nursing has been called the first formal professional model in hospital nursing (Zander, 1992).

The advantages of primary nursing include a focus on the client's needs, greater nurse autonomy, and greater continuity of care. Primary nursing eventually came to be associated with all-RN staffing but has moved away from that position. Problems in the implementation of primary nursing have included the wide variation in its operationalization and implementation. The result has been confusion and lack of a structure to enable primary nurse autonomy. Under cost-containment pressure, an all-RN staff is difficult to justify. Total accountability may create burnout, and a poorly prepared RN may feel threatened by primary nursing.

Research conducted to compare team nursing with primary nursing care models found higher quality of nursing care, higher levels of nurse satisfaction, increased continuity of care, improved nurse retention, and positive client outcomes with primary nursing. Levels of client satisfaction were equal and cost comparisons were inconclusive between the two models (Gardner, 1991; Lee, 1993).

Private duty was a precursor of primary nursing emphasized the closeness of the nurse-client relationship, but primary nursing was more cost-effective. Primary nursing was a care model that evolved in reaction to the desire of RNs to return to more direct and active care instead of supervision of ancillary workers as in the team nursing care model. This approach promoted greater RN professional authority, accountability, autonomy, and continuity of care. Initially, an all-RN staff was thought to be needed. Compatible support systems were needed for a primary nursing care model to be effective. Primary nursing is highly sensitive to human resource distribution, skill mix, staff competency levels, and client care needs. However, as budget constraints, shortened lengths of stay, increased client severity, and pressures for cost containment in hospitals grew in the late 1980s and early 1990s, it was difficult to maintain primary nursing care models (Cohen & Cesta, 2005).

Case Management

Case management as a nursing model of care evolved in the late 1980s. It has been defined as both a process (it is a provider intervention) and a care delivery model. Case management has developed as a method to manage care. **Managed care** is care coordination that is organized to achieve specific client outcomes, given fiscal and other resource constraints. Managed care has been described as "the systematic integration and coordination of the financing and delivery of health care" (Grimaldi, 1996, p. 6).

The Case Management Society of America (CMSA) is the professional organization representing case managers in practice. It is a multidisciplinary organization. The CMSA definition of case management is "Case management is a collaborative process of assessment, planning, facilitation, care coordination, evaluation, and advocacy for options and services to meet an individual's and family's comprehensive health needs through communication and available resources to promote quality, cost-effective outcomes" (CMSA, 2012, p. 1). Thus there is a major professional organization that defines case management as a multidisciplinary provider intervention and promotes the knowledge base for practice.

In nursing, the ANA first defined *nursing case management* as a system of health assessment, planning, service procurement, service delivery, service coordination, and monitoring through which the multiple service needs of clients are met (ANA, 1988; Zander, 1990). Hospital acute care nursing case management is an attempt to reconfigure the delivery of hospital care away from previous care models. Case management and care coordination have been the care delivery models used for years by public health and community health nurses (Mikulencak, 1993). In these settings, case management has been centered on client needs, rather than the shift, unit, or system. Case management can occur inside or outside the hospital only, extend across the health care continuum, or be linked to a population focus (Lee, 1993; Lyon, 1993).

Case management is a system of client care delivery that focuses on the achievement of client outcomes within effective and appropriate time frames and resources. Case management has components of health services delivery, coordination, and monitoring through which multiple service needs of clients are met. Hospital-based acute care nursing case management was focused on an entire episode of illness, crossing all settings in which the client receives care. Care is directed by a case manager, who is not always a nurse, and can be unit- or population-focused.

Case management is frequently associated with the use of **structured care methodologies** (SCMs). SCMs are streamlined interdisciplinary tools used to "identify best practices, facilitate standardization of care, and provide a mechanism for variance tracking, quality enhancement, outcomes measurement, and outcomes research" (Cole & Houston, 1999, p. 53). Examples of SCMs are critical pathways, evidenced-based algorithms, protocols, standards of care, order sets, and clinical practice guidelines. The use of best evidence is considered the gold standard to reduce practice variation in an environment focused on patient outcomes. Critical paths outline time and the sequence of events for an episode-of-care delivery. Resources appropriate in amount and sequence to a specific case type and individual client are managed for length of stay, critical events and timing, and anticipated outcomes. A *critical path* is a written plan that identifies key, critical, or predictable incidents that must occur at set times to achieve client outcomes within an appropriate length of stay in a hospital setting. As a pathway, it is a tracking system for the timing of treatments and interventions, health outcomes, complications, activity, and teaching/learning.

In the face of strong economic external forces, acute care hospitals turned to case management to help reduce provider practice variation and to ensure the appropriateness of care. Case management was seen as a way to incorporate and build on the strengths of earlier care models yet provide a professional practice model for nurses through autonomous decision making and collaborative practice. The risk with case management models is that communication and coordination infrastructures may not be available or integrated for effectiveness. Converting case managers from a service-based approach to a unit-based model may not only improve efficiencies but also enhance integration into the patient care delivery model, improving communication and collaboration with the multidisciplinary health care team (Zander & Warren, 2005).

EVOLVING MODELS

Nursing shortages and health care reform will continue to have a strong impact on the creation of **current and evolving types** of patient care delivery models. Nurse staffing models were retooled in the late 1980s as a result of a severe nursing shortage and in an attempt to complement the work of the professional nurse with the use of nursing extenders (Eastaugh & Regan-Donavan, 1990; Lookinland et al., 2005). When managed care became predominant, fiscal restraint became a driver for restructuring, re-engineering, and redesign. Nurses were perceived as more "costly than cost-effective" as a result of their 24-hour responsibility for patient care and contribution to the overall labor budget (Hall, 1997). Many of the resulting structures for patient care were staff mix models, in which nurses were partnered with a variety of "extenders" or multiskilled workers. Outcome studies have clearly demonstrated the negative impact of "substitution models" in which extenders have not been used to complement nurses but, rather, served as replacements, thereby increasing RN/patient ratios (Aiken et al., 2002; Needleman et al., 2001). Unruh (2003) found that it was not the ratio of skilled to unskilled workers that influenced patient outcomes but, rather, the RNs' hours of care. It has not been determined which models are the most effective to fully utilize professional nursing skills in patient care while optimizing tasks that can be safely delegated (Duffy et al., 2007; Jennings, 2008; Lookinland et al., 2005).

Many of the models that evolved in the 1990s are identified in the literature as mixed models, or some form of second-generation primary nursing

or professional practice models that emphasize outcomes management, collaboration, the use of a variety of caregivers with variable competency and preparation, and integrated practice (Jones-Schenk & Hartley, 1993; Lengacher et al., 1993; Wolf et al., 1994; Zander, 1992). Concepts of accountability, cost containment, effectiveness, seamless continuum of care, integration, multidisciplinary collaboration, new roles, alteration in skill mix, and new assignment systems are key components. All sought to reconfigure nursing's work within resource constraints, care needs, and current ideas about professional nursing practice.

Patient- and Family-Centered Care

Patient-focused or patient- and family-centered care emerged as one method of patient care delivery to meet the needs of organizations that were reengineered to be more competitive and cost-effective. Pioneered by the Picker Institute in 1978 (Planetree, 2008), **patient-centered care** is defined as "the redesign of patient care in the acute care setting so that hospital resources and personnel are organized around the patient's health care needs" (Maehling, 1995, p. 62). It was part of a redesign effort to realign the structure and processes involved in delivering care to center around the patient to improve efficiency and resource use. Patients are aggregated according to care requirements or similar service demands (as opposed to similar diagnoses). Protocols or pathways (SCMs) form a central point of focus. With a patient and family-focused approach, there is an ongoing process to seek out and determine what is important to the person receiving care. This approach adopts the perspective of the person receiving care and strives to establish mutual goals between patient and provider to meet unique needs. To reach this complexity challenge, horizontal structures with an emphasis on relationships and effective working partnerships are built (Comack et al., 1999). The model is recommended by the Institute of Medicine (IOM) (2001) and has been expanded to include the aspect of the family as well as the patient.

The advantage of patient-focused care redesigns is that they center systems and services closer to the patient. This strong customer focus may increase quality, safety and patient satisfaction and conserve resources. However, implicit in these redesign efforts is a series of significant work group and culture changes affecting the financial operations and cost structure of hospitals. It also requires a commitment for initial allocation of resources to achieve ultimate financial and clinical outcomes. There are also concerns related to appropriate delegation, acceptance of assignments, and follow-up accountability (Duffy et al., 2007). The use of case managers addresses care coordination (Shirey, 2008).

INNOVATIVE AND FUTURE MODELS

Because the acute care environment is multifaceted around multiple levels and sites of care, patient types, diseases, and providers, a single organizational model for patient care delivery may be unrealistic. Deutschendorf (2003) proposed the development of unit-based models that incorporate an evaluation of structure and process criteria that influence direct and indirect patient care functions to determine an appropriate model.

The increase of health care errors noted in the IOM's report, *To Err Is Human: Building a Safer Health System* (Kohn et al., 2000), is a symptom of care delivery process and structures that have become dysfunctional, disorganized, and inappropriate as the health care environment has become increasingly complex. The IOM's 2001 report *Crossing the Quality Chasm: A New Health System for the 21st Century* described the need for sweeping change and redesign of patient care delivery systems to foster innovation and improve the delivery of care. It called for a comprehensive strategy and action plan that included high-functioning interdisciplinary teams that delivered safe, effective, patient-centered, timely, efficient, and equitable health care.

Affordable Care Act of 2010

Despite the dramatic activity from the public and private sectors and regulatory agencies demanding the demonstration of safety and quality outcomes, most hospitals and health systems made only incremental changes toward the kind of patient care redesign called for by the IOM (Kimball et al., 2007). Previous practice models that were either "nursing" or "medical" are single discipline–focused in an environment in which there are many structures of rationality and points of view. The focus on the hospital as the hub of all health care activity must be shifted to encompass the primary

care environment as well (Vlasses & Smeltzer, 2007). Emphasis on continuity of care through transitions of care with seamless communication and care coordination is a theme that must be addressed with future models to ensure quality and safety outcomes. This is the new imperative under the rapid changes in health care induced by the Patient Protection and Affordable Care Act (PPACA) of 2010.

Before the ACA, models that incorporated the principles of care coordination and integration began to emerge. In 2005, Partners HealthCare in Boston collaborated with Health Workforce Solutions to identify innovative models of patient care delivery that met the following criteria (Kimball et al., 2007):

- Primarily adult patients were served.
- Nurses served as primary caregivers.
- Acute care hospitals were involved.
- Technology, support systems, and new roles were integrated.
- Quality, efficiency, and financial outcomes were improved.

Their research identified 10 models meeting the stated criteria. All of them had common elements, which included an empowered RN role, heightened concentration on the patient and family, methods for smoothing patient transitions and handoffs across levels of care, optimizing technology, and outcomes management through performance measurement (Kimball et al., 2007).

The *12-bed hospital* is designed to improve communication and continuity through the development of 12- to 16-bed units, creating a feeling of a small hospital within a large one. A registered nurse functions as the patient care facilitator (PCF) for each unit and assumes 24/7 accountability for individualized patient care. The PCF is the primary point of contact for the interdisciplinary team, as well as the patient and family. The PCF mentors and educates new staff members and is responsible for achieving performance measures identified through a dashboard of quality, financial, and efficiency indicators. Initial outcome studies have suggested that patient satisfaction is improved, length of stay is shortened, and patient safety measures have reduced the number of falls with injury and the number of pressure ulcers (Kimball et al., 2007; Smith & Dabbs, 2007).

The *Partnership Care Delivery Model* is conceived as a multidisciplinary model of care that is patient- and family-centered, with all of the disciplines participating in collaborative practice. The term *partnership* implies that all disciplines are equally accountable for patient outcomes of care. The key components of this model include daily multidisciplinary rounds, partnerships with patients and families, education and support, and a systems approach to care delivery (Wiggins, 2006).

The *Transitional Care Model* incorporates the role of advanced practice nurses (APNs) to provide comprehensive care coordination and home follow-up of high-risk elders (Kimball et al., 2007). The APN, in collaboration with physicians and other members of the health care team, coordinates care during the patient's hospitalization, including discharge planning and the alignment of resources to facilitate post-discharge outcomes such as the reduction of readmissions and emergency department use. The APN not only provides a comprehensive assessment of the patient's health care status and development of plan of care in the acute care setting but also follows the patient into the home setting to ensure the continuation of the patient care plan. Outcomes achieved as a result of the implementation of the Transitional Care Model include decreases in time to discharge and total hospital readmissions, decreased total health care costs, and increased patient and physician satisfaction. Improving transitions of care is a focus of the National Transitions of Care Coalition (NTOCC, 2010) and is important because of the costs and poor outcomes associated with lack of care continuity (Naylor et al., 2011).

The *Patient-Centered Medical Home Model* (PCMH) was originally conceived by the American Academy of Pediatrics as a method to care for children with chronic diseases. The current model has been developed as a collaborative effort among several professional physician organizations to provide patient-centered care that is focused on prevention, health promotion, and coordinated care across the life span (Vlasses & Smeltzer, 2007). This model refocuses patient care from the hospital to the primary care setting. The interdisciplinary team is responsible for coordinating care across all levels of care and includes the provision of comprehensive health care services. Continuity and coordination across specialties, access to services, and patient responsibility for decision making are key components of this model. These models are being testing for efficacy and efficiency (Vlasses & Smeltzer, 2007).

"The Affordable Care Act is altering the way healthcare is delivered" (Katz & Frank, 2010, p. 82). The IOM's vision for the future, with a key feature being new models of care, has been carried forward in the ACA. The themes of integration and coordination of care, addressing needs in a comprehensive manner, with patients as key partners, and providing services efficiently are consistently present. Provisions of the ACA promote new models that will address these themes, such as ACOs. Care coordination is the linchpin. Propelled by the evidence-based recommendations of the IOM, the ACA is triggering a radical shift in the delivery of health care toward primary care–based and health promotion–focused systems. The focus has turned to how to prevent disease or chronic condition deterioration and unneeded ED visits and hospital admissions. Reimbursement structures and incentives to physicians are changing to incentivize new models. Meaningful changes in the workforce are a major implication. Evidence-based care delivery models, such as population health management programs (Rust et al., 2011), are likely to be the future models of care delivery.

LEADERSHIP AND MANAGEMENT IMPLICATIONS

Fundamentally, a care delivery system is the way clients' needs are matched to health care resources to achieve positive clinical outcomes. Through many complex relationships, the care delivery model influences the quality of nursing care provided and its cost. A number of nursing care models have been developed, and there is evidence of evolutionary changes yet repeating cycles. Traditionally, care delivery was provided within a pure nursing framework. Over time, nursing care delivery methods were changed and adapted to better fit external forces and the balance of the needs of clients and the needs of employing organizations. With these changes came variations in assignment systems, skill mix, and the role of the nurse. Nursing care delivery has become more complex as integration with other provider disciplines is essential to meet the client's needs through the entire continuum of care. Future trends point to greater integration and multidisciplinary team collaboration models for service delivery as health care reform drives changes in the organizations within the health care industry.

The current health care environment is dynamic and continues to change at a rapid pace. Health care costs continue to rise, and safety outcomes have not dramatically improved since the initial IOM report, *To Err Is Human* (Leape & Berwick, 2005). For nursing to ensure its status in health care, nursing leaders and managers must have a broad vision to facilitate the design of care delivery models that meet the objectives of cost containment, patient satisfaction, quality, and safety outcomes over the course of the care cycle (Vlasses & Smeltzer, 2007). Nursing leaders are in the perfect position to lead the changes essential in care delivery redesign.

Nursing, as a major percentage of the health care labor force, must be able to demonstrate its effectiveness in producing financial as well as clinical outcomes. Nurse leaders are responsible for creating the formal business plan, which includes quantitative analysis of costs and benefits with revenue and expense calculations (Morjikian et al., 2007). It is critical that caregiver costs, roles, and activities be clearly understood. The challenge to prove "value" will continue. Although outcome studies in recent years have clearly linked professional staffing ratios to clinical outcomes (Unruh, 2008), including patient morbidity and mortality, the focus on nursing recruitment and retention to alleviate the most recent nursing shortage has resulted in increased costs. Multiple studies have demonstrated the relationship of nursing satisfaction to work environment, leadership, and perceptions of autonomy, which include the method in which care is delivered.

Mentoring staff to participate in the creation of new care delivery methods is an aspect of effective leadership. Although there appears to be no one right model of care, nurses will be involved in the planning for care delivery, tinkering with improvements in the current model, exploring new models developed by others, or attempting to develop their own new model of care delivery. The leadership and management challenge is to balance risk taking and adoption of innovations with the pragmatic necessity to be systematic, evaluative, and realistic. Knowing and understanding organizational culture and formal and informal networks for getting things accomplished and having complete knowledge of the origin and purpose of policies, practices, and procedures are critical for nursing leaders to be seen as leaders in care delivery redesign (Morjikian et al., 2007).

The central components of practice that need to be considered in the construction of a patient care delivery model are the direct and indirect patient care functions; provider roles and responsibilities; competencies and experience; fiscal accountability and changes in reimbursement; patient characteristics, severity, and clinical service intensity; evidenced-based practice; and new medical information and technology (Deutschendorf, 2003; Wolf & Greenhouse, 2007). The American Organization of Nurse Executives (AONE) (2012) has developed a *Guiding Principles for the Role of the Nurse in Future Care Delivery* toolkit to help organizations design and build the best location-specific care delivery model. Nurses' autonomy and job satisfaction are affected by the work environment and the structure of the care model used. Leadership is needed to strike a balance between nurses' needs and preferences and those of clients, physicians, and organizations.

CURRENT ISSUES AND TRENDS

The challenges for patient care in the future are massive. The work environment of the nurse is dramatically different now from any other time. Cost containment and demands for quality and safety outcomes will continue to drive systems of patient care delivery. The need for structures to incorporate real-time interdisciplinary communication and care planning over all care transitions is essential to improve patient safety outcomes. The "age of information" will test the ability of the system to integrate discovery into safe practice. Even though studies (Aiken et al., 2002) have demonstrated the relationship between nurse-to-patient ratios and patient outcomes in ICUs and have resulted in increased focus on the nurse's work environment and value, dramatic evaluation must occur to create a vision for health care delivery models of the future. Professional nursing has an opportunity and an obligation to participate in shaping future models that address the changes in patient populations, as well as clinical and financial trends.

The AONE presented a strategy focused on the future development of care delivery models based on the complexities of the current and future health care milieu (Haase-Herrick & Herrin, 2007). Guiding principles address the following: nursing work as knowledge and caring, patient/client-directed care, access to new medical information and technology, "critical synthesis" of knowledge, understanding the relationships of care, and management of care throughout the continuum (Haase-Herrick & Herrin, 2007). Operationalization of the guiding principles can occur only after careful examination and creation of supporting organizational structures and processes.

Clearly, forces and pressures outside of professional nursing influence care models. It is not known which is the best model for each patient care setting, and research evidence to support specific inpatient nursing care models is seriously limited (Jennings, 2008). The evaluation of new patient care delivery systems must include specific quality, financial, and patient satisfaction outcomes. Nurses are urged to examine their client populations, come to grips with the business aspects of health care, and remain vigilant in analyzing emerging economic and clinical trends in order to be active participants in the creation of patient care delivery models of the future.

CASE STUDY

Overview

Memorial Medical Center was a 400-bed teaching hospital. The care delivery model for all areas was total patient care, with RNs of different experiences having shift responsibility for a group of seven to eight patients on medical and surgical floors. The third floor was a general medical unit with 72 beds. Patient diagnoses included cardiovascular (with telemetry monitoring), renal, pulmonary, oncology, and gastrointestinal diagnoses. An interim patient care manager had responsibility for the unit. Charge nurses were responsible for daily operations and frequently had patient assignments. Novice nurses accounted for 30% of the staff. Certified nursing assistants were occasionally assigned to a nurse but were more likely to be assigned tasks. Their responsibilities included basic custodial care and did not include simple technical skills. They were frequently assigned as "sitters," thus removing them from direct patient care.

There were many patient and physician complaints regarding the nursing care provided. Reporting of significant incidents and "near misses" had increased. The nursing director for the area conducted a comprehensive assessment of patient care to determine whether changes in the method of care delivery were needed.

Findings

It was found that patient care delivery at Memorial Medical Center was fragmented, with functions being performed among multiple caregivers with little communication. It was believed that staff did not have the opportunity to develop skills and expertise in specialty areas because of the scope of patient problems. Nursing assessments and reassessments were not timely or complete, and evidence of nursing care planning was limited in clinical documentation. Nurses were frequently unaware of the patient's diagnosis and medical plan of care. Nursing tasks were the focus of care, and evidence of critical thinking for decision making was lacking, especially among novice nurses. Care coordination was performed by the case manager but was not communicated to the point-of-care nurse. Discharge planning was usually not considered at time of admission and frequently delayed discharge. Communication of the plan of care from shift to shift and from caregiver to caregiver was inadequate because of a lack of continuity (with 12-hour shifts), problem identification, and prioritization. Multidisciplinary communication between providers (including physicians and nurses) was sporadic and incomplete. Nurses were not comfortable with delegation of tasks to the certified nurse assistants (CNAs) and frequently assumed nonnursing functions. There was no mechanism of oversight or support for novice or temporary nursing staff.

Care Delivery Redesign

The nursing director and the nursing vice president agreed that care delivery redesign was necessary to meet the objectives of quality patient care. The nursing director began by forming a team of multidisciplinary care providers and nursing staff who worked on the third floor. The group was surveyed as to their perceptions of patient care processes on the unit. Objectives for the redesign were constructed based on feedback from the staff, as well as a review of the literature. Staff members expressed anxiety regarding changes, but all agreed that transformation was necessary to improve the quality of care and working conditions.

It was determined that the third floor of Memorial Medical Center should be split into two separate units to maximize exposure to, and "knowing" of, specific patient populations. Patients were aggregated based on intensity of service, acuity, and diagnosis (cardiovascular/pulmonary and oncology/renal, with telemetry available on the cardiovascular unit). Staff

CASE STUDY—cont'd

members were assigned permanently on each unit based on preference but with an understanding that rotation to the sister unit was available after 6 months.

Because many members of the staff were inexperienced and temporary nurses were used to fill vacancies, it was decided to implement a modular approach to care delivery. A module consisted of 16 to 20 patients with an experienced nurse partnered with novice or agency nurses and 1 or 2 CNAs. Complete inter-shift report was taken by the module members, facilitating communication and continuity if one staff member was off the unit or not scheduled the following day. Daily multidisciplinary care-planning rounds, facilitated by nursing, were established for all patients and included participation from all members of the interdisciplinary team. The practice of hourly rounding and focused assessments was instituted to improve monitoring and surveillance of rapidly changing patient conditions.

A new level of CNA was established to increase simple skills that could be performed. This competency was validated in a skills lab. Skills were defined that could provide the most benefit to nurses and the least risk to patients (e.g., performance of electrocardiograms [ECGs]). Nurses and CNAs attended team-building workshops to facilitate understanding of delegation responsibilities and roles. A unit secretary position was approved for all shifts to assume clerical responsibilities for patient care.

The patient care manager remained responsible for both areas; however, a permanent charge nurse

position without direct patient care responsibility was established on each unit.

Evaluation

Process, quality, safety, and financial outcome indicators were established before redesign. Because clinical outcomes must follow successful implementation of processes, it was decided to measure process indicators for 6 months and then quality indicators at 6 months, 1 year, 18 months, and 2 years. At the end of the first year, nursing satisfaction and perceptions of quality care delivery were improved, including facilitation of assessment, monitoring, achievement of care goals, organization of care, delegation, patient teaching, documentation, and continuity. Agency usage was down, and attrition of new graduates was reduced by 20%. Patient satisfaction scores were beginning to demonstrate improvement with regard to pain management, discharge preparation, and meeting of care needs. Although the incidence of pressure ulcers remained constant, the number of patient falls was reduced.

It was demonstrated that careful and deliberate planning with the participation of stakeholders and end users can result in a successful project. Care delivery models can be established that maximize existing resources, ensure multidisciplinary collaboration, provide oversight and mentoring of staff, and ultimately result in improved patient quality outcomes.

CRITICAL THINKING EXERCISE

Nurse Manager Anthony Gardner finds himself in the nurse executive's (NE) office. Nurse Gardner has a problem with a staff nurse who was seen yelling at two nursing assistants in the middle of a crowded area. Nurse Gardner is asked to discuss what happened. Nurse Gardner says the staff nurse was irritated by the nursing assistants' loitering and yelled at them to get back to work. Nurse Gardner says he is too busy to spend all his time supervising nurses who have no sense of teamwork. The NE carefully explains that a staff opinion survey has uncovered that a significant proportion of the staff reported experiencing abuse or confrontation in the workplace, leading to conflict, tension, and stress. A major component of the reported abuse on this unit was "being yelled at." The NE explained that the hospital

has embarked on a new "healthy work environment" initiative and that written behavioral expectations and standards exist. The NE gives a copy of these standards and the "respect, communicate, and take responsibility" philosophy to Nurse Gardner.

1. Is there a problem?
2. What is the problem?
3. Whose problem is it?
4. What should the nurse manager do?
5. What interactions should have occurred before this point?
6. Whose values are in operation in this situation? Is there a clash of values?
7. If so, how should they be resolved?
8. Are there any legal considerations?

16

Evidence-Based Practice: Strategies for Nursing Leaders

Laura Cullen, Cindy J. Dawson,
Kirsten Hanrahan, Nancy Dole

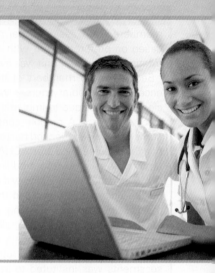

evolve WEBSITE

http://evolve.elsevier.com/Huber/leadership/

Nursing has a long history of using research to improve practice, beginning with Florence Nightingale's work, reemphasized with research utilization efforts beginning in the 1980s, and progressing to the current trend in using best evidence in guiding patient care. There is now a rising expectation by consumers as well as in regulatory standards that evidence-based knowledge be used in health care. Despite national and international policy and research agendas, provision of evidence-based care does not meet expectations (Burns, 2012; Jablonski & Ersek, 2009; Randall et al., 2010; Revello & Fields, 2012; Scales et al., 2011; Schmaltz et al., 2011; Williams et al., 2005), and a continuing gap exists between the conduct and application of research findings. Using the evidence-based practice process to answer clinical and operational questions can be challenging.

Nurses in leadership positions have responsibility for building and expanding the use of evidence-based practices in care delivery to improve patient and organizational outcomes. A number of models are available to provide direction for the evidence-based practice process for individual projects. Implementing evidence-based practice initiatives as an organizational program requires additional strategies for success. Less information is available to guide nurse executives in building evidence-based practice programs within health care organizations. Given this challenge, a building-block approach is outlined to provide guidance. Although the demand for evidence-based practice has grown, implementation science on which evidence-based practice work is based is still developing. The application of evidence-based practice is the responsibility of every nursing leader, especially in the nurse manager role. This chapter outlines successful strategies used to expand an evidence-based practice program.

DEFINITIONS

An understanding of evidence-based practice and related concepts requires requisite knowledge of a variety of terms. **Evidence-based practice** is a process of shared decision making in a partnership between patients and providers that involves the integration of research and other best evidence with clinical expertise and patient values and preferences in making health care decisions (Sigma Theta Tau International Research and Scholarship Advisory Committee, 2008). Evidence-based practice involves a process similar to

---

Photo used with permission from Photos.com.

research utilization. **Research utilization** encompasses critique of research studies, synthesis of findings, a determination of the applicability of findings, review for application with implementation of scientific findings in practice, an evaluation of the practice change, and dissemination of results to expand scientific knowledge. The shift from research utilization to evidence-based practice reflects the realization that not all clinical questions have been answered through research; thus other forms of evidence (e.g., lower rigor research, case studies, expert opinion) may be required to guide practice. An emphasis on use of evidence-based practice includes the application of the best available evidence and also represents a desire to improve patient outcomes with a consideration for patient values and preferences when making patient care decisions. Evidence-based practice is a broader, scientific process for improving health care quality and safety by building on what is learned from quality improvement, research utilization, and the conduct of research.

Other terms are related to evidence-based practice yet are distinctly different. **Best practice** is popular term, but the definition remains elusive. Common use of the term describes innovative practices that are recognized by peer organizations and that contribute to meeting quality or fiscal goals (e.g., American Society for Quality; Australian Government Department of Veteran Affairs, Guideline for the Provision of Community Nursing Care). Although "best practice" and "evidence-based practice" are sometimes used interchangeably, the extent that best practices are evidence-based is often unclear. To promote understanding when using scientific evidence as guidance, evidence-based practice is the clear term to use. A **clinical practice guideline** is a statement designed to assist providers and clients in making decisions about appropriate health care for specific clinical circumstances (Sackett et al., 2000). Guidelines are systematically developed, they link the evidence with health outcomes (benefits and harms), and they continue to require subjective judgments when making decisions for use (Institute of Medicine, 2011a; Woolf & Atkins, 2001). Guidelines are developed with the intent to influence clinical behavior by making clear practice recommendations. A rigorous scientific process used to combine findings from research (usually randomized controlled trials) into a powerful and clinically

useful report to guide practice is known as a **systematic review.** Standard components of a systematic review to consider are (1) process for initiating, (2) process for finding and assessing individual studies, (3) process for synthesizing the body of evidence; and (4) standard reporting format (Institute of Medicine, 2011b). Rigor used in development varies considerably among reports.

Translational research includes testing the effect of interventions aimed at promoting the rate and extent of adoption of evidence-based practices by nurses, physicians, and other health care providers and describing organizational, unit, and individual variables that affect the use of evidence in clinical and operational decision making (Titler, 2004; Titler & Everett, 2001). Translational research has provided guidance about effective strategies for implementing evidence-based practice. *Translational research* is often used interchangeably with *implementation science.* **Implementation science** includes scientific investigations that support movement of evidence-based, effective health care approaches from clinical knowledge into routine use; testing strategies to promote uptake and use of innovations; and explaining factors that promote and hinder use of scientific knowledge in health care delivery (Eccles & Mittman, 2006; Greenhalgh et al., 2005; Rubenstein & Pugh, 2006; Titler, 2007). After initial pilot implementation and evaluation, the process used to promote integration of evidence-based practice is called **reinfusion.**

Organizational context refers to the health system environment in which the proposed evidence-based practice is to be implemented. The core elements that help describe the organizational context include the prevailing culture of the system (e.g., patient-centered); the nature of human relationships in the system, including the leadership styles that are operational (e.g., team work, clear role delineation); and the organization's approach to routine monitoring of performance of systems and services within the organization (Kitson et al., 2008; Spyridonidis & Calnan, 2011; Stetler et al., 2009; VanDeusen et al., 2010).

Translational research has provided guidance about effective strategies for implementing evidence-based practice. **Academic detailing or educational outreach** is the use of a marketing strategy that uses presentations by a trained person who meets one-on-one with practitioners in their setting to provide information about the evidence-based practice. This may include feedback on the provider's performance. The detailer may be from inside or outside the provider's organization, and the information may be tailored to address site-specific barriers (Avorn & Soumerai, 1983; Davies et al., 1995; O'Brien et al., 2007; Sohn et al., 2004; Titler et al., 2002). The terms *academic detailing* and *educational outreach* are used interchangeably (Box 16-1).

Informal leaders who influence peers by evaluating innovations for use in certain settings and promoting clinicians' use of evidence in clinical decision making are referred to as **opinion leaders**. Opinion leaders are likeable, trustworthy, informative, and influential (Doumit et al., 2007; Majumdar et al., 2007).

Performance gap assessment is a strategy of demonstrating an opportunity for improvement at baseline and outlining current practice related to specific indicators (Bullock-Palmer et al., 2008;

BOX 16-1 STRATEGIES FOR USING ACADEMIC DETAILING OR EDUCATIONAL OUTREACH

As Outlined in the Literature*
- Meet one-on-one with practitioners
- Meet in/near the work setting
- Use two-way communication to increase involvement in educational interactions
- Establish the messenger's credibility and lack of conflict of interest
- Define the specific problems and objectives
- Provide information specific to the evidence-based practice topic using brief (e.g., 10-15 minutes) graphic materials to sustain interest
- Give both sides of controversial issues (for "inoculation" versus counter-argument)
- Troubleshoot implementation challenges
- Concentrate on a few key messages (include alternatives that are being discouraged)
- Provide positive feedback about key indicators that are specific to the practitioner or team
- Provide reminders, reinforcement, and rewards to sustain improvements

Adapted for Use in Practice
- Clearly articulate the goal (e.g., stroke certification to improve patient care and patient outcomes)
- Reaffirm the team's support for reaching that goal (e.g., recognition for previous support and commitment)
- Identify one key indicator (e.g., swallow screening) from the practice recommendations to address in achieving the goal
- Report the performance gap data demonstrating an opportunity for improvement (e.g., percent of swallow screens completed within 24 hours of admission)
- Outline the evidence for the issue, including the extent of existing research supporting the practice recommendation and gaps in current knowledge (e.g., limited evidence about elevating the head of bed for bedside swallow screening in selected stroke patients)
- Identify current strategies in place to meet the indicator goal (e.g., physician orders on admission, nursing assessment within 24 hours of admission, referral as indicated)
- Admit to the challenges in meeting the goal (e.g., busy workloads; timely differential diagnosis for type of stroke)
- Outline the unattractive alternatives to meeting the goal (e.g., nasogastric tube placement for oral intake; delayed administration of oral medications)
- State the desire to make the change systematic and with minimal impact on workload (e.g., standing orders to make the process easy for the clinicians)
- Brainstorm to identify innovative approaches to achieve the goal (e.g., location of standing orders within the documentation system)
- Develop an action plan with next steps, division of responsibility, and timeline, and again recognize efforts toward the goal and reiterate group decisions (e.g., stroke certification)

*Data from Soumerai S.B., & Avorn J. (1990). Principles of educational outreach ("academic detailing") to improve clinical decision making. *Journal of the American Medical Association, 263*(4), 549-556.

Oxman et al., 1995). This data-driven strategy is used early in the implementation to garner commitment for practice changes.

The best process to use when addressing clinical or operational issues depends on the question at hand and the extent of research or other evidence available on the topic. Several processes may be used to improve care, from quality/performance improvement to evidence-based practice or the conduct of research. For questions that can be addressed through quality improvement, improvements can be brought to the patient care level quickly and efficiently. Clinical questions with little or no research that include patient risk may be good questions to answer by conducting research.

MODELS

Work in nursing has led to the development of several evidence-based practice process models to guide nursing practice (Boyer et al., 2006; Goode et al., 2011; Logan et al., 1999; Rycroft-Malone & Bucknall, 2010; Rycroft-Malone et al., 2002; Stetler, 2001; Stevens, 2004; Titler et al., 2001). Evidence-based practice models have been used successfully to improve adoption of evidence-based practice recommendations (Block et al., 2012; Cullen et al., 2005; Dolezal et al., 2011; Hogan & Logan, 2004; Logan, et al., 1999) (Table 16-1). The Iowa Model (Titler et al., 2001) is one example used to guide clinician decision making in a variety of settings and is widely used.

TABLE 16-1 SELECT EVIDENCE-BASED PRACTICE PROCESS MODELS

MODEL	CITATION	SAMPLE REPORTS
Iowa Model	Titler, M.G., Kleiber, C., Steelman, V., Rakel, B., Budreau, G., Everett, L.Q., et al. (2001). The Iowa Model of evidence-based practice to promote quality care. *Critical Care Nursing Clinics of North America, 13*(4), 497-509.	Farrington, M., Lang, S., Cullen, L., & Stewart, S. (2009). Nasogastric tube placement in pediatric and neonatal patients. *Pediatric Nursing, 35*(1), 17-25.
Ottawa Model	Graham, K., & Logan, J. (2004). Using the Ottawa Model of Research Use to implement a skin care program. *Journal of Nursing Care Quality, 19*(1), 18-24.	Hogan, D.L., & Logan, J. (2004). The Ottawa Model of research use: A guide to clinical innovation in the NICU. *Clinical Nurse Specialist: The Journal for Advanced Nursing Practice, 18*(5), 255-261.
Stetler Model	Stetler, C.B. (2001). Updating the Stetler model of research utilization to facilitate evidence-based practice. *Nursing Outlook, 49*(6), 272-279.	Romp, C.R., & Kiehl, E. (2009). Applying the Stetler model of research utilization in staff development: Revitalizing a preceptor program. *Journal for Nurses in Staff Development, 25*(6), 278-284, quiz 285-286.
Model for EBP Change	Rosswurm, M.A., & Larrabee, J.H. (1999). A model for change to evidence-based practice. *Image: Journal of Nursing Scholarship, 31*(4), 317-322.	Boyer, D.R., Steltzer, N., & Larrabee, J.H. (2009). Implementation of an evidence-based bladder scanner protocol. *Journal of Nursing Care Quality, 24*(1), 10-16.
ARCC Model	Melnyk, B.M., & Fineout-Overholt, E. (2011). *Evidence-based practice in nursing & healthcare. A guide to best practice* (2nd ed.). Philadelphia, PA: Wolters Kluwer/Lippincott Williams & Wilkins.	Wallen, G.R., Mitchell, S.A., Melnyk, B., Fineout-Overholt, E., Miller-Davis, C., Yates, J., & Hastings, C. (2010). Implementing evidence-based practice: Effectiveness of a structured multifaceted mentorship programme. *Journal of Advanced Nursing, 66*(12), 2761-2771.

Source: Cullen, L., Tucker, S., Hanrahan, K., Rempel, G., & Jordan, K. (2012). *Evidence-based practice building blocks: Comprehensive strategies, tools, and tips* (1st ed.). Iowa City: Department of Nursing Services and Patient Care, University of Iowa Hospitals and Clinics.

The challenge for clinicians is to identify a model that guides practice and also promotes successful translation and implementation of evidence-based practice (Block et al., 2012; Cullen et al., 2012; Dolezal et al., 2011). Adoption of one evidence-based practice model across the organization and multidisciplinary initiatives (Gawlinski & Rutledge, 2008) is one strategy for promoting coordination of efforts. Evidence-based practice models tend to follow a basic problem-solving process and can be used parallel to other quality improvement processes (e.g., Six Sigma). Senior leadership support for evidence-based practice can be leveraged by outlining the similarities between evidence-based practice and existing quality improvement processes and structures and then synergistically blending them.

IMPLEMENTING EVIDENCE-BASED PRACTICE CHANGES

Implementation of evidence-based practice changes can be challenging in complex health care settings. Despite the research supporting the use of effective strategies for implementing evidence-based practice changes, the use of ineffective implementation strategies persists (Bloom, 2005). In fact, Bloom (2005) stated that use of these ineffective implementation strategies results in "reduced patient care quality and raises costs for all, the worst of both worlds" (p. 380). Education is an essential first step to develop an understanding of why and how the evidence-based practice is done, but education alone does little to change practice (Farmer et al., 2008; Forsetlund et al., 2009; Jablonski & Ersek, 2009; Nicol et al., 2009; Pipe et al., 2009; Prior et al., 2008). In addition to education, multifaceted interactive interventions are needed to communicate the practice change to clinicians (Greenhalgh et al., 2005; Titler, 2008).

The Diffusion of Innovations Model (Rogers, 2003) provides a theoretical framework that supports the hard work of implementing practice change in health care (Dobbins et al., 2002; Greenhalgh et al., 2005; Titler & Everett, 2001). Planning for implementation requires use of effective implementation strategies across phases of adoption. Although strong evidence supports the use of some strategies that promote the integration of evidence-based practice in health care, other strategies need further testing. The Evidence-Based Practice Implementation Guide (Figure 16-1) was developed to assist nurse leaders with planning and use of effective

implementation strategies that advance stakeholders (both people and systems) through a process of diffusion: creating awareness and interest, building knowledge and commitment, promoting action and adaptation, and integrating and sustaining use (Cullen & Adams, 2012). The Evidence-Based Practice Implementation Guide can be used with evidence-based practice process models as a planning tool. Multiple interactive and reinforcing strategies, as outlined, promote adoption of evidence-based practice recommendations (Prior et al., 2008). Strategies to capture a busy clinician's attention are important to include in the project implementation plan. Nurse leaders can identify additional strategies as they work across phases. Strategies are added to create a comprehensive implementation plan and momentum before, during, and after implementation.

A number of strategies have good evidence and are particularly effective. Academic detailing or educational outreach is an implementation strategy that is effective in promoting adoption of evidence-based practice recommendations (O'Brien et al., 2007) by increasing knowledge and commitment to the change. Academic detailing involves a multifaceted approach to discussions with practitioners. Use of academic detailing has been shown to be an effective way to communicate with practitioners. Clinicians tend to buy into the need for the practice change when there is a strong evidence base, the topic addresses an identified need, data demonstrate an opportunity for practice improvement within the clinical area, and the practice change offers a relative advantage. Localizing or adapting practice recommendations to fit the local setting and culture is an essential step in the process, often using the role of the opinion leader and team of local experts (Doumit et al., 2007; Titler, 2008). When done by an opinion leader, academic detailing with a performance gap assessment is a highly effective example of using multifaceted interactive strategies in promoting adoption of evidence-based practice. In practice, this approach can be used to increase knowledge and garner consensus from a multidisciplinary team.

Once the practice has been adapted and is ready for piloting, additional planning is needed for implementation and evaluation. Development of a fluid action plan can be highly effective in keeping the team on task and collectively moving forward (Cullen & Adams, 2012; Gifford et al., 2011; Schimizu & Shimanouchi, 2006). The following case example demonstrates the effectiveness of

Implementation Strategies for Evidence-Based Practice

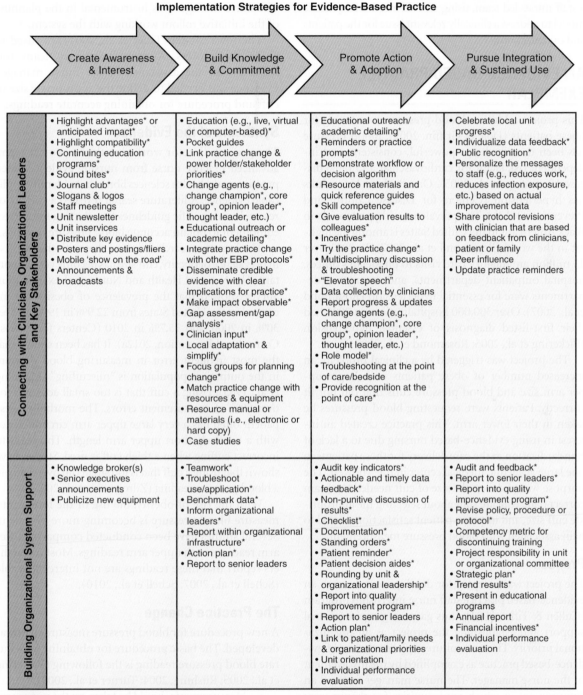

*=Implementation strategy is supported by at least some empirical evidence in healthcare.

FIGURE 16-1 Evidence-Based Practice Implementation Guide. (Reproduced with permission from Laura Cullen, MA, RN, FAAN [From Cullen, L., & Adams, S. (2012). Planning for implementation of evidence-based practice. *Journal of Nursing Administration, 42*(4), 222-230].)

a staff nurse–led team, using an evidence-based practice model to address a clinically relevant issue for the patients and organizations.

AN EVIDENCE-BASED PRACTICE EXEMPLAR

This project addresses blood pressure monitoring for obese patients (Dole & Griffin, 2009). Blood pressure has been described as a powerful, consistent, and in-dependent risk factor for cardiovascular and renal disease (Pickering et al., 2005). One in three U.S. adults has hypertension (Centers for Disease Control and Prevention, 2012b). The prevalence of hypertension in Black Americans in the United States is among the high-est in the world (Rosamond et al., 2007). In 2002 over 45 million ambulatory care visits to physician's offices, hospital outpatient departments, and emergency de-partments were for essential hypertension (Rosamond et al., 2007). Over 300,000 hospitalizations in 2005 had their first-listed diagnosis of essential hypertension (Pickering et al., 2005; Rosamond et al., 2007).

The project was triggered by a clinical problem, an increased number of obese patients with larger up-per arm size and blood pressure cuffs that did not fit correctly. Patients were requesting blood pressures be taken in their lower arm. This practice created an in-terest in using evidence-based nursing due to a lack of standardization in the care delivery for these patients in one large academic medical center in the Midwest. The purpose was to define the size of cuff needed to obtain correct data, educate staff about selecting the appropri-ate cuff size, and improve patient satisfaction related to pain associated with blood pressure measurement.

Process

The project was accepted for development through an evidence-based practice staff nurse internship program (Cullen & Titler, 2004), thus garnering organizational support and establishing the project as an organiza-tional priority. The unit culture supports the use of evi-dence-based practice as exemplified by the involvement of the nurse manager. The nurse manager fostered an environment in which opportunities for change were welcomed. In addition, the nurse manager ensured that non–patient care time was available for the staff nurse project director. The project director relied on the nurse manager for assistance with scheduling meetings, taking minutes, and providing follow-up on issues.

The nurse manager was instrumental in the planning of the initiative rollout working with the system.

The Iowa Model (Titler et al., 2001) was used to guide the process. A multidisciplinary team was formed with the assistance of the nurse manager. Evidence was needed to define the appropriate size of cuff and procedure for obtaining accurate readings.

Synthesis of the Evidence

The project director worked with the project team, advanced practice nurse from nursing evidence-based practice, and a health sciences librarian to identify appli-cable evidence. A literature search revealed a scarcity of research and specific guidelines for selecting the correct equipment to obtain accurate blood pressure readings.

The literature search did show that with the increase in prevalence of obesity, cuff size has become very impor-tant. The National Health and Nutritional Examination Survey showed that the prevalence of obesity has in-creased in the United States from 22.9% in 1994, to over 30% in 2000, and 35.7% in 2010 (Centers for Disease Control and Prevention, 2012a). It has been shown that the most frequent error in measuring blood pressure in the outpatient population is "miscuffing" (Manning et al., 1983). Using a cuff that is too small accounts for over 80% of measurement errors. The morbidly obese patient often has a very large upper arm circumference with a relatively short upper arm length. This leads to incorrect cuffing when a thigh cuff is used. Studies have shown that using a cuff that is too small can overestimate a blood pressure reading (Zdrojewski et al., 2005).

With the rise of obesity, the use of the forearm to measure blood pressure is becoming more prevalent. Several studies have been conducted comparing fore-arm readings with upper arm readings. Most research-ers report that these readings are not interchangeable (Schell et al., 2007; Schell et al., 2010).

The Practice Change

A new procedure for blood pressure measurement was developed. The basic procedure for obtaining an accu-rate blood pressure reading is the following (Pickering et al., 2005; Rushing, 2004; Turner et al., 2008):

- Measurements should be taken on the upper arm
- The cuff bladder length should be at least 80% of arm circumference and the width should be at least 40% of upper arm length
- The patient's arm is supported horizontally at the level of the heart

- If the patient is sitting both feet should be flat on the floor
- The nurse and the patient should not talk during the procedure
- Do not use the arm that has an IV or the side of a mastectomy
- The patient should be sitting 3 to 5 minutes before measurement

The practice change required purchasing new cuffs to meet the needs of patients with larger arm circumference. Longer and larger cuffs were purchased from the manufacturer of the automatic blood pressure monitors. These longer cuffs have nearly eliminated the use of the thigh cuff for upper arm measurements. The new procedure was rolled out from the internal medicine clinic to the cardiology clinic.

Implementation

Staff training began when the new cuffs were available for clinic use (Table 16-2). The longer blood pressure cuffs were readily accepted by the staff and patients. No problems occurred once a supply of cuffs was available

TABLE 16-2 IMPLEMENTATION STRATEGIES USED	
PLANNING PHASE	**STRATEGIES USED FOR BLOOD PRESSURE MONITORING IN AMBULATORY CLINIC**
Creating awareness and interest	• Highlight the advantages • Highlight compatibility • Report anticipated impact • Staff meetings • Unit in-services • Postings
Building knowledge and commitment	• Education • Pocket guide • Change agents • Trying the change • Disseminate credible evidence • Local adaptation • Match the practice change with the equipment available • Case study • Team work • Trouble shooting implementation
Promoting action and adoption	• Educational outreach • Practice prompts • Demonstrate workflow • Feedback evaluation results • Trying the change • Report progress & updates • Role-model the change • Troubleshooting by change champions at the point of care • Rounding by unit leaders • Report within quality improvement program • Report to senior leadership • Link to patient needs
Pursuing integration and sustained use	• Celebrate unit progress • Recognition for change • Report within quality improvement program • Revise policy • Presenting at educational programs

From Cullen, L., & Adams, S. (2012). Planning for implementation of evidence-based practice. *Journal of Nursing Administration, 42*(4), 222-230.

for the automatic blood pressure equipment. A policy was written on monitoring blood pressure on the obese arm in an outpatient setting and presented to the nursing policy committee. The committee requested that it be presented to the ambulatory nurse managers for their approval and resubmitted to the committee. The only suggestion was to revise the policy for both adult ambulatory and inpatient use. The revised policy was resubmitted and accepted.

Evaluation

The team selected process and outcome indicators for evaluation. The desired process was to select the correct size blood pressure cuff in order to have the most accurate readings. The pilot clinics were given the evaluation form after a three-month trial of the longer cuffs. A questionnaire was developed for the staff and patients to measure knowledge and satisfaction regarding the use of the correct size cuff. The results demonstrated satisfaction for both the staff (pre=2.75; post=3.56; scale: 1 to 44) and patients (pre=3.35;

post=3.4) with the appropriate size cuff. Nurses also report being better able to identify the correct cuff (pre=3.1; post=3.7) and having the proper cuff available (pre=2.4; post=3.6). Nurses report patients being more satisfied (pre=2.2; post=3.0).

By using the longer cuffs the automatic monitors did not reinflate to get a blood pressure reading. Over 94% of the patients questioned agreed that the longer blood pressure cuffs caused less pain then using a cuff that was the wrong size. Ultimately, the length of the visit decreased with use of proper equipment to obtain the blood pressure.

The success of this project in measuring a blood pressure for the adult patient was a valued patient and nurse satisfier. Accurate measurement of blood pressure is essential to diagnose patients, ascertain blood pressure related risks, and guide for medical management. Training the nursing staff in proper blood pressure measurement techniques should provide the clinicians with information to help with the proper management of cardiovascular health.

RESEARCH NOTE

Source

Gifford, W., Davis, B., Tourangeau, A., & Lefebre, N. (2011). Developing team leadership to facilitate guideline utilization: Planning and evaluating a 3-month intervention strategy. *Journal of Nursing Management, 19*(1), 112-132.

Purpose

Research demonstrates the importance of leadership in use of clinical practice guidelines, but the development of leaders and the skills they require are less clear. The purpose of this study was to describe planning and implementation of a leadership intervention aimed to facilitate the use of a clinical practice guideline for diabetic foot care. The intervention, to develop leaders, was planned using a synthesis of research and theory, along with data from qualitative interviews at two nonparticipating sites and chart audit data (Gifford et al., 2009). In this study, nurse managers and clinical leaders (n=15), responsible for supervising 180 staff nurses at two sites, participated in a 6-hour workshop and three teleconferences. The intervention was evaluated by workshop surveys and interviews.

Discussion

The intervention components that workshop participants rated highest (on a scale of 1 to 4; 1=not

at all relevant and useful, 4=extremely useful and relevant) were identification of target indicators (mean 3.7), chart audit findings about the research/practice gap (mean 3.5), and development of a team action plan (mean 3.5). Interviews with participants 3 months after the intervention showed that identification of target indicators and development of a team action plan continued to be the highest ranked activities (mean 8.1 and 8, respectively on a similar 10-point scale). Pre-workshop materials and barriers assessment activities were rated lowest (median 5.5). Limitations included the lack of assessment of baseline leadership knowledge and skills, and a small sample size.

Application to Practice

Leadership skills that support the adoption of clinical practice guidelines in clinical settings should be developed through a planned intervention that is tailored to the specific team and leadership. Access to clinical measures (data) is valuable for nurse leaders to identifying target outcomes, monitor progress, identify gaps, and benchmark. Action plans are useful tools for leaders to operationalize leadership strategies, actively engage staff, and monitor outcomes.

ORGANIZATIONAL INFRASTRUCTURE AND CONTEXT

Strategies for implementing evidence-based practices occur at both the unit/clinical level, as illustrated in the exemplar, and also at the organizational level. A strategic approach is needed for building evidence-based practice capacity (Cullen et al., 2005; Newhouse, 2007; Stetler et al., 2009; Titler, 2010; Titler & Moore, 2010). The Magnet Recognition Program® provides standards expecting evidence-based practice and innovation within organizations and uses evidence-based practice as a key component to drive elements of the 14 Forces of Magnetism *(www.nursecredentialing. org/MagnetModel.aspx)*. The Magnet standards can provide guidance when expanding and prioritizing an evidence-based practice program. The way to do this is for organizations to integrate evidence-based practice at the organization or health system level with leadership efforts focusing on the following (Titler et al., 2002, p. 26):

> *…four major building blocks: (1) incorporating evidence-based practice terminology into the mission, vision, strategic plan, and performance appraisals of staff; (2) integrating the work of evidence-based practice into the governance structure of nursing departments and the health care system; (3) demonstrating the value of evidence-based practice through administrative behaviors of the chief nurse executive; and (4) establishing explicit expectations about evidence-based practice for nursing leaders (e.g., nurse managers and advanced practice registered nurses) who create a culture that values clinical inquiry.*

Development of a mission and vision statement inclusive of evidence-based practice provides a foundation for this work at all levels of the organization and begins the process of building a culture in which evidence-based health care practices are the expected norm (Cullen et al., 2005; Newhouse, 2007; Stetler et al., 2009). The vision statement can stretch the current boundaries of evidence-based practice and promote work that leads staff to "reach" for a higher standard. An example of a vision statement might be that the organization will develop a center of excellence for evidence-based practice and be seen as a leader in use of evidence-based care delivery. To support the vision, an infrastructure for evidence-based practice is needed as another building block. The infrastructure should take advantage of the expertise currently available and not be added work in an already busy workplace (Newhouse, 2007). Additional expertise can be developed through consultation and collaborations within a practice network (see Table 16-2), partnerships with academic institutions, or hiring nurse scientists (Brewer et al., 2009; Debourgh, 2012; Granger et al., 2012; Missal et al., 2010; Weeks et al., 2011).

Staff with expertise in research and quality improvement processes likely will have the requisite skills to facilitate evidence-based practice. In many organizations, clinical experts who make up the clinical practice committee may have the right membership for further developing expertise in evidence-based practice processes. Critical skills include critique and synthesis of the evidence, development of an implementation and evaluation plan, statistical analysis for quality improvement, and reporting of results (Cullen et al., 2005; Cullen et al., 2010; Hart et al., 2008; Newhouse, 2007; Thiel & Ghosh, 2008). The right committee or council structure will vary in each organization but should reflect the expertise and functions needed to promote evidence-based practices.

The value of evidence-based practice must be evident through the behaviors of nursing leadership. Action steps for building a culture that values evidence-based practice can be included in the departmental strategic plan. Discussion during committee meetings can stimulate interest in and use of evidence-based practice; including an evidence-based practice item on each agenda is a key strategy. Accountability is outlined in committee functions (Cullen et al., 2005; Granger et al., 2012; Stetler et al., 2009). An organizational culture that promotes use of evidence values nurses questioning their practice, provides education about evidence-based practice, adopts an evidence-based practice model, and recognizes and rewards the work. Recruiting and hiring nurses with interest in evidence-based practice also will help build the desired culture. Orientation can contain basic evidence-based practice concepts and protocols, with new staff learning from colleagues who share experiences from evidence-based practice teamwork on their unit. This provides recognition for the work done, sets the expectation that evidence-based practice is important in clinical care, and demonstrates that nurses have authority over their practice. New graduates have developed skills that support evidence-based practice (QSEN, 2012). Nurses in new graduate residency programs can stimulate new or support existing evidence-based practice work, using their creativity, technical skills, and supported time. Evidence-based practice must be alive in daily practice, not just "pulled off the shelf" when organizational leaders appear in the clinical area. Another building block involves the use of evidence-based practice components in performance appraisals for all roles. Performance appraisals based on job descriptions with evidence-based practice components across all job classifications promote positive reinforcement and priority setting in the busy work environment.

The exemplar demonstrates ready adoption in a clinic. The organizational culture and infrastructure will impact adoption of evidence-based practices and patient outcomes (Brewer et al., 2009; Cummings et al., 2007; Dogherty et al., 2012; Stetler et al., 2009; Wallin et al., 2006). Organizational systems must be designed to support the incorporation of evidence-based practices into clinical work flow if adoption is to occur. Practice change is best facilitated when documentation, policies and procedures, and education include the essential components from the clinical practice guideline. Regardless of whether paper or electronic systems are used, documentation systems, designed to support clinical practice, must capture the essential elements of the guideline that practitioners are expected to perform. The documentation system can serve as a "trigger" to assess important risk factors (e.g., risk for falling, risk for pressure ulcer development), patient conditions (e.g., pain intensity, duration, or location), and outcomes of care (e.g., development of pressure ulcers or oral mucositis) (Durieux et al., 2008; Haynes et al., 2009; van Klei et al., 2012; Weiss et al., 2011). Electronic documentation systems may also provide the opportunity for decision support to assist clinicians with use of evidence-based practice guidelines.

The need for education regarding a practice change is fundamental. The organization can support the use of evidence-based practices by incorporating education about the evidence-based practice in orientation for new hires, competency review for current employees, and education for senior leadership. When working to sustain evidence-based practice, strategies are needed to hardwire the work into the organizational system. One strategy to promote integration

of an evidence-based practice is to incorporate the evidence-based practice into organizational policies and procedures. Clinical experts can provide an excellent critique of a new policy or procedure and make recommendations so policies link practices with the evidence and support the adaptation of guidelines for their organization.

Linking quality improvement and evidence-based practice is another strategy for building a strong organizational context. The quality improvement committee has standardized forms, a reporting system, and an established process for use of results to continuously improve practice until the practice reaches the established goal and becomes integrated. Using the quality improvement system for reporting evidence-based practice changes provides efficient communication within the existing organizational infrastructure. The quality improvement process also supports ongoing planning, monitoring, and reinfusion of the expected care delivery, supporting successful adoption and integration of evidence-based practices.

Successes need to be rewarded along the way. Celebrations help build a culture that supports and expects the use of evidence in practice. Rewards should include formal recognition from high-level organizational leaders, visibility for the team and project champions, accessibility to practitioners within the organization, and a clear articulation of the benefits of evidence-based practice. Celebrations provide the opportunity to put clinicians in the spotlight for doing great work. Recognition can clearly articulate the benefits to and commitment of the organization. Celebrating successes promotes buy-in and commitment of the organization to the evidence-based practice process and strengthens the foundation for future efforts.

LEADERSHIP ROLES IN PROMOTING PRACTICE

Leadership is needed across all organizational levels and roles when implementing evidence-based changes (Davies et al., 2006; Gifford et al., 2007; Gifford et al., 2011; Wallin et al., 2005). Many nursing roles are essential and complementary in the work of evidence-based practice. From the chief nurse executive through nurse managers, advanced practice registered nurses, and staff nurses, everyone has a role in evidence-based practice work that builds upon their knowledge and skills (QSEN, 2012). Nurse executives have organizational responsibility for creating a culture in which clinicians expect evidence-based practice, creating the capacity to accomplish evidence-based practice, and developing and sustaining a vision inclusive of evidence-based practice—all important building blocks for evidence-based practice. Innovative organizations with responsive leadership that support staff will promote use of evidence-based care (Estabrooks et al., 2007; Wallin et al., 2006). Allocating resources and time has been demonstrated to be important to promote evidence-based health care (Fleuren et al., 2004; Gerrish et al., 2011; Gerrish et al., 2012; Gifford et al., 2011; Mallidou et al., 2011).

Senior leaders have a responsibility to articulate the business case for evidence-based practice to governing boards. Communication with boards has been identified as an important strategy by the Institute for Healthcare Improvement (2012). Key messages to share with board members include reporting the linkages between evidence-based practice and the organization's mission, values, strategic plan, and committee's functional responsibility within the organizational and nursing infrastructure (Conway, 2008; Goeschel et al., 2010; Slessor et al., 2008). Reporting of project results is essential to garner continued support and recognition for the program. Using the existing reporting mechanisms, evidence-based practice can capitalize on existing structures and processes to gain support from senior leadership in future decision making. For example, a staff nurse–led project resulted in an estimated $1.9 million cost savings (Cullen et al., 2005) and an ergonomics program reduced work injury expenses by nearly three quarters of a million dollars (Stenger et al., 2007). These results were shared with the CEO to acquire new equipment and additional resources for continuing implementation and program development.

Reports will best capture attention when addressing three to five key talking points or take-away messages with clear links to organizational priorities and infrastructure. Reporting anticipated outcomes can be helpful early in the process. Outcomes that target patients and families, staff, and finances are valued by the organization and need to be considered in evaluation planning.

Outcomes targeting key initiatives would include patient satisfaction and other Center for Medicare & Medicaid Services (CMS) reportable measures (e.g., care for heart failure patients, practices preventing surgical site infections, pressure ulcer prevention) (AHRQ, 2002; CMS, 2011). Cost savings or cost avoidance may not be achieved with every project but should be calculated whenever possible. A large volume of cost data is available in the literature and can be used to calculate estimated cost savings. For example, data demonstrate that each decubitus ulcer adds $2384/case, at a cost of over $2.5 million in the United States (Pappas, 2008; Van Den Bos et al., 2011; Zhan et al., 2006). While hospital admissions increased 15%, acquired pressure ulcers increased 80% between 1993 and 2006 (Russo et al., 2008). In addition, pressure ulcers contributed to a threefold increase in length of stay and fourfold increase in mortality (Russo et al., 2008). The incidents and costs continue to exist despite an extensive body of research around prevention and treatment. If evidence-based practice changes reduced only 20 cases in 1 year, an estimated cost savings for that organization would be $47,680, not including the patient and family experience, which would be an additional highly valued impact. Reporting program and project results, linked within the organizational infrastructure, and capturing important outcomes assist the governing board in seeing the connection between these activities and the overall organizational mission. Nursing leaders have a responsibility to clearly articulate evidence-based practice work in a way that will be heard by decision makers.

The strategies discussed in building an organizational infrastructure for evidence-based practice are effective in developing the culture, building the capacity, and sustaining the vision at both organization and unit levels. The nurse manager is responsible, parallel to the nurse executive, for developing the unit culture. Developing a positive unit culture for promoting evidence-based practice impacts the outcomes of the unit (Hughes et al., 2009; Zohar et al., 2007). Managers' use of participatory leadership that is responsive to and supportive of staff will promote evidence-based care by staff nurses (Boström et al., 2007; Cummings et al., 2007; Gifford et al., 2007; Wallin et al., 2006). Creating action plans can facilitate leadership support and use of evidence-based practice (Gerrish et al., 2011) (see Research Note) The nurse manager can use the action plan to support evidence-based practice, set the expectations for the unit, discuss the importance of the work of evidence-based practice with the unit nurses and other disciplines, encourage and respond to new ideas, promote staff questioning practice, support the team with time to work on the project, be a project cheerleader, track progress, facilitate moving the project through appropriate committees, and allocate resources as needed. By encouraging nurses to attend and present at conferences, stimulating inquiry and participating in research, nurses on their unit will increase use of evidence-based practice on their unit (Boström et al., 2007; Cummings et al., 2007; Pepler et al., 2006). The nurse manager's commitment to improvement and performance feedback is critical to project success and can significantly affect project outcomes (Wallin et al., 2005; Wallin et al., 2006).

Advanced practice registered nurses may partner with project team leaders and play an important role in evidence-based practice project development. Capitalizing on their existing knowledge and skills will facilitate use of research findings in practice (Cullen et al., 2010; Gerrish et al., 2012; Newhouse, 2007; Pepler et al., 2006; QSEN, 2012). Advanced practice registered nurses can function as opinion leaders and facilitators. They have the ability to take on the most challenging steps in the process by leading a team, identifying potential roadblocks, facilitating problem solving during implementation and evaluation, reporting results, and providing expertise throughout the evidence-based practice process. Critique and synthesis of the evidence, development of an evaluation plan, and analysis of results are steps that utilize this expertise. Strong skills are needed for the facilitator to keep a team focused and moving forward. These nurses may also act as mentors for the team and the project director (Dogherty et al., 2012; Gerrish et al., 2012). The path to improving care can be bumpy, and teams will need encouragement to address the barriers and sustain the commitment and momentum all the way to through.

Staff nurses are ideally positioned to identify important and clinically relevant topics to develop into evidence-based practice improvements. Staff nurses are expert clinicians who have the skills to collaborate and problem solve, finding many creative solutions. They are critical to providing quality care through implementation of evidence-based practices. Staff nurses can function as change champions and core group members within their current functions. With

appropriate coaching and support, staff nurses also can function as an opinion leader or even project director (Cullen & Titler, 2004; Ploeg et al., 2010). As point of care clinicians, they are the key to quality and use of evidence-based practices.

Use of a bottom-up approach for topic selection by staff nurses (identified by nurses at the point of care) can facilitate adoption of the practice change. Clinicians will "pull" the practice change into their care instead of having the change "pushed" down from above or outside the organization (Kirchhoff, 2004; Stetler et al., 2009). Programs are needed to help staff nurses integrate evidence-based practice change into care delivery (Forsetlund et al., 2009; Jablonski & Ersek, 2009; Pipe et al., 2009; Wells et al., 2007). When staff nurses receive sufficient support, they are effective at integrating evidence-based practice changes into care and find the experience to be empowering (Block et al., 2012; Bowman et al., 2005; Dole & Griffin, 2009; Farrington et al., 2009).

One important role that will keep the project moving forward is that of the project director (Harvard Business Essentials, 2004). The project director is responsible for establishing meeting schedules and timelines with the group, running the meetings, maintaining the action plan, delegating work assignments, and overseeing the process and progress. The focus of the project director must always be on moving the project forward, despite challenges, as a key strategy for success. The project director may orchestrate discussions for identifying potential challenges, addressing those that cannot be avoided but continuing to move forward despite distractions. Staff nurses can function as project directors if they are given sufficient support and mentorship (Block et al., 2012; Bowman et al., 2005; Cullen et al., 2010; Dole & Griffin, 2009; Farrington et al., 2009). Staff nurses and nursing leaders work together with complementary skills and expertise to address challenges and issues inherent in evidence-based practice.

LEADERSHIP AND MANAGEMENT IMPLICATIONS

Regardless of job title, all nurses have a role in making evidence-based practice changes successful. A multifaceted approach is needed when integrating evidence-based practice at the unit/clinic or organization level. Change is difficult. Combining strategies to build on existing strengths should be considered (Cullen et al., 2012).

For example, educational offerings may already exist in familiar formats (e.g., posters, in-services); adding new approaches can stimulate interest (e.g., executive summaries, resource manuals, selected research references). Identifying those nurses and physicians who are innovative and influential among their peers to function as opinion leaders and change champions is important. A performance gap assessment can motivate participation. Academic detailing, along with audit and feedback, should be included throughout implementation. Simple solutions should be sought first; creativity becomes important when addressing barriers. Staff nurses can often bring fresh approaches to address challenges. Adding new graduates to the team creates a culture for evidence-based practice building upon the knowledge and skills gained through academic programs (QSEN, 2012) and resources from new graduate residency programs *(http://www.aacn.nche.edu/education-resources/ nurse-residency-program)*. Strategic planning is essential for provision of evidence-based health care and weaving evidence-based practice throughout the organization at all levels. Meeting these expectations is an essential component of a Magnet organization *(www. nursecredentialing.org/Magnet.aspx)*.

Leaders should use action planning to address building blocks when developing the organizational culture and capacity for evidence-based practice. Beginning with incorporating evidence-based practice into strategic documents, actions plans include the mission statement, vision, strategic plan, job descriptions, performance appraisals, and committee functions. Leadership that demonstrates and expects evidence-based practice will promote its use in clinical and operational decision making. Dialogue must be conducted during important meetings about use of evidence for decision making. Prioritizing and holding leaders and clinicians accountable for the work are essential. The use of multiple, interactive strategies will promote adoption of evidence-based practice at all levels in the organization. Nurse leaders also may notice an important urgency and increased volume of data analysis and nurse informatics resource needs as evidence-based practice becomes the norm.

CURRENT ISSUES AND TRENDS

Senior leaders have responsibility for developing an organizational culture promoting evidence-based health care. The organizational context is (Greenhalgh et al., 2005) resulting in a complex and dynamic culture that is unique to each practice setting. Research is needed to better understand the role organizational context plays in impacting adoption of evidence-based practice and effective strategies to impact the organizational context, thus encouraging adoption of evidence-based care delivery (Stetler et al., 2009; Titler, 2010). A related and emerging priority for implementation science is to better understand how nurse leaders can promote adoption of evidence-based health care to improve quality and reduce costs (Institute of Medicine, 2010; Luther & Savitz, 2012; Sandström et al., 2011).

Leadership is essential in developing an organizational culture promoting innovation and evidence-based practice. Leadership is one important contextual factor impacting an organization's ability to consistently use evidence to inform practice (Aarons, 2006; Davies et al., 2006; Fleuren et al., 2004; Vaughn et al., 2002; World Health Organization, 2007). An exhaustive body of research on barriers consistently finds that leadership support is essential for success. Leaders have a responsibility to provide resources, structures, and processes that move teams beyond barriers to facilitating evidence-based practice. A better understanding of specific leadership strategies is needed such as that spotlighted in the Research Note (Dogherty et al., 2012; Gifford et al., 2011).

Nursing leadership is needed to meet a growing demand for patient-centered care, expectations for improved quality and safety, increased provision of evidence-based practice, and increasing public accountability and transparency (Institute of Medicine, 2008; The Joint Commission, 2011). Pay for performance through CMS using value-based purchasing has grabbed the attention of health care leaders (AHRQ, 2002; CMS, 2011). This reimbursement structure reflects the importance of comparing key quality indicators to benchmarks and will likely expand to include additional quality indicators and private payer reimbursement structures. The financial pressure for provision of evidence-based practice will continue to grow.

Other recent developments at the federal level will also impact delivery of evidence-based nursing and have a long lasting imprint on health care. The Health Information Technology for Economic and Clinical Health (HITECH) Act was enacted as part of the American Recovery and Reinvestment Act to stimulate the economy and improve the delivery of health care (DHHS, 2009). The HITECH Act provides incentives for adoption and implementation of electronic health records (EHRs) while enhancing privacy and security for patients and providing incentives for practitioners and hospitals to engage in meaningful use. The first stage focuses on interoperability or sharing of health care information about immunizations, laboratory data and outbreak surveillance (CMS, 2010). The transition to using EHRs is a focus of health care leaders because of the expected contribution to safety through accessibility of stored health data, evidence-based clinical decision support, improved communication about patients' health and health care needs, and reduced risk for medical errors (Institute of Medicine, 2011b). The opportunity for enhanced data mining of large health care databases will be a boon for researchers (AHRQ, 2011) and nursing leaders to track and trend the provision of evidence-based health care. Nurses will play key roles in using these data to improve quality and manage cost.

Nursing leaders must stay abreast of resources and standards that are available to promote evidence-based care. National patient safety goals established by The Joint Commission include a growing number of evidence-based standards. Recent standards for catheter-association urinary tract infections reflect a growing intolerance for hospital acquired infections *(www.jointcommission.org/standards_information/npsgs.aspx)*. The Institute for Healthcare Improvement *(www.ihi.org/)* has easily accessed resources that promote collaborative learning while continually raising the bar for organizations and nursing leaders. The National Guideline Clearinghouse, sponsored by the Agency for Healthcare Research and Quality, provides a large repository for international guidelines, offering free access to guideline summaries and links to full reports *(www.guideline.gov)*. Nursing leaders have a responsibility to use these resources and to stay abreast of a changing health care agenda aimed at delivering increased quality and safety for patients and consumers while managing costs.

The trend for evaluating evidence and making recommendations has evolved in recent years. In the past, only meta-analyses and randomized trials were considered sufficient research or evidence base for making practices changes. Current inclusion of other research designs and other supportive evidence for making practice changes is growing. Increasingly, it is accepted that not all practices have a clear research base for making practices changes. Accordingly, the evidence hierarchy, or grading systems, have also changed. Whereas individual research studies were previously graded by research design, the current trend is toward grading the whole body of evidence practice recommendations (AHRQ, 2012; GRADE, 2012).

As the demand for evidence-based care has increased, there has been a proliferation of guidelines brought forth by federal agencies, specialty organizations, special interests groups, and organizations. Instead of independently exploring evidence, nurse leaders can utilize evidence-based recommendations from clinical practice guidelines and tailor them to the organization, population, or setting. Methodology for guideline development has varied. Nurse leaders must be able to evaluate clinical practice guidelines for rigor, bias, and generalizability before adopting them. New tools, such as the AGREE II (Brouwers et al., 2010), for evaluating clinical practice guidelines are evolving, and nurse leaders should become familiar with them. Standards for clinical practice guidelines (Institute of Medicine, 2011a) have recently emerged and will promote consistent, rigorous, and unbiased methods for guideline development.

Nursing has a long history of valuing provision of high-quality care and using the best evidence for care improvements. Despite the many years of work, there are many challenges to using evidence-based care in the current health care environment. Nurses in leadership positions have responsibility for supporting evidence-based clinical care as well as evidence-based operational decision making. Models outline the process for updating practices that are applicable when addressing clinical and operational issues. Implementation is one of the most challenging steps in the evidence-based practice process. Multiple reinforcing and interactive strategies are needed over phases for implementation. Effective, evidence-based implementation strategies can be combined to create a highly influential implementation plan.

Nursing leaders can build a strong program supporting evidence-based care delivery using a building block approach. Building on the organization's vision, mission, and value for high-quality care provides a foundation for success. Nurse leaders must connect their evidence-based initiatives to the organization's vision, mission, values, and infrastructure to garner support and resources for provision of the best care delivery. Implementing evidence-based practices is best accomplished by understanding the interplay between organization and unit factors that are supported through the organization infrastructure. The infrastructure supporting evidence-based practice is essential for creating the desired organization and unit culture and capacity. Communicating the business case for evidence-based practice will help nurses articulate their impact in a way that will be heard by senior leaders. Leadership is a vital ingredient to success. Complementary skills are needed within all nursing roles to create effective evidence-based practice teams. Every nurse has a responsibility to support evidence-based care delivery to improve outcomes for our patients and their families, staff, and the organization.

CASE STUDY

A member of your general surgery unit staff approaches you with a practice question. This senior nurse wants to know whether bowel sounds are a good indicator for return of gastrointestinal (GI) motility for her patients after abdominal surgery. As a nurse manager, you recognize this as an opportunity to build in evidence-based practice for your unit. The following benefits are anticipated:

- Improving care
- Empowering staff nurses
- Developing a unit culture that uses evidence in daily practice

What Are Your Next Steps?

You recognize that you will need a strong team, a review of the evidence, an implementation plan, and an evaluation method. Partnering with experts in the organization will best match the skills and expertise needed. The staff nurse raising the question is the unit quality improvement coordinator. She is already an opinion leader and is ideally suited to lead a team; you are committed to helping her. The team develops an action plan and divides responsibility for the project. Team members tackle each of the following: reviewing the literature, developing a questionnaire of current nursing practice within the hospital, notifying physicians of the practice up for review, developing a physician practice questionnaire, developing an educational poster based on the literature review, and developing strategies for implementing a potential practice change.

An early obstacle occurs when you have trouble finding nursing research on auscultation of bowel sounds. This is a good time to add a team member who can tackle the search, critique, and synthesis of the evidence. The nursing questionnaire is revised and sent to a national group of experts to determine current practice patterns. Certified wound, ostomy, and continence nurse practitioners are identified as appropriate experts to provide the team with the necessary guidance. Simultaneously, the physician's practice questionnaire is sent to general surgeons within the organization. A secondary analysis of basic science research, a small body of research and other literature, and the questionnaire findings indicate that bowel sound assessment is not the best indicator of return of GI motility following abdominal surgery. A change in practice is needed.

A traditional practice, such as bowel sound assessment, can be difficult to change. Multiple interventions are needed (Cullen & Adams, 2012). The team decides to use multiple strategies for implementation: educational posters, change champions, opinion leaders, resource manual, practice prompts, audit-feedback, and EHR documentation changes. Processes and outcomes are reviewed through the evaluation. The team reviews nursing knowledge, compliance with documentation of return of GI motility, nurses' perception of facilitators of the practice change, and rates of bowel obstruction and paralytic ileus. The data suggest that nursing documentation of return of flatus improves (60%; pre-group; 88%; post-group) and that documentation of first bowel movement also improves (60%; pre-group; 88%; post-group) and could be better, so a task force works with the nursing informatics group to revise the documentation process. Bowel obstruction rates are lower in the post-group (0%; compared to the pre-group 4%); and paralytic ileus rates decrease from 12.5% in the pre-group to 0% in the post-group, creating some confidence that eliminating bowel assessment is not causing any patient harm.

This project was successful in many ways, yet like so many evidence-based practice changes, additional work is needed. The unit quality improvement coordinator will now complete reinfusion and integration through the unit's quality improvement efforts. A fundamental practice question has been answered, and patient care improvements continue through the evidence-based practice process (Madsen et al., 2005).

CRITICAL THINKING EXERCISE

Katie Gardner is a nurse practitioner in otolaryngology–head and neck surgery at a Midwest tertiary care facility. Her patient population often requires an altered airway, including tracheostomy, for treatment. Tracheostomy care is a frequently challenging nursing intervention with conflicting practice information. Tracheostomy care policies and procedures are often based on experience and expert opinion. Tracheostomy care, as taught at Melissa's undergraduate program, less than 5 years ago, differs from current practices in the otolaryngology clinic. More recent research evidence is specific to patient populations that are intubated and differ from patients undergoing tracheostomy for head and neck surgery. One controversial example of practice variation is the instillation of saline before tracheal suctioning (Hudak & Bond-Domb, 1996; Rauen et al., 2008). Supporting research is dated but remains a classic. Unfortunately, the Hudak study has not been replicated (Hudak & Bond-Domb, 1996). Katie wants to take the lead in developing an evidence-based policy for tracheostomy care that is universal for patients with an altered airway due to tracheostomy.

What process does she follow? Please respond to the following questions:

1. What are the issues for pursuing an evidenced-based, standardized policy for tracheostomy care?
2. Is this a problem or knowledge focused project?
3. How can she determine if this is a priority for the organization?
4. What are the target patient populations?
5. Who are the stakeholders and potential team members?
6. Why is it important to involve a nurse manager?
7. Why is a review of current literature important?
8. How do you grade/score "classic" research studies and expert opinions?
9. What are the variations in practice? Are the variations based on evidence?
10. Why is it necessary to obtain the approval of the proposed policy from experts in nursing practice?
11. After developing an evidence-based recommendation:
    a. Who needs education and competency assurance?
    b. What are key process and outcome indicators to measure?
    c. How should the key indicators be measured?
    d. Who can assist with the ongoing compliance with the practice change?

Quality and Safety

Luc R. Pelletier

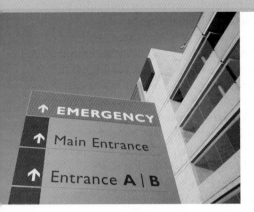

℮volve WEBSITE

http://evolve.elsevier.com/Huber/leadership/

In this era of health care reform, accountability is taking center stage. Health care quality and safety principles and practices form the foundation of an accessible, reliable enterprise. Health care quality is an art and science that continues to evolve. Its relevance was heightened with ongoing reports from the Institute of Medicine (IOM) and other national organizations related to health care and health care quality. Well before these reports were published, however, professional nurses assumed key roles in the business of measuring, monitoring, and improving health care quality and safety. The news of health care errors is not new. Nurses have typically taken a leadership role in performance and quality improvement and continue to do so in their roles as board members, executives, chief quality officers, health care quality professionals, enterprise risk managers, and safety officers. It is important to note that identifying opportunities for improvement and continuously improving services is everyone's job. Where once there was a dedicated quality department in an organization, now best-in-class health care organizations train everyone in performance improvement models and

Photo used with permission from Photos.com.

techniques. It would be difficult to describe the entire field of health care quality and patient safety in one chapter. In this chapter a large amount of information and emerging trends have been distilled, and specific content has been targeted toward nurse managers. This system overview includes industrial, health care, and emerging models of quality; the costs of poor quality; health care quality leadership and planning strategies; resources available to the nurse manager; health care safety; health care enterprise risk management; and education and policy initiatives to promote quality and safety in professional nursing.

DEFINITIONS

There are many concepts and terms related to health care quality and safety. Definitions are:

Benchmarking is a tool to assist in quality-of-care decision making. Most recently, it has been defined as "an improvement process in which an organization measures its strategies, operations, or internal process performance against that of best-in-class organizations within or outside its industry, determines how those organizations achieved their performance levels, and uses that information to improve its own performance" (Sower et al., 2008, p. 4). **Best-in-class**

291

is defined as "a standard that [an organization] should aspire to attain" (Sower et al., 2008, p. 5).

Continuous quality improvement (CQI) is defined by the American Society for Quality (ASQ) as "a philosophy and attitude for analyzing capabilities and processes and improving them repeatedly to achieve customer satisfaction" (ASQ, 2007). Further, the Agency for Healthcare Research and Quality defined CQI as "techniques for measuring quality problems, designing interventions and their implementation, along with process re-measurements" (Shojania et al., 2004, p. 16). **Evidence-based practice** is defined by Sackett and colleagues (1996) as "the conscientious, explicit, and judicious use of current best evidence in making decisions about the care of individual patients" (p. 71). More recently, evidence-based practices have been defined as "those clinical and administrative practices that have been proven to consistently produce specific, intended results" (Hyde et al., 2003, p. 15).

Health care quality indicators "provide an important tool for measuring the quality of care. Indicators are based on evidence of 'best practices' in health care that have been proven to lead to improvements in health status and thus can be used to assess, track, and monitor provider performance" (Hussey et al., 2007, p. i). A **patient safety practice** is "a type of process or structure whose application reduces the probability of adverse events resulting from exposure to the health care system across a range of conditions or procedures" (Shojania et al., 2001, p. 29).

A **performance measure** is "a quantitative tool (for example, rate, ratio, index, percentage) that provides an indication of an organization's performance in relation to a specified process or outcome" (The Joint Commission, 2011a, ¶ 113). A **performance measurement system** is "an entity composed of a set of process and/or outcome measures of performance; processes for collecting, analyzing and disseminating these measures from multiple organizations; and an automated database that together can be used to facilitate performance improvement in health care organizations. A measurement system must be able to generate both internal comparisons of each participating organization's performance over time, and external comparisons of performance among participating organizations" (The Joint Commission, 2011c, ¶ 1).

Quality refers to characteristics of and the pursuit of excellence. **Health care quality** is defined as "the degree to which health services for individuals and populations increase the likelihood of desired health outcomes and are consistent with current professional knowledge" (Lohr, 1990, pp. 128-129). **Patient engagement** is defined as "actions an individual must make to obtain the greatest benefit from the health care services available to them" (Center for Advancing Health, 2010, p. 2). A **performance/quality improvement program** is an overarching organizational strategy to ensure accountability of all employees, incorporating evidence-based health care quality indicators, to continuously improve care delivered to various populations. It is the organization's blueprint for achieving and maintaining performance excellence.

Risk adjustment is a process in which differences among clients or variables such as age or disease severity are weighted or adjusted for in outcomes analyses or benchmarking efforts (Maas & Kerr, 1999). **Enterprise risk management (ERM)** is defined as "a structured analytical process that focuses on identifying and eliminating the financial impact and volatility of a portfolio of risks rather than on risk avoidance alone. Essential to this approach is an understanding that risk can be managed to gain competitive advantage" (Carroll, 2003, p. 1). An **ERM program** is defined as "an organization-wide program to identify risks, control occurrences, prevent damage, and control legal liability; it is a process whereby risks to the institution are evaluated and controlled."

A **sentinel event** is "an unexpected occurrence involving death or serious physical or psychological injury, or the risk thereof. Serious injury specifically includes loss of limb or function. The phrase 'or the risk thereof' includes any process variation for which a recurrence would carry a significant chance of a serious adverse outcome. Such events are called 'sentinel' because they signal the need for immediate investigation and response" (The Joint Commission, 2012c, ¶ 2).

Standards are defined as written value statements. These statements form the rules that apply to key processes and the results that can be expected when the processes are performed according to specifications. The three basic types of standards for health care quality are (1) structure, (2) process, and (3) outcome standards (Katz & Green, 1997). **Total quality management (TQM)** is described as follows (ASQ, 2013): TQM is a term coined by the Naval Air Systems

Command to describe its Japanese style management approach to quality improvement. "Since then, TQM has taken on many meanings. Simply put, it is a management approach to long-term success through customer satisfaction. TQM is based on all members of an organization participating in improving processes, products, services and the culture in which they work. The methods for implementing this approach are found in the teachings of such quality leaders as Philip B. Crosby, W. Edwards Deming, Armand V. Feigenbaum, Kaoru Ishikawa, and Joseph M. Juran".

HEALTH CARE QUALITY IN THE TWENTY-FIRST CENTURY

Professional nurses have an obligation to reasonably ensure that the care they provide is evidence-based and that work processes are consumer-centric. Providing "quality" health care is "the degree to which health services for individuals and populations increase the likelihood of desired health outcomes and are consistent with current professional knowledge" (Lohr, 1990, pp. 128-129). Nurses, as leaders and managers, have served as health care quality professionals and have promoted standardization, measurement, and continuous quality improvement in a myriad of care delivery settings. Professional nurses have consistently held the practice of quality management in high regard and have the effective care of clients and families as their primary focus. Nurses are bound by their professional associatizon's *Code of Ethics* (Fowler, 2008) and scope of professional standards to participate in the continuous improvement of the services they provide. Specifically, in provision 3, the "nurse promotes, advocates for and strives to protect the health, *safety* and rights of the patient" (Fowler, 2008, p. 143). Recent health reform legislation serves as a "call to action" for professional nurses—from frontline clinicians to executives—to be actively involved in health care transformation. This includes ensuring that patients and families receive safe and effective health care (Institute of Medicine, 2011, p. 22).

Although the manufacturing industry has dutifully explored ways to enhance its business practices, health care has lagged behind, and only within the past 30 years or so has it embraced improvement concepts. Health care has borrowed and applied models of continuous quality improvement and TQM with principles and practices originally developed for the manufacturing industry. As industry has had its quality gurus, so too has the health care quality movement been fostered by health care professionals who have focused on continuous improvement.

Donald M. Berwick, MD, co-author of the book *Curing Health Care: New Strategies for Quality Improvement* (Berwick et al., 1990), was an early pioneer in identifying how the concepts of TQM programs could apply to health care. In 1991, the National Demonstration Project on Quality Improvement in Health Care was conducted as a collaboration between members of the John A. Hartford Foundation, the Harvard Community Health Plan, the Juran Institute, the Hospital Corporation of America, and other health care organizations (Institute for Healthcare Improvement [IHI], 2004). The goal was to apply the methods and tools of industrial quality improvement in a variety of organizations to determine whether they could apply to a service industry. Berwick was a principal investigator for this project. As a result of this endeavor, the IHI was founded and became an early advocate for the concepts of process improvement and team problem solving in health care organizations. In 2010, Berwick was appointed by President Obama as administrator of the Centers for Medicare & Medicaid Services. He served for 18 months and was responsible for introducing the "triple aim": improving the patient care experience, improving population health, and reducing health costs (Berwick et al., 2008). His administration was also responsible for initiating major transformative changes under the new health reform legislation.

In the mid-1990s, The Joint Commission (TJC) began incorporating the principles of continuous quality improvement into its revised standards. Starting in 1996, the Institute of Medicine (IOM), through its Committee on Quality of Health Care in America (CQHCA), has convened the nation's quality leaders and other public and private stakeholders to assess and improve health care for all. These leaders have promoted continuous quality improvement in health care through education, research, and evaluation. Through their dedication and insights, they have defined health care quality for this generation and those ahead. Tenets promoted by these health care

---

BOX 17-1   INSTITUTE OF MEDICINE'S SPECIFIC AIMS FOR HEALTH CARE QUALITY IMPROVEMENT

- *Safe:* "Patients should not be harmed by the care that is intended to help them, nor should harm come to those who work in health care" (IOM, Committee on the National Quality Report on Health Care Delivery, 2001, p. 47).
- *Effective:* "Refers to care that is based on the use of systematically acquired evidence to determine whether an intervention, such as a preventive service, diagnostic test, or therapy, produces better outcomes than do alternatives—including the alternative to do nothing" (IOM, Committee on the National Quality Report on Health Care Delivery, 2001, p. 49). Evidence-based practice requires that those who give care consistently avoid both underuse of effective care and overuse of ineffective care that is more likely to harm than help the patient (Chassin, 1997).
- *Patient-centered:* "Refers to health care that establishes a partnership among practitioners, patients, and their families (when appropriate) to ensure that decisions respect patients' wants, needs, and preferences; and that patients have the education and support they need to make decisions and participate in their own care" (IOM, Committee on the National Quality Report on Health Care Delivery, 2001, p. 50).
- *Timeliness:* "Refers to obtaining needed care and minimizing unnecessary delays in getting that care" (IOM, Committee on the National Quality Report on Health Care Delivery, 2001, p. 53).
- *Efficient:* "Refers to a health care system where resources are used to get the best value for the money spent" (Palmer & Torgerson, 1999, p. 1136). "The opposite of efficiency is waste; the use of resources without benefit to the patients a system is intended to help. There are at least two ways to improve efficiency: (a) reduce quality waste and (b) reduce administrative or production costs" (IOM, CQHCA, 2001, p. 54).
- *Equitable:* "Providing care that does not vary in quality because of personal characteristics such as gender, ethnicity, geographic location, and socioeconomic status" (IOM, CQHCA, 2001, p. 6).

From Pelletier, L.R., & Hoffman, J.A. (2002). A framework for selecting performance measures for opioid treatment programs. *Journal for Healthcare Quality, 24*(3), 25. Reprinted with permission from the National Association for Healthcare Quality.

---

leaders and organizations, and embraced by health care professionals, include the following:

- Processes and systems are the problems, not people.
- Standardization of processes is key to managing work and people.
- Quality can be enhanced only in safe, non-punitive work cultures.
- Quality measurement and monitoring is everyone's job.
- The impetus for quality monitoring is not primarily for accreditation or regulatory compliance, but rather as a planned part of an organization's culture to continuously enhance and improve its services, based on continuous feedback from employees and customers.
- Consumers and stakeholders must be included in all phases of quality improvement planning.
- Consensus among all stakeholders must be gained to have an impact on quality and safety.
- Health policy should include a focus on continuous enhancement of quality and safety.

A framework for understanding health care improvement has been proposed by the IOM Committee on Quality of Health Care in America (Box 17-1). These six aims for health care quality improvement propose that health care systems ensure that care is safe, effective, patient-centered, timely, efficient, and equitable.

COLLABORATION AND HEALTH CARE QUALITY AS PROFESSIONAL NURSING IMPERATIVES

Collaboration should be a goal of any interaction, regardless of the workplace or situation. Collaboration is an imperative set by the American Nurses Association (ANA). The ANA, in its release of a revised *Code of Ethics for Nurses with Interpretive Statements* (Fowler, 2008), proposed that "The nurse collaborates with other health professionals and the public in promoting community, national, and international efforts to meet health needs" (Provision 8, p. 143). Collaborative partnerships are part of this imperative and shape the way professional nurses act clinically and how they participate in performance and quality improvement efforts.

Collaboration is about relationships. Conflict is typically the result of an undeveloped or poor interpersonal relationship with a colleague. To overcome conflicts, it is necessary to strengthen, not shy away from, the relationship of the two opposing parties. The Pew Health Professions Commission (PHPC) talked about practicing relationship-centered care as one of 21 health profession competencies for the twenty-first century (O'Neil & PHPC, 1998, p. 23). Relationship-centered care in this context surely involves nurse and client/family interactions, but it also stresses the importance of collaborative interdisciplinary relationships. These 21 competencies are necessary ingredients for effective professional relationships and can become guideposts for successful professional working relationships within a continuous improvement framework.

The 21 competencies also include a professional nurse's responsibility and accountability to health care quality. The specific statements related to health care quality include "Take responsibility for quality of care and health outcomes at all levels," and "Contribute to continuous improvement of the health care system" (O'Neill & PHPC, 1998, pp. 29-43) (Box 17-2).

INDUSTRIAL MODELS OF QUALITY

Industrial models have heavily influenced the way quality is currently understood and measured in health care settings across the continuum. Industry leaders who have influenced nursing's understanding of health care quality include Walter Shewhart, Joseph Juran, Philip Crosby, and W. Edwards Deming. These leaders provided blueprints from which nursing performance and quality improvement programs have been derived.

Shewhart (Deming, 2000b) explored causes of variation in work processes. He quantified these variations, categorizing variables as common or special cause. His *Plan, Do, Check, Act (PDCA)* model is probably the most frequently used in health care quality settings today, as follows (Figure 17-1):

- *Plan* (identify an issue and plan a process improvement)
- *Do* (map the current and proposed process, collect data, and analyze the results)
- *Check* (propose a solution and check the results of the new process)
- *Act* (adopt, adapt, or abandon the solution)

BOX 17-2 TWENTY-ONE COMPETENCIES FOR THE TWENTY-FIRST CENTURY

1. Embrace a personal ethic of social responsibility and service.
2. Exhibit ethical behavior in all professional activities.
3. Provide evidence-based, clinically competent care.
4. Incorporate the multiple determinants of health in clinical care.
5. Apply knowledge of the new sciences.
6. Demonstrate critical thinking, reflection, and problem-solving skills.
7. Understand the role of primary care.
8. Rigorously practice preventive health care.
9. Integrate population-based care and services into practice.
10. Improve access to health care for those with unmet health needs.
11. Practice relationship-centered care with individuals and families.
12. Provide culturally sensitive care to a diverse society.
13. Partner with communities in health care decisions.
14. Use communication and information technology effectively and appropriately.
15. Work in interdisciplinary teams.
16. Ensure care that balances individual, professional, system, and societal needs.
17. Practice leadership.
18. Take responsibility for quality of care and health outcomes at all levels.
19. Contribute to continuous improvement of the health care system.
20. Advocate for public policy that promotes and protects the health of the public.
21. Continue to learn and help others learn.

From O'Neil, E.H., & the Pew Health Professions Commission (PHPC). (1998). *Recreating health professional practice for a new century: The fourth report of the Pew Health Professions Commission.* San Francisco: PHPC.

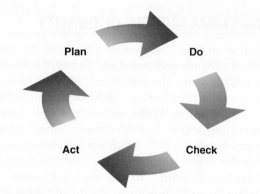

FIGURE 17-1 PDCA (Plan, Do, Check, Act) cycle.

Shewhart also provided the industrial community with statistical process control techniques that are used widely today. Deming (2000a, b) adopted his work and refined it.

Juran (1989) defined quality as "fitness for use." Quality, in his work, was defined as freedom from defects plus value and continuously meeting customer expectations. His approach to quality centered around the use of interdisciplinary teams that used diagnostic tools to understand why industrial processes produce a product not fit for use. His framework included a three-pronged approach: quality planning, quality control, and quality improvement. Quality planning:

> ...establishes the design of a product, service, or process that will meet customer, business, and operational needs to produce the product before it is produced. Quality planning follows a universal sequence of steps, as follows:
> - Identify customers and target markets
> - Discover hidden and unmet customer needs
> - Translate these needs into product or service requirements: a means to meet their needs (new standards, specifications, etc.)
> - Develop a service or product that exceeds customers' needs
> - Develop the processes that will provide the service, or create the product, in the most efficient way
> - Transfer these designs to the organization and the operating forces to be carried out (Juran Institute, 2009, ¶ 1-2).

Crosby viewed quality in production terms of zero defects and measured quality in relation to conformance to requirements. He believed that the results or products of a company are made by people. He focused on systems and the consequences of poor quality. He emphasized doing the right thing the first time to prevent waste. Waste and rework were seen as costly and good managers were those who prevented costly mistakes.

In addition to PDCA, Deming focused on statistical process control techniques and on continuous quality improvement through a culture of quality. He is credited as being influential in the success of Japanese industries. He proposed 14 points to help management staff understand and commit to quality. These points are listed in Box 17-3 (Deming, 2000a, b). These 14 points, although created just after World War II, have heavily influenced health care's adoption of quality principles.

BOX 17-3 DEMING'S 14 POINTS FOR QUALITY

1. Create constancy of purpose toward improving products and services.
2. Adopt the new philosophy.
3. Cease dependence on inspection to achieve quality.
4. End the practice of awarding business on the basis of cost alone.
5. Improve constantly and forever every process for planning, production, and service.
6. Institute training on the job.
7. Adopt and institute leadership aimed at helping people do their jobs better.
8. Drive out fear by promoting two-way communication.
9. Break down barriers between departments.
10. Eliminate exhortations for the workforce in such forms as posters and slogans; these methods tend to create adversarial relationships.
11. Eliminate numerical quotas for productivity; instead have leaders promote continuous quality improvement (CQI).
12. Permit pride of workmanship by removing the barriers that prevent this.
13. Encourage education and self-improvement for all workers.
14. Define management's commitment to CQI and their obligation to implement these points.

From Deming, W.E. (2000a). *The new economics for industry, government, education.* Cambridge, MA: MIT Center for Advanced Engineering Studies; and Deming, W.E. (2000b). *Out of the crisis.* Cambridge, MA: MIT Center for Advanced Engineering Studies.

STANDARDS OF QUALITY

Health care quality standards and measures can be grouped in three categories: structure, process, and outcome. Donabedian (1980) developed the initial theoretical model that identified that quality can be measured using these three aspects. Donabedian's (1980) framework of structure, process, and outcomes is the most widely referenced model of quality; professional nurses have used this model to develop performance and quality improvement programs and conduct evidence-based improvement studies and research. Standards essentially define quality, against which performance and outcomes are measured. Standards and measures are typically developed from benchmarking activities and reviews of best practices. Therefore the selection of standards and measures is a critical activity in the performance and quality improvement process. Actually, standards establish the baseline against which measurement and evaluation are conducted. Therefore it is critical to decide who determines standards and which standards are selected to define quality. Over the past 20 years, national groups have been formed to gain consensus on performance standards and measures. One such entity is the National Quality Forum (NQF), a not-for-profit, public-private membership organization created to develop and implement a national strategy for health care quality measurement and reporting.

Structure Standards and Measures

Structure standards, or structural measures, focus on the internal characteristics of the organization and its personnel. They answer the following questions. Is an infrastructure in place and tools accessible to allow quality to exist? Is the structure of the organization set up to allow for the effective, efficient delivery of services? For example, a structural standard for a long-term care facility might be to have an adequate mix of registered nurses and nursing assistants on site to ensure that comprehensive care is delivered. For specialized areas, structure standards may address whether there are enough specialists, "hospitalists" or "intensivists" to ensure quality care. Certain committees, policy statements, rules and regulations, or manuals, forms, or contracts may be needed. Structure standards regulate the environment to ensure quality. Human, organizational, and physical resources, as well as environmental characteristics, are examples of structure elements.

Process Standards and Measures

Process standards and measures focus on whether the activities within an organization are being conducted appropriately, effectively, and efficiently. Process measures focus on the behaviors of the professional nurse as a provider of care. The interventions recommended in a clinical practice guideline or best practice are examples of process standards. They relate to what the nurse will be doing and the process the nurse should follow to ensure effective, evidence-based care. Process standards look at activities, interventions, and the sequence of caregiving events, sometimes referred to as *work flow*. Typically, processes are assessed by audits, observational studies, or work flow analyses. Examples of process standards include the following: a nursing assessment is completed within 24 hours of admission; client calls are returned within 1 hour of the initial call; a face-to-face assessment is completed within 1 hour for seclusion and restraints.

Outcome Standards and Measures

Outcome standards and measures refer to whether the services provided by the organization make any difference: Were they effective? They answer important questions about the services that nurses provide and whether those services make a difference to the clients or to the health status of the population. Outcome standards address physical health status, mental health status, social and physical function, health attitudes/knowledge/behavior, utilization of services, and the client's perception and satisfaction with the care received. *Outcome* refers to a change in the current or future health status attributed to antecedent health care and client attributes of health care. Outcome standards present the possibility of measuring the effectiveness, quality, and time and resources allocated for care. Examples of outcome measures include the following: percentage of patients whose activities of daily living have improved by 80%; percentage of clients who have stopped smoking after 12 weeks of intensive psychoeducational therapy.

In measuring quality, both structure and process parameters are important but they are not sufficient in determining whether the care led to an effective outcome or whether the client learned, recovered, or improved his or her health status. Over the years, the emphasis on structure, process, and outcome aspects of health care has varied. Ultimately, various stakeholders are interested in knowing whether care resulted in a positive, expected clinical outcome, based on objective, measurable criteria.

When developing a performance and quality improvement program, nurse managers are cautioned to not start by creating new standards and measures. Rather, a literature review will undoubtedly yield measures from which to choose. These measures have typically been tested for reliability and validity and have been piloted in the field. National repositories of performance measures can be found at:

- American Nurses Association National Database for Nursing Quality Indicators®
- Agency for Healthcare Research and Quality
- National Quality Forum
- Leapfrog Group
- The Cochrane Library
- Specialty professional associations and societies

Selection criteria can then be adopted and measures chosen for a specific intervention or program. A number of selection criteria guideline statements have been developed, including the performance measurement evaluation criteria from the National Quality Forum (National Quality Forum, 2011). The performance measurement attributes common to these entities' guideline statements have been reported in the set of criteria proposed to be used for a national health care quality report (Institute of Medicine [IOM], Committee on the National Quality Report on Health Care Delivery, 2001). Common performance measurement selection criteria are listed in Box 17-4 (Pelletier & Hoffman, 2002). The adoption of these performance measurement selection criteria is the first step in developing a comprehensive performance measurement system.

More recently, an international working group on health care quality indicators defined the following as selection criteria (The Commonwealth Fund, 2004), which are similar to those previously cited:

- *Feasibility:* indicators already being collected by one or more countries
- *Scientific soundness:* indicators that are valid and reliable; existing reviews of the scientific evidence and approval by a consensus process in one or more countries

---

BOX 17-4   COMMON PERFORMANCE MEASUREMENT SELECTION CRITERIA*

- *Relevance:* The measure should address features of the health care system applicable to health professionals, policy makers, and consumers.
- *Meaningfulness and interpretability:* The measure should be understandable to at least one of the audiences. It should help inform them about the important issues or concerns.
- *Scientific or clinical evidence:* The measure should be based on evidence documenting the links between the interventions, clinical processes, and/or outcomes it addresses.
- *Reliability or reproducibility:* The measure should produce the same results when repeated in the same population and setting.
- *Feasibility:* The measure should be specified precisely. Collection of data for the measure should be inexpensive and logistically feasible.
- *Validity:* The measure should make sense (face validity), correlate well with other measures of the same aspects of care (construct validity), and capture meaningful aspects of care (content validity).
- *Health importance:* The measure should include the prevalence of the health condition to which it applies and the seriousness of the health outcomes affected.

From Pelletier, L.R., & Hoffman, J.A. (2002). A framework for selecting performance measures for opioid treatment programs. *Journal for Healthcare Quality, 24*(3), 26. Reprinted with permission from the National Association for Healthcare Quality.
*NOTE: Criteria are listed in order of their frequency, with the one mentioned most often listed first. The same label for a criterion can have different meanings depending on the framework, because the criteria are not standardized. The definitions, rather than the labels, were used to construct the figure. Feasibility was used as a category covering several criteria in some of the frameworks and as a single criterion in others. Parts of this figure were adapted from NCQA's list of desirable attributes for HEDIS measures (IOM, Committee on the National Quality Report on Health Care Delivery, 2001, p. 81).

- *Interpretability:* indicators that allowed a clear conclusion (a clear direction) for policy makers
- *Actionability:* measures of processes or outcomes that could be directly affected by the health care entity
- *Importance:* indicators reflective of important health conditions representing a major share of the burden of disease, health care costs, or policy-maker priorities.

EMERGING MODELS OF HEALTH CARE PERFORMANCE AND QUALITY ASSESSMENT AND MANAGEMENT

A number of industry-based models for quality management and measurement have been adopted by the health care industry over the past two decades. These include Six Sigma, Lean Enterprise, the Baldrige National Quality Award, ISO 9000, and the concept of high-performance organizations. These models are briefly described in the following sections.

Six Sigma

A strategy developed by Motorola and implemented successfully at General Electric (GE) and AlliedSignal Companies provided an innovative approach to reduce variation and error rates. Not surprisingly, the Six Sigma approach that these companies use is similar to tried-and-true approaches historically deployed by health care quality professionals, as previously described. In the Six Sigma breakthrough strategy, errors are measured in defects per million opportunities (dpmo). Six Sigma is achieved when the organization reaches an error or defect rate of 3.4 or less per one million. As a result of its implementation and investment of $6 million since 1995, GE boasted financial benefits of over $600 million in 1998 (Harry & Schroeder, 2000). AlliedSignal reported a 1.9% growth in operating margin in the first quarter, 1999, and "cumulative impact of Six Sigma has been a savings in excess of $2 billion in direct costs" (Harry & Schroeder, 2000, p. ix). The Six Sigma strategy (Harry & Schroeder, 2000) is remarkably similar to Juran's problem-solving strategy (Plsek & Omnias, 1989), which has been applied to health care. Table 17-1 illustrates these similarities (Pelletier, 2000).

Lean Enterprise

Lean Enterprise is a model of quality measurement that was originally associated with Deming but reintroduced to the United States by Womack in the mid-1990s (Jones & Womack, 2003). The premise of this model is that operational waste in an organization needs to be eliminated. Nightingale presents seven principles of lean thinking:

1. Adopt a holistic approach to enterprise transformation.
2. Identify relevant stakeholders and determine their value propositions.
3. Focus on enterprise effectiveness before efficiency.
4. Address internal and external enterprise interdependencies.
5. Ensure stability and flow within and across the enterprise.
6. Cultivate leadership to support and drive enterprise behaviors.
7. Emphasize organizational learning (Nightingale, 2009, p. 8).

Malcolm Baldrige National Quality Award Program

The Baldrige National Quality Award (BNQA) establishes a set of performance standards that define a total quality organization. Named after the Secretary of Commerce, the BNQA "was established by Congress in 1987 to enhance the competitiveness and performance of U.S. businesses" (National Institute of Standards and Technology, 2007, p. 1). The standards in seven areas of excellence are (1) leadership, (2) strategic planning, (3) customer and market focus (focus on patients, other customers, and markets), (4) information and analysis, (5) human resource focus, (6) process management, and (7) business results (organizational performance results). Organizations committed to quality improvement choose to adopt the BNQA approach as another means of defining and improving their organizational processes to achieve quality outcomes. Manufacturing, service, and small business were the original award categories, but in 1999, education and health care were added. With the trend in health care to adopt industry applications and measure sets for quality improvement, it was fitting that the health care industry was recognized as one that could benefit from participating in this program. It is appropriate for health care entities to strive

TABLE 17-1	COMPARISON OF SIX SIGMA BREAKTHROUGH STRATEGY AND JURAN'S PROBLEM-SOLVING STRATEGY		
SIX SIGMA BREAKTHROUGH STRATEGY		**JURAN'S PROBLEM-SOLVING STRATEGY**	
STAGE	**STEP (OBJECTIVE)**	**PHASE**	**STEP**
Identification	1. Recognize 2. Define (Identify key business issues)	Project definition and organization	1. List and prioritize problems 2. Define project and team
Characterization	1. Measure 2. Analyze (Understand current performance levels)	Diagnostic journey	1. Analyze symptom 2. Formulate theory of causes 3. Test theories 4. Identify root causes
Optimization	1. Improve 2. Control (Achieve breakthrough improvement)	Remedial journey	1. Consider alternative solutions 2. Design solutions and controls 3. Address resistance to change 4. Implement solutions and controls
Institutionalization	1. Standardize 2. Integrate (Transform how day-to-day business is conducted)	Holding the gains	1. Check performance 2. Monitor control system

From Pelletier, L.R. (2000). On error-free health care: Mission possible! (Editorial). *Journal for Healthcare Quality, 22*(3), 9. Reprinted with permission from the National Association for Healthcare Quality.

to achieve internationally recognized standards for performance excellence, which enable them to benchmark their "best practices" with others in the field. The first health care organization to apply and be awarded the BNQA in health care was the SSM system in St. Louis in 2002. The Alliance for Performance Excellence is a network of national, state, and local Baldrige-based organizations helping organizations achieve performance excellence using the Baldrige criteria (*www.baldrigepe.org/alliance/*). Various states have also developed quality awards based on the BNQA criteria. Health care Baldrige award recipients have been found to have the advantage of displaying faster 5-year performance improvement (Foster & Chenoweth, 2011).

ISO 9000

The International Organization for Standardization (ISO) is a network of 163 countries that have agreed on an international reference for quality requirements in business and service industries. The ISO 9000 series of standards are those that address quality management—that is, what the organization does to manage its systems and processes. Health care sector standards, originally developed in 2001, were updated in 2005 (Frost, 2005). The achievement of an ISO 9000 registration results when a company complies with its own quality system. Benefits of ISO include the following (ISO, 2011):

- Make the development, manufacturing and supply of products and services **more efficient, safer, and cleaner**
- **Facilitate trade** between countries and make it **fairer**
- Provide governments with a technical base for **health, safety, and environmental legislation,** and conformity assessment
- **Share** technological advances and good management practice
- Disseminate **innovation**
- **Safeguard consumers,** and users in general, of products and services

- Make life simpler by providing **solutions** to common problems

As many health care organizations are committed to the ongoing pursuit of quality, the ISO 9000 registration process provides another type of assessment and evaluation of an organization's quality systems and sets a benchmark for achievement that is internationally recognized.

High-Performance Organizations

As organizations continue to evolve their quality models, those that are in pursuit of continuous and ongoing improvement are embracing a concept referred to as *high-performance organizations (HPOs)*. These are organizations that may already be practicing Six Sigma or Lean Enterprise or have achieved recognition through ISO 9000 registration or Malcolm Baldrige compliance. HPOs are those that have a culture of "building and sustaining a customer focused, team based organization that pays as much attention to results as it does to process" (Ward, 2004, p. 3). Following are some of the attributes of an HPO:

- Leaders who communicate a strong and clear mission and vision to employees
- Strategic thinking that anticipates customer needs and market changes
- A commitment to ongoing identification of problems and a preoccupation for potential failures
- Resiliency
- Flexibility
- Creative and improvisational problem solving to address failures or "near misses"

HPOs apply the principles learned through the study of high-reliability organizations (HROs). These are organizations that require reliability to ensure stable outcomes in the face of variable working conditions. In 2009, The Commonwealth Fund offered recommendations "for a comprehensive set of insurance, payment, and system reforms that could guarantee affordable coverage for all by 2012, improve health outcomes, and slow health spending growth by $3 trillion by 2020" (The Commonwealth Fund Commission on a High Performance Health System, 2009, p. 3).

Magnet Designation

The American Nurses Credentialing Center's (ANCC) Magnet Recognition Program® recognizes health care organizations for "quality patient care, nursing excellence and innovations in professional nursing practice" (ANCC, 2012, ¶ 1). The Magnet model includes the following components: Through a secondary analysis of a four-state survey of 26,276 nurses in 567 acute care hospitals, Kelly and colleagues (2011) recently found that Magnet designated hospitals "have better work environments, a more highly educated nursing workforce, superior nurse-to-patient staffing ratios, and higher nurse satisfaction than non-Magnet hospitals" (p. 428).

COSTS ASSOCIATED WITH POOR HEALTH CARE QUALITY

The cost associated with medical errors "in lost income, disability, and health care costs is as much as $29 billion annually" (Quality Interagency Coordination [QuIC] Task Force, 2000, p. 1) and plagues every sector in the health care industry. A more recent estimate of the cost of poor quality health care has escalated to $1.2 trillion annually of the $2.2 trillion spent annually on health care (PricewaterhouseCoopers, 2008). The number of medical errors has been described as unacceptable by an IOM report *To Err Is Human: Building a Safer Health Care System* (Kohn et al., 2000), which has been referenced widely in the professional and consumer press since its release. The IOM report has reached the highest levels in the federal government, but response to its findings and recommendations was lackluster at first. The research associated with this report was preceded by other federal initiatives. Poor quality includes overuse, underuse, misuse, waste, and inefficiency. Several reports on health care quality and safety have followed this landmark report.

The IOM reports defined specific strategies that could inform the development and refinement of health care safety systems nationwide. An important component of these reports is the mention of the error-reduction techniques of other industries. The federal reports provided another opportunity to advocate for patients, families, and populations. They gave health care quality professionals the evidence and research with which to defend a quality management budget, enhance information systems and technologies to track errors, and further develop quality activities and studies using proven tools and techniques. The reports are also models in defining and describing cost/benefit analyses and return-on-investment scenarios for quality and performance improvement programs. In essence, they provided a business case for quality.

RESEARCH NOTE

Source

Cibulka, N., Fischer, H., & Fischer, A. (2012). Improving communication with low-income women using today's technology. *OJIN: The Online Journal of Issues in Nursing, 17*(2). Retrieved from *http://nursingworld. org/MainMenuCategories/ANAMarketplace/ ANAPeriodicals/OJIN/TableofContents/Vol-17-2012/ No2-May-2012/Articles-Previous-Topics/Communication- With-Low-Income-Women-and-Technology.html.*

Purpose

These nurse researchers investigated reasons for missed health care appointments and preferences for appointment reminders within an inner city obstetrics and gynecology clinic.

Discussion

The authors reviewed the literature on missed appointments and information technologies that could ensure that low-income women keep their medical appointments. Sixty low-income women, including African Americans, Whites, and members of other ethnic groups, with a mean age of 27 years, were interviewed by telephone. Forgetfulness was the most frequently cited reason for missing appointments. Almost all study participants indicated that they would like a text message reminder of upcoming appointments in addition to traditional telephone and/or postal letter reminders.

Application to Practice

Nurses have an opportunity to increase access to health care services to the disenfranchised. By applying performance and quality improvement principles, these nurses concluded that text messaging appointment reminders can decrease missed appointments among young, low-income women.

A technical report published by the IOM identified key characteristics that health care microsystems use to continuously enhance the services that they provide to individuals and communities (Donaldson & Mohr, 2000). After interviewing 43 microsystems, the researchers identified eight common themes: "integration of information, measurement, interdependence of care team, supportiveness of the larger system,

constancy of purpose, connection to community, investment in improvement, and alignment of role and training" (Donaldson & Mohr, 2000, p. 21).

The IOM report *Crossing the Quality Chasm: A New Health System for the 21st Century* (IOM, Committee on Quality of Health Care in America [CQHCA], 2001) recommended that Congress establish a Health Care Quality Innovation Fund "to support projects targeted at (1) achieving the six aims of safety, effectiveness, patient-centeredness, timeliness, efficiency, and equity; and/or (2) producing substantial improvements in quality for the [15] priority conditions" (p. 11). The overall goal of the funding would be to produce a "public-domain portfolio of programs, tools, and technologies of widespread applicability" (p. 11). The report recommended an initial investment of $1 billion over 3 to 5 years to support this goal. Health care organizations could take the lead either by enhancing the current resources dedicated to quality and performance improvement in their organizations or by using the funds to finance regional collaborative health care quality projects. These successes could then be described in the literature for wider application.

The third in a series of IOM quality chasm reports, entitled *Leadership by Example: Coordinating Government Roles in Improving Health Care Quality,* was released in 2002 (Corrigan et al., 2002). The original charge of the IOM Committee on Enhancing Federal Healthcare Quality Programs (CEFHQP) was to acknowledge that "The current federal quality oversight programs represent a patchwork of requirements and processes that have evolved over the last 30 to 35 years" (IOM, CEFHQP, 2002, p. 1). The committee was convened "to re-examine the various federal quality improvement and oversight programs to assess whether changes are needed to (1) provide adequate protection to beneficiaries, (2) provide strong incentives to providers to improve quality, and (3) improve the efficiency of the oversight processes by reducing redundancy" (IOM, CEFHQP, 2002, p. 1). In doing their work, the committee held workshops to obtain perspectives and information from various stakeholders with expertise in the fields of quality measurement, improvement, oversight, and research on ways to improve current federal programs (Medicare, Medicaid, Children's Health Insurance Program, Tricare, and Veterans Affairs). From his introductory remarks at the press briefing, the committee chair outlined the major findings of the study as follows (Omenn, 2002, p. 2):

- *There is a lack of consistency in performance measurement requirements both across and within these government programs.*
- *The programs are not using standardized measures.*
- *There is no well-thought-out conceptual framework to guide the selection of performance measures.*
- *Medicare, Medicaid, and the State Children's Health Insurance Program lack computer-based clinical data, which is seen as a major impediment.*
- *There is also a lack of commitment to transparency and openly sharing information on safety and quality.*

These findings were not a surprise to many nurses and health care quality professionals, who have been burdened with duplicative reporting for years. The positive message was that strong recommendations from this committee were sent to the federal government's leadership, asking them to attack these problems with a good deal of muscle to shape the measurement of performance for the whole health care sector. The charge was clear to the Secretaries of the U.S. Department of Health and Human Services, Department of Defense, and Department of Veterans Affairs (Omenn, 2002): "Work together to establish standardized performance measures, as well as public reporting requirements for clinicians, institutional providers, and health plans in each program. The standardized measurement and reporting requirements should replace the many performance assessment activities currently under way in various programs" (p. 3). Standardization of protocols and measures is not a new idea (Pelletier, 1998). Reducing administrative burden and duplicative reporting could easily put time back in the hands of clinicians to do what they do best: provide health care services to individuals, families, and communities.

LEADERSHIP AND MANAGEMENT IMPLICATIONS

Planning for Health Care Quality

An organization that adopts and nurtures a continuous performance and quality improvement culture (and rewards those who identify opportunities for improvement and their solutions) recognizes that change is an everyday event. One of the ways that change can be managed is to acknowledge it and make it a part of the organization's strategic planning process. Just as an organization defines its mission, vision, and core values, so too must change agents and teams define the purpose of the change (expected outcomes), the mission and vision of the change process, and the core values of the group that will be responsible for managing the change.

An organization's mission is a concise statement that answers the question: What business are we in today (Pelletier, 1999a)? Some companies refer to their mission as a *purpose*. Sharp HealthCare, a not-for-profit integrated regional health care delivery system based in San Diego, CA, that was the recipient of the Baldrige Award in 2007 stated that its mission is "to improve the health of those we serve with a commitment to excellence in all that we do. Our goal is to offer quality care and programs that set community standards, exceed patients' expectations and are provided in a caring, convenient, cost-effective and accessible manner" (Sharp HealthCare, 2012, ¶ 1). The Visiting Nursing Service of New York's (VNSNY) mission is "to promote the health and well-being of patients and families by providing high-quality, cost-effective health care in the home and community; to be a leader in the development of innovative services that enable people to function as independently as possible in their community; to help shape health care policies that support beneficial home- and community-based services; to continue our tradition of charitable and compassionate care, within the resources available" (VNSNY, 2012).

An organization's vision should accurately depict what the company is striving to become. The vision statement should be able to stand on its own and be understandable to people new to the enterprise. Sharp HealthCare's vision is "to be the best health system in the universe" (Sharp HealthCare, 2012, ¶ 2). VNSNY's vision is "To be the #1 home health care organization in the nation and reshape the health care system to improve the health and lives of those in our communities."

It is critical for mission and vision statements to be communicated effectively and widely to internal stakeholders (employees and management personnel) and to external stakeholders (investors, clients, patients, vendors, and accreditation agencies). In this way, the statements keep employees on a path to an attainable goal. Nurse managers need to be familiar with the organization's mission and vision statements. Representatives from various stakeholder groups, including patients and consumers, need be included in the development of these statements. Mission and vision statements need to be reviewed and updated periodically to accurately reflect what leadership, staff, and stakeholders believe is the purpose and future direction of the organization. This is important because mission, vision, and values form the foundation for quality and its management and improvement. Departmental mission and vision statements must be aligned with the organization's statements.

Just as a nurse's professional behavior is based on personal values, so too must an organization describe the core values that are the foundation of the enterprise or endeavor. Strategic planning often includes the development of core value statements that are in alignment with the mission and vision statements of the organization. "Value statements become part of an organization's culture; they act as a quick reference or navigation device—just as mission and vision statements do" (Pelletier, 1999b, p. 2). Marcus and colleagues (1995) defined values as "interests that reflect fundamental purpose and integrity: issues to which you hold fast as a matter of principle, with little room for compromise" (p. 430). Furthermore, "Values

are operational qualities used by organizations to maintain or enhance performance" (Harmon, 1997, p. 246).

Values consciously and unconsciously guide a professional nurse's personal and professional behavior. His Holiness the Dalai Lama and Cutler (1998) said the following about values: "Higher stages of growth and development depend on an underlying set of values that can guide us. A value system that can provide continuity and coherence to our lives, by which we can measure our experiences. A value system that can help us decide which goals are truly worthwhile and which pursuits are meaningless. Values help us with the challenges of everyday life" (pp. 192-193).

Nurses' personal and professional values come from the experiences they have shared with others in interpersonal exchanges at work and at home. To identify a group's core values, ask and record the responses to these questions: Which three people have had the greatest influence in your personal and professional life? What are the three most important values these influential people taught you? The answers to these questions can help inform the development of mission, vision, and core value statements. An example is a set of core values or "core principles" from the Mayo Clinic, as outlined in Table 17-2.

TABLE 17-2   MAYO CLINIC VALUE STATEMENTS

Value statements	These values, which guide Mayo Clinic's mission to this day, are an expression of the vision and intent of our founders, the original Mayo physicians and the Sisters of Saint Francis.
Respect	Treat everyone in our diverse community, including patients, their families and colleagues, with dignity.
Compassion	Provide the best care, treating patients and family members with sensitivity and empathy.
Integrity	Adhere to the highest standards of professionalism, ethics and personal responsibility, worthy of the trust our patients place in us.
Healing	Inspire hope and nurture the well-being of the whole person, respecting physical, emotional and spiritual needs.
Teamwork	Value the contributions of all, blending the skills of individual staff members in unsurpassed collaboration.
Excellence	Deliver the best outcomes and highest quality service through the dedicated effort of every team member.
Innovation	Infuse and energize the organization, enhancing the lives of those we serve, through the creative ideas and unique talents of each employee.
Stewardship	Sustain and reinvest in our mission and extended communities by wisely managing our human, natural and material resources.

From Mayo Foundation for Medical Research and Education. (2012). *Mayo Clinic mission and values*. Rochester, MN: Author. Retrieved March 30, 2012, from *www.mayoclinic.org/about/missionvalues.html*.

CURRENT ISSUES AND TRENDS

A Nurse Manager's Health Care Quality Toolbox

Along with the paradigm shift from quality assurance to organizational performance improvement, came the expectation that accredited organizations become skilled at the art and science of continuous performance and quality improvement. This included the concepts of leadership involvement, a commitment to customers' needs (i.e., patients and families), an understanding of the principle of process versus people, a devotion to data collection and analysis as the foundation for problem solving, and the view that multidisciplinary teams working within the processes under study were the experts and therefore best equipped to drive change and improvement.

Nurse managers in accredited organizations are expected to learn these principles and tools for quality improvement, educate staff in these tools and techniques, identify improvement opportunities on their units, and be able to speak to process changes that occurred as a result of data analysis. They were also tapped to participate in organization-wide improvement teams designed to address overarching problem resolution or process redesign projects. Many of the early quality leaders received training in facilitation and group meeting techniques, in addition to the performance and quality improvement (PQI) tools. This enabled them to promote the team-based model of cross-functional problem solving that became the standard for most organizations. Skills and expertise in the concepts of team building, conflict resolution, statistical process control, customer service, and process improvement continue to be needed by nurse leaders in the new millennium.

Health care quality professionals and nurses involved in performance and quality improvement activities have an enormous set of resources available to them as they plan for an enterprise-wide quality program. Tools and techniques that nurses can readily use are illustrated in Table 17-3. Figures 17-2 through 17-7 illustrate examples of templates and forms to be included in a nurse manager's quality "toolbox."

TABLE 17-3	A NURSE MANAGER'S HEALTH CARE QUALITY TOOLBOX	
TOOL	**DESCRIPTION OF THE TOOL**	**EXAMPLE**
Data-collection tools	Check sheets and checklists facilitate the gathering of data for eventual analysis and reporting. Good data collection tools can help to count and categorize data.	Sample data collection sheet for a nurse manager's quality toolbox (see Figure 17-2).
Control chart	This tool includes data points and their placement on a graph to depict variation. Its purpose is to illustrate whether the process variation is expected ("common cause") or an unexpected or unusual variation ("special cause"). Included are three lines—the mean, an upper control limit (UCL), and a lower control limit (LCL). Generally, a process is considered "out of control" when the data points stray outside of the control limits or a series of data points follow a defined pattern that illustrates a lack of control in the process.	Sample control chart for a nurse manager's quality toolbox (see Figure 17-3).
Cause-and-effect (or fishbone) diagram	This tool resembles diagramming sentences. The "effect" is illustrated in a box at the end of a midline (or "head" of the fish). The "causes" are generally four or five categories of elements that might contribute to the effect (e.g., machines, methods, people, materials, measurements) and the specific activities. Under each of these category headings, individual items that might lead to the effect are listed. By diagramming all of the possible contributors, the predominant or root causes may be found more readily.	Sample cause-and-effect diagram for a nurse manager's quality toolbox (see Figure 17-4).

Continued

TABLE 17-3 A NURSE MANAGER'S HEALTH CARE QUALITY TOOLBOX—cont'd

TOOL	DESCRIPTION OF THE TOOL	EXAMPLE
Detailed flowchart	Using various shapes, this tool is used to depict a work process, from start to finish, illustrating all of the processes' action steps, decision points, hand-offs, or waiting stages. Flowcharts form the cornerstone of process improvement planning and analysis. The entire process must first be accurately defined to identify problems or process improvement opportunities.	Sample detailed flowchart for a nurse manager's quality toolbox (see Figure 17-5).
Pareto chart	This bar graph can help depict the "80/20" rule. In the nineteenth century, it was used to show that 80% of the wealth was held by 20% of the people. In health care, typically 20% of the issues cause 80% of the problems. The use of this tool allows a performance improvement team to focus on the "vital few" causes of the problems in a process under study.	Example of a Pareto chart for a nurse manager's quality toolbox (see Figure 17-6).
Scatter diagram	This graph describes the relationship between two variables that are continuous. It is used when the potential causes of effects under study cannot be easily categorized, such as in a Pareto chart or cause-and-effect diagram. Data points are plotted along the vertical and horizontal axes of the graph, and a correlation between the two variables can either be weak or strong, based on the pattern of the data points.	Example of a scatter diagram for a nurse manager's quality toolbox. (see Figure 17-7).

Data Collection Sheet

Organization/Unit: _____   Date: _____

Process: _____

MEASURE	DATE	TIME	WHERE	WHEN

FIGURE 17-2 Sample data collection sheet for a nurse manager's quality toolbox.

Control Chart

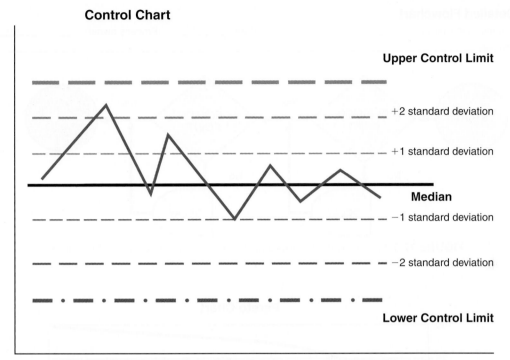

Upper Control Limit

+2 standard deviation

+1 standard deviation

Median

−1 standard deviation

−2 standard deviation

Lower Control Limit

FIGURE 17-3 Sample control chart for a nurse manager's quality toolbox.

Cause-and-Effect Diagram

Organization/Unit: _____   Date: _____

Process:_____

Environment

Personnel/
people

Cause

Subcause

Clear
description
of problem,
undesired
outcome,
result, or
effect

Equipment/
machinery/
hardware

Policies/
procedures/
protocols

Time

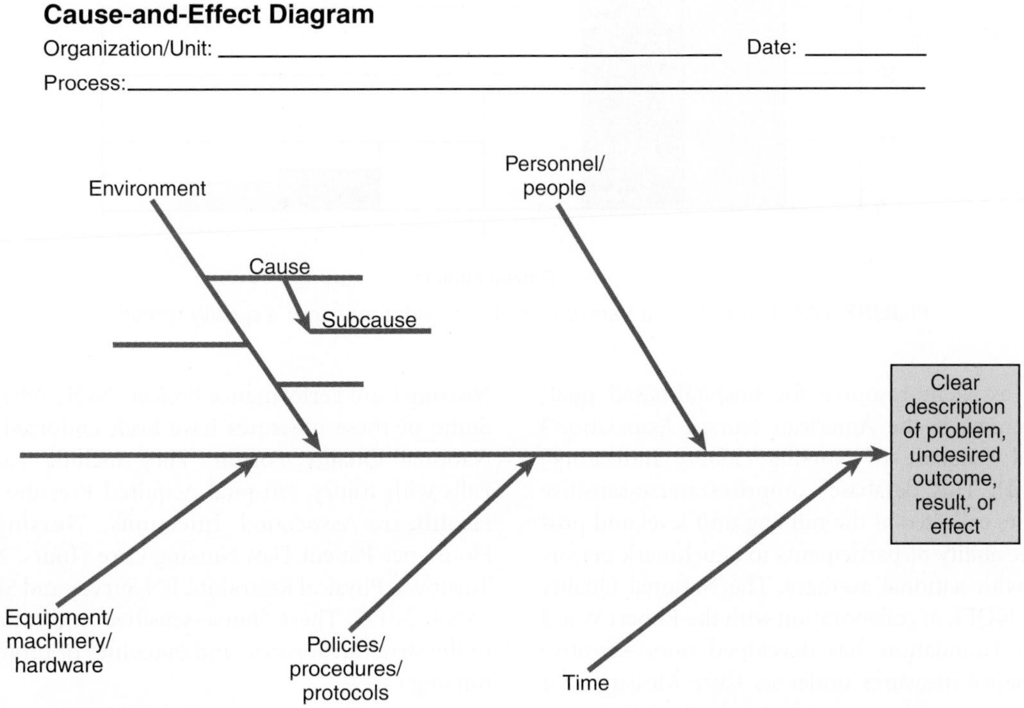

FIGURE 17-4 Sample cause-and-effect diagram for a nurse manager's quality toolbox.

Detailed Flowchart

Organization/Unit: _____   Date: _____   Process owner: _____

Process:_____

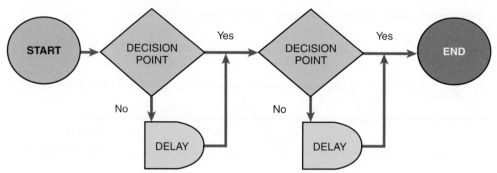

FIGURE 17-5 Sample detailed flowchart for a nurse manager's quality toolbox.

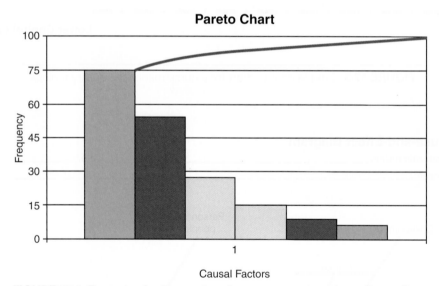

FIGURE 17-6 Example of a Pareto chart for a nurse manager's quality toolbox.

One excellent resource for hospital-based quality programs is the American Nurses Association's National Database of Nursing Quality Indicators® (NDNQI). This database comprises nurse-sensitive indicators collected at the nursing unit level and provides the ability of participants to benchmark performance with national averages. The National Quality Forum (NQF), in collaboration with the Robert Wood Johnson Foundation, has developed nurse-sensitive performance measures under its Core Measures for Nursing Care Performance Project (NQF, 2004, 2011). Some of these measures have been endorsed by the National Quality Forum. They include Falls and Falls with Injury, Hospital-Acquired Pressure Ulcers, Healthcare-Associated Infections, Nursing Care Hours per Patient Day, Nursing Care Hours, Nursing Turnover, Physical Restraints, RN Survey and Skill Mix (ANA, 2012). These "nurse-sensitive" indicators refer to the structure, process and outcomes of professional nursing care.

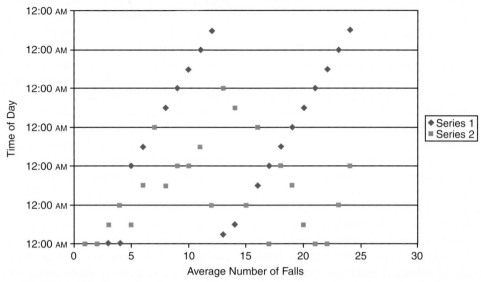

FIGURE 17-7 Example of a scatter diagram for a nurse manager's quality toolbox.

In addition, the Internet can provide professional nurses with administrative and clinical tools to support a quality and performance improvement program, regardless of the delivery setting.

A health care quality glossary can also assist professional nurse managers in navigating the health care quality field. A glossary of frequently used terms is discussed in the Definitions section.

HEALTH CARE SAFETY AND HEALTH CARE ENTERPRISE RISK MANAGEMENT

Accreditation and Regulatory Influences on Quality

Health care organizations have always been required to meet standards for federal and state reimbursement regulations (Medicare and Medicaid) and state licensure rules and regulations in order to operate. These regulations have traditionally defined requirements for quality. However, the private accreditation process has probably had the most significant impact on the development of quality improvement systems in health care. It has been through organizations such as The Joint Commission (TJC), The American Osteopathic Association's Healthcare Facilities Accreditation Program (HFAP), the Commission on Accreditation of Rehabilitation Facilities (CARF), the National Committee for Quality Assurance (NCQA), and others that performance standards have been promulgated and universally adopted. In each of these accreditation processes, the concept of system-wide quality improvement provides the framework for the standards. Although accreditation is not mandatory, eligibility to participate in and receive reimbursement from managed care organizations or federal and state program funding sources is often tied to the achievement of accreditation by one or more of the voluntary accreditation organizations.

Of all of these voluntary accreditation programs, TJC has had the greatest degree of impact on the health care industry. Founded in 1951, it led the way in establishing a set of performance standards for hospitals to follow to become accredited. Over the years, its accreditation standards and programs have evolved to reflect the myriad of types of providers that now constitute the health care system, thus expanding its role beyond hospital accreditation. Currently, TJC sponsors accreditation programs for organizations that provide services in the areas of ambulatory care, assisted living, behavioral health, critical access hospitals, health care networks, hospitals, home care, laboratory, long-term care, and office-based surgery.

Throughout its evolution, TJC has continually adjusted its performance standards for quality. During the 1980s and the early 1990s, TJC promoted a "10-Step Process for Quality Assurance" that provided the framework for quality in hospitals. In 1994, TJC identified the need to enhance overall quality of care via an improvement in its own accreditation processes, and it completely revised the accreditation standards for all programs. Instead of chapters organized by department, the new approach revised and reorganized the requirements into *cross-functional processes of care and services* (e.g., Patients Rights, Patient Assessment, Patient Family Education), to more appropriately reflect the manner in which care is delivered. A new chapter entitled "Improving Organizational Performance" was introduced that created specific standards focused on quality that were based on the principle of continuous improvement rather than on pre-established thresholds for performance of individual health care quality indicators. This change reflected the influence of the industrial quality movement on health care in the early 1990s.

With this major restructuring of TJC standards, the new era of thinking in terms of *process improvement* rather than *quality assurance* began, not only for TJC-accredited organizations but also for other accrediting bodies. The description for this organization-wide programmatic approach, or *performance improvement (PI)*, established the expectation that quality initiatives in the organization were no longer the responsibility of a single quality assurance nurse or department but, rather, the responsibility of the enterprise's leaders. Standards in the newly developed "Leadership" chapter established the expectation that the outcomes of performance improvement measures be elevated to review by the administrative and clinical leaders of the organization. This review of performance measurement at senior levels of the organization provides the information that leaders require to provide oversight to the quality of care being provided to all patients and families (customers).

The Joint Commission PI standards delineate specific requirements for data collection in high-risk areas such as medication management, restraints, and blood transfusions. Beyond these mandatory quality indicators, the leaders of each organization are expected to set their own priorities for measurement that reflect the types of services provided to the various populations served by the organization. The PI and Leadership standards also expect that the outcomes of data analysis and the actions taken to address improvement opportunities should be communicated to staff. It is in this arena that a nurse manager can make the PI process "come alive" for nursing staff. Staff can relate to and understand data outcomes that are based on measurement of the everyday processes in which they work. The nurse manager should involve staff in identifying relevant and significant data collection measures for their unit/department that will have a direct impact on changing and continuously improving care processes. A sample data collection sheet is displayed in Figure 17-2.

Nurse managers need to stay abreast of changes in the standards of their organization's primary accrediting and state and federal regulatory agencies to ensure that quality outcome measures for their units/departments remain current and viable. In addition to keeping up with these requirements, and as previously described, many hospitals are pursuing or have plans to pursue Magnet recognition of their hospital's nursing practice as awarded by the American Nurses Credentialing Center through its Magnet Recognition Program® (American Nurses Credentialing Center, 2012). To be positioned to score well on an application for the Magnet Recognition Program, nurse leaders must take an active role in the development of robust and effective quality measures. A step further might be to participate in local, regional, and national committees that set performance standards. This can be done through professional associations such as the American Nurses Association, the National Association for Healthcare Quality, and the American Society for Professionals in Patient Safety. Certification programs are available through these professional associations.

As new standards are introduced, either through participation in voluntary accreditation programs or because of regulatory requirements, policies and procedures at the unit/department level must be updated and/or revised. Staff must be educated about the impact and meaning of the standards that are applicable to the care they provide. Documentation requirements may change, and this may affect the outcome of clinical data measures and/or reimbursement.

Nurse managers need to provide leadership in adopting and adapting to ongoing changes in these arenas. Many organizations do not have the luxury of devoting one individual or department solely to managing accreditation or regulatory compliance processes. At best, in those organizations that have dedicated individuals or departments for this purpose, they serve as facilitators for the accreditation and licensing processes. Since 2006, TJC surveys have been conducted on an unannounced basis. This requires that managers throughout the organization be in a continual state of readiness (i.e., to have their departments and staff in compliance with all applicable standards at all times). Thus the onus of responsibility and accountability for continuous readiness has moved from a single regulatory or quality department to all leaders and managers in the organization.

Data Collection and Public Reporting of Quality Outcomes

By 1998, The Joint Commission developed a requirement for accredited organizations to participate in their ORYX®, an antecedent to a core measure initiative. This program required accredited health care organizations to select six outcome measures that reflected the operations of their organizations and to choose a performance measurement vendor to aggregate and analyze the data and submit them on a quarterly basis to The Joint Commission. Similarly, since 1991, the Healthcare Effectiveness Data and Information Set (HEDIS) outcomes have been an integral part of the NCQA accreditation process for managed care plans. Of note, CARF has required both program evaluation and quality outcomes measurement as components of its accreditation process since the 1980s, about a decade before the other accreditors.

One drawback to The Joint Commission's initial ORYX® process, and that of the quality reporting required by other accreditors, was an inability to compare performance outcomes across and among health care organizations. This was due primarily to the variability allowed in selection of measures and reporting systems. Also, as most organizations that analyzed their ORYX® data discovered, there was a limitation in identifying improvement opportunities with data that were purely outcomes-based. In further refinement of its ORYX® process, The Joint

Commission devised its Core Measures program. The initial measures were acute myocardial infarction (AMI), community-acquired pneumonia (PN), and heart failure (HF) and comprised 10 process measures, often referred to as the "starter set." In July 2002, accredited hospitals were required to begin collecting data on the core measures (with some exceptions, such as pediatric and psychiatric hospitals) and submit the data to The Joint Commission. Although participation in the ORYX® program was mandatory for each organization to be accredited, the results of Core Measures were not initially made public. The current core measure sets include: Substance Use, Tobacco Treatment, Venous Thromboembolism, Pneumonia Measures, Immunization, Acute Myocardial Infarction, Children's Asthma Care, Heart Failure, Surgical Care Improvement Project, Hospital-Based Inpatient Psychiatric Services, Perinatal Care, Stroke and Hospital Outpatient Department (TJC, 2012a). See Table 17-4 for sample core measures from the HospitalCompare database.

Since the 1980s, CMS has mandated that the cost and quality of services provided to its Medicare recipients be evaluated through its peer review organizations (PROs). These PROs evolved into state and regional quality improvement organizations (QIOs) that have continued their statutory mandate through the "Statement of Work" projects. At the time of this publication, hospitals are working under the "9th Scope of Work." The *Specification Manual for National Hospital Inpatient Quality Measures* is a guide that combines both the CMS measures and The Joint Commission Core Measure sets "to achieve identity among common national hospital performance measures and to share a single set of common documentation" (TJC, 2012b).

CMS has historically mandated data submission programs for non-hospital health care organizations to qualify for participation in their Medicare programs. For long-term care facilities, CMS has required the submission of data through its Minimum Data Set (MDS) program. For home health care, CMS requires submission of data to the Outcome and Assessment Information Set (OASIS) that includes clinical quality, cost, and administrative measures. In both these initiatives, the results for individual health care organizations also were not originally made public. In fall

TABLE 17-4 SELECTED HOSPITAL MEASURES REPORTED ON THE HOSPITAL COMPARE WEBSITE

Hospital Process of Care Measures

HOSPITAL MEASURES	UPDATE FREQUENCY	CURRENT COLLECTION DATES FOR AVAILABLE MEASURES	
		FROM	THROUGH
Surgical Care Improvement Project Process of Care Measures			
Outpatients having surgery who got an antibiotic at the right time—within 1 hour before surgery (higher numbers are better)	Quarterly	July 2010	June 2011
Outpatients having surgery who got the right kind of antibiotic (higher numbers are better)	Quarterly	July 2010	June 2011
Surgery patients who were taking heart drugs called beta blockers before coming to the hospital, who were kept on the beta blockers during the period just before and after their surgery	Quarterly	July 2010	June 2011
Surgery patients who were given an antibiotic at the right time (within 1 hour before surgery) to help prevent infection	Quarterly	July 2010	June 2011
Surgery patients who were given the right kind of antibiotic to help prevent infection	Quarterly	July 2010	June 2011

From U.S. Department of Health and Human Services. (2010). *HospitalCompare database*. Retrieved March 21, 2012, from *www.hospitalcompare.hhs.gov/staticpages/help/hospital-resources.aspx*.

2001, the U.S. Secretary of Health and Human Services announced the Bush administration's commitment to quality health care through the publication of consumer information, along with quality improvement data, through CMS's QIOs. Their program, "The Quality Initiative," began in 2002 with the Nursing Home Quality Initiative (NHQI) and continued in 2003 with the Home Health Quality Initiative (HHQI). Its purpose was to allow consumers to make informed choices about their health care providers and encourage providers to improve their care. In 2004, The Quality Initiative was broadened to include renal dialysis or end-stage kidney disease (ESRD) and has now expanded to a Physician's Quality Reporting Initiative (PQRI).

In 2011, CMS developed the Hospital Value-Based Purchasing Program, which applied beginning in fiscal year 2013 to payments for discharges occurring on or after October 1, 2012. Under the program, CMS will make value-based incentive payments to acute care hospitals, based either on how well the hospitals perform on certain quality measures or how much the hospitals' performance improves on certain quality measures from their performance during a baseline period. The higher a hospital's performance or improvement during the performance period for a fiscal year, the higher the hospital's value-based incentive payment for the fiscal year would be (Centers for Medicare & Medicaid Services, 2012).

Initially, health care providers were resistant and concerned about issues such as data integrity and the lack of risk adjustments that would ensure that the results were comparable. They were convinced that, without safeguards built into state reporting systems, their organizations might look "bad" to the public. Data analysis systems have certainly evolved and improved over the years to address these concerns. A majority of states have now enacted legislation requiring public reporting; and with federal reporting requirements increasingly linked to reimbursement, providers must participate in data submission for public reporting or risk losing accreditation, income, and community status. As an example, organizations must be diligent in documentation of initial assessments, because care for patients with poor outcomes (e.g., skin breakdown) that are not recorded as being "present on admission" (POA), will no longer be reimbursed. Terms like "never events" represent a category of adverse outcomes that, in the view of insurers, should never happen and for which they are no longer willing to pay.

Nurse managers need to be cognizant of the variety of measures being collected for state, federal, and accreditation purposes that apply to their units and patients. These managers and their staffs often have to participate in the data collection effort and discuss outcomes at quality improvement committees. Managers are held accountable to implement corrective action plans focused on their unit/department to address issues of noncompliance with quality indicators such as Core Measures (e.g., not documenting education about smoking cessation for AMI patients). In the future, patients and families may inquire about the organization's publicly reported outcomes, so it is imperative that managers are conversant with this topic.

Health Care Safety and Quality Improvement

A landmark report from the IOM launched a major national focus on the safety of health care systems and processes. In fact, the conclusion that 98,000 deaths in health care organizations were preventable was considered a call to action, not only by health care providers but also by business and government. Not surprisingly, health care safety became the focus as a key component of the accreditation process. Soon after the millennium, new standards were established by The Joint Commission and other accrediting, regulatory, private, and public organizations to address the issue of health care safety within health care organizations.

In July 2001, new standards were introduced that required all hospitals accredited by The Joint Commission to establish and implement a formal patient safety program. Additional standards to integrate health care safety programs into organization-wide processes have been added over time. The components of a health care safety program are listed in Box 17-5. Those individuals and organizations committed to health care safety initiatives believe that a rigorous, ongoing, and proactive approach to the identification

---

BOX 17-5   COMPONENTS OF A HEALTH CARE SAFETY PROGRAM

- Leadership commitment as evidenced through the allocation of resources for health care safety
- Assignment of individual(s) to manage the program
- Interdisciplinary (cross-organizational) participation, coordination, and communication about safety activities
- Education and involvement of patients and families in health care safety issues
- Disclosure of unanticipated outcomes of care to patients and families
- Education of staff on safety-related topics and training in team communication techniques
- Data collection and analysis in safety-related areas, including the following:
  - Incident/variance reporting
  - Medication errors, near misses
  - Infection surveillance and prevention
  - Facility/environmental surveillance
  - Staff willingness to report errors
  - Staff perceptions of and suggestions for improving safety
  - Patient and family perceptions and/or suggestions for improvement regarding safety
- Definition of terms related to safety, including sentinel events, "near misses" and what is reportable, and the development of policies and procedures to address each category of event
- Management of sentinel events
- Adherence to The Joint Commission National Patient Safety Goals
- Establishment of a risk reduction process to include Healthcare Failure Modes Effects Analysis (HFMEA)

of risks will result in the prevention of errors as well as provide the framework to respond most effectively when errors do occur.

Just as a paradigm shift was required to move from a quality assurance mindset to performance improvement, the new paradigm for health care safety requires that organizations create a non-punitive culture for error reporting. This is application of the "process or system, not people" philosophy in its truest form. Systems that single out caregivers who commit errors must be eliminated. More important, nurse managers must learn the principles of the non-punitive approach (i.e., they applaud and commend staff for reporting errors or "near misses"). In fact, in some industrial models, those managers or staff who detect and report errors or system failures in their areas are rewarded. An example of the effectiveness of this approach is reported in a study conducted by Harvard Business School professor Amy Edmondson. She found that the nursing units in one hospital that were considered to be the best performing were those that had higher detected rates for adverse drug events (Hesselbein & Johnston, 2002). Certainly, the conclusion was not that more errors were committed on this unit but that the staff's willingness to report errors contributed to the improvement of the unit's overall processes, resulting in a positive reputation within the hospital.

Personnel management regarding safe practices has generated a concept of *fair and just culture* (Marx, 2007). In a fair and just culture, everyone throughout the organization is aware that medical errors are inevitable, but all errors and unintended events are reported—even when the events may not cause patient injury. This culture can make the system safer as it recognizes that competent professionals make mistakes and acknowledges that even competent professionals develop unhealthy norms (shortcuts or routine rule violations), but it has zero tolerance for reckless behavior. Three principles of a just culture can be stated as follows:

- A fair and just culture is not an effort to reduce personal accountability and discipline. It is a way to emphasize the importance of learning from mistakes and near misses in order to reduce errors in the future.
- In a fair and just culture, an individual is accountable to the system, and the greatest error is to not report a mistake and thereby prevent the

system and others from learning. Policies that would discourage any health care provider from self-reporting errors are therefore at odds with the goals of a fair and just culture.
- A new culture of patient safety is successfully created when all serve as safety advocates regardless of their positions within an organization. Providers and consumers will feel safe and supported when they report medical errors or near misses and voice concerns about patient safety (Marx, 2007).

Health care organizations that embrace a fair and just culture identify and correct the systems or processes of care that contributed to the medical error or near miss. Managers believe that protected by a non-punitive culture of medical error reporting, more health care professionals will report more errors and near misses, which will further improve patient safety through opportunities for improvement and lessons learned (California Patient Safety Action Coalition, 2008; Marx, 2007). The American Nurses Association has endorsed just culture as a means of ensuring safe care (American Nurses Association, 2010).

An example of a large organization that has created health care safety programs and initiatives since the IOM reports were released is the Veterans Affairs (VA) National Center for Patient Safety. The VA National Center for Patient Safety (NCPS) is committed to the reduction of error and improvement of quality through proactive approaches to risk reduction (U.S. Department of Veterans Affairs, 2004). This is accomplished through focusing on prevention, creating non-punitive environments, and conducting safety research through such concepts as human factors analysis and studying high-reliability organizations (HROs) in other industries such as aviation and nuclear energy. The VA has created numerous educational programs through the NCPS and freely shares them with all health care providers who want to learn about health care safety tools and techniques. They have taken the lead in adopting the methodology and tools of Healthcare Failure Modes and Effects Analysis (HFMEA).

The National Quality Forum (NQF) is a consortium of public-private organizations that work collaboratively to address health care quality and safety. In 2003, the NQF published a list of 30 consensus standards to address safe practices that, if implemented, would yield improvements in the safety of health care. Examples of this initial list included establishment of a culture for safety, adoption of protocols to prevent wrong-side surgery, and implementation of effective admission assessments to identify and treat underlying conditions early in the care process. The NQF Safety Practices were updated in 2006, and a total of 34 practices were included in 2009 Safe Practices. New Safe Practices in the 2009 set were added in areas such as pediatric imaging, glycemic control, organ donation, catheter-associated urinary tract infection, and multidrug-resistant organisms. A number of previously endorsed practices were updated based on new evidence, including the pharmacist's role in medication management and pressure ulcers and an entire chapter on health care–associated infections (NQF, 2012). Current safety topics that the NQF has endorsed and recommend include implementation of effective "hand-off" communication, initiation of rapid response teams, and management of methicillin-resistant *Staphylococcus aureus* (MRSA) infection.

Nurse managers can personally create an environment that is devoted to health care safety by doing the following:

- Learning the concepts and tools related to risk identification, analysis, and error reduction
- Adopting and embracing the concept of non-punitive error reporting
- Advocating for the establishment of a non-punitive culture if it is not currently a strong ideal within the organization
- Encouraging staff to be constantly vigilant in identifying potential risks in the care environment
- Creating a sense of partnership with patients and families to promote communication about safety concerns and soliciting their suggestions to correct and prevent potential risks
- Becoming a role model for staff and peers in practicing health care safety concepts.

Sentinel Events

One element included in The Joint Commission standards for both the Leadership and Performance Improvement chapters addresses a key component in health care safety—that of the organizational response to sentinel events. A sentinel event is defined by The Joint Commission as follows: "A sentinel event is an un-expected occurrence involving death or serious physical or psychological injury, or the risk thereof. Serious injury specifically includes loss of limb or function. The phrase 'or the risk thereof' includes any process variation for which a recurrence would carry a significant chance of a serious adverse outcome. Such events are called 'sentinel' because they signal the need for immediate investigation and response. The terms 'sentinel event' and 'medical error' are not synonymous; not all sentinel events occur because of an error and not all errors result in sentinel events" (TJC, 2012c, ¶ 2).

In 1999, The Joint Commission began requiring health care organizations to respond to sentinel events in a systematic and formal way (i.e., expecting that a Root Cause Analysis [RCA] be conducted by the staff involved with the event). Time frames for concluding this analysis and guidelines for conducting a "credible" process were outlined in the standards. Organizations not familiar with the quality tools for conducting RCAs (primarily flowcharting and cause-and-effect diagramming) had to quickly learn them. The purpose of the RCA is to "drill down" to the most common cause(s) for the event and determine what process improvements can be made to prevent the sentinel event from occurring in the future. Controversy over whether a sentinel event was reportable to The Joint Commission and what information could be shared with the accreditor from a risk management and legal perspective resulted in the creation of a number of alternatives for submission of the required RCAs. The detailed requirements for reporting and submitting RCAs are contained in the Sentinel Event policy and can be found on The Joint Commission website (*http://www.jointcommission.org/ Sentinel_Event_Policy_and_Procedures/*). Specific sentinel event outcomes are considered "reviewable" by The Joint Commission. Reviewable sentinel events are events that have resulted in an unanticipated death or major permanent loss of function, not related to the natural course of the patient's illness or underlying condition, or one of the following events (even if the outcome was not death or major permanent loss of function):

- *Any patient death, paralysis, coma, or other major permanent loss of function associated with a medication error*
- *A patient commits suicide within 72 hours of being discharged from a hospital setting that provides staffed around-the-clock care*

- *Any elopement, that is, unauthorized departure, of a patient from an around-the-clock care setting resulting in a temporally related death (suicide, accidental death, or homicide) or major permanent loss of function*
- *A hospital operates on the wrong side of the patient's body*
- *Any intrapartum (related to the birth process) maternal death*
- *Any perinatal death unrelated to a congenital condition in an infant having a birth weight greater than 2500 grams*
- *A patient is abducted from the hospital where he or she receives care, treatment, or services*
- *Assault, homicide, or other crime resulting in patient death or major permanent loss of function*
- *A patient fall that results in death or major permanent loss of function as a direct result of the injuries sustained in the fall*
- *Hemolytic transfusion reaction involving major blood group incompatibilities*
- *A foreign body, such as a sponge or forceps, that was left in a patient after surgery (TJC, 2011b, p. SE7).*

Organizations that have initiated comprehensive and robust health care safety programs are committed to the process of ongoing risk identification and prevention. These organizations encourage the staff to identify potential errors and report any "near misses" that occur. Even if an adverse event is not considered "reviewable," such organizations conduct RCAs on these identified risks to prevent similar errors from occurring in the future.

The Joint Commission accreditation standards also now require that organizations go a step beyond the RCA process in their health care risk reduction and management programs. A set of standards in the Leadership chapter requires the leaders to ensure that an integrated patient safety program is implemented. This includes the establishment of an interdisciplinary group to manage the program, definition of the program's scope, integration of the program into all components of the organization, systems to immediately respond to system or process failures, systems for reporting these failures both internally and externally, defined processes for response to unanticipated adverse events, proactive risk assessment programs, systems to support and care for staff who have been involved in an adverse event, and at least annually, a formal process for reporting to the organization's governing body on the program's components (TJC, 2012d).

One of the methods for proactive risk assessment that accredited hospitals are expected to implement is the process of HFMEA. The expectation is that an HFMEA will be performed on at least one identified high-risk process annually. The HFMEA is conducted by an interdisciplinary team of professionals who own the process being studied and is facilitated by someone with knowledge and skills in quality improvement tools. The HFMEA begins with flowcharting the steps of the process being studied. The team assesses risk points within the process steps, and these key risk points are ranked in terms of their impact on the potential failure of the system. Scores for severity and probability are calculated to give a "hazard" score to the identified breakdown, and detectability of the failure mode is factored into the analysis of its impact on the overall process. The team then "designs out" the most critical of the potential failures and recommends process improvements for prevention of the failures. Once these prevention strategies are identified, action plans for implementing them are reported to the enterprise leaders and endorsed for implementation (see the VA National Center for Patient Safety website for a detailed description of the HFMEA and tools at *www.patientsafety.gov/CogAids/HFMEA/index.html#page=page-1*).

National Patient Safety Goals

Since the late 1990s, The Joint Commission has been collecting data on sentinel events and the outcomes of their RCAs for the purpose of sharing those data with health care organizations to prevent similar sentinel events from occurring. The results of the aggregation of this data collection are published by The Joint Commission in a series of newsletters entitled *Sentinel Event Alerts*. These *Sentinel Event Alerts* address events such as wrong-sided surgery, infant abduction, infection control issues, fires, and medication error events, among others. The original intent of these alerts was for health care organizations to review the "lessons learned" from those facilities that had experienced these sentinel events and to incorporate the recommendations for prevention described in each publication. This process was entirely voluntary and initially not tied to the accreditation process. However, certain sentinel events continued to plague the health care industry (e.g., wrong-sided surgery, suicide risk, patient falls, and the frequency of certain deadly medication errors). With the emphasis on health care patient safety (including the adoption of their own set of patient safety standards), the impact of the IOM report, and the industry-wide emphasis on error prevention as a backdrop, The Joint Commission formalized the information contained in their sentinel event database into a new accreditation requirement called the *National Patient Safety Goals.*

In 2002, The Joint Commission's Board of Commissioners approved an initial list of six National Patient Safety Goals (NPSGs) that represented the most commonly occurring and/or serious events from its sentinel event database, combined with the recommendations of an interdisciplinary task force. Each goal had evidence-based or expert-based recommendations to define how to successfully implement the goal. The Joint Commission Board reevaluates the goals annually. New goals are added to the list if necessary, and/or existing goals may be replaced with new goals that reflect processes in which there are safety concerns (e.g., hand hygiene, goals for medication reconciliation and hand-off communications, and a goal for anticoagulation therapy). Annually, the updated lists are published in the summer, with an implementation date of January 1 of the following year, providing a 6-month time period in which accredited organizations must design and implement the processes necessary to become compliant with the new standards. Each organization must demonstrate compliance with all applicable NPSG recommendations during the time of their accreditation survey. These goals have become the underpinning of the survey process. Those organizations that effectively implement the NPSGs find that they are more apt to have a successful survey outcome in this era of unannounced surveys.

Nurse managers can serve as role models by fully embracing the NPSGs on their units/departments and communicating their belief that implementation of these standards leads to safer patient care.

The Accountability Imperative and Patient Engagement

Health care reform brings a heightened focus on accountability. A critical component of reform includes an emphasis on patient-centered care and patient engagement. Patient engagement is defined as "actions an individual must make to obtain the greatest benefit from the health care services available to them" (Center for Advancing Health, 2010, p. 2). Emphasis is on the actions of patients and families versus the interventions of health professionals. Engaging the patient in shared decision making has been shown to produce better health outcomes (Glascow, 2002). Patient engagement in this context involves an active process of synthesizing health information, recommendations of health care professionals, and personal beliefs and preferences to manage one's illness. Nurse managers will continue to play an important role in designing care delivery systems that promote patient and family engagement.

Health Care Enterprise Risk Management

Enterprise risk management (ERM) is defined as "a structured analytical process that focuses on identifying and eliminating the financial impact and volatility of a portfolio of risks rather than on risk avoidance alone. Essential to this approach is an understanding that risk can be managed to gain competitive advantage" (Carroll, 2003, p. 1). Risk management is an integral component of an organization's quality improvement and health care safety programs. An *ERM program* is defined as an organization-wide program to identify risks, control occurrences, prevent damage, and control legal liability; it is a process whereby risks to the institution are evaluated and controlled. ERM domains include the following:

- **Operational:** Derived from the organization's core business, including its systems and practices. Examples include clinical services and outpatient care.
- **Financial:** Risks related to the organization's ability to earn, raise or access capital as well as costs associated with its transfer of risk. Examples include bonds and insurance premiums.
- **Human:** Relates to the risk related to recruiting, retaining and managing its workforce. Examples include worker's compensation, employee turnover and absenteeism, unionization, and discrimination.
- **Strategic:** Risks related to the ability of the organization to grow and expand. Examples include joint ventures, mergers, profitability, customer satisfaction, and financial performance.
- **Legal/Regulatory:** Risks related to health care statutory and regulatory compliance, licensure and accreditation. Examples include Health Insurance

Portability and Accountability Act compliance, Occupational Safety and Health Administration regulations, Medicare-deemed status, and The Joint Commission accreditation.

- **Technological:** Risk associated with biomedical and information technologies, equipment, devices and telemedicine. Examples include clinical information systems such as computerized physician order entry, radiology picture archiving and communication systems and off-site monitoring of critical care units (American Society for Healthcare Risk Management, 2006, p. 2).

ERM is a process whereby risks to the institution are evaluated and controlled to *reduce* or *prevent future loss.* Before the advent of comprehensive performance improvement and health care safety programs, one of the primary purposes of risk management was to prevent financial loss resulting from malpractice claims. The Joint Commission has traditionally required a risk management program for the entire organization as a part of its quality improvement efforts. Because a risk management program is structured to identify, analyze, and evaluate risks, these programs have now been incorporated as key components in organization-wide health care safety and PI programs. A risk manager is one of the "first responders" in a serious or sentinel event situation. Risk managers should facilitate the process by which the organization's definition of risk categories is established (i.e., what constitutes a "near miss," what is reportable on an incident report, what is included in the organizational definition of sentinel event). A new concept called "enterprise risk management" addresses the evaluation of all risks confronting an organization in order to maximize safety and risk reduction. The idea is to prevent undesirable events from happening and to minimize the impact of unpreventable risks. The concept of enterprise risk management dovetails with the overall requirements of a comprehensive organization-wide approach to health care safety.

The Chief Risk Officer (CRO) manages the ERM program. Key tasks of the CRO include:

1. Chairs the enterprise risk management committee
2. Develops a framework for the organization's risk management activities
3. Ensures that the organization is in full compliance with regulations
4. Does policy assessment
5. Assures business continuity (ability to sustain operations in the event of a disaster) through risk assessment, planning, financing, and risk transfer
6. Identifies and monitors emergent risks
7. Extends risk principles into the wider business strategy
8. Develops the data strategy required to build an accurate picture of operational risk; uses models to describe and quantify
9. Educates the investment community on the organization's risk management strategy
10. Does disclosures (internal and external)
11. Informs the board of significant risk issues
12. Delivers an integrated picture of risk across the enterprise
13. Determines the organization's tolerance for risk
14. Evaluates insurance coverage
15. Develops alternative risk strategies
16. Trains and communicates with the workforce on risk management policies and structures (American Society for Healthcare Risk Management, 2006, p. 12).

As a tool for ongoing risk identification and reporting, *incident or variance reports* form the core of organizational reporting from a risk management perspective. The purpose of an incident/variance report is to provide a factual accounting of an incident or adverse event to ensure that all facts surrounding the incident are recorded. A successful incident reporting process is one in which 100% of all appropriate incidents/adverse outcomes are reported to the risk manager. This goal is more apt to be achieved in those organizations that have adopted a non-punitive culture for reporting errors. The data contained in an incident/variance report also alert the risk manager about facts and circumstances that may contribute to a potential malpractice or lawsuit claim. The incident/variance reporting system provides the CRO with the opportunity to investigate all serious situations immediately. Data from incident reports are collated, analyzed, and used by leaders to identify risk areas that have ongoing trends or to point to areas that have emerging risk potential. These data can inform the choices that the organization's leaders make in the selection of processes to target for HFMEA projects or to "drill down" further via an RCA to study an adverse outcome or "near miss" more fully. Aggregated data from the organization's health care risk management program are reported through the performance improvement and health care safety reporting systems to coordinate information about overall organizational risks. Performance measures of action plan elements resulting from an RCA or HFMEA can be incorporated into a unit's/department's set of quality measures. Nurse managers can set the expectation for 100% reporting of risk events and "near misses" on their units/departments. Through diligent follow-up and the adoption of a non-punitive culture, managers can set the tone for a truly proactive ERM program.

In addition to internal reporting, many states (most via their health care licensure agencies, such as a department of health) have implemented mandatory adverse event reporting requirements, resulting in a new role for many health care risk managers. In organizations in these states, often the risk manager is accountable for the reporting of incidents that are on the mandated list. Most of these mandatory reporting programs also require the submission of formal RCAs as a follow-up to the initial report, including actions taken and assessment of the effectiveness of those actions. If the regulatory agency determines that the organization has not appropriately responded to the identified risks, it may result in further requirements for reporting and follow-up. This expanded role of the health care CRO in external reporting creates a need for collaboration with the quality professionals in the organization. Working together as a team, the risk manager and quality manager will often share responsibilities for facilitation of RCA and HFMEA teams to meet all of the internal and external accreditation and regulatory reporting requirements.

The most frequently cited factor in medical errors is poor or inadequate communication. TeamSTEPPS®, an evidence-based teamwork system, was designed for health care professionals by the U.S. Department of Defense and the Agency for Healthcare Research and Quality to improve communication and teamwork skills among health care professionals (AHRQ, n.d.). The program provides a comprehensive suite of ready-to-use materials and a training curriculum to successfully integrate teamwork principles into all areas of a health care system.

Educating Nurses About Quality and Safety

Academia has confronted the challenge of educating nurses about quality and safety by developing formal curricula. Quality & Safety Education for Nurses (QSEN), funded by the Robert Wood Johnson Foundation, is a comprehensive resource for faculty to help new health care professionals learn the knowledge and skills necessary to lead and support quality and safety initiatives in health care organizations (QSEN, 2012). These resources are free and regional education sessions have provided the opportunity for the content to spread throughout nursing academia. In acknowledging that nurses play a critical role in improving the safety and quality of patient care, the Agency for Healthcare Research and Policy published a comprehensive compendium of health care quality resources in their book *Patient Safety and Quality: An Evidence-Based Handbook for Nurses*. Readers are provided with proven techniques and interventions they can use to enhance patient care outcomes (Hughes, 2008). The Institute for Healthcare Improvement provides an "open school" for health professionals to learn about quality and safety. The IHI Open School for Health Professions is an interprofessional educational community that gives students the skills to become change agents in health care improvement (Institute for Healthcare Improvement, 2012).

Advancing Quality and Safety Policy

The Nursing Alliance for Quality Care (NAQC) was established in 2010 at the George Washington University School of Nursing as a "bold partnership among the nation's leading nursing organizations, consumers, and other key stakeholders" (NAQC, 2010, p. 1). **NAQC's mission** is to "Advance the highest quality, safety, and value of consumer-centered health care for all individuals—patients, their families, and their communities" (NAQC, 2010, p. 1). NAQC members include the following: American Association of Colleges of Nursing, American Academy of Nursing, AARP, American College of Nurse-Midwives, American Nurses Association, American Organization of Nurse Executives, American Academy of Nurse Practitioners, Association of Nurses in AIDS Care, Association of periOperative Registered Nurses, Consumers Advancing Patient Safety, Mothers Against Medical Error, National Council of State Boards of Nursing, National League for Nursing, National Organization of Nurse Practitioner Faculties, and the National Quality Forum. The group proposes to set policy related to nursing's pivotal role in health care transformation.

Clearly, nurses have been accountable for health care quality and safety since the profession's inception. Over the years, nurses have assumed roles in various health care settings for oversight of quality and performance improvement, as well as health care risk management. The IOM reports, the CMS requirements for public data reporting, and recent health care reform legislation initiatives have raised public awareness about quality and safety outcomes in health care organizations. These quality and safety issues have challenged health care quality professionals and nurse managers for decades. A heightened public awareness, combined with increasingly stringent standards for reporting quality and safety outcomes, is driving the need for health care organizations to address these issues. Professional nurses, in direct care, managerial, and executive roles, need to continue to be at the forefront, leading the charge in adoption of quality and safety initiatives that continuously enhance the quality of care and services provided to patients/clients, families, and communities.

CASE STUDY

Nurse Anthony Gardner has been asked by senior leadership to spearhead a group to evaluate patient falls to decrease their frequency and ideally prevent them from occurring. Based on the ERM data available from incident/variance reports, he selects nurses and nurses' aides for his team from the patient care units in which patient falls are most prevalent. He adds a pharmacist and physician to the team to represent the interdisciplinary aspects of the fall issue. He also recruits a family member of one of the patients on an Older Adult Unit to provide their perspective. Nurse Anthony then applies the Plan, Do, Check, and Act (PDCA) process to his project on patient falls.

In the "Plan" phase, he and the team use flowcharting to visually illustrate the steps that occur when a patient falls. Next, the team brainstorms a list of all of the problems that are associated with a patient fall. From this list, Nurse Anthony directs the team to categorize these factors into five or six groups, using an affinity diagram. Once the categories are defined, the team uses a cause-and-effect (fishbone) diagram to identify all of the potential causes that lead to the eventual effect of a patient fall. From this fishbone diagram, specific factors are considered as potential root causes (e.g., no fall assessment, bed too high, patient confusion, slippery floors, poor lighting, medications that can cause dizziness, no assistance with ambulation, staffing and staffing mix, call bells not answered promptly).

Nurse Anthony suggests collecting more data on each of these potential root causes. He further suggests that the data be stratified by patient age and gender, time of day, patient diagnoses, patient location, and staffing. He and the team design a data collection tool that will allow all of the data to be collected on one form.

After the data are collected, the team uses a Pareto chart to visually illustrate the most frequently occurring problems in descending order. By using this technique, they find that inadequate patient assessment and reassessment, call bells not answered promptly, and beds too high are the most common factors in patient falls. They also use Pareto charts to further define the stratification categories. When using this tool, they find that women older than 75 years with postoperative hip surgery seem most likely to fall on the evening shift. Most of the occurrences are on 4 South (the postsurgical unit).

During the "Do" phase, Nurse Anthony and the team design an assessment tool for the Older Adult Unit staff to collect data on all of the key factors identified earlier. For the trial, however, only the rooms of those female post–hip surgery patients older than 65 years are designated with a special symbol (a falling leaf) created by the team to represent a fall risk. Stickers with this symbol are also put on the call bell system lights for these rooms. Staff members are educated to the issue regarding quick call bell response and are requested to be especially vigilant in responding to the rooms with the special stickers. The data are collected for a 4-week trial period.

In the "Check" phase, the team reconvenes to evaluate the data collected in the trial. The data demonstrate a 37% reduction in patient falls from the same month in the previous year—just from addressing call bell response and none of the other factors.

Because the data on a sole factor demonstrated such a clear improvement, the team proceeds with development of a fall protocol, incorporating action plans to implement interventions for the other key factors identified earlier. The trial is expanded to another unit. When the data are analyzed for these two units and compared with the two other units with high fall occurrences, it is clear to the team that the protocol is having a positive

CASE STUDY—cont'd

impact on patient fall reduction. Throughout the process, nursing staff on the two trial units are solicited for feedback on the project, and their recommendations are incorporated into the protocol.

In the "Act" phase, the new Fall Prevention Protocol is adopted. Before its official "launch" in the organization, physicians, pharmacists, and nursing personnel are educated on the protocol. Data are collected not only on the outcomes but also on compliance with the interventions included in the protocol. After 3 months, the data demonstrate that those units with the lowest frequency of falls were those that had adopted the new protocol with enthusiasm and commitment. Nurse Anthony shares the data with the Nursing Leadership group, using control charts to demonstrate the outcomes. Based on the results, and in consultation with the Chief Risk Officer and the Performance and Quality Improvement Council, the group expands the definition of Fall Risk to include those patients who experienced a "near miss" (i.e., a fall in which the patient was assisted when falling and did not reach the floor). Data will now be collected on these patient occurrences and on their contributing factors. In so doing, leaders believes that overall patient safety can be further enhanced. Nurse Anthony and his team receive an award at the hospital's annual Health Care Quality Day for contributing to significant improvements in patient safety and quality of care.

▌ CRITICAL THINKING EXERCISE

Nurse Manager Todd Kennedy has just completed an online course on change and negotiation in health care. He has also served as the nursing department's quality improvement champion for 6 months, and he has been given accountability for program development. Nurse Jonathan Applington thinks that some of the health care quality indicators that nursing is using are out of date and may not be evidence-based. Furthermore, he does not see that the indicators address critical issues that the American Nurses Association (National Database of Nursing Quality Indicators), the Centers for Disease Control and Prevention (CDC; Handwashing Guidelines), and The Joint Commission have been emphasizing, especially in the areas of infection control and safety. He wants to ensure that the program is current, evidence-based, and responsive to accreditation and other regulatory standards.

1. What should Nurse Todd do first to address this issue?
2. Describe the written materials he must prepare.
3. What sources can Nurse Todd investigate to find national standardized performance measures related to nursing?
4. Because the nursing quality management program does not currently have mission and vision statements, what is the process he should employ to develop them?
5. How should Nurse Todd address resistance to change in this situation?

18

Measuring and Managing Outcomes

Sean P. Clarke, Lianne Jeffs

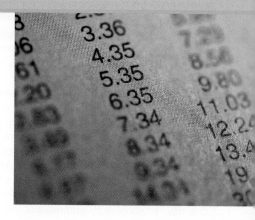

evolve WEBSITE

http://evolve.elsevier.com/Huber/leadership/

Today's health care organizations are required to respond to patient and societal demands while simultaneously improving quality and efficiency (Naranjo-Gil, 2009). Over the last decade, great progress has been made towards developing health care performance measurement and quality improvement frameworks (Clancy, 2007; Klassen et al., 2010). The American Academy of Nursing Expert Panel on Health Care Quality identified performance measurement as an integral component in transforming health care (Lamb & Donaldson, 2011). As part of this panel's call to action, a series of target papers are being developed and include: measuring episodes of care, care coordination, economic value of nursing, nurses' workload, and patient engagement. Nurse leaders have special opportunities to demonstrate nursing's contributions given the current focus on quality measures (process and outcomes) and initiatives attempting to link performance measures and reimbursement policies (Kohlbrenner et al., 2011). Meanwhile, the field of outcomes research continues to evolve. Outcomes research aims at a better understanding of the end results of health care practices

Photo used with permission from Photos.com.

and interventions such as the impact of care that are most important to patients, families, payors, and society. Key examples of these outcomes are health status, ability to function, quality of life, and mortality.

In this chapter, some basic ideas about outcomes and outcomes management will be reviewed, along with what outcomes research is, how it is conducted, and how it can be used by managers. Particularly important for managers are the implications of outcomes research for measurement and analysis of indicator data and the management of practice settings for nurses and other professionals.

DEFINITIONS

Key terms related to outcomes and their measurement and management include *outcomes, indicators, outcomes management, outcomes research, nursing outcomes research,* and *risk adjustment*. Simply put, an **outcome** is the result or results obtained from the efforts to accomplish a goal (Huber & Oermann, 1998). When most nurses consider outcomes, they think of the consequences of a health care intervention or treatment. The term *outcomes* has also been defined as the conditions in patients and others that health care delivery aims to achieve (Peters, 1995). Donabedian (1985) described outcomes as changes in the actual or potential health status of individuals, groups, or communities.

Indicators are "valid and reliable measures related to performance" (Oermann & Huber, 1999, p. 41). They are the specific tools used to make quality visible to stakeholders in health care. Outcomes are measured (quantified) by observing or describing indicators. Recently, the Agency for Healthcare Research and Quality (AHRQ, n. d.) developed a set of three broad categories of desirable attributes of a quality indicator: (1) importance; (2) scientific soundness, including clinical logic and measurement properties; and (3) feasibility.

Because quality is so important yet can be so elusive to define, a variety of accrediting and regulating bodies and a number of trade and professional associations, as well as health care quality assessment organizations (sometimes in alliances), have developed standardized health care performance indicator data sets to measure outcomes. For example, the AHRQ has developed a series of Patient Safety Indicators (PSIs) that include eighteen preventable adverse events and complications that patients may experience in their contacts with the health care system. A recent study explored using the AHRQ's PSIs to identify nursing-specific opportunities to improve care (Zrelak et al., 2012).

There are growing efforts to develop indicator sets involving nursing-specific or nursing-sensitive outcomes in an attempt to quantify nursing's contribution to quality and safety (Doran et al., 2011; Loan et al., 2011; McGillis-Hall, 2002; Naranjo-Gil, 2009). For example, the American Nurses Association (ANA) developed the National Database of Nursing Quality Indicators (NDNQI) based on their Nursing Quality Indicators initiative (ANA, 1996; NDNQI, n.d.). According to the ANA, outcome measures or indicators measure how nursing care affects clients (e.g., urinary tract infection incidence 72 hours after admission as an indicator of nosocomial infections potentially related to nursing care).

Indicators are used to measure all three of Donabedian's (1985) aspects of quality: structure, process, and outcomes. Donabedian's framework is useful to understand the relationship between outcomes and the structure and processes that have produced them. This suggests that nurse managers and leaders should attend to structure and process factors as precursors to patient outcomes (Donabedian, 2005).

Outcomes management, as originally described by Ellwood (1988), is a process used to assist managers and others make rational patient care–oriented decisions based on what is known about the effect of those choices on patient outcomes. To understand outcomes, the entire care process needs to be carefully examined, and variations must be analyzed. **Outcomes management** is defined as "a multidisciplinary process designed to provide quality health care, decrease fragmentation, enhance outcomes, and constrain costs. The core idea of outcomes management is the use of care process activities to improve outcomes" (Huber & Oermann, 1998, p. 4).

Outcomes research is a field (or subfield) in health services research that examines the extent to which services achieve the goals of health care. What makes outcomes research distinct from other bodies of research that examine end points in patients (i.e., much clinically-oriented research) is that outcomes researchers seek to tease out the effects of patient-level care and systems-level environments from the background demographic, psychosocial, and clinical characteristics of patients as influences on end points. The purpose is to understand which patients or clients fare well and which do not in relation to treatments selected and/or the organizational context of care delivery (Kane, 2006; Mitchell et al., 1998). An example of a provider characteristic that might be investigated as a predictor of patient outcomes might be the professional background of providers (e.g., physicians versus advanced practice nurses; RNs versus LPNs/LVNs).

Nursing outcomes research is a subspecialty within the larger field of health outcomes research that focuses on determining the effect of different contexts and conditions, related specifically to nurses and nursing care, on the health status of patients. Nursing outcomes researchers are interested in the structures or management strategies for nursing care delivery, as well as the mix of health care workers best equipped to care for them. Other types of outcomes research are intended to determine the types of patients who benefit most from certain nursing interventions.

OUTCOMES MANAGEMENT

The process of managing outcomes includes the following five steps:

1. Data are collected about outcomes.
2. Trends are identified from data analysis.
3. Variances are investigated.
4. Appropriate service delivery changes are determined.
5. Changes are implemented and reevaluated.

In managing outcomes, the information derived from measuring client outcomes is collected, trends are identified, variances are examined, and appropriate care needs are determined to improve care to an individual, group, or population. Goals of this process include quality improvement and risk reduction. Variance analysis is one outcomes management tool. A variance is a deviation from what is expected. For nurses, this may mean a departure from the anticipated clinical trajectory. Variances may be positive or negative but are most useful for trends analysis.

Outcomes research and measurement examines the effectiveness of nursing care in improving client outcomes. Outcomes data and information about factors or approaches that promote favorable outcomes can help nurses assist clients and their families in meeting health needs and care needs across the continuum of care. Reading outcomes research can also help nurses to locate and select interventions that are the most useful in accomplishing the desired improvement in the client's health status. Identifying the most effective interventions can provide invaluable information for patient self-management (Oermann & Huber, 1997, 1999).

As in any area of clinical care or the management of health services, ideally practice is at least partially guided by research evidence. Although outcomes research has a great deal in common with other forms of research, it involves some special elements. In particular, outcomes researchers are especially concerned about understanding "real" differences between expected and observed outcomes and between outcomes on different units, in different institutions, or at different points in time.

Outcomes research can provide key data for managerial decision making to improve quality of care. Data derived from outcomes research can be used to answer the following types of questions:

- What mix of staffing skill level and education is appropriate to achieve optimal outcomes for a clinical population with a particular level of patient acuity?
- What level of technology and ratio of technology and staff achieve the best outcomes for high-risk patients?
- What is the optimal organizational structure to maintain efficiency, safety, and patient satisfaction at institutions that provide high volumes of services?

Although the answers to each of these questions depend on individual and institutional contexts and economic considerations, data from outcomes research can be used to inform decision making.

INFLUENCES ON OUTCOMES

It is critical that all consumers of outcomes data, including managers, understand how to interpret measures. Clinicians and other workers attempt to foster positive patient outcomes and avoid negative ones. However, the specific treatments delivered to patients are only one factor influencing how well patients do. A model of factors influencing outcomes is useful as a guide for managers. Kane (2006) summarized the factors influencing outcomes and expressed this in the form of a mathematical "function" as follows:

Outcomes=f(patient clinical characteristics and risk factors, patient demographics, organizational characteristics of the setting, treatment, random chance)

Nurses and nurse leaders are obviously most interested in the effects of treatment on outcomes. For nurses, the focus is usually the process of nursing care on outcomes, but that often encompasses the actions of the entire multidisciplinary health team. However, correctly interpreting health outcomes data across settings or providers (whether in practice or in research) and attributing differences and outcomes to the right causes or sources requires attention to two major challenges. The first lies in ensuring that consistent definitions and data collection processes have been identified, and accurate measures of the phenomena of interest are used. This includes the outcomes, treatment, and any other risk factors thought to influence outcomes. The second challenge, shared with all research dealing with dependent variables influenced by many factors, is that of risk adjustment (Iezzoni, 2003). Risk adjustment involves accounting for patient factors, the intrinsic risks that a patient brings to the health care encounter in the form of clinical and/or demographic factors, before drawing conclusions about the meaning of different values for indicators. Comparisons of outcomes across settings or time periods are meaningful only when potentially important differences in the characteristics of patients involved are taken into account.

MEASUREMENT OF OUTCOMES

Jennings and colleagues (1999) have presented a framework classifying outcome indicators into three categories by stakeholder perspective: patient-focused, provider-focused, and organization-focused. Patient-focused outcomes can include such indicators as disease status, symptom experience, or pain. Other outcomes indicators incorporate a broader impact of disease and its management on clients' lives. These perceptual outcomes include quality of life, functional status, health status, and patient satisfaction. There are also provider and organizational outcomes. Provider-focused outcomes include such phenomena as nurse burnout, turnover, and job satisfaction. Organization-focused outcomes may include patient or provider outcomes that are aggregated to the organizational level, such as rates of hospital-wide inpatient or 30-day mortality, errors, and other adverse events. Cost indicators are commonly measured at the organizational (hospital-wide) or unit level. A number of health system level outcomes are also receiving increased attention and include measures of successful movements of patients across settings (i.e., care transitions) (Naylor et al., 2011) and readmission rates (Epstein, 2009; van Walraven et al., 2011).

ELEMENTS OF OUTCOMES RESEARCH

Various types of indicators can be used to aid managers in decision making, highlighting improvements in structures and processes of nursing care and justifying various investments in human and material resources in their settings. Indicators can also be used in formal research studies that examine the factors associated with the quality of care.

Variable Selection

When reading outcomes research, managers should be aware that researchers are often faced with considerable challenges when selecting outcome measures. The specific measures used should influence how managers interpret and apply study findings. For instance, outcomes can either be generic or broadly applicable to many patient groups or be condition-specific, but they must be defined clearly. An outcome that is not clearly defined is impossible to interpret, and any conclusions or decisions by managers based on those research data may be flawed. Managers should also consider the sources of data used. For example, consider a study examining the association of workload with nurse injuries. It would be important to know whether the injury data were gathered from nurse self-reports, an injury data-base, manager reports, insurance records, or some other source and to be aware of the potential limitations or biases of each of these sources.

Risk Adjustment

Analyses of outcomes across groups are meaningful only if those analyses account for relevant individual differences in the patient populations being served. Risk adjustment can be a complicated exercise but an important one because, if given inadequate attention, patterns and associations that are found related to differences across units, hospitals, or time periods may or may not be validly interpreted as reflecting variations in quality of care. One caution is important. Certain types of outcomes are so dramatic and so closely tied to systems failures (e.g., transfusion errors, severe pressure ulcers) that risk adjustment is unlikely to alter the interpretation of the relevant indicators. The literature contains some excellent references that discuss the state of the science in risk adjustment techniques (Iezzoni, 2003; Kane, 2006).

LEADERSHIP AND MANAGEMENT IMPLICATIONS

Today's health care leaders are charged with the ensuring high-quality services that achieve a variety of desired outcomes. Outcomes research can provide nurse leaders with an evidence-based foundation for leadership decisions around allocating resources and monitoring of patient safety (Albanese et al., 2010; Doran et al., 2011). Broad concepts from outcomes research can help nurse leaders analyze and interpret their own data and assist them to make better decisions in establishing environments for delivering care that favor good results.

Managers and executives today have a wealth of information available to them, and they are charged with determining which data indicate a need for action. A significant body of literature in nursing outcomes research that continues to grow is a valuable point of reference for managers. There is, for instance, a large and expanding body of literature suggesting that lower staffing levels and skill mix in acute care hospitals are associated with increased risk of negative outcomes (Clarke & Donaldson, 2008). Low staffing levels have often but not always been associated with a number of unfavorable outcomes, including increased surgical mortality, failure to rescue, and rates of complications due to errors in care such as urinary tract infections, intravenous line infections, decubitus ulcers, and patient falls (Kane et al., 2007). However, the specific context of the care environment and the patient population of interest call for continual monitoring of outcomes against internal and external benchmarks. Several data systems support the monitoring of nursing-sensitive outcomes. For example, the ANA has developed a proprietary national database of quality indicators and measures called the National Database for Nursing Quality Indicators (NDNQI). NDNQI participants contribute unit-specific data on nursing-sensitive indicators that are then benchmarked across peer units elsewhere (Gallagher & Rowell, 2003). Similar databases were established for the military and veterans' health systems (VANOD and MilNOD) and a similar initiative that began in California (CalNOC) continues to recruit participants from across the United States and internationally. The National Quality Forum (NQF) endorsed and later re-endorsed a set of voluntary consensus standards for nursing-sensitive care that quantify the contribution of nursing to patient safety, health care outcomes, and the professional work environment (Frith et al., 2010; NQF, 2004, 2009; Naylor, 2007). Also, agencies as diverse as the Centers for Medicare and Medicaid Services (CMS), The Joint Commission, and the Magnet Recognition Program® of the American Nurses Credentialing Center incorporate outcome-based reporting requirements into their processes.

Nurse leaders have a crucial role in identifying outcomes sensitive to nursing care, acquiring computerized data support for tracking them, and participating in multidisciplinary teams toward comprehensive outcomes management. The collection, reporting, and benchmarking of nursing-sensitive patient outcome data can make a powerful contribution to quality of care (Patrician et al., 2011). In some organizations, nurse leaders are using patient outcome data to drive patient care improvement strategies (Donaldson et al., 2005; Jeffs et al., 2011; Smith, 2007). Managers and executives in practice struggle with decisions regarding the minimum number of data elements needed to satisfy payers and regulators in relation to the challenges of being sufficiently comprehensive and inclusive in measure selection. In terms of a guide or framework for selecting groups of outcomes for tracking purposes, balanced scorecard and dashboard approaches are gaining popularity. Dashboard approaches seek to identify the key factors for which a nurse manager needs to frequently monitor data to manage quality and costs. The balanced scorecard uses four areas for data evaluation—internal business processes, learning and growth, customer, and financial—and directs managers to select indicators from each of these areas (Park & Huber, 2007).

CURRENT ISSUES AND TRENDS

More than ever, the consequences of decisions in health care involving nursing services need to be clarified, investigated, and matched to desired outcomes. The importance of evidence-informed decision making based on reliable outcome data is paramount, especially in times of financial constraint (Jeffs et al., 2009). Cost-containment strategies have often involved a single-minded focus on decreasing staff coverage or reducing the proportions of registered nurses in staff mixes without forethought to the potential consequences for patient outcomes. Outcomes research will be vital for understanding the consequences of deploying various configurations of staff in different circumstances, especially if circumstances arise where traditional models of care are no longer viable because sufficient numbers of the certain types of nursing staff are no longer available or affordable. Again, it is vital that management decision making be evidence-based wherever possible in order to optimize quality of care, as called for by the Institute of Medicine.

Outcomes research also shapes the policy environments and constraints in which managers operate. Since 1999, when California Governor Gray Davis signed Assembly Bill 394 (AB 394) into law, which requiring the State Department of Health Services to adopt regulations establishing minimum nurse-to-patient ratios, there has been widespread discussion of similar legislation at both state and federal level across the United States. The legislative intent behind the California initiative was to improve quality of care, patient safety, and nurse retention. Then and now, proposals to regulate nurse staffing in some way (requiring the reporting of staffing levels, submission of staffing plans, or mandating specific ratios) cite the body of evidence from outcomes research demonstrating links between low nurse staffing and poor outcomes. Evaluation of the impacts of the California experiment continues, and results in terms of net benefits to patients and the state's health care system have been decidedly mixed (Donaldson & Shapiro, 2010); nonetheless, the continued dialogue shows both widespread concern regarding safety outcomes and significant pockets of support for tracking and regulating structural elements in hospitals like staffing.

Another trend is the exponential growth of aging patients coping with multiple conditions and chronic diseases. This cohort continues to be the major expenditure of health care costs and at risk for experiencing negative outcomes (e.g., medication errors, increased length of stay in hospital, unplanned readmissions) due to poorly executed care transitions (Naylor et al., 2011, Naylor, 2012). There are promising innovative solutions aimed at improving integration and continuity across episodes of care. One leading example, the Transitional Care Model (TCM), is a delivery system innovation that is designed to increase alignment of the care system with the preferences, needs, and values of high-risk individuals and their family caregivers and achieve higher-quality outcomes while reducing health care costs (Naylor, 2012). Implementation of the TCM has been associated with the following favorable outcomes: (1) reductions in preventable hospital readmissions; (2) short-term improvements in physical health, functional status, and quality of life; (3) increased overall satisfaction with the care experience; and (4) reductions in total health care costs.

Another trend receiving growing attention is the pay-for-performance reimbursement systems that tie a preestablished portion of payment of services to achieving specific levels of measurable, targeted outcomes or attaining the highest scores on specific measures. Where particular nursing services and interventions are linked to improvements and consistency in achieving outcomes that are pay-for-performance indicators, managers and institutions have tangible incentives for altering organizational structures and practices to achieve better outcomes (Kohlbrenner et al., 2011). However, there are continuing concerns that pay-for-performance initiatives, in health care as well as in other sectors such as education, may produce serious unintended consequences (Clarke et al., 2008) and may not ultimately improve patient outcomes (Jha et al., 2012).

As consumers, regulators, and payers increase their focus on outcomes, nurse managers must proactively engage in outcomes management and participate in the ongoing development and implementation of nursing-sensitive quality indicators. Awareness of advances in outcomes measurement and the results of outcomes research is essential and will continue to be critical for effective nursing leadership.

Nursing outcomes offer insights and challenges for managers to use evidence in shaping practice environments to ensure best practices and positive patient outcomes. A wealth of research-based and research-informed measures and databases are available to managers to assist in databased decision making and outcomes management. As health care systems become more outcomes-driven, nurse managers and leaders must be involved, and where appropriate, spearhead the development of outcomes tracking and management systems.

RESEARCH NOTE

Source

Naylor, M.D., Aiken, L.H.A., Kurtzman, E.T., Olds, D.M., & Hirschman, K.B. (2011). The importance of transitional care in achieving health reform. *Health Affairs, 30*(4), 746-754.

Purpose

Transitions, or "handoffs," are vulnerable exchange points that contribute to unnecessarily high rates of health services use and health care spending, and they expose chronically ill people to care of poor quality. Transitional care programs help hospitalized patients with complex chronic conditions—who are often the most vulnerable patients—transfer from one type of care setting or level of care to another. The purpose of this systematic review was to identify and synthesize available evidence regarding transitional care for populations with adult chronic illnesses.

Discussion

Twenty-one randomized clinical trials of transitional care interventions targeting chronically ill adults were reviewed. Outcome measures included a variety of primary and secondary outcomes in five categories: health outcomes; quality of life; patient satisfaction or perception of care; resource use (including readmis-sions); and costs. Among these studies, the end point for assessment of the interventions' effect ranged from 1 month to 12 months (mean=5.4 months). Nine interventions demonstrated reductions on measures related to hospital readmissions (total all-cause read-missions, time to first readmission, or length of re-admission stay)—a key focus of health reform. Most of the interventions had sustained impacts on read-missions through at least thirty days after discharge. Many of the successful interventions shared similar features, such as comprehensive discharge planning and follow-up interventions with home visits, assigning a nurse as the clinical manager or leader of care and including in-person home visits to discharged patients.

Application to Practice

Based on these findings, the authors recommend several strategies to guide the implementation of transitional care. Nurse leaders must invest in transitions programs supported by evidence, implement scientifically sound measures to monitor impacts across the full range of transitional care processes and outcomes, and educate all health care professionals to develop necessary knowledge and skills to deliver effective transitional care.

CASE STUDY

Nurse Maria Garcia manages a primary care clinic, where several years ago nurses noticed a problem with women's health care. Little counseling regarding menopause and health care was being provided. Nurse Garcia and her colleagues see menopause counseling as a prime opportunity for nurses to deliver needed preventive and wellness care. Furthermore, the National Committee for Quality Assurance (NCQA) that accredits managed care organizations includes responses to user surveys regarding menopause counseling in its HEDIS data set, which is its national database of standardized performance and accreditation information for benchmarking. Nurse Garcia wants to take the menopause counseling program to "the next level." However, several questions, which were asked at the beginning of the program, remain: How much does this cost? Which personnel should be involved? What should be included in the program? Which patients should be targeted?

1. What is the problem?
2. Why is it a problem?
3. What are the key issues?
4. What should Nurse Garcia do first?
5. How should Nurse Garcia handle this situation?
6. What outcomes should be used to monitor this ongoing program?
7. What outcomes measures or indicators are relevant?

CRITICAL THINKING EXERCISE

Nancy is an advanced practice nurse with expertise in pressure ulcer and ostomy care on the general surgical unit at Mt. St. Elsewhere Hospital. She has been asked by her clinical director and the quality improvement director for the hospital to develop a strategy to address the increase of pressure ulcers reported in the hospital's recent quality scorecard. Data on pressure ulcers are captured in what is abstracted from the patients' charts and analyzed in an aggregate format. In addition to hospital reporting, the hospital's pressure ulcer rates are publicly reported and benchmarked with other hospitals in their state. Patients on Nancy's unit had not only a very high number of ulcers but also a high number that were not documented on admission, suggesting that they occurred during the patients' hospital stays. This finding is concerning from a quality of care perspective and financially as added hospital days and costs related to nosocomial pressure ulcers are not billable to the Medicare program and other health insurance carriers. To assist Nancy in determining the indicators to be measured to evaluate the impact of a targeted pressure ulcer intervention, she needs to consider the following questions:

1. Using the AHRQ criteria, how could Nancy ensure the indicators selected to measure the impact of the pressure ulcer intervention are sound measures? In answering this question consider drawing up a list of potential explanations that reflect a real decline in quality of care related to pressure ulcer prophylaxis on Nancy's unit or an artifactual one (related to something other than quality of care).

2. What are the structure, process, and outcomes elements associated with pressure ulcer incidence?

3. What would Nancy want to clarify about these data and how they were collected before getting too far into a discussion about next action steps?

4. If Nancy or her colleagues wanted to compare the unit's rates of pressure ulcers with those of other units or hospitals (or even to last year's figures), what cautions should be applied? Where would they go to find benchmarks?

5. Drawing on your background and a search of the Internet, what investments of resources could be attempted to change this situation?

6. How would Nancy and her colleagues know if the approaches in No. 5 worked? What kinds of data would you suggest they gather?

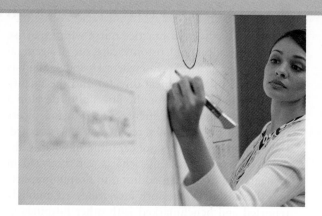

evolve WEBSITE

http://evolve.elsevier.com/Huber/leadership/

Strategic management (Coulter, 2009; Dess et al., 2011; Pearce & Robinson, 2012; Sare & Ogilvie, 2009) involves conducting an environmental scan, knowing the competition, establishing goals, setting targets, developing an action plan, implementing the plan, and evaluating success. This approach has long been used in business to ensure a competitive advantage over similar enterprises. It has become imperative for health care organizations to function as businesses. Those that do not do so fail to remain viable for long.

Issues in the health care industry, including the Hospital Consumer Assessment of Healthcare Providers and Systems (HCAHPS) and the Hospital Value-Based Purchasing Program, among others, require strategic management to obtain and maintain a competitive advantage. The success of an enterprise depends on its competitive advantage—that is, how well it does something compared with similar efforts and how well it is able to continuously achieve superior performance. Collins and Porràs (2004) and Peters and Waterman (2004) studied a number of best-run companies and identified strategic management approaches that these companies used that

made them successful and allowed them to dominate the market. In 2011, Collins and Hansen described the principles that ensured the success of enterprises in an unpredictable, chaotic environment, such as health care.

Strategic management involves strategic planning and implementation. It provides a "blueprint" for operating a business, establishing a competitive position, ensuring customer satisfaction, and reaching strategic objectives or goals. Although most strategic management occurs at the "macro" level (i.e., the executive levels of the health care institution), it can benefit the "micro" level, such as the nursing division, department, or unit, as well. Strategic management prepares nurses to adapt to the current health care environment. Strategic management helps nurses achieve their goals, whether related to the workplace or to the profession.

DEFINITIONS

Thinking and behaving strategically are prime methods for nurses to be proactive in a complex, fast-changing, rapid-cycle environment. The concept of strategic management includes strategic planning (The Association for Strategic Planning [*www.strategyplus.org/*]), and also focuses on strategy implementation. The terms associated with an organization's use of strategy include *strategic management, organizational vision or mission, strategy, strategic plan,* and *objectives.* **Strategic management** is defined as the management of an organization based on its vision or mission. **Organizational vision** or **mission** is a guiding framework that describes what the organization views as its business and future direction. **Core values** define the characteristics or values that underlie the organization's activities. The **core purpose** is the reason the organization is in business. **Strategy** is a competitive move or business approach designed to produce a successful outcome. **Tactics** are operational choices for action that are made to implement a strategy. A **strategic plan** is a document that specifies a plan for actualizing the mission. A strategic plan may also involve a *business plan* or an *action plan* (either as part of the strategic plan or as an adjunct to it) that consists of the who, what, by when, where, and in general terms, the costs involved in implementing the activities identified as objectives in the strategic plan. **Objectives** are defined as the targets an organization wants to achieve. These can be financial or performance-based with short-range or long-range targets.

STRATEGIC PLANNING PROCESS

Strategic management generally begins with a strategic planning process, triggered by recognition of the need for an organization to establish its competitive position in the marketplace or to address some other believed need (e.g., seeking Magnet recognition from the American Nurses Credentialing Center Magnet Recognition Program®, [2008], applying for the Malcolm Baldrige National Quality Award, or simply to establish future directions). The following are questions to be answered in the strategic planning process:

- Where are we currently?
- Where do we want to go?
- How will we get there?

The components of the nursing process—assessment, planning, implementation, and evaluation—are similar to those employed in strategic management, as follows:

- Developing a strategic mission or vision
- Setting objectives
- Developing strategies to achieve the objectives

- Implementing the strategies
- Evaluating the results

The strategic plan provides a framework for strategic management, considering both external and internal environmental factors.

Developing a Mission and Vision

The first step of the strategic planning process is to identify the organization's vision or mission. This requires a determination of what the organization is, what business it is in and for whom, and where the business seeks to be in the future. The mission statement reflects the vision of what the organization seeks to do and to become; it provides a clear view of what the organization is trying to accomplish, and it indicates its intent to carve out a particular position in the industry or field.

The core values of an organization and its core purpose inform its mission statement. The core values held by an organization are those that are held whether or not circumstances (either internal or external) change. These core values are so embodied in the culture of the organization that even if they were seen as a liability, they would not be abandoned. These core values do not change even if the industry in which the organization operates changes. Thus, in health care, the organization that has as its core values excellent customer service, integrity, and social responsibility would retain those core values despite internal changes (e.g., changes in chief executive officers [CEOs]) or external changes (e.g., reimbursement, the nursing shortage).

The organization's core purpose is the reason the organization exists. The core purpose, like the core values, is relatively unchanging. The core purpose provides direction to the organization and contributes to the articulation and implementation of its mission.

In the strategic planning process, a facilitator or the planners themselves address questions that assist the planners to arrive at a specific vision and mission including the following:

- What business are we in now?
- What business do we want to be in?
- What do our customers expect of us now?
- What will be the customers' expectations in the future?
- Who are our customers now?

- Who will be our customers in the future?
- Who are our current stakeholders (other than customers)?
- How will those stakeholders change in the future? What about their expectations?
- Who are our primary competitors currently?
- Who will be our competitors in the future?
- What about partners, now and in the future?
- What will be the effect of technology?
- What are the available and the needed resources, both human and financial?
- What is happening in the environment both internally and externally, now and in the future, that may affect us?

It is assumed that the core values and the core purpose of the organization have been defined previously; but if not, planners should develop these using questions such as the following:

- What are the values on which we base our work?
- How central or essential are these to the organization?
- Would these values be supported if circumstances changed? If the industry in which we currently operate changes?

The core purpose can be explicated by asking and answering questions such as what business are we in and what business do we want to be in? The core purpose can be refined by asking "why," so that the initial response, "We are in the business of health care," may be further refined to "We want to contribute to the community in which we exist." Thus asking "why" may result in the core value of social responsibility and the core purpose of providing needed health care services to the community in which the organization is located.

Generally, addressing the strategic planning process questions involves considering both external environmental factors (e.g., activities of regulatory bodies) and internal environmental factors (e.g., financial and human resources). The assessment of future environmental impact takes the form of assumptions. These assumptions encompass the sociodemographic, political, economic, and technological aspects of the external environment. Of course, these assumptions are merely "best guesses," because it is impossible to predict the future with any certainty.

Responses to these questions by the principals involved in an organization (e.g., executive management, supervisory staff, department heads) will shape an organization's strategic plan and, as a result, its strategic management. Involving individuals at all levels of the organization (e.g., staff nurses, clerical workers) in addition to those at the top of the hierarchy will ensure a variety of perspectives and more "buy-in" to the final product.

Crafting a vision with the input of many individuals has the advantage of being a result of many perspectives, and it also engages those individuals in helping make the vision a reality. When everyone involved in an institution shares the same vision, individuals know where the organization is going and can be instrumental in helping it get there through their daily activities. As the old saying goes, "If you don't know where you're going, then any path will take you there." Conversely, if all of the individuals in the institution know where they are going, there is a greater likelihood they all will take the same path.

Setting Objectives

Once the organization's mission and vision have been established, the next step in strategic planning is to develop the ways and means to get there. Thus strategic goals and objectives are crafted. These objectives generally define the "who," "what," and "where" of the strategies to be implemented. Focusing the objectives allows individuals to recognize where the organization currently is, where it wants to go, and how much time it will take to get there. Absence of strategic objectives results in individuals trying to move in too many directions without a coordinated plan or not moving at all because of confusion about the organization's direction.

The strategic objectives provide a way of converting the rather abstract mission of an organization into concrete terms—targets of performance that, taken together, will achieve the mission. Objectives also offer a way of measuring progress toward achieving the organization's mission. These objectives generally are written to reflect not what *is* but what *should be*— activities that encourage the individuals implementing them to be creative, to stretch beyond their current limits, and to challenge themselves to improve their performance. These objectives must be achievable, however, lest individuals lose faith that they can accomplish them. If the strategic objectives are challenging but achievable, they will prevent employees of an institution from becoming complacent or settling for the status quo.

Objectives generally are written in terms of financial outcomes that relate to improvements in an organization's fiscal health and those that will result in a stronger position for the institution in the industry. For example, a for-profit hospital may set a financial objective to increase earnings growth by a specific percentage each year. A specific strategic objective might be to achieve lower overall costs than competitors or to attain technological advantage.

Developing an Implementation Strategy

The third step in the strategic planning process is to decide how to achieve the financial and strategic objectives that were established, how to obtain a competitive advantage over rivals in the field or industry, how to respond to changing conditions both externally and internally, how to defend against adverse conditions, and how to grow the business to increase market share. The strategies must be planned in advance and must also be adaptable to outside influences. Thus objectives are the targeted results and outcomes, and the strategy is how to achieve that outcome. The strategy must be deliberate and purposeful (planned and intentional) and also flexible enough to respond to events that are unanticipated when the strategy is developed. For example, new opportunities may arise that were unknown at the time a strategic objective was developed; these opportunities could greatly increase an organization's competitive position. Changes in a product line or service provided by an organization may necessitate a change in a strategic objective.

Basically, an organization's strategy consists of how it treats its customers and stakeholders; how it responds to changes in the industry and marketplace; how it capitalizes on new opportunities; how it manages its operations; how it grows and develops; and how it achieves its financial and strategic objectives. The challenge is to involve key people in the organization in developing this strategy so that these individuals can champion the implementation of the strategy. The desired outcome is to ensure that the strategy is timely, responsive, innovative, creative, and designed to take advantage of opportunities as they arise.

The benefits of strategic management cannot be overemphasized. In today's business climate, particularly in the health care environment, survival is tenuous and success is fraught with difficulty. A good management strategy helps an organization remain strong enough to withstand competition, overcome obstacles, and achieve peak performance. The organization's strategy must be flexible to respond appropriately to the following:

- Evolving needs and preferences of customers and stakeholders
- Advances in technology
- Changes in political climate and regulatory requirements
- New opportunities
- Altered market conditions
- Disasters and crises

The organization's strategic plan must include these aspects: where the organization is currently and where it is headed, how it plans to get to its desired future through short-term and long-term performance targets (i.e., strategic objectives), and what will be done to achieve these outcomes. The strategic plan encompasses the organization's mission and vision, strategic and financial objectives, and a strategy for achieving the objectives.

Implementing the Strategy

Once the strategy has been delineated, the next step is to implement it. Implementation involves trying out the activities in a way that determines how best to close the gap between how things are done and what it takes to achieve the strategy. For example, given an objective related to improvement of the financial bottom line, the first step is to determine current cost and then compare it with desired cost to decide what needs to be changed to reach the desired lower cost.

Strategy must be implemented proficiently and efficiently, as well as in a timely manner, if it is to be effective. For this to occur, the organization must attend to its capabilities, the reward structure, available support systems, and the organizational culture. If any of these characteristics are not in place, implementation of the strategy will surely fail. If, for example, employees are not rewarded in ways that are meaningful to them to implement a strategy, it is highly unlikely that they will initiate or maintain efforts to implement the strategy. If the organizational culture does not support innovation or risk taking, or if the prevailing attitude is "if it's not broken, don't fix it," then efforts to improve performance or outcomes will be doomed.

Implementing strategy is closely linked to an organization's operations; it involves managing, budgeting, motivating, changing culture, supervising, and leading. Strategic planning and implementation are managerial processes that accomplish the following:

- Demonstrate leadership in implementation of strategy
- Reward those who carry out strategy successfully
- Allocate necessary resources to activities critical to strategy
- Formulate policies and procedures that support identified strategy
- Initiate continuous quality improvement activities
- Develop and reward best practices
- Maintain a culture that supports strategy

Evaluating Effectiveness

The final step in strategic management is to evaluate the outcomes of the strategic planning process and the implementation of strategy. This evaluation component is an ongoing process; it is not a static endeavor. Because of the nature of health care environments, things change and it is necessary to constantly evaluate performance and strategy, use the data collected to decide how things are going, and make changes as indicated. Changes that may need to be made range from adjusting the organization's long-term direction, raising or lowering performance expectations, or modifying a strategy, depending on what the situation requires.

It may be—and often is—necessary to make mid-course corrections to the strategic plan, the strategic objectives, or the strategy. The evaluation process should facilitate identification of the areas in which changes need to be made. The need for changes should not be interpreted as failure of the process; rather, elements of the plan may flounder for a variety of reasons, such as diminished focus on the strategic plan, lack of commitment on the part of employees (who may not have initially been part of the process of developing the plan), and the inability to create a balance between staying the course and making corrections in midcourse.

Part of the evaluative process of a strategic plan is an annual review of the plan, of the assumptions underlying it, and of the feedback received from performance data, activity reports, market indications, and customer surveys. Also, an environmental scan and analysis should be undertaken to ensure that the conditions that affect the organization, its mission, vision,

and strategic plan have not changed to a level sufficient to necessitate change in the organization itself.

Environmental analysis incorporates an internal analysis such as a review of the mission statement and value system, as well as an external analysis. The analysis needs to review four areas: **s**trengths, **w**eaknesses, **o**pportunities, and **t**hreats (SWOT) (Fine, 2011). The SWOT method is one of the most popular ways to develop strategic plans for an organization. In this approach, strengths and weaknesses internal to the organization are identified. These strengths and weaknesses generally are related to resources, programs, and operations in key areas of the organization, examples of which are the following:

- *Operations:* efficiency, capacity, processes
- *Management:* systems, expertise, resources
- *Products:* quality, features, prices
- *Finances:* resources, performance

Once identified, these components are analyzed for the purpose of drafting a picture of the critical features of the organization, its achievements and failures, and its good points and bad points.

The external components are described as opportunities and threats, and they are identified in the same manner as the internal factors. Opportunities and threats may include changes in the following:

- Industry
- Marketplace
- Economy
- Political climate
- Technology
- Competition

Once identified, these strengths, weaknesses, opportunities, and threats must be analyzed for their impact on the organization. Next, priorities must be established for the critical issues so that strategies are based on the priority issues. For example, a change in the market for the organization's services may be a threat but a low priority, so the organization determines it is not essential to target resources (e.g., human, financial) to deal with the threat when a higher priority is to take advantage of an opportunity involving technology. The SWOT analysis often leads to future strategies in which the organization determines to do the following:

- Build on strengths
- Resolve or minimize weaknesses
- Exploit opportunities
- Avoid threats

The strategies identified through the SWOT analysis can be shaped into a strategic plan on which strategic management is based. The more carefully the analysis is done, the more reliable the strategic plan. A plan based on faulty assumptions or careless analysis will not serve the organization well and, indeed, may lead eventually to its demise.

ELEMENTS OF A STRATEGIC PLAN

Most strategic plans result in a written document. This document can be written by the individuals involved in the strategic planning process or, more likely, by the individual who facilitated the strategic planning process (e.g., consultant, employee). Generally, strategic plan documents contain the following sections:

- *Executive summary:* A two- to three-page encapsulation of the essence of the plan, written in language understandable by all potential readers, because many will not venture beyond the first few pages of the document
- *Background:* A description of the institution, its history, and current state, including its accomplishments, as well as the situation that prompted the strategic planning process
- *Mission, vision, and values:* Should describe the philosophy of the organization
- *Goals and strategies:* Should describe the target objectives and the strategies identified to ensure achievement of the objectives
- *Appendixes:* All the documentation related to the strategic planning process so that the reader obtains a sense of the background information used by the strategic planners to arrive at the strategic plan

Appendix materials can include the following elements:

- Annual reports of the institution
- SWOT analysis results
- Financial information
- Environmental scan results
- Staffing information
- Current and projected programs and services

Other materials can be included as desired. Caution should be exercised, however, to not include confidential data that should not be viewed by individuals outside of the organization.

The strategic plan should be disseminated widely throughout the institution. It is not necessary to reproduce the document in its entirety for everyone in the institution. A decision needs to be made about which parts of the strategic plan are appropriate for the individuals who will receive them. Some will need the entire plan; others may need only the executive summary; and still others may need only the goals and strategies.

In any case, the strategic plan should be communicated to stakeholders: board members, management, and staff. Copies should be included in orientation programs for new employees. The institution's vision and mission, including the core values, should be displayed in public areas (e.g., waiting rooms, cafeteria), as well as in areas reserved for employees. The core values can be listed on employee identification badges and printed in all marketing materials for the organization. The strategic plan tenets should be incorporated into all of the institution's policies and procedures.

Copies of the plan can also be provided to trade or professional organizations with which the institution is associated. The public relations or community outreach department in the institution can use the strategic plan as the basis for a media campaign to educate the community and other stakeholders and audiences about the institution's vision and mission. Patients can be provided with a condensed summary of the strategic plan on admission, particularly those sections related to their care. Patients should be informed of the institution's core values as well.

IMPLEMENTATION OF THE STRATEGIC PLAN

At this point, strategic management often fails. Strategic plans are developed and then allowed to languish as the necessary commitment to implementation is not realized for whatever reason. Often the reason is conflicting priorities. Executives and staff in health care organizations have a myriad of tasks facing them, and implementing strategic objectives adds another burden to an already overwhelming workload. To overcome this obstacle, the strategic plan must be integrated into the organization's daily activities. Everyone must be committed to implementing the strategic plan, from the leaders to the staff at all levels and in all departments. Focusing on the strategic plan and its meaning to the viability and future of the institution is imperative.

It also is necessary to develop an action plan based on the strategic plan. Those individuals who will be responsible for implementing the strategic objectives need to develop this plan. The action plan should include the following elements:

- A priority order for achieving the strategic objectives or outcomes
- The determination of who (individual or group) will be responsible for achieving these objectives
- An indication of available or necessary financial support
- A timetable outlining when achievement of the objectives can be expected

It may also be advisable to include interim activities and time frames if the strategic objective is long-term or complex, so that progress can be monitored.

The action plan breaks the strategic plan into manageable components, particularly for those individuals who were not directly involved in crafting the strategic plan. The action plan, then, must become a living document so that it is constantly referenced, consulted, and discussed. The action plan should be reviewed and updated at intervals. Actions that have been completed or those that do not move the organization toward achievement of its goals should be deleted, and new actions based on existing environmental conditions should be added. It may also be necessary to readjust the time line for completion of some activities in response to external or internal factors that affect the ability to accomplish the desired activities.

Ensuring that the action plan remains at the forefront of daily activities, whether in an institution as a whole, a department, or a unit, often requires a "champion." This is an individual who is passionate and committed to the process and who can inspire others also to be. Often, a champion appears as the strategic planning process unfolds; generally, this individual contributes freely, is engaged in the work groups, and expresses interest in the process. Champions can be selected as well, but those who volunteer are usually more enthusiastic about the work than those who are "drafted."

LEADERSHIP AND MANAGEMENT IMPLICATIONS

Strategic management is useful for nursing leaders and managers because it can be used to analyze the environment for opportunities and threats; to set measurable, achievable goals and plans; and to help determine the future of the nursing area, such as a department or unit. Success in strategic planning and implementing that strategic plan will position nursing well in an institution. The process provides an opportunity for nursing to shine, because the similarities between the nursing process and the strategic planning process allow nurses to shortcut the learning curve and begin to move forward with the implementation phase while others may still be grappling with the planning process. Nursing skills and abilities make it relatively easy to plan strategically; and nurses, as 24-hour workers, can approach implementation as an ongoing, continuous, and seamless process. Nurses' involvement with continuous quality improvement and performance improvement systems provides a basis for participation in strategic planning that is systematic and thorough.

Implementation of the organization's strategic plan can be useful in unifying staff on a nursing unit or in a department. Collaboration and cooperation among staff generally are required to accomplish strategic objectives. Working together to accomplish a strategic objective keeps staff engaged. Involvement in decisions that ultimately will affect them is essential and often results in positive spin-offs; for example, staff members feel a sense of ownership in the process and pride in their accomplishments.

CURRENT ISSUES AND TRENDS

The current issues in nursing may seem an awful lot like the "past" issues and ones that have been discussed for years; an example is entry into practice, which has been debated for nearly 50 years. However, the progression of time as well as current trends in health care augurs for some resolution; and if the profession does not resolve the problem on its own, outsiders fairly certainly will. The recent appearance of two publications underscores the urgent need to move forward to resolve this issue.

In their book, *Educating Nurses: A Call for Radical Transformation,* Benner and colleagues (2010) challenged nursing education programs to upgrade classroom education to prepare nurses for complex clinical environments, urged that the baccalaureate in nursing be established as the minimal educational level for entry into practice, and suggested that all nurses obtain a master's degree in nursing within 10 years after graduation. The Institute of Medicine (2011)

RESEARCH NOTE
Source
Conway-Morana, P.L. (2009). Nursing strategy: What's your plan? *Nursing Management, 40*(3), 25-29.

Purpose

The purpose of this article was to describe the process of "bringing vision to an operational reality."

Discussion

The author asserts that it is the responsibility of nurse leaders to develop strategic plans for nursing departments that augment the hospital's strategic plan. The author then lists the steps that must be taken: reaffirming the nursing department's mission and its vision, assessing the environment, gauging the political climate, and evaluating the workforce. These efforts are not undertaken in isolation but in concert with institutional strategic planning efforts.

Next, the author discusses setting priorities and organizing the strategic plan around financial metrics such as cost per admission, patient days, and length of stay; the plan also can be organized on the basis of customer metrics such as patient and physician satisfaction, or name recognition. The plan can be organized on the basis of the pillars of quality, service, cost, people, and growth (Studer, 2003). Nursing departments in the process of seeking American Nurses Credentialing Center (ANCC) recognition from the Magnet Recognition Program® may choose to organize the strategic plan according to the 14 Forces of Magnetism.

The author asserted that the nursing strategic plan must complement the organization's strategic plan, incorporate the views of stakeholders, and be communicated to others within the institution. Finally, the author stated that the strategic plan should be evaluated on an ongoing basis.

This article clearly reflects the steps in the strategic planning process, and the author uses a case study to illustrate how the plan is operationalized. The implementation of the action component of strategic planning is what strategic management is all about (Coulter, 2009). Strategic plans do no one any good when relegated to a shelf and ignored after being developed.

Application to Practice

This article and others in the literature, as well as a myriad of books on the topic, demonstrate the process of strategic planning to achieve specific goals and strategic objectives and tactics that can be used to achieve the goals. In addition, the author described the individual(s) or group(s) responsible for executing each of the tactics and the time line for expected completion of these actions.

Institution-wide involvement in strategic planning provides an opportunity for nurses to actualize and practice autonomy, be recognized for their contributions, and lessen the feelings of being disenfranchised. Although admittedly a lot of work, the benefits of engaging in strategic planning and then implementing that plan far outweigh the disadvantages.

A strategic plan should be realistic and make sense to nurses at all levels. Participation and input help shape the organization's future and that of the nurses employed in the institution.

---

issued a report, *The Future of Nursing; Leading Change, Advancing Health,* which called for an improved educational system that promotes seamless academic progression.

Other issues and trends in nursing include evidence-based practice, the impact of technology, the emergence of the Doctor of Nursing Practice (DNP) degree, the growing ethical demands of practice, workplace culture, and others as identified by nurse leaders (Sigma Theta Tau International, 2011). Though the nursing shortage is still an issue in the profession, its significance is eclipsed by these and many of the other issues affecting nursing and the health care industry.

However, strategic planning is not reserved for activities such as seeking recognition through the ANCC Magnet Recognition Program® or for ameliorating workforce issues in a particular institution. Any business venture will benefit from having a strategic plan. The plan provides for assessment of the environment, including current and future opportunities, and identification of specific, measurable, realistic ways of taking advantage of those opportunities. Most important, perhaps, the strategic plan answers the question, "What business are we in?" Clearly defining a mission and vision will help a nursing unit or department focus its efforts on its core business.

Strategic planning and strategic management are necessary components of business in today's competitive and highly unstable environment. Strategic planning is a process similar to the nursing process, with defined and specific steps to be taken to ensure that a comprehensive and thorough process occurs. Strategic management involves implementation of the strategic plan to ensure that the organization is responsive to changes in its environment, as well as to internal events.

Strategic planning and strategic management are not reserved exclusively for organizations. Individuals, such as nurses, can use these techniques to determine their own direction and establish objectives to ensure that they meet the goals they have set for themselves. Nurses in all areas of practice and in all employment settings can use the principles of strategic planning to explore programs, projects, and services and to advance their careers. Nurses who are involved in any aspect of an institution's strategic planning efforts should incorporate those activities into a personal portfolio (Oermann, 2002) and use those activities to reflect their competence and expertise as well as their own professional development.

CASE STUDY

Nurse Michele Smith is a staff nurse on a medical-surgical unit. She is a recent graduate of a baccalaureate program and is concerned with the interdisciplinary relations between nurses and other health care professionals. Michele believes that disruptive and bullying behaviors are undermining a culture of safety on the unit, contributing to preventable adverse patient outcomes, causing patient dissatisfaction, and contributing to staff turnover.

Michele approaches her supervisor, the nursing professional development specialist who managed her nursing orientation program, and her preceptor. During this meeting, the three nurses discussed the strategic planning process. Michele used materials from a leadership course in her nursing education program and facilitated the group work to address the following questions:

Where are we currently?

Where do we want to go?

How will we get there?

At the conclusion of the meeting, everyone agrees that there is indeed a problem on the unit and that resolution is possible if everyone works together to define the problem and seek solutions. The nursing supervisor seeks permission to hold an off-unit retreat for the staff to obtain their buy-in and commitment to work on the problem.

In the meantime, the group agrees to conduct a formal SWOT analysis, contact a professional facilitator from the local university to participate in the staff retreat, and conduct a literature review on the topics of disruptive behaviors, bullying in the workplace, and interprofessional relationships:

The group divides the tasks among themselves and agrees to meet again within a month to share progress and determine the next steps in the strategic planning process.

CRITICAL THINKING EXERCISE

With the support of the nursing leaders in the hospital, Michele Smith arranges for a nurse faculty member with a Doctor of Nursing Practice (DNP) degree to facilitate a retreat of medical-surgical unit nursing staff to develop a plan to deal with the disruptive behaviors she has noticed on the unit. In addition to covert or overt acts such as gossiping, nonverbal aggression, withholding information, and ostracism, Michele has noticed that some nurses have kept quiet about an improper medication order because of an intimidating physician or colleague (Institute for Safe Medication Practices, 2008). Michele hopes the strategic planning session with her colleagues will provide a necessary resource for addressing and preventing this violence in the workplace. In casual conversations with several of them, however, she is met with concerns about "telling on each other," and denials that a problem exists.

1. What are the issues that are present in this situation?
2. How should Nurse Smith approach the problem?
3. What are the elements of strategic planning and strategic management that might be helpful?
4. Why might these particular elements of strategic planning and strategic management be helpful here?

Confronting the Nursing Shortage

Linda L. Workman

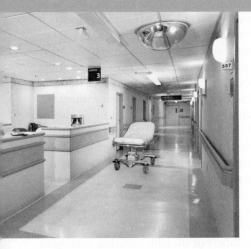

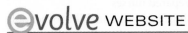 WEBSITE

http://evolve.elsevier.com/Huber/leadership/

DEFINITIONS

A nursing shortage is a condition in which the delicate balance of nurse supply and nurse demand is not at equilibrium. A **nursing shortage** is defined as a situation in which the demand for employment of nurses (how many nurses employers would *like* to employ) exceeds the available supply of nurses willing to be employed at a given salary. A nursing shortage is not just a matter of understaffing; in fact, understaffing can occur in conditions of shortage, equilibrium, or surplus, depending on local factors such as tight budgets or poor working conditions. The hallmark of a nursing shortage is the discrepancy between the supply and demand for registered nurses (RNs).

A nursing shortage can be identified by opinions of nurses, the public, or experts. Nurses or the public may believe there is a shortage based on a variety of factors. Experts generally use indicators such as employer reports, vacancy rates, turnover, recruitment difficulty, staffing levels, RN supply per population, or forecasting models to determine a nursing shortage.

Issues surrounding the nursing shortage have highlighted the important leadership and management

Photo used with permission from Photos.com.

interventions related to recruitment and retention of nursing personnel. **Civility** is authentic respect for others requiring time, presence, engagement, and intention to seek common ground. **Incivility** is low-intensity deviant behavior with ambiguous intent to harm the target, characteristically rude, discourteous, and displaying a lack of respect for others. **Recruitment,** defined as replenishment, is the process used by organizations to seek out or identify applicants for potential employment. The impact is to ensure that an adequate number and quality of workers are available for selection and employment. **Retention** is the ability to continue the employment of qualified individuals, that is, nurses and/or other health care providers/associates who might otherwise leave the organization. The impact of this action is to maintain stability and enhance quality of care while reducing cost to the organization. **Selection** is defined as the job of determining the most qualified candidate for a job. This process includes reviewing, sorting, ranking, and offering of candidates recruited for a job. **Staff vacancy** is defined as an employee position—full-time or part-time equivalent—that is budgeted but not filled. **Transformational leadership** refers to a leader who inspires and transforms followers by raising their sense of the value of the task and their sense of importance (Bass, 1998). Bass (1998) outlined four components of transformational leadership: (1) charisma or idealized influence, (2) inspirational motivation, (3) intellectual stimulation, and (4) individualized consideration. **Turnover** is defined as the loss of an employee because of transfer, termination, or resignation. The turnover rate is derived by dividing the total number of nurses who left a work unit in 1 year by the total number of nurses employed on that unit. **Transfer** is the movement of an employee whose performance is satisfactory from one area to another within the same institution or corporation. **Termination** is the discharge of an employee who is performing at a less-than-satisfactory level or is not a good match for the organization. **Resignation/voluntary turnover** is the failure to retain an employee who is performing at or above satisfactory level. Although all turnovers have an associated cost to the organization, the most costly are those dealing with termination and resignations.

BACKGROUND

Historically, the nursing shortage has been cyclical, vacillating between a supply shortage and a demand glut as noted in the nursing timeline discussed later. However, never before has the problem reached the magnitude that is presented by the United States Registered Nurse Workforce Report Card and Shortage Forecast, published in the January 2012 issue of the *American Journal of Medical Quality* (Juraschek et al., 2012), predicted to last through 2030. Cycles of nursing shortages and surpluses have been the focus of study and discussion for many decades. Multiple factors contribute to these phenomena. Just as numerous factors contribute to the nursing shortage, multiple possible solutions are needed to resolve it. An analysis of these factors will highlight the nursing shortage as a current and future issue, then leadership and management implications will be discussed.

The nursing shortage cycles over the past few decades have been primarily driven by the following six factors:

- Aging of current nurses in the workforce and their preparation for retirement
- Lower numbers of students entering nursing as a career and a shift in need for both BSN and MSN/DNP prepared nurses
- Aging of nursing faculty and inability of schools of nursing to meet education demands
- Aging of the American population and struggles to expand capacity to meet demand for care
- Significant changes in health care delivery system as the nation moves into health care reform

Figures 20-1 and 20-2 show nursing supply and demand models.

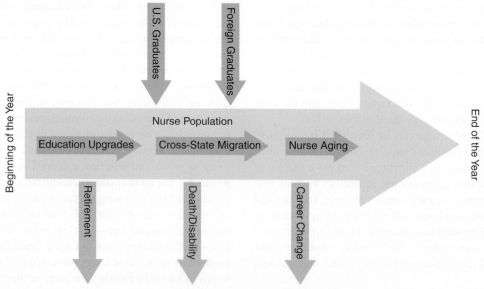

FIGURE 20-1 Overview of the nursing supply model. What is behind the Health Resources and Services Administration's projected supply, demand, and shortage of registered nurses? (Data from *http://dwd.wisconsin.gov/healthcare/pdf/behind_the_shortage.pdf*. Retrieved October 7, 2012.)

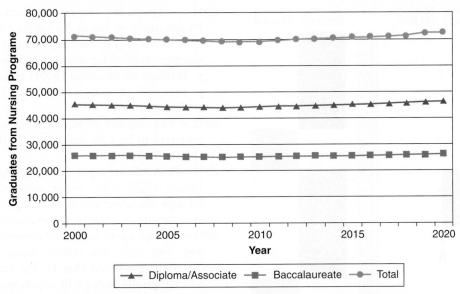

Source: Analysis of the 2000 SSRN.

FIGURE 20-2 National baseline projections of annual nursing school graduates. (Retrieved October 7, 2012, from *http://www.medaidesillinois.org/pdf/whynow/hrsa_graphs.pdf*)

The RN Workforce

The 3.1 million U.S. registered nurses make up the largest health care occupation in the United States, holding about 2.6 million jobs in 2008, with about 63% of jobs in hospitals and more than 1 in 5 (21%) working part-time (American Nurses Association [ANA], 2011; Bureau of Health Professions [BHPr], 2010; Bureau of Labor Statistics [BLS], 2007). Despite large numbers, the supply of RNs has not been in balance with demand, nor has it been stable over time. Since the early 1900s, the U.S. nursing shortage and surplus has gone through phases. Although the length of each phase varies, clearly the alternation between shortage and surplus has been more frequent since the mid-1960s. Shortage phases have lasted longer, with only brief periods of surplus. Figure 20-3 shows the cycles of nursing shortages and surpluses from 1901 to 2012. However, the game changed in 2007 with the onset of the second recession in the new millennium that lasted longer than all previous recessions since World War II and resulted in high unemployment (Buerhaus et al., 2009a). These cycles are interrelated with social and economic forces, shifts, and changes. For example, the nursing shortage from about 1915 to 1920 resulted from the inability to recruit qualified and suitable students, because students provided most of the service on hospital wards (King, 1989). A little more than a decade later, in the context of the Great Depression (1929-1932), a surplus prevailed (Carlson et al., 1992). The 20 years after World War II (1945-1965) saw yet another nursing shortage (Grando, 1998).

NURSING SHORTAGE TIME LINE OF EVENTS AND PREDICTIONS

1964 – Nurse Training Act financial aid program increases nursing enrollment and lowered job vacancy rates for next 6 years

1970 – Job vacancy rate steadily climbs through 1980, sparking the next shortage (Carlson et al., 1992)

1981 – Recession converts the vacancy rate to a surplus

1985 – Implementation of diagnosis-related groups (DRGs) passes and more patients are housed in hospitals prompting the next decline

1986 –Through 1992, hospital RN vacancy rate at national level of 11% (Buerhaus et al., 2005)

1992 – Managed care, capped reimbursements, cost containment, and downsizing hit the hospital industry again, boosting a nursing surplus

1998 – Cycle again shows evidence of reversal into shortage and marks the beginning of the shortage lasting into 2008

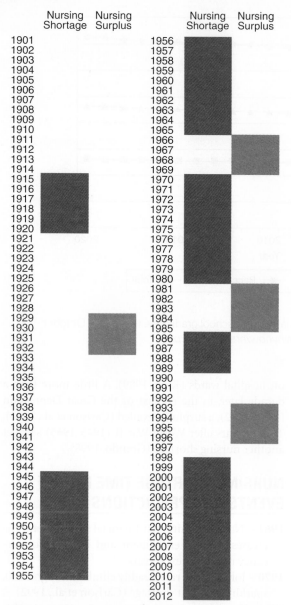

FIGURE 20-3 Nursing shortage and surplus cycles. (Copyright © Diane L. Huber, 2012. All rights reserved.)

2000 – Average age of registered nurses is 45.2 years, with only 9% younger than 30 years

2001 – Recession: hospital RN vacancy rate at a national average of 13%, ranging up to 20%
- 126,000 full-time equivalent (FTE) RN positions unfilled (BHPr, 2006)

2001 – American Nurses Association/American Organization of Nurse Executives (ANA/AONE) held Nursing Professional Summit to analyze shortage and develop strategic plan for future
- Institute of Medicine (IOM) releases *Crossing the Quality Chasm: A New Health System for the 21st Century*

2002 – The number of new licenses in nursing is projected to be 17% lower in 2020 than in 2002 (BHPr, 2002)

2002 – ANA releases report, *Nursing's Agenda for the Future: A Call to the Nation,* addressing shortage through education and workforce policy

2003 – Nursing shortage predictions continue

2004 – Average age of registered nurses is 46.8 years, and now only 8% report, being under age 30; BHPr predicted that by the year 2015, all 50 contiguous states will experience a nursing shortage

2005 – The average age of nurse educators is 55 years (Davidhizar, 2005)

2006 – In April, the BHPr's Health Resources and Services Administration (HRSA) released projections of shortfall of more than 1 million nurses by 2020 (BHPr, 2006)

2006 – International Council of Nurses (ICN, 2007a) report indicated that an aging population is a worldwide issue through first quarter of the twenty-first century, projecting more than 1 billion people over age 60 years, with Japan, Italy, Greece. and Switzerland at highest risk with 31% older than 60 years

2007 – Great recession hits and lasts into 2012. According to the U.S. Government (BHPr, 2006; BLS, 2007) more than 1 million nurses will be needed by 2016. Projected shortage growth:
- 405,800 in 2010
- 683,700 in 2015
- 1,016,900 in 2020

2007 – The American Association of Colleges of Nursing (AACN, 2007) *2007 Survey on Faculty Vacancies* report showed a national nurse faculty vacancy rate of 8.8%, which equates to approximately 2.2 faculty vacancies per school.

2007 – 71.4% of U.S. nursing schools turning away 40,285 qualified applicants to baccalaureate and graduate nursing programs because of faculty shortages

2007 – Buerhaus and colleagues revise and reduce their prediction of shortage for 2020 from 1 million to 800,000

2008 – Recession results in unprecedented rise in hospital employment of nurses, with estimates at 243,000 FTEs and more than 100,000 RNs older than age 50 years (Staiger et al., 2012), with average age of 46 years

2009 – Since 2002, RN FTEs increase 62% for nurses ages 23 to 26 years to approximately 165,000 (Auerbach et al., 2011)

2010 – 12.7% of U.S. population currently age 65 years or older

2010 – Enactment of the Patient Protection and Affordable Care Act to transform health care delivery

2011 – Enrollments in entry-level baccalaureate programs in nursing increased by 5.1% (AACN, 2011)

2011 – Institute of Medicine (IOM) releases *The Future of Nursing: Leading Change, Advancing Health,* calling for increased numbers of advanced-degree educated nurses to promote patient safety and quality of care (IOM, 2011)

2012 – AACN 2011-2012 Survey reports that 75,587 qualified applicants from baccalaureate and graduate nursing are turned away because of insufficient number of faculty, clinical sites, classroom space, and clinical preceptors and budget constraints

2012 – Current nursing workforce average age now is 44.2 years (Auerbach et al., 2011)

2012 – Nursing workforce now projected to grow at roughly the same rate as the population through 2030 (Auerbach et al., 2011)

2012 – Bureau of Labor Statistics (BLS) identifies registered nursing as one of the leading occupations in terms of job growth through 2020 (AACN, 2012a, b)

Clearly, the cycling through shortages and surpluses increased in frequency in the last quarter of the twentieth century. No doubt, as the shortage/surplus cycles have increased in cycle time, planning change in the nurse labor force has become more difficult. Projecting the future demand for nurses requires careful attention to social and economic forces and is tied to an increase in chronic illnesses, an expanding geriatric population, and promotion of a national health care program ensuring access for all Americans. The current shortage is of particular concern because of the 78 million baby boomers who will be retiring by the year 2015, a factor expected to cause health care demands to soar.

FACTORS CONTRIBUTING TO THE NURSING SHORTAGE

The nursing shortage is a national and international phenomenon. The causes are complex and interactive. There is no one simple, quick fix. For an analysis of the causes of the nursing shortage, it is best to examine and understand the factors that contribute: those impacting nursing supply and those influencing demand for nursing services into the future.

Supply

Factors that affect nursing supply include the following:
- *Nursing education:* Those impacting the number of new nursing graduates
- *Demographics:* Those affecting the nature of the current RN workforce, thus the number of practitioners who can continue to work
- *Work environment:* Those influencing the ability of the workplace to recruit and retain nurses

Nursing Education

The ability of the educational system to produce new graduates is affected by limited enrollment, a shift from associate degree to baccalaureate-prepared RNs, and a shortage of nursing school faculty, compounded by an insufficient number of clinical sites, classroom space, and clinical preceptors, as well as budget constraints (AACN, 2011-2012). Adding complexity, the average age of nurse faculty (60% age 50+ years; ANA, 2011) suggests a probable large surge of retirements in the near future. AACN's report, *2010-2011 Salaries of Instructional and Administrative Nursing Faculty in Baccalaureate and Graduate Programs in Nursing,* shows the following average ages of doctoral-prepared and master's-prepared nurse faculty:
- Professors: 60.5 years (PhD); 57.7 years (master's)
- Associate professors: 57.1 years (PhD); 56.4 (master's)
- Assistant professors: 51.5 years (PhD); 50.9 years (master's)

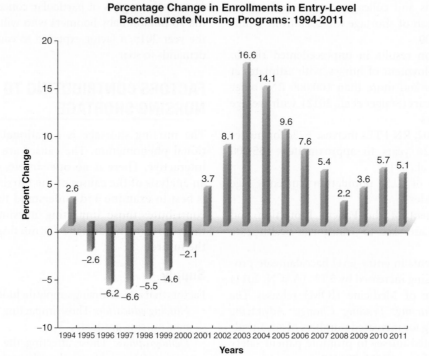

FIGURE 20-4 Percentage change in enrollments in entry-level baccalaureate nursing programs: 1994-2011. (From American Association of Colleges of Nursing (AACN). (2011). *2011 Survey overview: Percentage change in enrollments in entry-level baccalaureate nursing programs: 1994-2011.* Washington, DC: Author. Retrieved October 6, 2012, from *http://www.aacn.nche.edu/Media-Relations/EnrollChanges.pdf*)

The overall numbers of nursing school enrollments is not growing fast enough to meet projected demand (Figure 20-4) for RN and APRN services into the next two decades. Even though the AACN reported a significantly higher percentage of increase (5.1%) in enrollments for entry-level baccalaureate nursing programs in 2011, the increase is not sufficient considering the implementation of the Affordable Care Act of 2010 and the impending increase of more than 32 million Americans accessing heath care services.

Clearly there is strong interest among new nursing students and across the RN workforce in advancing education. The question now becomes what is the ability of higher learning institutions to handle the high number of applicants? In the 2010-2011 academic year, the data indicated that only 39.5% of applications were accepted for entry, whereas 75,587 qualified applicants were turned away, primarily because of shortage of faculty and resource constraints. The average eligibility rate for applications submitted into entry-level baccalaureate programs was approximately 50% overall, creating a shortfall on eligible admissions of 10.5%. The top reasons given by nursing schools for **not** accepting all qualified applicants into entry-level baccalaureate programs include insufficient clinical teaching sites (65.2%), a lack of faculty (62.5%), limited classroom space (46.1%), insufficient preceptors (29.4%), and budget cuts (24.8%). (The graphed data on turnaways can be found at *http://aacn.nche.edu/media-relations/TurnedAway.pdf*.)

The AACN survey also noted an increase in total enrollments into nursing programs, with an increase of 10% from 2010, across all baccalaureate, masters, and doctoral programs in 733 nursing schools (87.5%) in the United States. AACN reports that 80,767 students graduated from baccalaureate programs last year: "Given the call by the IOM for nurses to increase their education, AACN was pleased to see growth in degree-completion programs for RNs looking to earn their bachelor's or master's degree" (AACN, 2012a). For the ninth straight year, enrollment in RN-to-baccalaureate programs increased by 15.8% within a total of 814 advancement degree programs available nationwide. There are also 62 new advancement degree programs in development, marking a 7% increase in available programs.

Demographic Factors

The Bureau of Health Professions (BHPr, 2004) projected that the number of licensed RNs would remain relatively constant (2.7 million) between 2000 and 2020. The number of licensed RNs was projected to increase slightly through 2012, but "today the youngest cohorts of nurses in the workforce are projected to be the largest in history by the time they reach middle-age and will provide 30 percent more FTE RNs than the baby-boomer cohorts who are now nearing retirement" (Auerbach et al., 2011).

Aging of the RN Workforce. Understanding the demographic nature of the RN workforce requires an examination of the factors affecting the number of practitioners who may continue to work, that is, the aging of and the changing composition of the RN workforce.

The current nursing shortage may last longer because of the large number of RNs approaching retirement age and the growth and aging of the U.S. population. For example, the report by the Bureau of Health Professions (BHPr) (2006) titled, *The Registered Nurse Population: Findings from the March 2004 National Sample Survey of Registered Nurses,* showed that the average age of registered nurses was 46.8 years in 2004 compared with 45.2 years in 2000. According to the BHPr's (2010) report, *The Registered Nurse Population: Initial Findings from the 2008 National Sample Survey of Registered Nurses,* the percentage of nurses under age 40 years grew to 29.5% of RNs, increasing their numbers by nearly 18% from the same age group in 2004. This is a very positive finding, although as it was noted by Buerhaus and colleagues (2009a), the same survey sample revealed that most surveyed RNs were white females working in hospitals located in urban and suburban areas where the average nursing age only decreased by 2 years in 2008 compared to 2006. Only 19% of RNs were under age 35 years, and 4 in 10 RNs continued to

fall between the ages of 35 to 49 years and 50 years and over (Figure 20-5).

The aging of the RN workforce is affected by the following two factors: the higher average age of recent graduates, and the aging of the existing pool of licensed nurses.

- The "graying" factor makes the nursing shortage an even greater issue, as the RN loss is projected to be 128% higher in 2020 than in 2002. The graying of the existing licensed pool is evident in the following data. According to the 2008 National Sample Survey of Registered Nurses released in September 2010 by the federal BHPr, the average age of the RN population in 2008 was 46 years of age, up from 45.2 years in 2000.
- With the average age of RNs projected to be at 44.5 years in 2012, nurses in their 50s are expected to become the largest segment of the nursing workforce, accounting for almost one quarter of the RN population (Buerhaus et al., 2009c).
- Within the next 8 years, the Bureau of Labor Statistics (BLS) projects the need for 1.2 million additional nurses to fill new positions and replace those retiring from the profession.

Historically, when the unemployment rate was high, the RN workforce tended to be larger than predicted, and when unemployment was low, the RN supply decreased more than expected. An increase of 1 percentage point in the unemployment rate was associated with 1.2% increase in the size of the RN workforce (Staiger et al., 2012).

Although these figures are daunting, Auerbach and colleagues (2007) revised their forecast, noting a smaller shortage than originally projected based on trend analysis through 2005. The results of this analysis indicated that there was a larger-than-expected increase in overall interest in nursing as a second career choice, especially among people in their late 20s and early 30s. Based on the influx of nurses, their projection was that the shortage would be approximately 800,000 by the year 2020.

Clearly, recruitment and retention will be major factors in the future. Multiple approaches will be needed, coming from both political arenas and the marketplace if the shortage is to be averted or minimized in the future. Actions noted by Auerbach and colleagues (2007) for addressing the shortage were directed toward workforce planning by policy makers.

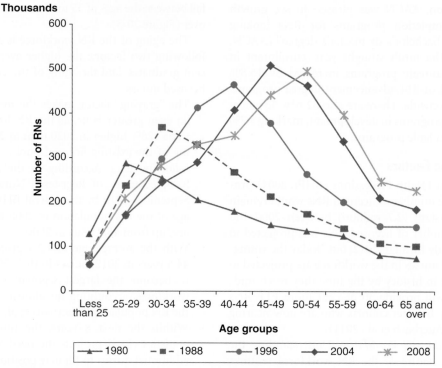

Source: 1980-2008 National Sample Survey of Registered Nurses

FIGURE 20-5 Age distribution of the registered nurse population, 1980-2008 (Source: 1980-2008 National Sample Survey of Registered Nurses. Bureau of Health Professions (BHPr). (2010). *The registered nurse population: Findings from the 2008 National Sample Survey of Registered Nurses.* Rockville, MD: U.S. Department of Health and Human Services, Bureau of Health Professions, Health Resources and Services Administration. Retrieved from *http://bhpr.hrsa.gov/healthworkforce/ allreports.html* and *http://bhpr.hrsa.gov/healthworkforce/rnsurveys/rnsurveyfinal.pdf*)

They recommended that initiatives include strategies for engaging high school and college graduates to select nursing as a career, finding ways to increase nursing education program capacities, providing incentives for hospitals to continue efforts to retain older RNs, and clarifying how the use of foreign nurses will be addressed. They further noted that, in order to increase educational program capacity, faculty would have to be recruited and developed and paid a salary that is equivalent to their hospital RN counterparts.

Work Environment Factors

RN employment overall has risen from 2 million in 2001 to 2.35 million in 2007 and 2.6 million in 2008, with 63% of this increase occurring in hospitals.

There were an estimated 3,063,163 licensed registered nurses living in the United States in March of 2008; this is an estimated increase of 5.3% since 2004. However, nearly all of this employment increase was supplied by older RNs and non-U.S. born nurses, the two most rapidly increasing segments of the nursing workforce today (Buerhaus, 2008).

In general terms, a nursing shortage has been shown to have adverse effects, including decreased access to care, decreased job satisfaction, and increased turnover. For example, an inadequate number of nurses to staff the operating room results in decreased OR capacity, which in turn increases wait time for surgical procedures. The concern about the effect of RN shortages on the quality of patient care is growing. The meta-analysis conducted by Kane and colleagues (2007) found that the shortage of RNs and the increased workload can negatively impact the quality of patient care. Duffield and colleagues (2007) found that stabilizing the work environment, whether by low nurse turnover, stable nurse leadership, or adequate competent staff, enhances patient outcomes.

Nurse vacancy and turnover rates are predictors of nursing shortages as well. The average nursing vacancy rate reported in 2008 was 8.1% (American Health Care Association, 2008) which represents a nearly 50% decrease from 16.1% in 2005. The turnover rate is slowly decreasing: 15.5% in 2003, and 13.9% in 2005 (AACN, 2008). However, the turnover rate for first-year nurses remains high; one survey reported 27.1% in 2007 (PricewaterhouseCoopers, 2007); another revealed 13% turnover and also found 37% of first-year nurses reporting that they felt ready to change jobs (Kovner et al., 2007).

Several work environment factors have been cited as reasons for increased turnover (Buerhaus et al., 2000; Tri-Council for Nursing, 2004), including workload, autonomy, relations with managers, and compensation. Such factors influence job stress, in turn leading to job satisfaction or dissatisfaction (Hayhurst et al., 2005) and ultimately turnover and intent to stay.

Workload. One of the findings of a study by Aiken and colleagues (2002) was that nurses with the highest nurse-to-patient ratios (fewer nurses for the number of patients) were more likely to describe feelings of burnout, emotional exhaustion, and job dissatisfaction than nurses with lower ratios (more RNs for the number of patients). In addition, 43% of nurses who reported high levels of burnout and dissatisfaction intended to leave their jobs within a year. In contrast, only 11% of nurses who did not complain of burnout or dissatisfaction expressed intent to leave their current jobs. Buerhaus and colleagues (2005) found that insufficient staffing is raising the stress level of nurses, impacting job satisfaction, and causing nurses to leave the nursing profession.

Autonomy. Professional autonomy, or control over the practice environment, was identified as the strongest predictor of nurses' identification with the organization (Apker et al., 2003). Nurses who did not believe their jobs provided sufficient freedom were less likely to experience feelings of affiliation and loyalty toward their employers.

Relations with Managers. The manager's leadership style was found to be a significant predictor of nurses' job satisfaction (Duffield et al., 2007; Weberg, 2010) and retention. Duffield and colleagues (2007) found that nursing leadership at the unit level is important for job satisfaction and intention to leave, which in turn has an impact on safety and patient outcomes. Weberg's (2010) study showed significance between transformational leadership and increases in satisfaction and well-being with decreasing burnout and overall stress in staff nurses.

Compensation. An increase in salary for nurses relative to the salary in other occupations increases the attractiveness of nursing as a profession. An increase in salary now correlates more to the education level, expertise, and/or higher certification of the nurse as an individual. The impact of the recessionary decade increased the supply of nurses through several mechanisms. Part-time RNs were motivated to work more hours or full-time; older RNs delayed retirement or returned to work from retirement. Licensed RNs working in non-nursing jobs returned to nursing, and young people decided to enroll in nursing programs, a demand occupation with future stability (Staiger et al., 2012).

Changing Composition of the RN Workforce. The reliance on older RNs and on internationally educated RNs has increased significantly in the past 12 years. Older RNs comprised 44.7% of the total RN population in 2008, compared with 41.1% in 2004 and 33.4% in 2000. The percentage of RNs who were 60 years and older increased from 13.6% in 2004 to 15.5% in 2008, and the average age of the RN population in 2008 was 46 years of age compared to 46.8 in 2004 (BHPr, 2010).

Between the years of 2001 and 2008, employment of older nurses in hospital settings fluctuated with the economy from boom to bust and accounted for 59% of the total increase in RN employment. During this same period, the nonhospital employment settings accounted for 18% of RN employment growth as well, but all growth in this period was represented by the older RN group over age 50 years (Buerhaus et al., 2009a). During this same period, the growth of middle-aged nurses (ages 35 to 49 years) was negative, with a substantial loss in nonhospital settings, thus overwhelming the hospital employment segment. Organizations reported that the shortage had a serious impact on nurse staffing, including increased overtime usage, higher stress, restricted expansion, changes in recruiting and hiring practices, decreased quality of care, and increased difficulty in scheduling coordination (May et al., 2006).

This shortage is further being fueled by the international demand for nurses. According to Daniel and colleagues (2000), international recruitment of nurses once again surfaced as a way of addressing the nursing shortage, specifically in the United States, United Kingdom, Canada, and Western Europe. The International Council of Nurses (ICN) (2007a) reported worldwide population aging projections in the first quarter of the twenty-first century. The results clearly indicated that an aging population is an issue around the world, with greater than 1 billion people older than 60 years. The distribution of this population includes approximately 700 million in developing countries (which will increase nearly 240% from the 1980 levels). Included in this latter group are five of the ten largest populations in the world—China, India, Indonesia, Brazil, and Pakistan. This projection also indicated that the four countries with the oldest populations (with 31% older than 60 years) in the world—Japan, Italy, Greece, and Switzerland—also would be severely affected. Given the global magnitude of this shortage, few countries have nurses in excess; as a result, recruiting nurses internationally often creates an even more severe shortage in their home country.

International Recruitment

According to McHugh and colleagues (2008), the U.S. recruits more internationally educated nurses (IEN) than any other country. This is evident in that the number of IENs working in the United States has tripled since the 1990s. In March of 2008, an estimated 170,235 RNs living in the United States received their initial nursing education in another country or U.S. Territory, claiming 5.6% of the total nursing population. Approximately half of the IENs were originally from the Philippines (48.7%), 11.5% from Canada, and 9.3% were from India (BHPr, 2010). In 2008 alone, a record number of 48,000 RN FTEs were filled by foreign-born nurses (Buerhaus et al., 2009a). According to McHugh and colleagues

(2008), major barriers to recruitment of IENs have been related to both limited visas and ethical concerns related to depletion of nursing resources in other countries.

International recruitment has been of major concern to the International Council of Nurses (ICN) for more than a decade now. In 1999, the ICN released a position statement, *Nurse Retention, Transfer and Migration*, now updated as *Nurse Retention and Migration* (ICN, 2007a). In this document, the ICN linked the nursing shortage (inadequate supply of nurses) to lack of quality in health care. The statement addressed the individual nurse's rights, as well as positive and negative issues related to migration. It also delineated roles that national nurses associations should take to raise nurse awareness of potential constraints and ensure that countries seeking to recruit nurses had policies and practices relative to fair and humane treatment of nurses. The ICN supports the migration of nurses as a short-term strategy for addressing the nursing shortage, viewing nurse migration as a way of increasing the nurse's career opportunities and personal self-interests. Nurse migration is further viewed by the ICN as a way of increasing multicultural practice and learning opportunities within the nursing profession. This is especially true as nurses have identified two major reasons for leaving their home country—economic security and professional opportunity—although personal safety/security in the workplace and/or country has also been noted. However, concerns related to recruitment practices led the ICN in 2001 to issue a position statement on ethical nurse recruitment, now updated (ICN, 2007b).

In 2004, the ICN and its sister organization, the Florence Nightingale International Foundation, investigated global nursing shortage issues related to international recruitment. This global analysis aimed to identify the policy and practice issues and solutions to be considered by governments, international agencies, employers, and professional associations when addressing the supply and use of nurses. To date, this initiative has produced an overview paper and white papers addressing such issues as migration, recruitment and retention, policy and planning, the work environment, and problems specific to Latin America and sub-Saharan Africa. Those papers are available on ICN's website (*www.icn.ch*).

Principles are relevant because they address changes that need to take place to ensure that nurses are treated fairly and equitably in the international marketplace. Unethical recruitment of nurses in the past has led to nurses being exploited and misled into accepting job responsibilities and work conditions incompatible with their qualifications, skills, and experiences. The ICN condemns the recruitment of nurses into countries where authorities support human rights violations. Sparacio (2005) addressed the complexity of international recruitment and the ethical impact of "brain drain" on the country from which nurses are being recruited. The California Nurses Association (CNA) and National Nurses Organizing Committee put forward a resolution, which was adopted by the CNA's 2005 House of Delegates, outlining a code of practice for international nurse recruitment (Dumpel, 2005). This code was directed at the concerns and unlawfulness of international recruitment relative to the health care impact. The code specifically targeted human rights issues relative to accessibility and quality of care within the home country.

Although international recruitment of nurses has greatly increased in the United States in recent years, few studies have been conducted to examine the adaptation, socialization, and true "lived experience" of the IEN or foreign-born nurse working in the United States. (Jose, 2011). Even though the core values of professional nursing are universally the same, the delivery of quality nursing care is dependent upon contextual factors such as shared common language and understanding among co-workers, patients, and families (Blythe & Baumann, 2009). Recent literature suggests that overall socialization into current American culture can add additional psychological stressors and possible retention issues in the long run for international recruits. Successful adjustment of IENs in the United States is important to ensure quality patient care and financial stability for recruiting health care agencies. Jose (2011) examined the socialization of foreign-born nurses working in the United States for less than 5 years and found six common themes among them: (1) dreams of a better life, (2) a difficult journey, (3) a shocking reality, (4) rising above the challenges, (5) feeling and doing better, and (6) readiness to help others. Considering that the "American way" is most often viewed through the media in other countries, it is often misperceived as a journey to immediate affluence without the struggles. For nurses coming into this country without any prior cultural or workplace socialization, culture shock is detrimental to them and to the recruiting organization. In light of this situation, more health care organizations are using intermediary recruitment agencies to provide preliminary workforce orientation and life skills planning. Kawi and Xu (2009) similarly found that the positive work ethic of IENs and their persistence and willingness to learn and adapt will ultimately prevail in their adjustment to their new U.S. workplace and add value to the nursing workforce.

Demand

The recent increase in demand for RNs is projected to continue as a result of accelerating demand for health care services. This demand is affected by population growth, a rising proportion of people older than 65 years, with Americans 65 years and older representing nearly 20% of the population by 2030 (IOM, 2011), socioeconomic and cultural shifts, and advances in technology.

Changing Demographic Nature of the Population

Population growth and aging baby boomers are the major factors changing the demographic nature of the population, which in turn are affecting the demand for RNs. According to the Bureau of Health Professions (2004), the U.S. population will grow 18% between 2000 and 2020, which equates to an additional 50 million people requiring health care. Increased life expectancy resulting from advances in science and medicine accounts for most of this population growth, as well as the increase in the proportion of the population older than 65 years. A rapid increase in the elderly population began around 2010, when those at the top end of the baby boom generation reached age 65 years (Figure 20-6). The subgroup of people 65 years and older will grow 54% between 2000 and 2020, which equates to an additional 19 million people in this age group. This is equivalent to a tsunami wave that cannot be stopped yet has huge implications for health care delivery financing.

Individuals older than 65 years, particularly those ages 85 years and older, have the greatest per capita

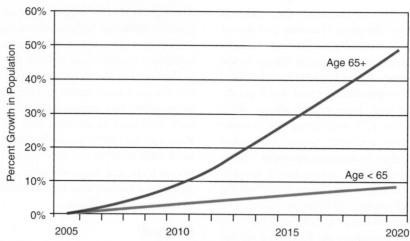

FIGURE 20-6 Population growth, 2000–2020. (From Bureau of Health Professions. [2006]. *The registered nurse population: Findings from the 2004 National Sample Survey of Registered Nurses.* Rockville, MD: U.S. Department of Health and Human Services, Health Resources and Services Administration. Retrieved November 20, 2008, from *http://bhpr.hrsa.gov/healthworkforce/rnsurveys/rnsurvey2004.pdf.*)

demand for health care and thus the greatest need for the services of RNs. These individuals tend to have (1) a higher incidence of chronic conditions such as arthritis (50%), hypertension (36%), and heart disease (32%); and (2) a higher occurrence of multiple conditions requiring more regular care. Thus with living longer and current rates of obesity comes the increased prevalence of chronic medical conditions. As a result, this population uses a larger portion of the available health care services and resources. They visit physicians twice as often as those younger than 65 years, account for 38% of hospital discharges (they represent 13% of the population), and have annual per capita health care expenditures of $5400 compared with $1500 for those younger than 65 years.

Health Delivery System

Health delivery systems form the structure around how care is delivered, where it is delivered, and how it is paid for. For example, Medicare and Medicaid reimbursement, The Patient Protection and Affordable Care Act, along with regional and local customs and cultures influence the demand for nursing services. It is commonly known that socioeconomic determinants such as culture, income, educational level, and age affect an individual's health practices, which in turn affect the person's health status and subsequent

use of and access to health care services. Increased acuity of patients puts more demand on critical care services such as emergency and intensive care areas, thereby increasing the need for nurses. A combination of decreased supply and increasing demand creates a nursing shortage potential situation, which varies by geographic region. Urban and suburban hospitals reported higher vacancy rates than did rural hospitals, and individual and multihospital systems reported higher average RN vacancy rates than did integrated delivery systems.

AMERICAN NURSES ASSOCIATION'S CALL TO ACTION

In September 2001, the American Nurses Association (ANA)—in conjunction with the American Organization of Nurse Executives (AONE), Sigma Theta Tau International (STTI), 60 other professional nursing organizations, and 19 steering committee organizations—held a summit meeting to begin to analyze the nursing shortage problem and to develop a strategic plan entitled *Nursing's Agenda for the Future: A Call to the Nation* (ANA, 2002). The outcome of this meeting was a vision statement and 10 domains for action. The vision statement was as follows (ANA, 2002):

*Nursing is **the** pivotal health care profession, highly valued for its specialized knowledge, skill and caring in improving the health status of the public and ensuring safe, effective, quality care. The profession mirrors the diverse population it serves and provides leadership to create positive changes in health policy and delivery systems. Individuals choose nursing as a career and remain in the profession because of the opportunity for personal and professional growth, supportive work environments and compensation with roles and responsibilities. (p. 7)*

The 10 domains that emerged from this summit were derived from the research literature and the Institute of Medicine's study, *Crossing the Quality Chasm: A New Health System for the 21st Century,* published in 2001. The domains are as follows (Institute of Medicine, 2001, p. 7):

1. Leadership and planning
2. Delivery systems
3. Legislative/regulatory/policy
4. Professional/nursing culture
5. Recruitment/retention
6. Economic value
7. Work environment
8. Public relations/communication
9. Education
10. Diversity

In addition to the vision and domains, a short-term plan was developed that outlined the desired future state, strategies for achieving the desired state, objectives to support the primary strategy, and the co-champions for each. The project was comprehensive given that the nursing shortage and its impact on health care are complex. The group recognized that in order to actualize the *Nursing's Agenda for the Future: A Call to the Nation* by 2010, extensive partnerships would be required to bring about strategic change, and change would have to occur, for example, in health care leadership, health care organizations, academic programs, health care policy, governmental agencies, health care and professional regulatory agencies, governmental and private funding, professional practice groups, and consumer groups.

The ANA (2002), as part of the *Nursing's Agenda for the Future: A Call to the Nation,* developed a "Desired Future Statement (Vision)" for each of the 10 domains.

The statement for the domain of "Recruitment and Retention" clearly delineated the comprehensiveness of the undertaking, as follows (ANA, 2002):

Nursing is comprised of a diverse body of individuals committed to promoting and sustaining the profession through addressing diversity, image, education, funding, practice models and environments, and professional development. (p. 17)

The vision was derived from the nursing research literature and incorporated the recurring themes related to recruitment and retention. Five strategies were formulated to achieve this vision. The strategies also addressed the two-pronged recruitment issue of the shortage (supply-side economics) and recruitment of (1) students for nursing education programs, and (2) qualified nurses for health care agencies. The strategies also targeted retention issues to be addressed within health care agencies and academic programs focusing on the development of career-based opportunities within health care, development and funding of creative educational initiatives, creation of a desirable and appealing image for nursing as a career choice, formulation and implementation of professional practice models, work environments that ensure career satisfaction, and development of comprehensive recruitment and retention strategies that will appeal to a diverse customer group/population (ANA, 2002). These global strategies were then broken down for the primary strategy in each of the domains, with work on the remaining strategies to be developed. The ANA also identified strategies that could be used to enhance student and faculty recruitment and/or retention (Table 20-1).

To meet the demand for nurses now and in the future, actions need to be taken that are directed at what drives young people and career switchers to choose nursing as a career. Erickson and colleagues (2004) reported on an initiative undertaken by Partners Healthcare in Boston. The goal was to gain insights into the dynamics of career selection by young people and career switchers. To determine this information, a consulting firm was hired to conduct focus groups and telephone interviews. Specific questions used in this qualitative approach focused on the following: How were decisions made relative to choosing a career? How did significant influences in one's life affect career choice? What was the individual's perception

TABLE 20-1 STUDENT-RELATED AND FACULTY-RELATED STRATEGIES FOR RECRUITMENT AND RETENTION

RECRUITMENT AND RETENTION STRATEGIES	STUDENTS	FACULTY
Develop professional mentoring models	X	
Create a specific curriculum to address diversity	X	X
Obtain funding to support minority enrollment	X	
Develop and distribute promotional and recruitment materials to attract individuals from diverse backgrounds into nursing	X	
Recruit retired nurses to form professional mentoring corps	X	
Provide joint educational and service standardized internships and residencies	X	X
Co-op program/student clinical assistant (SCA) program	X	
Negotiate professional paid development opportunities with employers	X	
Create a website for leadership development that can be used by education, service, and professional organization members	X	X

and image of nursing? As a result of this study, vital information was identified reflecting differences in the two groups. Outcomes of the study included two major marketing strategies that would promote the image of nursing as a career choice: "Be Somebody" and "Valuable Partner." In addition, the following nine strategies for promoting nursing as a career were identified (Erickson et al., 2004, p. 86):

1. Classroom ambassadors program
2. Job-shadowing experiences
3. Bring-your-child-to-work day
4. Volunteer health care settings opportunities for students and adults
5. Part-time employment opportunities for students and adults
6. Presentation to clubs/organizations regarding nursing
7. Participation at community health fairs
8. Advertising campaigns directed at job satisfaction, making a difference in people's lives, flexible scheduling, and competitive salary and benefits
9. Advertising that directs people to dynamic, comprehensive websites that offer positive, motivating information about nursing and its reward

RECRUITMENT

Recruitment is about the replacement of non-retained staff and the hiring of staff to fill newly created and/or expanded positions. With the changes that have occurred in health care over the past two decades, the concept of recruitment has begun to focus more and more on the identification and development of pre-employment hires. This means marketing the agency to potential pre-nursing students and active nursing students. Recruitment therefore has become more complex and more linked to partnerships than ever before. These partnerships are not only with schools of nursing but also with elementary and secondary schools and other community agencies. Co-op programs and/or student clinical assistant (SCA) programs (Henriksen et al., 2003) and other related preceptor programs create a model for attracting and retaining new graduates. These and other student-related activities blend the student-employee role, thus changing recruitment to a retention strategy once the student gets linked in a nursing capacity to the health care facility.

Following work with the AONE and American Association of Colleges of Nursing, Johnson & Johnson (J&J) (2012) launched a multi-year nursing initiative, *The Campaign for Nursing's Future,* in February 2002. This campaign grew out of J&J's concern over the nursing shortage, both current and future, and was designed to enhance the image of the nursing profession, recruit new nurses and nurse faculty, and help retain nurses. The campaign was international and covered a broad spectrum of activities that were directed at enhancing the image of nursing as a profession (e.g., fund-raising for scholarships [student and faculty]; research, awards, and support to nursing schools program expansion; national television, print, and interactive advertising; development and maintenance of a website; and production and distribution of recruitment and retention materials). These activities clearly put nursing forward in the public arenas and raised the status of nursing as a profession. According to Donelan and colleagues (2010), this campaign has had a positive effect on nursing recruitment and enrollment in schools of nursing. The campaign was a major initiative in the private corporate sector and has provided valuable insights into ways to examine challenges confronting the nursing workforce.

Clearly, recruitment needs both long-term and short-term strategies. Although the long-term plan is extremely important, most of the organization's resources tend to go to short-term initiatives—filling vacant and/or newly created positions. The recruitment focus of this chapter is directed at short-term strategies.

Recruitment of Professional Nurses: The Evidence-Based Magnet Recognition Program®

The evidence-based Magnet Recognition Program® has a long history of research behind its recognition criteria. In 1983, a study was conducted (1) to identify variables in hospital organizations and their nursing services that create a magnetism that attracts and retains professional nurse staff, and (2) to identify particular combinations of variables that produce nursing practice models within hospitals in which nurses receive professional and personal satisfaction to the degree that recruitment and retention of qualified staff are achieved (McClure et al., 1983). The study included 41 of 165 hospitals from 10 geographic regions (designated by the Bureau of Labor Statistics). The hospitals were nominated by Fellows in the American Academy of Nursing (AAN). Each AAN Fellow was asked to nominate 6 to 10 hospitals of varying sizes in their region of the country that demonstrated success in recruiting and retaining staff. The final selection of the institutions for inclusion in the study was done after a review and ranking of the top 10 choices in each region based on established criteria and recruitment and retention data provided by each institution. Originally, 46 hospitals were chosen, but 5 were unable to participate. The results of the study clearly showed that the three major variables of administration, professional practice, and professional development, with related attributes, positively affect hospitals' ability to recruit and retain registered nurse staff.

This study was one of the first to describe organizational and leadership factors that are important to the recruitment and retention of nurses in the workplace. As noted by the variables just mentioned, the nurses specifically wanted a leadership and organizational structure that supported participatory involvement, as well as flexibility for work scheduling and personal/professional development. In addition, nurses wanted to work in an institution that had a clearly defined professional practice model that used the skills and knowledge of the professional nurse. Nurses were also interested in working in an organization that allowed them to be "able to practice nursing." Managerial visibility and support were viewed as strengths in promoting autonomy. Nurses also wanted to have control over their practice (autonomy) and collaborative relationships with physicians relative to care management. This study and the follow-up study conducted by Kramer and Hafner (1989) 5 years later were the basis for the ANA'S Magnet Recognition Program®.

The America Nurses Credentialing Center (ANCC) implemented the Magnet Recognition Program® in the 1990s, with the first award going to the University of Washington Medical Center in 1994. According to the ANCC as of July 30, 2012, recognition has since been awarded to 395 health care organizations in 50 states, District of Columbia, Virgin Islands, Puerto Rico, and Guam, as well as three in Australia and one each in Singapore and Lebanon, for their excellence in nursing service. This clearly indicates the importance placed on this program nationally and internationally relative to recruitment and retention by hospitals and other health care organizations.

Human Resources, Managerial, and Staff Roles Associated with Recruitment

Recruitment initiatives in the past several years have used strategies targeted at nurse satisfiers as reported in the nursing and health care literature. Satisfiers have included strategies such as professional practice model usage, preceptor/mentorship opportunities, increased flexibility in work scheduling, low patient-to-RN ratios, a collaborative practice environment, Magnet recognition status, environment of respect and value, and a competitive compensation

BOX 20-1 RECRUITMENT STRATEGIES

- Flexible hours
- Competitive salaries
- Bonus pay
- Relocation pay
- Fixed shifts
- Weekend option program
- Part-time pay with bonus hours
- Flexible benefits packages
- Scholarships for BSN or graduate studies
- Tuition benefit plan
- Educational loan repayment
- Residency programs and RN specialty internships
- Onboarding
- Refresher courses—return to work
- Professional development opportunities
- Career opportunities
- Specialty certification reimbursement
- Low nurse-to-patient ratios; higher numbers of RNs for the patient load (workload staffing)
- Shared governance/leadership models
- Care delivery model that promotes professional care at the bedside
- Clinical ladder/career ladder
- Free parking
- Magnet Recognition Program®
- Culture of safety: zero tolerance for incivility
- Research/evidence-based practice
- NCLEX review course
- Qualified managerial support
- Clinical support: staff educators, clinical nurse specialists
- Workforce diversity
- Interdisciplinary collaboration opportunities

1. Posting position
2. Advertising
3. Screening
4. Interviewing
5. Selecting
6. Orienting
7. Counseling/coaching
8. Evaluating performance
9. Developing staff

Position Posting

Position posting for recruitment begins after determination of vacancies based on position controls developed for each of the clinical/service areas. The vacancies are identified based on the full-time equivalent (FTE) status for each of the positions. Once the positions have been identified and the shift/holiday schedules are determined, the first step is to post them internally for staff review and selection. The length of this posting time is determined by each organization and/or respective collective bargaining contracts. Positions not filled within a defined period are then posted externally to the organization. Based on the need and/or limited number of nurses in a given specialty, recruitment agencies may be contacted at this time to conduct a regional, statewide, or national search for the position.

Advertising

Advertising includes the development of an institutional advertisement outlining the positions or job opportunities within an organization. The advertisement addresses the area of need and specific information that would be likely to attract an employee (RN) to the position. The HR department determines distribution sites, with input from the specific departments. Sites may include professional journals or newspapers, local or regional newspapers, radio, or the organization's website. An advantage of online advertisement is that the application process can be made available at the same time, making it a one-stop process for the person seeking employment.

If the recruiter is planning to attend special events, information about the position will be taken for posting along with the application forms. In addition, information about the organization and related benefits and specialty strengths will be highlighted. A shortcoming that needs to be addressed related to

model. Strategies commonly used that are related to nurse recruitment of new and experienced nurses are identified in Box 20-1.

In the context of a nurse shortage, recruitment is a major human resources (HR) strategy. Because the organization needs to find and hire the best qualified nurses who also "fit" with the culture and are willing to work for a specific salary and work conditions, both recruitment and retention are important. Both managers and staff contribute to successful recruitment and retention. A complex and detailed process is followed for effective recruitment and retention. The nine major processes or phases of recruitment are as follows:

advertising is that organizations often spend a considerable amount of money on advertising only to miss the most important aspect, that of a quick, effective, courteous follow-up with potential candidates (Curran, 2003). Positive results from expensive advertising and recruiting efforts can be lost depending on how the institution follows up with candidates. For example, if potential candidates for a position have been encouraged to apply through advertising and recruitment efforts and then log on to an institution's website and find that they cannot complete an application for the job, in frustration they may decide not to pursue the job (Curran, 2003). In addition, if candidates cannot obtain a response about the status of their application after submitting it, they may decide that they do not want to work for this type of institution. If recruitment and advertising efforts are to be productive, these kinds of flaws in the system must be avoided.

Screening

Screening is the process in which the application is reviewed before determining whether the nurse meets the pre-established criteria for the position. During this activity, the reviewer selects who should be interviewed. According to Nall (2012), all applicants should be reviewed for gaps in employment and skill experiences, as well as for a match with the job description for the position under review. It is important to remember that if an organization is classified as an *equal opportunity employer,* the reviewers are required to follow the guidelines established by the federal government. Most application processes are currently completed and reviewed online, thus increasing the pool of applicants that in turn requires more recruitment time in screening. Review of large applicant pools may result in delays in responding back to the applicants. Electronic applications, however, are easier to file and sort relative to identified areas of interest by the applicant.

Interviewing

Interviewing is the time for clarification of information presented in the application and dossier submitted by the applicant. The job description is the basis for a hiring interview. The interview can be conducted in person or over the telephone, in a group/committee or one-on-one meeting. For best results, predefined

questions should be used to interview all candidates for the position. Also, questions should be directed at the work expectations outlined in the position description and/or practices. Open-ended and follow-up questions are recommended. For example, the following questions or discussion points can be posed:

- *Tell me about your current position.*
- *What do you like least about it?*
- *What do you like best about it?*

To get more in-depth responses and to determine behavior-specific examples, questions can be framed as follows:

- *Think of a time in your experience when X was needed, and describe how you did X.*
- *How did you handle X?*

It is appropriate to ask the candidate about aspects of his or her actions and decisions related to the job, such as the following:

- *Given the varied work hour requirements, how would you handle this?*
- *What problems do you see the work hour requirements presenting?*
- *Based on the work requirements relative to lifting, how would you go about transferring a patient whose body weight is more than 350 pounds?*

The information obtained through this process will help the committee or manager assigned to the recruitment process determine the applicant's "fit" with the unit and/or organizational culture, as well as providing consistent data for comparison of candidates. Use of formalized questions is often referred to as a *structured interview* or *targeted selection process* (Lipsey, 2004). The targeted selection process is built on analysis of work per job, organizational values, clear identification of competencies for key positions, and development of interview skills and confidence of the interviewers. Using the targeted interview ensures that all candidates are interviewed based on the same criteria. In addition, during the targeted interview process, the interviewer asks questions that are directed at having the candidates describe typical situations that they have encountered in previous jobs. Use of the targeted interview method allows the interviewers to gain data from the candidates to more fully evaluate their values and practice patterns. It further allows for objective comparison of candidates based on their responses, and it decreases personal biases and assumptions. It prevents interviewers from veering off target and/or asking of questions that may be inappropriate or illegal. Questions that should be avoided during the interview relate specifically to personal information about the candidate, such as the following: age, marital status, living arrangements, children, limitations or disabilities, religion, substance abuse, and membership in professional organizations.

Selecting

Selecting is the determination of who will be offered an opportunity for employment (termination of the recruitment process). A committee or manager may complete the selection process. For best results, data used in the screening and interviewing phases should be used when comparing candidate responses and other related data. The selection process also involves the formal activity of making an offer to the candidate. Who performs this activity varies according to institutional policy, but it usually involves either the manager or HR personnel. At the time the job offer is made, the employee is informed of the position/job being offered, the FTE allocation (full-time [FT] or part-time [PT]) for the position, and the salary offer and benefits. Regardless of who makes the final offer, HR plays a role in determining the salary range.

Selection of an employee who is a match with the core values of an organization has been shown to have important implications. It facilitates ease of employee transition into the new role and fit with staff in the unit and organization. Employee fit and related retention have also been shown to have an impact on cost savings within the organization. According to Lipsey (2004), return on investment of hiring the right versus the wrong person (poor performer) is more significant than just the costs of simple replacement of an employee. The costs of hiring the wrong person are associated with not only the recruitment, replacement, and hiring expenses, but also the secondary costs. Secondary costs of hiring a poor performer include increased dollars wasted on training and development, decreased productivity and increased errors, lost opportunities to improve processes and/or outcomes, decreased or poor staff morale that results from staff struggling to pick up slack of the poor performer, and dissatisfied customers. The secondary costs have a significant impact on the organization and workers and are often much greater than those associated with the initial recruitment process.

Orienting

Orienting is an important activity for bringing new employees into the organization, department, and unit. It is the employee's introduction to the culture and values of the organization and discipline. Changes in orientation format and content have occurred as a result of study outcomes that have shown the relationship between job satisfaction and staff retention. The newest approach to orienting is referred to as "onboarding" (Lee, 2008). The approach is directed at fully engaging and integrating the employee into the organization by focusing on how to assist him or her in successfully preparing for the job. Onboarding expands the orientation beyond the employee's initial introduction to the organization and role expectations by providing ongoing coaching and mentorship through a defined program (Lee, 2008). These programs usually last from 3 months to 1 year. This approach is consistent with expectations expressed by the new nurse graduate (Pine & Tart, 2007), especially those in the Generation Y group (Hart, 2006). Onboarding, including new graduate residency program, is also consistent with a Magnet culture (Halfer, 2007). Onboarding has also brought about a change in learning; it has moved from a fairly passive, didactic experience to an interactive process built around self-learning and renewal.

Many hospitals have adopted residency and/or internship programs with RN preceptors working one-on-one with the new graduate (Park & Jones, 2010). The success of these programs has been closely tied with retention. Halfer (2007) reported 17.2% increase in retention with $707,608 cost savings. Pine and Tart (2007) reported that residency programs have been shown to have a positive return on investment (ROI); for example, over a 1-year period the program decreased turnover by 37% and ROI was 325.5%. Lastly, Mills and Mullins (2008) reported 15% increase in retention over 3 years. Intangible benefits associated with these programs include improved morale, increased nursing and health team satisfaction, increased confidence, and improved quality of care (Halfer, 2007; Mills & Mullins, 2008).

Counseling and Coaching

Counseling and coaching are strategies used to promote a sense of community for new and ongoing employees. These strategies create a professional and social network for new employees, an attribute identified in Magnet-recognized institutions. Use of these strategies also creates a sense of a non-punitive culture in which staff can learn and grow. Graduate nurses have indicated the need for positive support and timely verbal feedback from preceptors to gain the confidence and competence needed during their transition into the RN role; although this is not always received (Duchscher, 2009; Park & Jones, 2010). According to vanWyngeeren and Stuart (n.d.), healthy working relationships and group cohesion enhance retention for both new and experienced employees. For this to happen, the leaders at all levels need to work with employees to ensure group cohesiveness in a family-like environment.

Performance Evaluation

Performance evaluation is a mechanism for giving feedback to employees, both new and experienced. In addition to new employees receiving ongoing evaluation during their onboarding by an assigned preceptor/coach, they are expected to receive an initial performance evaluation within the first 60 to 120 days, depending on the policies of the organization. This feedback is directed at the individual employees' progress relative to their onboarding program (formative evaluation). During this evaluation, the employee and managerial staff also should take the time to evaluate the employee's "fit" with the organizational and departmental culture (summative evaluation). Strategies to address further needs and/or employment status should be decided at this time. A full performance evaluation then occurs at the end of the orientation period and annually thereafter. Feedback regarding ongoing performance needs to be provided to employees on a regular basis. Performance evaluation needs to focus on the employee's achievement toward defined goals, with feedback directed at the individual's contribution to the development of peers and clinical and/or leadership practices. The meeting can be conducted using a formal or informal process, one-on-one or in a group. According to Hall and colleagues (2011) and Palumbo and colleagues (2009), performance feedback/evaluation has been tied to staff satisfaction and intent to stay.

Staff Development

Staff development has been identified in the literature as an important factor in job satisfaction. It provides employees with an opportunity to improve their practice, level of competency, or other areas of self-interest. Programs for staff development are usually determined based on annual staff surveys. Programs are usually posted for staff selection, and the institution provides scheduling flexibility and funding for employees to participate.

Staff development, as defined in the Magnet studies (Halfer, 2007; Kramer & Hafner, 1989; McClure et al., 1983), was identified as having four areas of professional development beyond orientation. The four areas included in-service education, continuing education, formal education, and career development. Professional development was valued for its economic potential. However, other attributes identified were personal and professional growth opportunities, career advancement opportunities, and preceptor skill development. Nurses in these institutions viewed education as being valued. Administrative support was provided and available, as were clinical and managerial resources. Professional development opportunities overall were shown to have a positive influence on nurse satisfaction. Ongoing staff development at all levels of employment has been shown to increase retention and enhance staff entry into clinical ladder programs (Halfer, 2007; Pierson et al., 2010).

RETENTION: NEW GRADUATES AND EXPERIENCED REGISTERED NURSES

Renewed attention has been directed at retention of nurses in a multigenerational workforce over the past 10 to 20 years (Palumbo et al., 2009). The turnover rate of a new graduate ranges from 22.6% to 60% in the first year (Mills & Mullins, 2008; vanWyngeeren & Stuart, n.d.), the average age of the nurse is 45 years, and nurses begin to phase into retirement beginning at age 55 years. In light of these facts, it is little wonder that nursing has begun to focus attention on expanding retention programs beyond the promotion of job satisfaction, safety, respect, and financial security (401 [k] plans, gain sharing, IRAs) (Kramer & Hafner, 1989; Palumbo et al., 2009) to the development of infrastructure services that meet the diverse needs of current employees. The primary focus of these changes is to promote nurse autonomy and the nurse role on the interdisciplinary team while providing services that will enhance the work and life of the nurse both inside and outside of the organization. Today more than ever it is imperative that nurses and other health care workers experience a sense of community in the workplace because many spend more time at work than at any other single place.

With four generational groups now in the workplace, it is important that managers and staff consider differences when developing strategies for change or rewards. Each generation has its own perspective, and diversity exists even within each generation. Therefore it is imperative that generational groups have representation or opportunity for input in planning and decision making. In addition, it is important to develop a variety of alternatives from which employees can select rather than targeting a single approach. General strategies commonly used for nurse retention of new and experienced nurses are identified in Box 20-2. According to a study conducted by Palumbo and colleagues (2009), although common retention expectations have been identified as important to nurses of all ages, several difference were noted related to the perceived significance of various retention strategies reported by generational groups (Box 20-3).

There often were inconsistencies between what the nurses saw as important retention factors and HR/institutional offerings provided by the various organization. Although the study by Palumbo and colleagues (2009) was specifically related to a 12-institution sample in a small rural state, it has implications for consideration on a broader scale, given that all institutions/agencies are currently

---

BOX 20-2 RETENTION STRATEGIES USED TO RETAIN NEW GRADUATES AND EXPERIENCED NURSES

Positive Organizational Culture
- Values driven
- Culture of safety
- Streamlined processes
- Physician-nurse collaborative partnership
- Creation of community culture
- Magnet culture/designation
- Volunteer opportunities, inside and outside of organization
- Diverse workforce

Onboarding Supports
- Mentoring/precepting
- Social supports
- Internship/residency program
- Support services: discussion groups and social networking opportunities

Compensation/Financial Incentives
- Competitive salaries
- Financial support associated with credentialing and professional development opportunities
- Part-time pay with bonus hours
- Bonus pay
- Bonus pay for recruitment of employees
- Profit/gains sharing
- Child/elder care
- Phased retirement
- Increased vacation/paid time off (PTO) offerings

Professional Development Opportunities
- Career/clinical advancement programs
- Ongoing educational offerings/opportunities
- Scholarships for BSN/graduate programs
- Provisions for sabbatical
- Specialty training opportunities

Flexibility in Work Opportunities
- Flexible hours/schedules
- Fixed shifts
- Shift bidding
- Weekend options

Leadership Opportunities
- Creation of autonomous self-managed units
- Shared governance/leadership model
- Succession planning/development
- Precepting roles: staff and students

Technology
- Specialty equipment for use in care delivery
- Initialization of new technology into practice
- Technology/skill development support and training as integral part of roles

Miscellaneous Services
- Free parking
- Concierge services

BOX 20-3	RETENTION FACTORS RELATED TO RETAINING MULTIGENERATIONAL WORKFORCE			

	SIGNIFICANCE BY AGE		
RETENTION FACTORS	**<40**	**40-54**	**≥55**
Recognition and respect	X	X	X
Having a voice	X	X	X
Receiving ongoing feedback about performance	X	X	X
Compensation	X	X	X
Employee health and safety	X	X	X
Job design	X	X	X
Training and development	X	X	X
Flexible work options	X	X	X
Retirement options	X	X	X
Recruitment of older nurses			X

From Palumbo, M.V., McIntosh, B., Rambur, B., & Naud, S. (2009). Retaining an aging nurse workforce: Perceptions of human resource practices. *Nursing Economic$, 27*(4), 221-232.

working with generationally diverse groups. In addition, Leiter and colleagues (2010) have shown a difference in Generation X's and boomers' perceptions related to negative encounters (incivility) in the workplace. Although both generations reported significant levels of exhaustion, cynicism, turnover intention, and physical symptoms related to the incivility by supervisor, co-worker, and team, the greatest distress was found in Generation X. Exhaustion and turnover were strongly associated with supervisor incivility, whereas cynicism was strongly associated with supervisor and co-worker incivility. Greater incivility from co-workers and supervisors was found for Generation X than for boomers. Although significant efforts have been directed at the recruitment and retention of new graduates, in the past few years, equal effort has been directed at the retention of experienced older nurses because of their depth of knowledge relative to the organization and their clinical expertise. Retention factors related to the older nurse have been shown to vary significantly from that of the new graduate, as older nurses find it harder to manage the physical demands of hospital work and are focusing on establishing financial security for retirement. To meet the needs of the older nurse, organizations have had to rethink the rules and roles that have been in place. According to Mion and colleagues (2006), a number of changes to be made in the area of retention include the following (Park & Jones, 2010; Pierson, et al., 2010):

- Scheduling—decreasing frequency of rotations, reducing length of shifts, using sabbaticals
- Assignment requirements—geographic location, assignment consistency, work with preceptor
- Practice models—using specialty roles (e.g., wound nurse, audit nurse, admission and/or discharge nurse, telephone triage)
- Technology usage—lifting equipment, ergonomic computers and electrical devices, soften hard floor surfaces, cell phones, tracking systems, improved lighting
- Streamline processes—revised documentation systems, bed utilization programs, online continuing education, computer training, and multi-site computer access
- Communication and recognition opportunities—membership on unit-based and organizational committees, participation in shared governance activities, volunteer roles as institutional representatives, ambassador programs
- Educational opportunities—ongoing development, tuition reimbursement, scholarships, and so on

These and other changes are important if experienced nurses are to be retained at the bedside (Park & Jones, 2010; Pierson et al., 2010).

Probably the single most important factor in retention of nurses, however, is managerial leadership (Acree, 2006; Kleinman, 2004). The two leadership styles that predominate in the literature today are *transformational* and *transactional*. Acree (2006) presented Bass's definition of transformational and transactional leadership and noted that transformational leadership consists of four major components: "idealized influence (charisma), inspiration (engagement and confidence building), intellectual stimulation (problem awareness/solving) and individualized consideration (supportive, encouraging, and provision of developmental experiences" (p. 35). "Transactional leadership has two major components: contingent reward (reward for an agreed-upon effort) and management by exception (leader intervention only if something goes wrong or standards are not met)" (p. 35). Managerial use of transformational leadership has been shown to have the greatest impact on nurse job satisfaction. This is no surprise given the need for ongoing support, recognition, and life-balance expressed by both new graduates and experienced nurses. To provide this level of leadership, organizations will need to commit to the ongoing development of nurse managers and promote the cultural changes needed by nurse managers to actualize this level of leadership. Decreased cost has also been associated with effective recruitment strategies, consistent with the Magnet Recognition Program® (Halfer, 2007; Pine & Tart, 2007; vanWyngeeren & Stuart, n.d.).

TURNOVER: COST AND MANAGEMENT STRATEGIES

Turnover of qualified staff not only is disruptive to the care community in which the nurse works (Atencio et al., 2003; Hunt, 2009; Kuhar et al., 2004; Manion & Bartholomew, 2004;) but also is extremely costly to the organization (Jones, 2004a, b). According to Hunt (2009), the literature indicates that the total/real costs associated with nurse turnover have been evaluated using various approaches, such as direct and indirect, visible and invisible, and pre-hire and post-hire. The most common factors used in determining nurse turnover costs include the following (Hunt, 2009, Jones & Gates, 2007):

- Advertising and recruitment
- Vacancy costs
- Hiring
- Orientation and training
- Decreased productivity
- Termination
- Potential patient errors/decreased quality of care
- Poor work environment and culture
- Loss of organizational knowledge
- Increased accident and absenteeism rates
- Increased nurse and medical staff turnover

According to Hunt (2009, p. 2), "the average hospital is estimated to lose about $300,000 per year for each percentage increase in annual nurse turnover." Hunt further cited one 9000-person health care organization that lost over $15 million per year because of nursing turnover. Other figures for the average cost for a medical/surgical RN are reported to be $42,000, but it can be as high as $85,000 for specialty RNs. Often agency/traveler nurses are used as temporary coverage. Although the cost of this practice appears to meet institutional needs and comes at an estimated cost of 1.5 times the salary of a permanent employee, the practice often further perpetuates turnover. Residency programs for new graduates have been shown to have positive impact on retention and cost. The average rate of turnover is 15%, or approximately 195,000 RNs at an estimated yearly cost of $9.75 billion (AONE, 2010). Clearly, money spent for replacement could have been used by the organization to improve their competitive advantage, nurse satisfaction, and consumer perception of workforce quality and expansion of services. Figure 20-7 shows the cost per RN hire. Figure 20-8 displays a formula for calculating turnover.

$$\frac{\text{Total cost (e.g., recruitment, training, coverage)}}{\text{Total RNs hired}} = \text{Cost per RN hired}$$

FIGURE 20-7 Cost per RN hired. (Derived from Hoffman, P.M. [1984]. *Financial management for nurse managers.* Norwalk, CT: Appleton-Century-Crofts.)

$$\frac{\text{Number of terminations per year}}{\text{Average workforce per year}} \times 100 = \% \text{ Turnover}$$

FIGURE 20-8 Turnover formula. (Derived from Hoffman, P.M. [1984]. *Financial management for nurse managers.* Norwalk, CT: Appleton-Century-Crofts.)

RESEARCH NOTE

Source

Laschinger, H.K.S., Leiter, M., Day, A., & Gilin, D. (2009). Workplace empowerment, incivility, and burnout: Impact on staff nurse recruitment and retention outcomes. *Journal of Nursing Management, 17*, 302-311.

Purpose

Given the reported nursing shortage at the time of the study, as well as the projected future shortage and the cost associated with recruitment of staff, the authors believed it was important and timely to begin to scientifically evaluate factors that might impact retention of staff. The aim of the study was to examine the influence of empowering work conditions and workplace incivility on nurses' experiences of burnout and important nurse retention factors identified in the literature.

Discussion

Organizational empowerment and incivility have received increased attention as factors related to employee empowerment, work satisfaction, organizational commitment, and turnover intentions. Incivility has been viewed as a precursor to employees' intent to stay within an organization. These factors are important because they are closely tied to the successful retention of nurses within the health care setting. Failure to retain nurses is not only extremely disruptive in the workplace, it is extremely costly. In addition to financial costs, studies have shown that incivility and lack of empowerment among nurses has been correlated with manifestation of negative psychological and physical health of the employee: decreased overall health, burnout, depression, anxiety, low self-esteem, and emotional exhaustion (Leiter et al., 2008; Nedd, 2006; Vahey et al., 2004). Changes in employee health status play out in numerous ways, such as increased use of sick time, loss of productivity, negative effect on patient and staff safety, and decrease in quality of care.

Laschinger and colleagues used Kanter's model of structural empowerment to study the relationship of empowerment, incivility, and burnout to retention outcome. Workplace civility components included supervisor and co-worker. Burnout components included exhaustion and cynicism. Retention outcomes included job satisfaction, organizational commitment, and turnover intentions. The study was conducted in five organizations in two provinces in Canada and consisted of 1106 hospital employees. Staff was surveyed using six instruments: Conditions for Work Effectiveness Questionnaire II (CWEQ-II), Workplace Incivility Scale, Emotional Exhaustion and Cynicism subscales of the Maslach Burnout Inventory-General Survey, job satisfaction measures, Affective Commitment Scale, and Turnover Intentions. The job satisfaction questions looked at participants' satisfaction with co-workers, supervisors, pay and benefits, feeling of accomplishment from doing the job, and job overall. Data analysis consisted of hierarchical multiple linear regression analyses, used to test the influence of empowerment, incivility and burnout on the three retention outcomes: job satisfaction, organizational commitment, and turnover intentions.

The findings indicated that 67% and 77% of the nurses experience incivility from their supervisors and co-workers, respectively. Nurses also reported relatively high levels of emotional exhaustion, low levels of cynicism, moderately high levels of job satisfaction, moderate levels of organizational commitment, and low levels of turnover intentions. The analysis further revealed that empowerment, workplace incivility, and burnout jointly explained a strong relationship to the three retention outcomes: job satisfaction, organizational commitment, and turnover intentions. Empowerment, supervisor and co-worker incivility, and burnout were strong predictors of job satisfaction. Predictors of organizational commitment included: empowerment, incivility, and burnout; whereas predictors of empowerment included cynicism and supervisor and co-worker incivility. Overall, the findings indicated that nurses were relatively positive in terms of retention factors: job satisfaction, organizational commitment, and turnover intentions.

Application to Practice:

Although the nurses in this study did not report high levels of workplace incivility, the majority did experience some uncivil behaviors, and their perceptions of workplace incivility was significantly related to feelings of empowerment, burnout, job satisfaction, organizational commitment, and turnover intentions. An empowering practice environment and low levels of incivility and burnout were found to be significant predictors of nurses' experience of job satisfaction and organizational commitment and their intentions to leave their workplaces. According to Leiter and colleagues (2010) these finding are consistent with the results from their study, which measured generational differences, between Gen Xers and boomers, in distress, attitudes, and incivility among nurses. There is a difference between Gen Xers and boomers; the former encountered more incivility from co-workers and supervisor. The importance of Laschinger and colleagues (2009) and Leiter and colleagues (2010) studies are that they provide organizations with strong evidence of the

Continued

RESEARCH NOTE—cont'd

need to create a positive work environment and to promote worker engagement and manager support, as these are all key factors in staff and employee retention of staff and employee and patient safety. It further gives nurse administrators clearly delineated factors to address in developing a culture of retention. These factors are consistent with practices identified as a "Magnet culture."

A culture of civility is important for promoting employee health, employee safety, and patient safety and quality of care, because dealing with uncivil behavior leads to nurse exhaustion and burnout. Other key findings in the study were the importance of the manager role in the establishment of the milieu that fosters nurse engagement, ongoing professional development, positive collegial working relationships, and adequate resources that ensure highly skilled nurses remain engaged in their work. According to Weberg (2010), transformational leadership has been shown in the literature to positively impact burnout, exhaustion, increased well-being, and job satisfaction in the health care setting. Fostering empowerment and civility in the workplace are also closely tied to resources management—human and cost.

LEADERSHIP AND MANAGEMENT IMPLICATIONS

According to the IOM (2011), nurses are critical to the delivery and transformation of health care services in the United States. To fulfill the future demands in health care, the IOM indicated that the following four actions need to be addressed (see p. 4):

1. *Nurses should practice to the full extent of their education and training.*
2. *Nurses should achieve higher levels of education and training through an improved education system that promotes seamless academic progression.*
3. *Nurses should be full partners, with physicians and other health professionals, in redesigning health care in the United States.*
4. *Effective workforce planning and policy making require better data collection and an improved information infrastructure.*

According to Auerbach and colleagues (2011), the nursing shortage remains but has stabilized somewhat with the addition of nursing programs, both online and campus-based, offering traditional BSN, accelerated BSN, MSN, DNP, and PhD. Although it should be noted that the nurses and nurse educators are moving into retirement faster than they can be replaced, it is imperative that academic programs redesign their programs/offerings, find ways to move students through each of the programs more quickly, and find ways to increase the number of students who enter programs.

Given the recommendations/challenges outlined in the IOM (2011) report specific to educational advancement of RN to 80% BSN by 2020 and expansion of practice to the full extent of their education with realignment of non–value added tasks assigned to other workers (IOM, 2011), it is unclear whether the shortage of RNs exists at the current projected levels. However, this issue needs to be further addressed. Using an economic model (supply and demand), history would suggest that with increased labor available in the workforce (supply), opportunities and pay would diminish. If this happens, nurses will once again begin to withdraw from the marketplace, creating another nursing shortage.

Although nursing and health care organizations are moving forward to address the current shortage, efforts also need to be directed at the development of new practice models and changes in organizational systems, processes, and practices that enhance nurses' ability to successfully perform their work. Changes in health care and nurse reimbursement systems will also need to be addressed.

According to the literature, to truly address and effectively manage the changes needed relative to this current nurse shortage, partnerships will have to be formed among health care organizations, educational programs, professional organizations, and collective bargaining groups. To achieve the desired outcomes, extensive data analysis, strategy design, and policy changes will be required (Aiken, 2011; Buerhaus et al., 2009a; IOM, 2011).

In addition, administrations will need to evaluate their organizational structure and scope of assignment for managerial staff, because nurses repeatedly report that lack of managerial presence and support are significant dissatisfiers (Weberg, 2010). Managerial staff needs to be aware of the ongoing support and development requirements of new nurse graduates. Managers need to work with experienced staff to create mentorship and/or preceptor models that promote the development of new graduates. Managers further need to work with support staff (staff educators and clinical specialists) to develop unit-based registered nurse staff with skills and knowledge about how to manage workload and be accountable for outcomes while promoting growth of non-nurse caregivers and other support staff (Halfer, 2007; Palumbo et al., 2009).

To meet the current and future demand for nurses and to create stability in the workplace, greater efforts will have to be directed at recruiting minorities, including males, into the profession (Buerhaus et al., 2009a). Nurse managers need to explore all opportunities to fill vacant positions. Special attention will need to be directed at retention of qualified, experienced staff. This can be accomplished in a number of ways. One approach that is strongly supported in the literature is to survey staff and to plan institutionally-based recruitment and retention strategies jointly with staff (Kuhar et al., 2004).

CURRENT ISSUES AND TRENDS

Job dissatisfaction has been linked with nurse turnover or intent to leave (Aiken et al., 2002; Laschinger et al., 2009; Leiter, et al., 2010). Driving change through the creation of a Magnet culture has been shown to have significant impact on nurse practices and beliefs within an organization. Halfer (2007) described how use of the Magnet model to develop a new graduate internship program in an acute care pediatric medical center impacted retention of new graduates, yielded $707,000 savings annually, resulted in improved staff satisfaction (far exceeding national norms), and became a magnetic attraction for ongoing recruitment. According to Jenkins and Jarrett-Pulliam (2012),

there is a strong synergistic relationship between Magnet organizations and accountable care organizations (ACO). Although these organizations appear to have different commitments—excellence and recognition in Magnet organizations, and quality and reimbursement in ACOs—Jenkins and Jarrett-Pulliam (2012) noted that both are built on models of shared characteristics that in the end will prove a source of success for the creation of both ACOs and Magnet organizations. The authors identified 10 characteristics derived from the two organizations (Box 20-4).

The similarities of these two groups are driven by common characteristics in that both require excellent nursing and professional staffs in order to bring about the desired outcomes of improved staff and patient/family satisfaction and ongoing coordination of care across the continuum. Certainly none of these outcomes can be accomplished without strong leadership and accountability, data/research, and fiscal management. Nursing has lead the way in navigating a serious nursing shortage through commitment to quality of care. It would be nearsighted for health care providers not to blend the two models in promoting health care changes.

The frontline nurse manager is the linchpin for ongoing recruitment and retention of both new graduates and career nurses. Although it has been reported in numerous studies that frontline managers are key to successful recruitment and retention of staff and quality of care at the point of service (Leiter et al., 2010), currently this role is more important than ever, given that for the first time in history there are four generations of workers at the point of care. According to Kleinman (2004), research studies have consistently indicated leadership behaviors that positively influence staff nurse retention. These behaviors include support and consideration of staff, high visibility, and willingness to share leadership responsibility. Additional behaviors noted by Laschinger and

BOX 20-4 **CHARACTERISTICS OF MAGNET AND ACO ORGANIZATIONS**	
Patient-centeredness	Evidence-based practice (EBP) and research
Leadership	Innovation
Relationships	Quality and efficiency
Workforce investment	Fiscal management
Accountability	Outcomes

colleagues (2009) and Leiter and colleagues (2010) include civility and structural empowerment. According to the *AONE Guiding Principles for the Newly Licensed Nurse's Transition into Practice* (AONE, 2010), nurse managers are identified as the key driver for ensuring the experience of the newly licensed nurse is successful. The success of nurse managers is related to understanding and using of transformational leadership skills (Weberg, 2010).

To achieve the outcomes previously noted, it is imperative that additional focus be given to the role of the nurse manager. Although this role is pivotal to staff retention, staff satisfaction, quality of patient care, and achievement of organizational goals, the number of qualified nurse managers in acute care institutions is decreasing (Zastock & Holly, 2010). According to AONE (2002), vacancy rates for nurse managers are on average as high as 8.3% nationwide. Factors shown to impact nurse manager retention include aging and retirement, demands related to span of control (number of direct reports), decreased resources, decreased clinical involvement, increased staff diversity, increased coordination across differing nursing units, issues with assistive personnel, changing regulatory requirements, and need for new management skills coupled with increasing complexity of hospitalized patients and widespread use of personal communication devices. The latter, enabling constant communication through cell phones, e-mail, and pagers, leads to a sense of being "on" 24 hours a day, 7 days a week (Zastock & Holly, 2010). Clearly these issues need to be addressed to retain the number of nurse managers needed within health care institutions. Mackoff and Triolo (2008a, b) have developed a model of manager engagement that looks at both work entry into the organization and into the nurse manager position as a way to enhance effective communication and organizational support.

The current nursing shortage is driven by a number of factors such as inadequate supply of students, increased aging of the registered nurse workforce, increased demand for nurses within and outside of health care, and generational differences in nurses related to their intention to stay in nursing (Palumbo et al., 2009). In addition to the shortage of nurses, health care is facing a reduction in all health care workers, both professional and nonprofessional.

Nursing care has been strongly linked to both quality and cost; yet organizations are struggling to establish an environment and culture that promote job satisfaction and retention of nurses (Aiken, 2008). Onboarding of new graduates and experienced staff is a major factor in enhancing staff satisfaction and intent to stay (Park & Jones, 2010). Strategies that improve the work life of older experienced nurses will facilitate them staying in the workforce longer (Palumbo et al., 2009).

As identified in the literature, nurse managers play a key role in both retention and recruitment of staff. The nurse manager's leadership style plays a major role in setting the tone for the unit and/or establishing a culture of retention. According to Laschinger and colleagues (2009), structural empowerment and creation of a culture of civility are important managerial and organizational behaviors related to staff satisfaction and intention to stay. It is clear from the literature that considerable work needs to be done within nursing services and health care administration to establish a community/culture of caring and safety/security for nurses and other health care providers. People, for the most part, want to be able to go to work each day with a sense of pride and respect for their contributions. In return, they expect to be treated with respect and have a sense of security within the job and work environment. It is projected that this area of study and the application of related strategies will be a major thrust in the future. This approach is consistent with the Magnet Recognition Program® of the ANA, the AHA (2002) report, *In Our Hands,* and the IOM (2001) report, *Crossing the Quality Chasm.*

It appears that market and political forces have begun to create pressure in an attempt to help mitigate the nursing shortage and its impact on health care. These actions have been directed at the supply end, through funding availability for students who choose nursing as a career, nursing program expansion, and faculty funding. In addition, more efforts are being directed at the retention of experienced bedside nurses and managerial staff. As the full impact of the Affordable Care Act plays out into the near future, demand for unmet health care needs from the 30 to 40 million uninsured Americans may become the more predominant market force. Nurses, and the health care delivery system, will feel the impact.

What is the Cost of Retention to the Organization and to the Employee?

Mr. Jamar, a 42-year-old African male of Muslim faith (which he and his family maintained strong ties with) was hired as a new graduate on a medical-surgical unit of an academic pediatric medical center. The unit into which he was hired was predominately composed of white females ages 23 to 50 years, with one Asian and several African-American nurses. Upon hire, Mr. Jamar started orientation and was viewed as open, receptive, and knowledgeable. He was also a critical thinker and an excellent cultural resource.

Before accepting the position, he came into the United States through normal immigration. He and his family left their home in Africa because of oppression. At the time of his arrival in New York, he and his family had very limited resources. He took numerous jobs to support his family and paid his way through nursing school. He initially completed his LPN program, was licensed, and worked as a LPN for 4 years while he completed the Associate Degree Nursing program.

Upon completion of orientation and starting work at the unit level, things began to change. Mr. Jamar was assigned a preceptor for unit-based orientation. During the initial time with his preceptor, he continually asked questions in an effort to learn about the care needs of patients and technical procedures. By week four of coming to the unit, Mr. Jamar began to experience a sense of isolation. Most of the staff did not acknowledge his presence and were often terse with him when he asked questions. His sense of isolation prompted him to request of meeting with the Unit Educator to discuss his orientation and staff responses. At this time he was informed that there were no problems and to just keep up his practice and orientation. Shortly thereafter upon entering a room in which an infant had been crying for some time, Mr. Jamar asked the mother to feed the baby, by saying "you must feed your baby." The mother later reported Mr. Jamar to the preceptor stating that she was dissatisfied with the way he had spoken to her. She said that he had spoken in a terse tone. The preceptor shared this complaint with Mr. Jamar and told him to watch the tone he used in providing instructions to patients/families. He was further told that his cultural mannerisms were not consistent with this country/region. This incident was followed by further isolation of Mr. Jamar by the other staff. They distanced themselves from him, acted covertly uncivil, did not

acknowledge him when he asked questions, or just shrugged their shoulders in response. Mr. Jamar was taken off guard by all of these actions. He believed that all he had done was to tell the mother that she needed to feed the baby. Also, Mr. Jamar had received numerous compliments from other patients/families he had cared for.

In an attempt to further clarify what was going on, Mr. Jamar requested a meeting with the Nurse Manager and Unit Educator to discuss their perceptions of his practice and work progress. He also contacted the Staff Development Educator and his Nurse Recruiter who had worked with him in institutional orientation to try to get clarification of unit expectations.

At Mr. Jamar's request, the Nurse Manager and Unit Educator met with him to discuss his practice. At the meeting he was informed that his practice was inconsistent with the unit expectations and that they thought he had had a medication error. No written information was provided to Mr. Jamar at that time. The Nurse Manager orally communicated to Mr. Jamar that he should go home for 3 days since he was scheduled off for those days and told him that when he returned they would let him know if he would be allowed to stay. Following the meeting Mr. Jamar contacted the Nurse Recruiter to see what was going on. He was still in his probationary period and was concerned about losing his job. The fear of losing his job was both an embarrassment and concern. He was concerned about possible loss of income for him and his family and position within his cultural community. Upon return to work following his 3 days off, Mr. Jamar was terminated by the Nurse Manager and Nurse Educator. The reason given for the termination was that his practice was inconsistent with unit expectations.

The medical-surgical unit to which Mr. Jamar had been hired had been running a high census for over 6 months, with numerous staff working overtime and time and a half for 10 months. The position had been posted but not filled for 5 months, although recruitment efforts had been ongoing. Mr. Jamar had been in orientation for 10 weeks and so was not yet counted in the staffing numbers. His work time and salary were recorded as an educational, nonproductive cost that had to be absorbed in the unit budget for replacement and training. With the termination of Mr. Jamar, the recruitment and onboarding process would have to start all over.

CRITICAL THINKING EXERCISE

You are the nurse manager on the medical-surgical unit described in the case study. You have been the nurse manager for 6 months and became the manager because two units were merged following new facility construction. You have many pressing priorities. Analyze the case study by reviewing the processes that might have seriously impacted the retention of this nurse and what actions you would take in the future. Address the following questions:

1. Consider Mr. J.'s demographic profile and analyze it from a manager's point of view:
   a. Could the interviewing process have impacted this outcome?
   b. What onboarding process would you have put in place?
   c. Describe the point at which intervention should have occurred?
   d. How did unit culture and staff behavior affect this case?
   e. What predictive and preventive actions need to occur for future hiring considerations?

2. As a manager, reflect on your considerations around this case:
   a. What impact did this case have on staff? (Include Mr. J. in staff considerations.) (trust, safety, transparency, ethical, moral)
   b. What impact did this case have on patients and families? (trust, safety)
   c. What impact did this case have on the organization? (risk, financial loss)
   d. Was the onboarding of Mr. J. directed at the appropriate level of valuing and professional development? If not, what actions should be changed?

3. Considering the need for staff to feel connected:
   a. How do you as a manager create the shared environment that promotes:
      i. Staff safety
      ii. Continuous learning and improvement
      iii. Collegiality
      iv. Civil work environment
      v. Appropriate interviewing, hiring, and onboarding
   b. Examine biases in this case:
      i. Mr. J.'s culture and unit impact
      ii. Staff/educator/preceptor cultural knowledge and actions to support
      iii. Manager supportive and deficient actions

4. What would you change or do differently with the next hire?

Staffing and Scheduling

Sharon Eck Birmingham, Beth Pickard,
Lori Carson

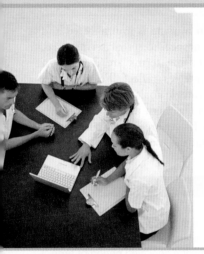

℮volve WEBSITE

http://evolve.elsevier.com/Huber/leadership/

Nurse staffing methodology should be an orderly, systematic process, based upon sound rationale, applied to determine the number and kind of nursing personnel required to provide nursing care of a predetermined standard to a group of patients in a particular setting. The end result is prediction of the kind and number of staff required to give care to patients. This prediction of the number and kinds of personnel to give patients nursing care 24 hours a day, 7 days a week…is no small task. The aim is to provide, at a reasonable cost to the general public the agency serves, a standard of nursing care acceptable to its clientele and the nursing staff serving it (Aydelotte, 1973, p. 3)

Nurse staffing methodology eloquently articulated by Aydelotte in the early 1970s continues as a critical issue affecting the quality, safety, and cost of U.S. health care today (Aiken et al., 2002; Aiken et al., 2003; Blegen & Goode, 1998; Hinshaw, 2006; Institute of Medicine [IOM], 2004; Kane et al., 2007a, b; Kovner & Gergen, 1998; Litvak et al., 2005; Needleman et al., 2002; Needleman et al., 2006; Needleman et al., 2011; Unruh, 2008). Nursing is

Photo used with permission from Photos.com.

essential in the delivery of health care to society. Nursing's Social Policy Statement reflects the societal contract for the provision of safe and quality nursing care and services for all people in every health care setting (American Nurses Association [ANA], 2010a). The major goal of staffing management is to provide the right number of nursing staff with the right qualifications to deliver safe, high-quality and cost-effective nursing care to a group of patients and their families as evidenced by positive clinical outcomes, satisfaction with care, and progression across the care continuum (Eck Birmingham, 2010; Warner, 2006).

Staffing management is one of the most critical yet highly complex and time-consuming activities for nurse leaders at every level of the health care organization today (Abdoo, 2000; Sullivan et al., 2003). How well or poorly nursing leaders execute staff management impacts the safety and quality of patient care, financial results, and organizational outcomes, such as job satisfaction and retention of registered nurses (RNs) (Beyers, 2000). The purpose of this chapter is to assist students and nursing leaders at all levels to understand the complex issues associated with staffing management in patient care. A framework for staffing management is presented, and critical components of the staffing management plan are described. New evidence that fosters an understanding of the effects of RN fatigue, independent of staffing, on quality is presented. Technology tools for frontline nursing leaders to foster the alignment of roles and accountability for staffing management are discussed. Additionally, the IOM (2010) report on the future of nursing articulates many recommendations to strengthen the advancement of evidenced-based staffing and they are explored here.

DEFINITIONS

Staffing terminology in nursing is multifaceted and often confusing, with a specific set of terms used. The most common staffing terms are defined in Box 21-1. Staffing strategies reflect the hospital's mission, and annual strategic goals and are executed to meet the staffing management plan of an organization. Chief nursing officers are accountable to establish and translate staffing management strategies

---

BOX 21-1 STAFFING TERMINOLOGY

Human Resources Staffing Strategy

A set of actions undertaken to determine human resources needs, recruit and select qualified applicants, and meet the needs of the organization (Fried & Johnson, 2002).

Nurse Staffing Management Plan

A structured approach to the process of identifying and allocating unit-based personnel resources in the most effective and efficient manner (Kirby & Wiczai, 1985; Nash et al., 2000).

Nurse Staffing

Staffing refers to the process of assessing and allocating the direct care nursing staff on a shift to a patient care unit.

Skill Mix

Skill mix is the proportion of direct-care RNs to total direct care nursing staff; expressed as a percentage of RNs to total nursing staff (Unruh, 2003). For example, a medical surgical patient care unit may have a skill mix of 60% RNs and 40% unlicensed assistive personnel (UAP). A skill mix ratio is typically budgeted for at the patient care unit level, but must also be examined at the shift level during the scheduling process.

Staffing Pattern

A staffing pattern lists the total number of direct care staff by skill level scheduled for each day and each shift. For example, for a 12-hour day shift for a pediatric unit on Mondays, there may be six RNs and two UAP for direct care. An additional RN assigned to care for children being admitted or discharged may be scheduled from 3 to 6 PM, during this peak time where children are returning from the operating room or going home.

Scheduling

Scheduling is the process of assigning individual personnel to work specific hours, days, or shifts and in a specific unit or area over a specified period of time (Barnum & Mallard, 1989).

Staffing Effectiveness

Staffing effectiveness is an evaluation of the effect of nurse staffing on quality patient, financial, and organizational outcomes.

Nurse-to-Patient Ratio

The RN-to-patient ratio reflects the actual patient care assignment or a state-mandated regulatory requirement for an RN-to-patient assignment. The number of RNs assigned to care for a certain number of patients is stated as a ratio. For example, 1:2 is a common ratio for one RN to care for two patients in an intensive care unit and may be changed based on the condition of the patients.

Skill Level

Skill level is the licensure (e.g., RN, LPN, LVN) or certification (e.g., UAP, NA) of a direct care staff member.

Nursing Workload

Workload is defined as the intensity (in terms of effort required) of the work a nurse performs within a given period (Unruh, 2008). Because so many variables affect workload, there are efforts to better explicate and measure workload, such as nursing intensity (Moore & Hastings, 2006) and nurse dose (Brooten & Youngblut, 2006; Huber, 2008).

Nursing Direct-Care Hours

Direct-care hours is the number of nursing staff hours that are assigned to provide direct care to a patient or groups of patients for a specified period; the most common direct-care staff include the RN, LPN/LVN, and UAP.

BOX 21-1   STAFFING TERMINOLOGY—cont'd

The hours are typically calculated per patient day or nursing hours per patient day (NHPPD).

Average Daily Census

The average daily census (ADC) is calculated by dividing the number of patients cared for per day over a certain period by the number of days in a period. It may be an actual ADC or a budgeted ADC.

Admission, Discharges, and Transfers

Admission, discharges, and transfers (ADT) refers to the patients who are admitted, discharged, and

transferred. The ADT factor has also been referred to as a churn or turnover of patients. ADT is associated with increased care or workload to meet the standard of care for the patient, and with safe and effective RN-to-RN communication or handoff regarding the patient condition and plan of care.

Average Length of Stay

Average length of stay is the average number of days the patient is in the hospital. It is determined by dividing the total number of patient days by the total number of admissions.

Data from Finkler SA, Kovner CT, and Jones CB: *Financial management for nurse managers and executives*, 3rd edition, Philadelphia, 2007, Saunders.

for the overall patient care divisions. The nurse managers accountable for a patient care unit or area execute the staffing management strategies, to yield an optimal health experience and clinical outcomes for patients and their families; a healthy, satisfying work environment; and cost-effective staffing model for the organization. Nursing leaders at all levels are challenged to clearly identify the leadership roles that are accountable for staffing management and adopt technologies that provide the real-time tools to execute, measure, and achieve the desired outcomes.

FRAMEWORK FOR STAFFING MANAGEMENT

Staffing management is complex and challenging because of the numerous dependencies and interrelated organizational processes. A conceptual framework provides logic and order to complex processes for administrators and scientists to consider (Edwardson, 2007). A conceptual framework for staffing management is proposed and illustrated in Figure 21-1.

This conceptual framework is adapted from Donabedian's (1966) framework for the evaluation of quality of care: relating various structures (e.g., hospital characteristics) that impact various processes (e.g., actual staffing) and subsequently influence various outcomes (e.g., patient quality, patient satisfaction, and staff satisfaction). Multiple staffing studies have adapted this framework to organize the variables of interest (Cho, 2001; Eck, 1999; Edwardson, 2007; Kane et al., 2007a, b; Mark et al., 2007; Mark et al., 2004).

In the proposed framework, structures represent the various nursing strategies, both internal and external to the organization, which directly influence an organization's ability to effectively manage processes for staffing. The processes are a series of defined stages with outputs that directly affect subsequent stages of staffing. Finally, the outcomes of staffing management are multidimensional and measured in terms of organizational outcomes including patient, fiscal, and staff outcomes. The staffing management framework is not intended to address all possible variables but, instead, is intended to provide a guide for nursing leaders to assess staffing management in their organizations.

STRATEGIES INFLUENCING STAFFING MANAGEMENT

It is important for all nursing leaders to remain current on both the internal and external influences affecting staffing management. Briefly presented are (1) professional resources and recommendations, (2) nursing care delivery models, (3) state legislative mandates, (4) The Joint Commission (TJC) regulation, and (5) nurse union agreements.

American Nurses Association Principles for Nurse Staffing

The American Nurses Association (ANA) has published guiding documents that serve as resources to understand the complex staffing issues associated with creating a nursing unit schedule, an organization-wide staffing plan, or meeting staffing

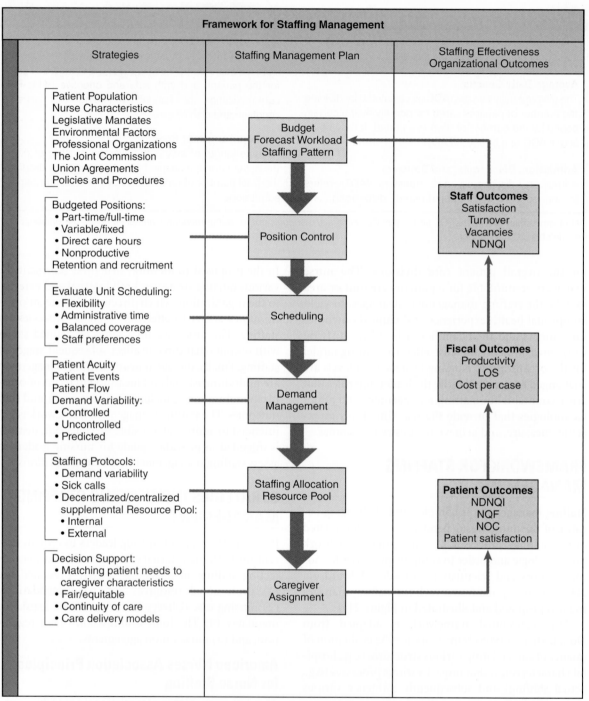

FIGURE 21-1 Framework for staffing management. *LOS,* Length of stay; *NDNQI,* National Database of Nursing Quality Indicators; *NOC,* nursing outcomes classification; *NQF,* National Quality Forum.

legislation. *Principles for Nurse Staffing* (ANA, 1999) was developed by an appointed expert panel to guide nurse staffing. The nine principles are organized into three categories pertaining to the patient care unit, the staff, and the organization (ANA, 1999). The nine principles capture the complexity of nurse staffing and offer an excellent guide for dialogue among nursing leaders. Principles related to the patient care unit are the following (ANA, 1999, p. 2):

A. *Appropriate staffing levels for a patient care unit reflect analysis of individual and aggregate patient needs.*

B. *There is a critical need to either retire or seriously question the usefulness of the concept of nursing hours per patient day (HPPD).*

C. *Unit functions necessary to support delivery of quality patient care must also be considered in determining staffing levels.*

Principles related to nursing staff are the following (ANA, 1999, p. 2):

A. *The specific needs of various patient populations should determine the appropriate clinical competencies required of the nurse practicing in that area.*

B. *Registered nurses must have nursing management support and representation at both the operational level and the executive level.*

C. *Clinical support from experienced RNs should be readily available to those RNs with less proficiency.*

Principles related to the organization are the following (ANA, 1999, p. 2):

A. *Organizational policy should reflect an organizational climate that values registered nurses and other employees as strategic assets and exhibit a true commitment to filling budgeted positions in a timely manner.*

B. *All institutions should have documented competencies for nursing staff, including agency or supplemental and traveling RNs, for those activities that they have been authorized to perform.*

C. *Organizational policies should recognize the myriad needs of both patients and nursing staff.*

These principles reflect values of the patient, nurses, work environment, and outcomes at the unit or practice level. The ANA recommends a professional model in which the staffing factors taken into account include the number of patients, acuity levels of patients, contextual issues such as unit geography and technology availability, and the level of preparation, experience, and competency of caregivers. The demand for this work was evident when the published principles were rapidly integrated and adopted into health care organizational policies, collective bargaining language, and state staffing legislation.

As the nursing shortage intensified, the ANA (2005) responded with an updated *Utilization Guide for the ANA Principles for Nurse Staffing*. This report highlighted several policy perspectives: (1) the value of direct-care nurses' input into an organization's staffing plan; (2) the value of direct-care nurses' input into the selection and implementation of patient classification or acuity systems; and (3) the value of both the clinically skilled and experienced RN who is familiar with the specific patients and nursing staff rendering their professional judgment regarding staffing decisions. This guide is an excellent document relevant for all nursing leaders and staffing committees for dialogue and planning.

Patient Acuity

Technology advancements foster adoption of the ANA staffing principles for annual budgeting and in everyday practice. Unfortunately, most patient classification systems aimed at adjusting staffing for acuity have been plagued with an inability to accurately and reliably measure patient care variability. Further, they have lacked organizational credibility and added burden to the direct care nurse. In recent years, health care reform and meaningful use legislation (HITECH act) has catapulted the advancement of health information technology to widespread adoption of electronic medical records (EMR) in the United States *(www. hipaasurvivalguide.com/hitech-act-summary.php)*. These advances additionally offer nursing leaders technologies that leverage the automated patient assessment information entered into the patient EMR by nurses to generate accurate measurements of patient acuity (Eck Birmingham et al., 2011). The electronic patient assessment information is translated into not only workload information at the patient level, but also standardized outcomes of care (Moorhead et al.,

2008) that may assist the nurse and care team in tracking patient progression to the anticipated Medicare Severity Diagnosis Related Groups (MS-DRGs) and length of stay (Eck Birmingham, 2010). The objective patient acuity information generated as a by-product of routine clinical documentation allows frontline charge nurses to make informed patient care assignment decisions. From the chief nurse's perspective, new acuity technologies help build the business case for acuity-adjusted staffing for both improved quality and cost outcomes (Dent & Bradshaw, 2012).

Nursing Care Delivery Models

Nursing care delivery models significantly influence staffing management. A nursing care delivery model "is defined as a method of organizing and delivering nursing care in order to achieve desired patient outcomes" (Deutschendorf, 2010, p. 444). Examples of nursing care delivery models include patient-focused care, team nursing, private duty nursing, total patient care, functional nursing, primary nursing, and various combinations.

Manthey (1990) and Person (2004) described the four fundamental elements of any nursing care delivery model as follows: (1) nurse/patient relationship and decision making; (2) work allocation and patient assignments; (3) communication among members of the health team; and (4) management of the unit or environment of care. Translating the nursing care delivery model's elements and inherent values to staffing management is a key role for nursing leaders (ANA, 2004). One common element among care models is the value of the nurse and patient/family relationship. Patient assignment technology offers charge nurses access to real-time data in order to match the right nurse (i.e., competency, expertise) with the right patient and provide continuity of care during an episode of care. A second common trend is the evolving role of the charge nurse as the frontline leader with responsibility to coordinate patient flow with expert communication among health care team members. Increasingly a charge nurse is appointed as a resource, managing patient flow and supporting novice nurses, and thus does not assume a direct care assignment.

Three nursing care delivery models, relationship-based care, the synergy model, and case management are briefly described next and depict how each model influences staffing management. Relationship-based care (RBC) is a common model used in care delivery (Koloroutis, 2004). Person (2004) articulated continuity of care as central to the RBC model, and this model also integrates Jean Watson's theory of caring (Watson, 2002).

The synergy model for patient care is presented by the American Association of Critical-Care Nurses (Hardin & Kaplow, 2005). The core concept of the model is also based on the nurse-patient relationship and acknowledges that the needs or characteristics of the patients and families drive the competencies of the nurse. Synergy, or optimum outcomes, results when the needs and characteristics of the patient clinical unit, or system, are matched with a nurse's competencies (Kaplow & Reed, 2008). Patient assignment technology may assist in defining, and therefore aligning, patient needs with the nurse's abilities, a concept central to the model.

A third example is case management, defined by the Case Management Society of America (CMSA) as "a collaborative process of assessment, planning, facilitation, care coordination, evaluation, and advocacy for options and services to meet an individual's and family's comprehensive health needs through communication and available resources to promote quality, cost-effective outcomes" (CMSA, 2012, p. 1). Case management can be coupled with demand management to best coordinate care and resources to achieve positive patient outcomes, transitions of care coordination, and hospital reimbursement (Pickard & Warner, 2007).

Complementing these models, the American Association of Colleges of Nursing (AACN) has recommended a new professional nurse role, the clinical nurse leader (CNL), into current care delivery models (AACN, 2003, 2007). The CNL role integrates various aspects of previous roles known in nursing, such as the case manager and clinical nurse specialist. The CNL vision statement is as follows: "The CNL champions innovations that improve patient outcomes, ensure quality care and reduce healthcare costs. The CNL integrates emerging nursing science into practice and leads this effort to enhance patient care. A recognized leader in all settings, the CNL is an advocate for reforming the healthcare delivery system and putting best practices into action" (AACN, 2003, p. 2).

The staffing management plan should reflect the values and roles established in the care delivery model that will ultimately influence the patient and organizational outcomes. Both the care delivery model and staffing plan within the context of patient populations in the health care organization are critical to the overall annual strategic plan for nursing.

American Organization of Nurse Executives

The American Organization of Nurse Executives (AONE), a subsidiary of the American Hospital Association, is a national organization whose mission is to represent nurse leaders. More than a decade ago, this key leadership group published *Staffing Management and Methods: Tools and Techniques for Nurse Leaders* (AONE, 2000), which presents an introduction to evolving staffing measures. It has a chapter dedicated to staffing management approaches in each of four hospital types: the large academic medical center, an integrated health care system, a small community hospital, and a rural hospital setting. The final chapter discusses how various innovations in information systems support nurse staffing.

More recently, AONE's 2008 Legislative Agenda for public policy and advocacy included several key points relevant to staffing management. The policy agenda aims to: "Develop, evaluate and support legislation that will foster the nurse executive's leadership role in the management of the care environment, especially in areas related to staffing, information technology and patient care services" (AONE, 2008, p. 1). The agenda does not support mandates, such as overtime or staffing ratios, and recommends working with state and federal legislators to shape policies that promote flexibility and recognize the volatility of the patient care environment.

Staffing Recommendations by Professional Organizations

Several professional nursing specialty organizations have published position statements for nurse staffing to offer evidence-based guidelines for specialty practice. Nursing leaders in specialty practice should encourage identification and discussion of the position statement during the annual staffing plan review. For example, the National Association of Neonatal Nurses (1999a, b) has a staffing position statement and recommended staffing ratios that are also described in the "Guidelines for Perinatal Care" (American Academy of Pediatrics [AAP] & the American College of Obstetricians and Gynecologists [ACOG], 2007). The ratios delineate care provided for women and newborns in the antepartum, intrapartum, and postpartum settings, as well as the newborn nursery. In recently revised guidelines, the Association of Women's Health, Obstetric and Neonatal Nurses (AWHONN, 2010)

describes the specific staffing recommendations for women in the various stages of normal labor and labor with complications.

Similarly, the Association of periOperative Registered Nurses (AORN, 2005) has a position paper addressing key staffing issues in the operating room (OR), and the Emergency Nurses Association (ENA, 2003), has published recommendations for staffing. Finally, the American Academy of Ambulatory Care Nursing (AAACN, 2005) has published an annotated bibliography summarizing the ambulatory nurse staffing literature. Haas and Hastings (2001) have outlined the methods for determining staffing requirements, skill mix, and productivity in the ambulatory care setting. Adoption of staffing recommendations in clinical settings by the relevant professional organizations is endorsed in the Principles of Nurse Staffing and frequently seen written into the staffing plans.

The Joint Commission Staffing Regulation

Private regulatory agencies, such as The Joint Commission (TJC), are widely used by hospitals today to conduct external reviews for quality and safety. The Joint Commission noted the following (TJC, 2006):

> *The goal of the human resources function is to ensure that the hospital determines the qualifications and competencies for staff positions based on its mission, populations, and care, treatment and services. Hospitals must also provide the right number of competent staff members to meet the patients' needs. (p. HR-1)*

TJC human resources standards clearly outline the complex requirements associated with staffing management today and include, but are not limited to, the adequacy of staff numbers, mix of staff levels, licensure, education, certification, experience, and continuing education.

Collective Bargaining Agreements and Staffing Management

Provisions in the ANA Code of Ethics articulate the rights of nurses to address work conditions through collective action (ANA, 2010b). Porter (2010) described a successful model of professional practice labor partnerships. The two largest nursing and health care unions are (1) the United American Nurses (UAN), a branch of the ANA; and (2) the

Service Employees International Union (SEIU) District 1199. Nursing unions are organizations that represent nurses for the purpose of collective bargaining, which has been defined as "the performance of the mutual obligations of the employer and the representative of the employees to meet at reasonable times and confer in good faith with respect to wages, hours, and other terms and conditions of employment... such obligation does not compel either party to agree to a proposal or require the making of a concession" (National Labor Relations Board, 2012, section 8b, paragraph 7d).

In nursing, there is a process of negotiation between the health care employer and the union representatives of nurse employees to reach a written agreement regarding certain terms of employment. The mandatory terms of employment vary widely, but they include subjects such as, but not limited to, wages, hours, overtime, low census call-off procedures, recall, floating, use of unlicensed assistive personnel (UAP), seniority, sick leave, discharges, and leaves of absence. These employment subjects have significant implications for staffing management and vary in their specificity regarding nurse staffing and scheduling. Nursing leaders working in settings with collective bargaining units need to have detailed knowledge of the relevant contractual implications for staffing management and incorporate them into the staffing technologies for compliance monitoring.

LEADERSHIP AND MANAGEMENT IMPLICATIONS

Legislative Impact on Staffing Management

Nurse dissatisfaction and concern for adequate staffing to provide quality nursing care to patients and their families arose from hospital cost-reduction initiatives throughout the 1990s. Armed with quality-of-care concerns, nurses began to organize and craft proposed staffing legislation in many states. The historical context that led to quality-of-care concerns continues to impact legislation today. Throughout the 1990s, hospital administrators relied on consultants to implement work redesign to promote patient-focused care as a method of cost reduction. The central labor reduction approach

in patient-focused care was reducing the number of RNs and increasing the number of UAP. This approach for decreasing nursing RN skill mix was implemented in a "one size fits all" approach across organizations and often lacked evaluation of the skill mix change and other changes on the quality of care and nurse job satisfaction and retention (Eck, 1999; Norrish & Rundall, 2001). This was most apparent in California where a leaner RN skill mix was tried by Kaiser Permanente Northern California in the early 1990s. Skill mix was reduced from 55% RNs to 30% RNs in 1995 (Robertson & Samuelson, 1996). The changes in skill mix led to widespread real and perceived increases in RN workload, patient safety concerns, and nurse and consumer complaints (Norrish & Rundall, 2001; Seago et al., 2003).

Despite patient complaints and reports of nurse dissatisfaction, little was done until 1999. Only then did the California legislature pass Assembly Bill 394 (AB 394) to mandate minimum nurse staffing ratios and acuity adjusted staffing. The mandating of minimum nurse-to-patient ratios legislated in California ignited great debate, controversy, and study. Nurse scientists and policy experts have presented compelling arguments against mandated ratios and explicate that the local nursing leaders are in the best position to determine the actual staffing required by the particular patient population (Clarke, 2005). The bold action, however, of the California state legislative mandate stimulated focused attention on addressing nurse staffing issues.

Since the late 1990s, state legislation regarding nurse staffing issues has been commonplace, and over 25 states have various regulations. Primary trends of the enacted state legislation include limiting or precluding mandatory overtime, requiring staffing committees with direct-care nurse input, whistleblower protection, mandated public access to staffing information, and a requirement that implementation of patient acuity methodologies must adjust for staffing workload (White, 2006). State nurse staffing legislation has a significant impact on staffing management via regulation. The economic downturn in 2008 following the end of the Bush administration, however, shifted political attention to jobs and the economy and has stalled further legislative nurse staffing mandates.

THE STAFFING MANAGEMENT PLAN

The staffing management plan provides the structured processes to identify patient needs and then to deliver the staff resources as efficiently and effectively as possible. An effective plan first focuses on stabilizing the unit core staffing. A staffing pattern, or core coverage, is determined through a forecasted workload and a recommended care standard (e.g., HPPD). Hiring to the associated position complement and developing balanced and filled schedules, without holes, are essential building blocks for efficient and cost-effective daily resource allocation. Daily staffing allocation requires managing a variable staffing plan, measuring and predicting demand, and then providing balanced workload assignments to ensure that the correct caregivers are best matched to patient needs (Warner, 2006). A successful staffing management plan incorporates the policies inherent to the organization, patient care unit, and nurse population including union and contracting affiliations. Kane and colleagues (2007a, b) suggested that nurse staffing policies should address both patient care units and organizations, such as shift rotation, overtime, full-time/part-time mix, and weekend staffing. The traditional emphasis in staffing planning has been on hospital settings. However, with shifts to primary care as the predominant site, staffing planning is equally critical.

Forecasted Workload and Staffing Pattern (Core Coverage)

Forecasting nursing workload for each patient care area is typically carried out at least once a year and as part of the annual budgeting process or when the patient characteristics, services, and/or volume changes. The amount of work performed by a unit is referred to as its *workload,* and workload volume is measured in terms of units of service. The unit of service is specific to the type of unit, such as the number of patients, patient days, deliveries, visits, treatments, encounters, or procedures.

Once the unit of service is determined, the number of units of service that will be provided in the coming year must be forecasted. Total patient days are commonly used in inpatient hospital areas. This is calculated by multiplying the average length of stay (ALOS) and the average daily census (ADC). The workload standard commonly used is nursing care hours per patient day (NHPPD), although the validity of this measure is disputed.

However, not all patients require the same number of care hours, and the total number of patient days may be inadequate for planning purposes. Finkler and colleagues (2007) suggested using adjusted units of service. For example, a nursing unit can be adjusted using a system for classifying patients, such as a patient acuity system, based on the resources each classification category is expected to use. Segregating patients into acuity classifications allows the staffing pattern to be developed based on the resource requirements of the specific mix of patients forecasted for the unit. Similar calculations can be made in ambulatory and primary care by using a method to classify patients into different categories to estimate the average resource required for patients in each category (Finkler et al., 2007).

In addition to adjusting workload based on acuity, patient turnover on the unit is an important factor in patient care workload measurement. Reduced length of stay, or higher patient turnover, requires intensive periods of higher resources for patient admissions, transfer, discharge, and other 1:1 activities, such as when the RN with an unstable patient is off the patient care unit, that will impact overall workload.

Outside of state-mandated nurse staffing ratios, there is no one "gold care standard" or recommended process to determine nursing workload. Inconsistent operational definitions and methods of measuring care have been a challenge both for benchmarking resources across organizations and for research analysis related to adequate nursing care (Kane et al., 2007a, b). Therefore each organization must document and provide rationale regarding how staffing standards are determined within each patient care area.

Once the annual workload is forecasted, the skill mix required on each shift is determined. There are two general staffing methods: (1) with *fixed staffing,* staffing is built around a fixed projected maximum workload requirement, and the staffing pattern is based on maximum workload conditions; (2) with *variable staffing,* units are staffed below maximum workload conditions and staff is then supplemented when needed. An effective staffing pattern requires clear definitions for productive time, non-patient care or "nonproductive" time (i.e., benefits time, work for the organization, knowledge-related projects), worked time, paid full-time equivalents (FTEs), and hours per unit of service. In addition, staff roles must be clearly defined as to whether they are fixed or variable. The necessary number of FTEs to yield the desired care standard for the forecasted number of patients in each department must be calculated. In addition, the number of FTEs to replace staff members when they use non-patient care, such as benefit time, must be accounted for in the model. Finkler and colleagues (2007) described the method for calculating a staffing pattern as follows:

1. Determine the number of paid hours per FTE.
2. Determine the percentage of productive hours to total paid hours.
3. Multiply the number of paid hours per FTE by the percentage of productive hours to find the number of productive hours per FTE.
4. Divide required care hours by productive hours per FTE to find the required number of FTEs.
5. Divide the required care hours by the number of days per year that the unit has patients to find care hours/day.
6. Divide that result by hours per shift to find the number of person shifts needed per working day.
7. Assign staff by employee type and among required shifts per day.

Box 21-2 refers to a sample variable staff calculation. Table 21-1 provides a sample staffing pattern that includes the final step of allocating total FTEs across shifts and by skill mix. In many patient care areas, the

---

BOX 21-2 VARIABLE STAFF CALCULATION

2080 paid hours per FTE
80% productive hours to total paid hours
$2080 \times 0.8 = 1664$ productive hours per FTE
71,830 care hours $\div$ 1664 = 43.17 FTEs
71,830 care hours $\div$ 365 days per year = 197 hours of care per day
197 hours of care per day $\div$ 8-hour shifts = 24.6 person shifts

---

staffing pattern may be different by day of week. For example, a post-surgical unit may have a lower patient census on weekends because of the lack of a surgical schedule; thus a different staffing pattern may apply (McKinley & Cavouras, 2000).

Position Control

Once the staffing pattern for each unit has been established, the next step to ensuring safe staffing coverage is to provide a structured measurement and evaluation of position control. Future schedule coverage and adequate staffing first require that unit staff are available to work the needed shifts. Therefore the hours of care requirement on a unit must be converted to the correct number of full-time positions. Position control is the process of providing and measuring the correct FTE, or complement, to adequately staff a given area. Full-time and part-time

---

TABLE 21-1 SAMPLE STAFFING PATTERN FOR A WEDNESDAY FOR AN INTERMEDIATE CARE NURSERY (40 BEDS)

STAFF TYPE	7AM–7PM SHIFT	7PM–7AM SHIFT	SKILL MIX	TOTAL
Fixed 8-hour day staff				
Nurse manager	1			1
Nurse educator—shared	0.5			0.5
Lactation specialist	1			1
Variable staff				
Charge nurse	1*			1
RN	8	7	75% RN	15
LPN/LVN	0	1	5% LPN	1
UAP	2	2	20% UAP	4
HUC	1	1		2

HUC, Health unit coordinator; *LPN/LVN,* licensed practical nurse/licensed vocational nurse; *RN,* registered nurse; *UAP,* unlicensed assistive personnel.
*Charge nurse on day shift without a direct-care assignment.

mix, shift lengths, weekend commitments, and available contingency, or flex staff, are components to be analyzed to produce the ideal complement. The correct complement of full-time and part-time employees requires an understanding of the institution's non-patient care time and other budgeted activities (e.g., new staff orientation, continuing education) that are not included in the direct patient care hours required for the staffing pattern. Brown (1999) provided an example equation to determine adequate FTEs needed to staff a sample medical-surgical unit, as shown in Box 21-3. An ideal measure of nursing staff adequacy, which considers intensity, was presented by Unruh and Fottler (2004, slide 3). They suggested that a staffing adequacy measure should indicate the volume of nurses of a certain skill level needed for a given volume of patients and the given intensity of nursing care required for those patients during their stay (Box 21-4).

Once position control is established to support the staffing patterns, vacancy and turnover rates need to be managed. A strategy for covering future vacant positions should be identified to prevent the use of

more costly, last-minute staff resources. An organization reported actual cost savings by over-recruiting by 1.0 FTE in the ICU area, which resulted in lower use of more expensive contingency and external staff resources (Cipriano & Cutruzzula, 2007). With fiscal and human resources support, managers need to recruit and retain the FTE complement of the full-time and part-time mix needed for each staffing level. This will then increase the available resource pool to respond to higher-than-budgeted patient volume. Filled positions are the foundation for adequate, balanced work schedules.

Scheduling

Best practice for scheduling is a system that is automated, provides data driven targets for core coverage, and engages staff members to participate in working specific shifts, hours, and days in their clinical area. The schedule typically spans a period of 4 to 6 weeks into the future. Staff members are usually hired by the organization with a commitment to work a particular number and type of hours (e.g., 36 hours, rotating day and night shifts). Organizations that focus on retention strategies

---

BOX 21-3   CALCULATING MEDICAL-SURGICAL STAFF COVERAGE

Given:

Average daily census = 33.4
Nursing hours per patient day = 4
Constant representing 7 days per week with an FTE working 5 days = 1.4
Average nonproductive time = 1.14
The potentially productive hours in 1 workday for 1 staff person for 1 shift = 7.5

Then:

$$\frac{33.4 \times 4 \times 1.4 \times 1.14}{7.5} = 28.4 \text{ total caregiver FTEs needed to staff the unit per shift}$$

Adapted from Brown, B. (1999). How to develop a unit personnel budget. *Nursing Management, 30*(6), 34-35.

BOX 21-4   AN IDEAL MEASURE OF NURSING STAFF ADEQUACY

$$\frac{\text{\# of RNs}}{\text{\# of Patient days} \times \text{Intensity of RN care for those patient days}}$$

Adapted from Unruh, L., & Fottler, M.D. (2004, June 6–8). *Patient turnover and nursing staff adequacy*. San Diego: Academy Health Annual Research meeting. Retrieved September 15, 2012, from *http://www.academyhealth.org/Events/content.cfm? ItemNumber=621*.

that include balanced, flexible, and predictable work schedules will have a competitive edge in recruiting top talent (PricewaterhouseCoopers, 2007).

An assessment of scheduling procedures should include the manager's role and time spent in scheduling. A recent strategy to better align the nurse manager's role to the accountabilities included providing support through technology, staffing office assistants, and staff members on scheduling committees. The manager's role is accountable for the oversight of the scheduling process and approval of the final complete schedule. The final schedule then needs to be accessible electronically to all staff members, whether at work or remotely from home or on their cell phone. Maintaining a consistent annual schedule of the precise dates for each scheduling request period and for when the final schedule is available is a best practice for staff satisfaction and work-life balance. The managerial role shifts from time-consuming scheduling "tasks" to a role approving a complete schedule that meets the guidelines of the organization and the Principles for Nurse Staffing (ANA, 1999).

The definition or perception of a "complete" schedule is likely as variable as nursing staff member satisfaction with staffing. Direct care nurses, however, expect when a schedule is electronically submitted to their home computer or cell phone that is it complete. Specifically, the staff expects that RNs, LPNs/LVNs, UAP, unit secretaries, and key staff are scheduled to their target number for every shift of the schedule. Sharing the patient census and acuity trends by month, day of week, and time of day with the staff will foster mutual understanding in how targets are established. Dialogue about nurse staffing for patient care is credible when it is data-driven. Direct care nurses expect that there will be a clinical expert on every shift and that new graduates are distributed across shifts with their preceptors. These are a few examples about how nursing leaders at all levels may engage staff to develop value statements and data-driven guidelines that serve to explicitly and transparently articulate the organization's scheduling process. Many scheduling committees have developed such documents in the past few years to reflect values such as a shared commitment to safe and excellent nursing care for all patients and families, support for staff member pursuit of BSN education, fairness in scheduling the major holidays (Thanksgiving, Christmas, and New Year's),

fiscal stewardship to not pre-schedule overtime, guidelines for numbers of staff vacations at one time by role, clarity in self-service dates for scheduling and communication, fatigue management guidelines, and a fair on-call schedule.

Demand Management

Demand management as a discipline focuses on (1) measuring, predicting, and understanding demand for an institution's products and services; and (2) deploying resources and management to ensure that demand is met in the way the consumer's wants and needs are satisfied. For health care, a key component of the "product and service" equation is high-quality, safe patient care, with the goal of having the patient leave the hospital in the shortest amount of time and at the lowest cost, given high-quality and safe care (Pickard & Warner, 2007).

An often overlooked strategy for creating predictable and cost-effective staffing is the need to staff according to real-time patient information or to make staffing decisions that facilitate individual patients moving through their stay as quickly as possible with high-quality, safe care. Because most staffing plans staff to average forecasted care levels, periods of higher patient volume and/or acuity levels, or peaks, may create serious stressors for both patients and nurses. Litvak and colleagues (2005) described the following three types of stress intrinsic to daily operations:

- Flow stress, representing the rapid rate of patients presenting for hospital care
- Clinical stress, which is expressed in the variability in type and severity of disease
- Stress caused by competing responsibilities of health care providers

System stress introduced by demand for nurses to care for more or sicker patients has been shown to be a leading cause of adverse patient outcomes (Litvak et al., 2005). When variability is minimized and/or better predicted, a hospital has greater resources for the remaining patient-driven peaks in demand, over which it has no control. Effective staffing requires an assessment of demand variability or the required hourly nursing care for each day on each unit. Ways to control variability, hence decrease peaks and valleys, include better planning for scheduled events such as elective OR procedures, integration to patient flow and bed management systems, better control over bed assignments based on current unit workload, and improved planning for discharges—all of which decrease the demand and stress for nursing resources. Computer technologies that continuously track and predict demand assist managers with variability analysis and prospective planning for predicted variability. These data support managerial decisions for non-traditional shorter shifts for the care areas that have high requirements at select predictable portions of the day. Predictive modeling can forecast unplanned patient and staff events, such as admissions by day of week and unplanned sick calls (Warner, 2006). Several examples driven by data may include: higher C-section rates in a labor and delivery unit may necessitate two RNs in the OR; infant births that are higher in the evening than during the day may require a shift of resources from days to evenings; or late afternoon patient transfers from the recovery room after neurosurgery on Tuesdays and Thursdays may require an increase in RN staff for those days and specific hours in a neurosurgical ICU.

Pickard and Warner (2007) outlined the essential components for effective demand management as the following 10 principles:

1. Being based on patient outcomes (how well he or she is progressing)
2. Being focused on the individual patient
3. Incorporating progress goals for each patient throughout his or her stay with which actual progress may be compared
4. Continuously measuring progress in real time, so that decisions can be made as the patient's needs change (rather than once a shift or once a day, which inherently bases decisions on information than is typically 8 to 16 hours old)
5. Being projected into the near future (several days ahead) to allow time for optimal staffing decisions to be made while there is still time for numerous choices among available caregivers and cost-effective options
6. Being able to be embedded in a decision support system
7. Being acceptable to all stakeholders, especially administration and finance, to avoid organizational polarity
8. Producing a need for care in terms of not only quantity and skill but also the caregiver attributes necessary to provide optimal care for the patient

9. Using outcomes-driven acuity system, based on an established taxonomy for assessing and documenting patient care on outcomes
10. Incorporating all presently and planned electronically available data, to reduce nursing time in data gathering and provide as much real-time, valid data as possible

"Incorporating these elements is not a simple task, but doing so offers significant advantages and benefits. By focusing on the individual patient, with individual outcome progress goals for each patient, hospitals can achieve results not previously addressed with traditional models" (Pickard & Warner, 2007, p. 3). In addition, this allows organizations to be informed and responsive when a select population of patients typically cared for in one location is housed in a new location. These results include (1) best-practice staffing protocols based on "true (outcomes-oriented) demand" and the optimal staffing levels to move a patient through each phase of his or her stay as quickly as possible, (2) early identification of patients who are not moving through their hospital stay as planned, and (3) improved near-term projection and prediction of staffing needs.

Staffing Allocation and Resource Pool

Even with the best planning and most accurate prediction of supply and demand, uncontrolled events such as unexpected high demand and sick calls are intrinsic to the health care environment. Key to effective staffing are protocols and processes for daily staffing decision support that are aligned with a budget-sensitive variable staffing plan. In a decentralized model, individual department managers and directors are responsible for daily staffing allocation. Units with decentralized staffing are typically units whereby volume and/or acuity may be most unpredictable and the nursing competencies are unique to that area (e.g., emergency department, labor and delivery, critical care). However, a decentralized model places a higher level of staffing responsibility on managers, which may take them away from other more strategic responsibilities.

In contrast, centralized staffing is filtered through a central staffing office, which maintains responsibility for ensuring adequate staffing for multiple units. Centralized staffing offers the benefit of being able to view supply and demand from an enterprise perspective. With patient acuity, nursing competencies, and available staff viewed across multiple units, staffing resources can be optimized by increasing staff in one area and reducing staff in another to accommodate variable patient demand. Staffing protocols for obtaining supplemental staff can be standardized, such as procedures for using internal staff, per diems, and external sources (e.g., travelers and agency). The staffing office can relieve nurse managers and/or charges nurses of the time-consuming administrative task of responding to sick calls and obtaining supplemental staff. In addition, the central staffing office provides a command center with protocols and information to manage disasters in which staff must be quickly obtained and deployed.

The downside to relying solely on a centralized staffing office is that it can become too remote from the unit, thus losing some of the intelligence that may be considered when making staffing decisions (Lauw & Gares, 2005). Policies and procedures clearly define the roles and responsibilities and communication among areas. But as with any of these staffing models, the key to eliminating chaotic, last-minute staffing decisions is adopt predictive tools and move more of the staffing decisions to the near future, or the next 2 to 4 days (Pickard & Warner, 2007). Assessment and analysis of staffing needs in the near future provides more available options, including more competent staff, at optimal costs.

Computerized staffing systems play a pivotal role in providing a "single version of the truth" and offering decision support such as staffing variances across units, workload indicators, employee competencies, and decision costs. Information for staffing decisions must be readily available and accurate. Staffing systems serve as a communication tool for all staffing "stakeholders" including employees, unit managers, centralized staffing office, and executives. Staffing systems also offer automated open-shift management, which posts open shifts electronically to qualified staff. Protocols direct which personnel are the best qualified and the most cost-effective to fill needed shifts. The staffing system measures and reports the staffing management performance at both unit and organization levels, providing staffing effectiveness data for the organization.

Access to nurses outside the unit to cover transient shortages is critical to meet last minute, unplanned nurse shortages, such as sick calls, and high patient demand. Supplemental staffing resources, frequently referred to as the *staffing pool,* are defined as a group of nurses who supplement the core unit staffing. This includes per diem nurses, float pool nurses, part-time nurses desiring additional hours, seasonal nurses, agency nurses, and traveling nurses. The scope of clinical competency, pay rates, and contractual arrangements vary among these internal and external pools of nurses as well. For example, select nurses may be competent to work on all of the adult medical-surgical units, whereas other specialty nurses may be competent to work in several areas, such as perioperative practice sites, or only one area, such as labor and delivery, the emergency department, or the dialysis unit.

Supplemental staffing resource guidelines need to be established to direct the use of additional resources detailing the data for decision making and algorithms for staffing. These guidelines are designed to prevent depleting supplemental resources for core staff coverage and, instead, to reserve them for unexpected intervals of high acuity or transient shortages. For example, a guideline may direct the use of a part-time nurse who has signed up to work extra shifts to fill a sick call, then to use a supplemental float pool nurse, and finally to use an external agency nurse if previous resources are unavailable. The option for overtime is also a consideration based upon policy regarding the fatigue associated with excessive hours in a day or days in a row worked and cost. The costs associated with each resource progression are then inherently built into the staffing decision model. Additional strategies for covering long-term family medical leaves are also needed to meet core coverage. Strategies for covering these longer term shortages are critical; otherwise, a manager is depleting the resource pools intended for last-minute and transient shortages.

Operational metrics for the supplemental resource pool are not only defined for daily staffing allocation but also may be defined during the scheduling stage. The operational total nurse vacancy rate for scheduling purposes is defined as all budgeted nurse positions that are vacant during the scheduling period, including the unfilled or vacant positions and positions for which nurses are on short-term or long-term leaves of absence (e.g., Family and Medical Leave Act [FMLA], workers' compensation) (Jones et al., 2005). For example, if a unit has an operational RN vacancy rate of 5% to 10%, it may be approved to cover the shortage with part-time nurses working additional shifts and possibly overtime, but would not be approved for agency nurses. Alternatively, a unit with a 22% operational RN vacancy rate may be approved for longer term contracted higher labor expense (e.g., travelers). Defining operational vacancy rates and incremental resource actions are important aspects of consistently managing staff shortages and ensuring a standard of care delivery. As such, protocols driven by operational vacancy rates generate consistency in how higher labor costs are aligned with the greatest need. In addition, wages, benefits, transfers, and work policies of supplemental internal float pools should be carefully designed so that the stability of unit-based core nursing staff is not compromised.

Patient Assignments

Nurse managers are responsible not only for forthcoming schedules and immediate staffing but also for ensuring that the patient care "assignments reflect appropriate utilization of personnel, considering scope of practice, competencies, patient/client/resident needs and complexity of care" (ANA, 2004, p. 9). The patient assignment is defined as the task of assigning the scheduled staff to specific patients for the shift duration. Nurse managers typically delegate assignment making to the charge nurse on the patient care area (ANA, 2004; Sherman, 2005). The charge nurse is responsible for matching the qualified caregivers to meet the patients' needs and for providing a balanced workload across caregivers. Often the nursing care delivery model articulates the value of nurse-to-patient continuity across time. A balanced workload enables nurses to provide reasonable equity in nursing care delivery to patients and their families. In addition, the staff members expect the charge nurse to create equitable assignments as a valued measure of fairness in workload distribution. Many organizations require an annual charge nurse competency and peer feedback demonstrating effective assignment making.

In the staffing management framework, the patient assignment is the point at which individual patients are linked with individual nurses. Welton (2010) has identified this as a critical new level of analysis to examine the relationship between staffing and clinical quality and cost that may better inform operational decision-making.

ORGANIZATIONAL OUTCOMES

Staffing Effectiveness

Hospital organizations examine the relationships between staffing and nurse-sensitive outcomes to meet The Joint Commission (TJC) staffing effectiveness requirements. TJC human resources standards state (TJC, 2006):

> Staffing effectiveness is defined as the number, competency and skill mix of staff in relation to the provision of needed care and treatment. Effective staffing has been linked to positive patient outcomes and improved quality and safety of care. This standard is designed to help healthcare organizations determine and continuously improve the effectiveness of their nurse staffing (including registered nurses, licensed practical nurses and nursing assistants or aides) through an objective evidenced-based approach. (HR-6)

This standard describes the required data collection of clinical quality and human resource indicators, analysis, trending over time, and subsequent improvement plans as deemed appropriate.

The Staffing Evidence on Quality

Over a decade of rigorous studies and a recent summary of current research conducted by the Ruckelshaus Center at The University of Washington concluded that, "fewer patients per nurse or more nursing hours per patient day is associated with fewer adverse outcomes–in particular mortality, failure to rescue, and some specific adverse events among surgical patients" (Mitchell, 2008, p. 30). Comprehensive reviews of staffing evidence and sentinel works are available (Aiken et al., 2002; Aiken et al., 2003; Blegen & Goode, 1998; Needleman et al., 2002, 2006, 2011; Unruh, 2008). These studies and a meta-analysis by Kane and colleagues (2007a, b) demonstrate the strong evidence linking inadequate staffing with adverse events and failure to rescue. Frith and colleagues (2010) found that higher RN staffing was associated with a reduced length of stay (LOS) among community hospitals. These findings suggest the direct fiscal impact to hospital margin by nurses today (Bogue, 2012).

Hospitals routinely employ supplemental nurses to provide additional resources to cover transient shortages; however, little is known about this nurse workforce and its relationship to quality of care. Aiken and colleagues (2007) examined the characteristics of supplemental nurses and the relationships of the supplemental staff to nurse outcomes and adverse events. Their findings suggest that widely held negative perceptions of temporary nurses may be unfounded. Both national and the state of Pennsylvania RN survey data in 2000 showed that an estimated 6% of hospital staff were employed by supplemental staffing agencies. The supplemental nurses were equally, if not more, educated than the permanent staff, and the supplemental nurses were not associated with a negative impact on quality-of-care indicators. The employment patterns of nurses and their effect on cost and quality is an important area for further study.

Given the slow economic recovery, it is possible that there will be a slow rate of retirement among nurses from the baby boomer era. This workforce cycle will once again heighten emphasis on nursing turnover. Significant nurse turnover measurement and costing is available to assist organizations in managing turnover (Jones, 2004, 2005; Jones & Gates, 2007). In 2008, the cost to replace one RN was reexamined and adjusted for inflation and was estimated to range between $82,100 and $88,100 (Jones, 2008).

Nurse leaders at all levels are called to action to incorporate relevant scientific findings into staffing administrative policy and practice and to lead the evaluation of all innovations in care delivery. Balancing these decisions with and conducting cost-effectiveness analyses is the current challenge for organizations and future research (Jones & Mark, 2005; Pappas, 2007).

RESEARCH NOTE

Source

Trinkoff, A.M., Johantgen, M., Storr, C.L., Gurses, A.P., Liang, Y., & Han, K. (2011). Nurses' work schedule characteristics, nurse staffing and patient mortality. *Nursing Research, 60(1)*, 1-8.

Purpose

The purpose of this study was to determine if, in hospitals where nurses report more adverse work schedules, there would be increased patient mortality when controlling for staffing. The conceptual framework for the study was based on balance theory, a human factors theory that job performance is affected adversely by excessive job demands (Gurses & Carayon, 2007). This cross-sectional study was conducted from a 2004 survey among 633 nurses working in 71 acute care hospitals in North Carolina and Illinois. Work schedule measures were adapted from the internationally applied Standard Shiftwork Index, a self-report tool for the hours actually worked. The mortality measures were the risk-adjusted AHRQ inpatient indicators, and the staffing data were from the AHA Annual Survey of Hospitals.

Discussion

The IOM (2004) report, *Keeping Patients Safe: Transforming the work Environment for Nurses*, cited extended RN work hours as a source of fatigue. National trends demonstrate the prevalence and the popularity of 12-hour shifts, but these shifts often extend past 12 hours, and nurses may work several consecutive 12-hour shifts on successive days. Extended work schedules for nurses can cause fatigue and performance deficits because of increased exposure to job demands and insufficient recovery time (Geiger-Brown & Trinkoff, 2010). In order to retain the best staff, nurse executives must balance the demand for the 12-hour shift with concerns for patient safety.

Results showed that the work schedule was related significantly to patient mortality when staffing levels and hospital characteristics were controlled. Pneumonia deaths were significantly more likely in hospitals where nurses reported long work hours (13 or more hours in a stretch) and lack of time away from work (less than 10 hours between shifts; worked on a scheduled day off or vacation day). Abdominal aortic aneurysm was also associated with a lack of time away from work for nurses. For patients in congestive heart failure, mortality was associated with working while sick, whereas acute myocardial infarction mortality was associated with weekly burden (hours per day; number of days in a row). In addition to staffing, the nurses' work schedule was associated with patient mortality. This finding suggests an independent effect of schedule on patient outcomes.

Application to Practice

A national dialogue reviewing the evidence and change strategies has begun, but on a limited scope because of the concerns of nursing satisfaction and retention. Based on the evidence, health care organizations have adopted fatigue guidelines. For example, Dr. Bob Dent, the Chief Nurse Executive at Midland Memorial in Midland, Texas, engaged all the health care professionals at his facility in dialogue regarding the issue, the evidence related to staffing, and the implications of fatigue on quality of care and staff risk of drowsiness. The result was an evidence-based guideline (see Box 21-5).

BOX 21-5 GUIDELINE: FATIGUE MANAGEMENT FOR DIRECT PATIENT CAREGIVERS

Purpose:

To provide a strategy that recognizes and manages the potential negative consequences of sleep deprivation and sustained work hours on patient outcomes and staff well-being.

Guideline:

The direct patient caregiver is responsible and accountable for individual practice and understanding the consequences of fatigue in preserving integrity and safety. Guidelines for length of hours worked, and number of hours worked in a patient care assignment during a period of seven days will be followed.

Definitions:

On-call: A designated period of time, outside of the designated hours assigned, or of the designated hours of operation, when direct patient caregivers are available to respond to patient care needs for unplanned circumstances or urgent or emergent conditions.

Call hours worked: Actual time the on-call personnel are called into the hospital to work.

Extended work period/sustained work hours: Work periods of more than 12.5 hours with limited opportunities to rest or sleep.

Extended hours worked per week: Any hours in excess of 60 hours per week.

Fatigue: A response to predefined conditions that has physiological and performance consequences. It is identified as deterioration in human performance arising as a consequence of changes in the physiological condition. Contributing factors include, but are not limited to, time on task, time and duty period duration, time since awake when beginning the duty period, acute or chronic sleep debt, circadian disruption, multiple time zones, and shift work.

Circadian rhythms: 24-hour cycles of behavior and physiology generated by an internal biological clock located in the hypothalamus. It regulates the daily cyclical patterns of sleep and wakefulness. It compels the body to fall asleep and wake up and regulates hour to hour waking behavior reflected in fatigue, alertness, and cognitive ability.

Off duty: A period of uninterrupted time during which an individual is free from work-related duties.

Guidelines:

1. Except in emergency situations, direct patient caregivers should not work in direct patient care assignments more than 12.5 consecutive hours in a 24-hour period, not more than 60 hours in a seven-day period, and not scheduled more than three consecutive 12-hour shifts. Working outside of these parameters requires manager and/or director approval.

2. Off-duty periods should be inclusive of an uninterrupted sleep cycle, a break from continuous professional responsibilities, and a period of time of not less than 8 hours to perform activities of daily living.

3. Arrangements will be made in relation to the hours worked, to provide additional time off for direct patient caregivers working a longer shift, an extra shift, or hours worked on call to accommodate an adequate off-duty recuperation period.

4. The number of shifts or on-call shifts assigned during a 7-day period should reflect the previous guidelines as to number of sustained work hours and adequate recuperation periods.

5. An individual's ability to meet an increased work demand should be taken into account.

6. All direct patient caregivers should uphold their ethical responsibility to patients and to themselves to arrive at work adequately rested and prepared for duty.

7. In extreme conditions, such as surge management or a disaster, staff may be asked to work additional hours, following the previous guidelines for fatigue management.

8. Leaders have a responsibility to monitor staff fatigue, provide breaks, and release staff as soon as possible.

Source: Midland Memorial Hospital (used with permission of Dr. Bob Dent).

CURRENT ISSUES AND TRENDS

The landmark IOM (2011) report on the future of nursing made eight key recommendations, including effective workforce planning and policy making, that require better data collection and information infrastructure. The report findings also advocated that nurses practice to the fullest extent of their education and be full partners with physicians in the delivery of care and its redesign. The ability to execute the IOM's recommendations is strong because of the collective national attention and action coupled with economic restraints that challenge the status quo. Simpson (2012) articulated the technology adoption required to place evidence for "better practices" at the point of care now and shorten the 17-year lag period between knowledge generation and integration into everyday practice. This includes not only clinical evaluation but also the ongoing systematic evaluation of the impact of staffing on patient outcomes (ANA, 2010c).

For more than 20 years, Magnet designation has been associated with healthier work environments (better staffing, excluding California where there is state-mandated ratios; lower burnout; lower turnover; and improved RN-MD collaboration) (Kelly et al., 2011) and higher quality patient care. With the revision of the Magnet model in 2008 and increased focus on outcomes, achieving Magnet designation has been increasingly associated with quality. It is now incorporated into the scoring for *US News and World Report*'s Best Hospitals in America Honor Roll and earns full credit for Safe Practice Standard #9 Nursing Workforce in the Leapfrog Hospital Survey, which scores hospitals on their "commitment to staffing with highly trained nurses."

Given the advent of value-based purchasing (VBP) and the Centers for Medicare & Medicaid Services (CMS) provision 1533-F, health care leaders have been incentivized to focus on improving care processes. CMS provides health care coverage for 80 million Americans via Medicaid, Medicare, and state children's programs and represents the largest payer in the world, administering over $800 billion in benefits annually. Many of the clinical processes and patient satisfaction measures under VBP are directly affected by the quality and quantity of nursing care, and the outcomes will have a significant impact on the key metrics that will drive hospital reimbursements (Bogue, 2012).

Since CMS provision 1533-F became effective October 1, 2008, hospitals are not being reimbursed for hospital-acquired conditions (HACs)—that is, conditions such as skin pressure ulcers, urinary tract infections, ventilator-acquired pneumonia, and falls with injury that occurred within the hospital stay and were not present on admission (POA). Among the 14 HACs in the provision, at least 9 of the conditions are sensitive to nursing care intervention. Thus hospitals have new financial incentives to support both nursing education and appropriate staffing to prevent HACs, reduce costs, and increase reimbursement. In addition, the Patient Protection

and Affordable Care Act mandates 1% of hospitals' Medicare payment will be at risk under value-based payments starting in 2013, and increased to 2% in 2017. Penalties for certain 30-day admissions also began in 2012. The LOS and readmissions financial penalties are the most compelling incentives for hospitals to support the appropriate amount of nursing care that is of high quality because of the known positive effect of nursing care and coordination on patients' transitions of care and acute care LOS (Frith et al., 2010). The nurse's inherent role in discharge planning with the interdisciplinary team, linkages to community services, and effective medication, symptom, and disease management teaching in all care settings is becoming increasingly important to organizational outcomes.

There are national policy initiatives to identify and make visible nursing care in the U.S. health care reimbursement system. It has long been known that nursing care has been historically bundled within the "room-and-board" hospital charges, which do not capture the variability in nursing care costs (Thompson & Diers, 1985). Given the variability in nursing care intensity and cost of nurse staffing, this traditional costing system has resulted in cost compression and distortion in the current inpatient prospective payment system (Dalton, 2007). A proposed solution separates nursing care from the room and board charges and accounts for this care as a variable, direct cost within the billing system based on actual nursing time delivered to patients (Welton & Harris, 2007; Welton et al., 2006). This proposal has generated national dialogue among health care leaders with CMS that would make nursing care visible as part of reimbursement reform. Welton (2010) suggested a new value-based nursing care model including (1) allocating nursing cost and intensity to each patient, (2) new metrics that link nursing-specific outcomes to individual patients, and (3) moving the focus from staffing to the assignment of caregivers to individual patients. Simpson (2012) further called to action the adoption of technology at the point of care to achieve value-based nursing care. These current issues in health care policy raise the visibility and importance of nursing care in society, and create a climate to advocate for safe, cost-effective, high-quality nursing care for all.

CASE STUDY

Susan Smith is the new nurse manager of a large surgical intensive care unit (SICU). When she began her new job, she was faced with constant last-minute staffing shortages requiring excessive overtime and agency use. Nursing staff were working multiple overlapping shift lengths to fill the continual shortages. Staff morale was low with high turnover and high absenteeism, and organizational loyalty was lacking among the nursing staff. Nurse Smith visited nearby intensive care units and collaborated with colleagues looking for best practices to stabilize the unit's staffing.

Based on her findings, Nurse Smith first analyzed her core coverage and developed a staffing pattern that met forecasted patient care needs. She determined that overlapping shifts did not provide balanced coverage during a 24-hour period and developed a staffing pattern using 12-hour shifts. She then converted her staffing pattern to full-time positions to determine whether the current and open positions provided the unit-based staff needed to cover a 4-week schedule. The position control showed that the budgeted unit position, if filled, did provide the total positions needed to schedule and staff the unit. However, based on the literature review, Nurse Smith decided to convert some of the full-time positions to part-time to provide more flexibility in scheduling. With a high vacancy, Nurse Smith consulted and worked with the human resources department to develop new strategies for recruiting ICU nurses and for obtaining ICU competency certification for a core group in the organization's supplemental resource pool. She also obtained budget authorization to obtain two full-time ICU travel nurses for a 2-month interval, which was less costly than agency use. This also helped establish full unit-based coverage for the initial schedule until the vacant positions were filled.

Nurse Smith surveyed the current nurses to determine satisfaction with current staffing and ideas for improvement. She determined two consistent findings among the staff. The first finding was that nurses described being stressed by high workload demands and left with a feeling of not providing adequate care. A unit-based committee was formed to evaluate patient care assignments and developed a standard procedure for ensuring workload assignments were manageable and safe. Improved communication with the operating room for transfers into the unit provided better planning for scheduled admissions, preventing episodes of high nursing intensity with admissions. Protocols were established for when workloads were exceeding unit-based standards for safe, quality care.

The second finding was that nurses were tired of the excessive calls to their homes to sign up for extra shifts. By using best practices from other units, staffing decisions were moved from last minute to evaluating staffing 2 to 3 days in advance. By using new computer technology, open shifts were posted in advance for staff to sign up for extra shifts. Staff also provided their availability to fill shifts on short notice so that only those nurses who were available were called. Staff found they were willing to sign up for availability if it prevented the last-minute unexpected calls. The result of this forward-looking planning was consistent with the literature noting that nurses want control over their work schedule and the ability to balance work with their lifestyle.

Within 3 months, vacant positions were filled and the supplemental travelers were no longer required to fill core staffing. Agency usage was eliminated, and overtime decreased. Initial schedules were posted only with all shifts filled. ICU-competent nurses from the supplemental resource pool were used only to fill last-minute sick calls. A second nursing survey was conducted that showed increase in staff satisfaction, which also had a positive impact on nursing turnover.

CRITICAL THINKING EXERCISE

Nurse Manager (NM) Lisbeth Klein is preparing annual goals for her upcoming one-on-one meeting with her pediatric director of nursing. Lisbeth has been the nurse manager for this level three 40-bed neonatal intensive care unit (NICU) in an academic medical center for the past 7 years. Two years ago, her hospital was awarded Magnet designation and her staff contributed significant evidence of high quality evidenced-based practice and the generation of research regarding neonatal pain control. However, this past year there were reported union discussions among the adult medical-surgical nurses. She examined her past fiscal year administrative data: average patient LOS exceeded budget by 1.7 days after adjustment for gestational age; 16 babies were diverted to surrounding hospitals because of full capacity; family satisfaction with infant care scores remained >95%. Only two central line infections were reported for the year, and no peripheral IV infiltrates resulted in injury. With an 85% response rate, nurse satisfaction survey (n=86) results dropped significantly from the previous year regarding the satisfaction with their schedule. Several comments were written in the survey about the lack of consistent UAP available for supply stocking and assisting with infant feeding and bathing. The personnel expenses exceeded budget by $177,000 after adjustment for high volume and acuity. The fiscal variance was explained by 3 months of traveler contracts for two RNs, OT over budget by $52,000, maternity leaves, and one long-term medical LOA.

1. What are the opportunities for the NM in the upcoming year?
2. What information might assist the NM?
3. What are the ways the staff might be engaged?
4. What neonate (patient) and family issues are involved?
5. What staffing management issues are involved?
6. What clinical, financial, and organizational outcomes might demonstrate improvement?

Budgeting, Productivity, and Costing Out Nursing

Mary Ellen Murray

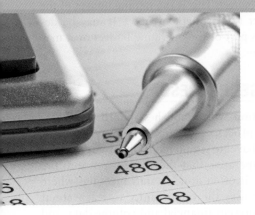

evolve WEBSITE

http://evolve.elsevier.com/Huber/leadership/

National Health Expenditures (NHEs) are a measure of spending for health care in the United States. In 1998, NHE exceeded $1 trillion for the first time. By 2020, NHE are projected to increase to $4.6 trillion (Keehan et al., 2011). Considered from another perspective, this amount of money in 1998 represented 13.1% of the gross domestic product (GDP), the value of all the goods and services produced in the United States in 1 year. By 2020, NHE is projected to represent 19.8% of the GDP. By 2014, when major coverage expansions from the Affordable Care Act begin, national spending growth is expected to reach 8.4%.

The magnitude of these expenditure increases emphasizes the need for nurses, as members of the largest health care profession, to understand the implications of these data for clinical practice. Understanding budgeting, productivity, and costing out nursing and relating that knowledge to the management of professional nursing is a leadership skill that will serve the nursing profession in an era of accelerating health care expenditures.

Photo used with permission from Photos.com.

BACKGROUND

All nurses will be involved in budgeting for nursing services in different ways and to different degrees. Staff nurses in particular often report, "I just want to take care of patients—don't bother me with money matters." Some nurse administrators have said, "Show me your budget and I will tell you your values." Nurses at all levels need to understand that "finance is not a dirty word" (Sorbello, 2008). Given that health care resources are limited, nurses do compete for these resources and need to understand financial management. In many organizations, staff nurses are expected to be aware of their unit's financial performance and the impact their decisions may have on it. Staff nurses' involvement is essential to the ability to contain costs at the unit level because they make many decisions about supply and resource use.

Budgeting is a major aspect of an organization's or unit's planning processes. A budget is a plan that is specified in dollar amounts. This plan becomes a guiding framework for organizational activities. It conveys management's intentions and financial expectations regarding revenues and expenditures. An organization-level budget compares expected revenues with

387

expected expenses to forecast profit (margin) or loss (deficit). Budgeting is a cyclical process of planning, implementing, and evaluating.

Budgets are designed to be planning documents. However, one often hears the statement, "We don't have the budget for that," or, "The budget won't allow it." It is crucial for managers to understand that the budget is a tool, created by humans. To be useful, it must be flexible and have processes in place to modify it when necessary. Individuals and organizations should not become so constrained by the approved budget that they hesitate to take appropriate actions or make appropriate decisions that vary from or were unanticipated in the budget process.

DEFINITIONS

A **budget** is defined as a written financial plan aimed at controlling the allocation of resources. It functions as both a planning instrument and an evaluation tool useful for financial management. A budget is used to manage programs, plan for goal accomplishment, and control costs. **Expenses** are defined as the costs or prices of activities undertaken in the organization's operations. **Revenue** is defined as income or amounts owed for purchased services or goods. *Total operating expenses* are the result of summing the costs of all resources used to produce services. **Total operating revenues** are the result of multiplying the volume of services provided by the charges (rate) for the services. **Income** (or profit) is the excess of revenues over expenses, or revenues minus expenses. A **variance** is the difference between the budgeted and the actual amounts. A variance may be favorable or unfavorable relative to the budget amount.

There are three main types of organizational budgets, as follows:

1. *Capital budget:* This budget is the plan for the purchase of major equipment or assets.
2. *Operating budget:* The operating budget is the annual plan for the unit's or organization's daily functioning revenue and expenses for a single year. For nursing units, this is a plan that lays out what it is going to cost to run the unit in the coming year. It includes such things as supplies, telephones, mailing, paper, and copy machines. In addition, there may be a cost allocation for such things as heat, light, and housecleaning.
3. *Personnel budget:* This is the staffing budget of the cost center (department or unit). It may be developed as part of the operating budget or it may stand alone.

THE BUDGET PROCESS

Each institution will establish standard budgetary formats and processes. Because employees of a cost center will have to implement the budget decision, it is imperative that they have input into the process. This is often done in staff meetings where the manager uses the opportunity to teach about the process, present financial and volume data, and solicit staff input.

The annual budgeting cycle process is complex and requires the completion of several related documents. It may be compared to income tax preparation where an individual gathers all the necessary data and receipts, completes all of the required forms, and submits them to the Internal Revenue Service. Like tax preparation, the budget process may require multiple revisions.

A typical budget process follows the priorities identified in the organization's strategic plan. This ensures that resources are aligned with key organizational initiatives. The budget process consists of the following three time periods:

1. *Preparation:* As a beginning point, the manager reviews the organization's strategic plan and the last year's budget for the cost center. The strategic plan will aid in writing a budget justification for any capital requests as well as linking to organizational priorities. The prior year's budget for the cost center will help the manager to identify volume projections and changes in the past year and potential changes in the coming year. In the hospital, patient days are the usual volume measurement. If the manager of a surgical unit knows that two general surgeons are being recruited to the organization, it is reasonable to project an increase in patient days. By reviewing the previous year's data, an informed projection can be made about the increase that can be anticipated. Similarly, the manager may be aware of factors that will decrease the volume of patient days, such as a new hospital being built in the suburbs. In ambulatory care, the volume unit of measurement is clinic visits. If a new nurse

practitioner is being hired, how would that impact the volume of visits projected?

2. *Completing the forms:* The manager will be given budget documents to use in preparing the cost center budget. These are usually spreadsheets sent electronically. They include embedded formulas that compute the summary statistics, thereby reducing human error. Firm due dates are assigned for the completion of this first draft of the budget. The finance department then "rolls up" the unit budget into the organizational budget.

3. *Revise and resubmit:* As budget documents go through review by senior management, requests tend to exceed the available resources. This necessitates review, adjustment, and appeal. This is when the competition for available resources enters the process. Managers may be asked to reduce their unit budget by a dollar percentage, leaving the question "where to cut" as the manager's decision. At other times, a manager may be directed to reduce the personnel budget by a number of full time equivalents (FTEs). This is the point at which the nurse manager must skillfully advocate for patient care, ensuring safety and quality. The nurse manager's knowledge of clinical care processes may be in conflict with directives of a financial administrator who lacks clinical expertise. This is the time when nurses must be prepared to "speak finance" in order to effectively respond to budget challenges. There may be multiple iterations of rebudgeting before the final budget is approved.

Capital Budget Development

Capital budget preparation is usually the first step in the annual budget cycle. The organization will define a capital expense in terms of a dollar amount and the anticipated life span of the purchase. For example, capital expenditures may be "items costing over $10,000 and having a life span of 5 years." Items of this magnitude are not placed in the operating budget.

The specific process used to create a capital budget will vary from organization to organization, but most organizations require extensive background material to support capital budget requests. The background or supporting material required will probably include the vendor quotes for costs of purchase, installation, staff education or training, and a justification or explanation of the reasons that the capital expenditure is needed. The justification must relate the expenditure to the organization's strategic goals or objective. For capital construction projects, architectural plans, regulatory considerations, and other supporting materials may also be required as part of the capital budget preparation process.

After each unit submits the capital expenditure list to the finance department, a compiled list is generated and typically prioritized by senior management. This is a period of intense negotiation. Given that there is rarely enough money to meet all of the requests, difficult decisions must be made.

Operating Budget Development

The *operating* budget covers a specific period, called a *fiscal year*. The fiscal year may begin July 1, may correspond to the calendar year beginning January 1, or may follow the federal government year that starts on October 1. Either way, it is the budget plan for day-to-day service delivery operations. It has at least has two parts: (1) the personnel budget, and (2) the expense budget for costs other than personnel. It includes historical or trend data, expenses, and revenues. Most nursing units in hospitals do not have a revenue budget but do use volume-based projections such as patient days.

The specific process used to develop operating budgets will vary considerably from one organization to another. The nurse manager's and/or nurse executive's role in developing operating budgets for nursing units and services will typically include input on or determination of volume projections, development of associated expense projections (including supplies, equipment, and salary/labor expenses), and some form of revenue projection. Many organizations develop and disseminate a set of budget assumptions that are to be used by managers and leaders in developing the operating budget. These assumptions may include such items as pre-established increases in labor or salary expenses based on contractual obligations, adjustments that must be made based on economic forecasts for supply charge changes (e.g., increased utility rates, increased cost of pharmaceuticals) or factors that will affect patient volume, such as the addition of a new service line.

The foundation of the development of the operating budget at the unit level is based on the projected volume of work for the coming year. The workload aspect often is measured in units of service. Key units of service need to be identified, the number of units predicted, and expenses and staffing calculated accordingly. Activity reports, such as historical census and average length of stay, identify trends related to volume of activity. The unit of service often needs to be adjusted to the case or patient mix, which is a proxy for severity of illness or need (Finkler et al., 2007).

Table 22-1 shows a sample volume budget flow sheet. Historical trend data are needed (e.g., occupancy percentages by time frames such as weekly or monthly) to determine growth projections and any impact of seasonality. The volume of services delivered for a year may be expressed as patient days, visits, procedures, or other units of service. Effects on volume are environmental effects such as reimbursement changes, new programs, process improvements, new technology, and marketing. If volume projections depend on another service or department, it is important for the two departments to communicate closely so that similar assumptions are used in establishing volume projections.

Once the volume projection has been completed, the manager can determine the *personnel services* (or *staffing budget*) portion of the expense budget. Calculation of staffing is complex and, given that staffing expenses generally are the largest portion of the nursing operating budget, nurse managers and nurse executives must have a consistent and well-defined approach to estimating staffing expenses. The methodology used will likely vary from organization to organization. Dunham-Taylor and Pinczuk (2006) described the following method that may be used to estimate staffing expenses.

First, the average daily census and occupancy (or utilization) rate are calculated using volume projections that have been developed. Next, the number of full-time equivalents (FTEs)—that is, the mix of full-time and part-time staff—needed to provide care for the expected volume is determined based on the unit's staffing plan. The staffing plan should include any needed adjustments for non-patient care, sometimes called "nonproductive" hours (vacation, staff education, or sick leave) based on benefit levels. The staffing plan should also specify the skill mix of direct care staff (registered nurse [RN], licensed practical nurse/licensed vocational nurse [LPN/LVN], nursing assistant [NA]) and the nursing hours per patient day (NHPPD) appropriate for the patient population on the unit. Costs for administrative and other fixed staff members, such as unit clerks, need to be included. Other labor costs, such as overtime, shift or other differentials and premiums, and fringe benefit costs, must also be factored into the personnel budget.

Table 22-2 displays a sample budget expense sheet for salaries, and Table 22-3 demonstrates how personnel budgets might be displayed. Salary increases might also be included as another column.

Supply budgets are a major component of the operating budget. Many supply items are variable (the amount used will vary based on the volume of service provided). Other supply costs are fixed and will be incurred at the same level no matter the volume of

TABLE 22-1 VOLUME BUDGET FLOW SHEET

MONTH	PATIENT DAYS BUDGETED	PATIENT DAYS ACTUAL	VARIANCE
January	300	310	10
February	310	315	5
March	310	330	20
April	300	290	(10)
May			
June			
July			
August			
September			
October			
November			
December			

TABLE 22-2 BUDGETED SALARY EXPENSE FLOW SHEET

EXPENSE ITEM	BUDGETED	ACTUAL
Salaries		
Regular		
Overtime		
On-call		
Vacation		
Holiday		
Illness		
Other		
Total Salaries		

TABLE 22-3	PERSONNEL BUDGET FLOW SHEET			
POSITION	NAME	FTE	HOURLY WAGE ($)	YEARLY SALARY ($)
RN	Smith	1.0	23.08	48,006
RN	Jones	1.0	26.92	56,000
LPN	Roe	0.5	13.94	14,498
CNA	Ash	1.0	10.57	21,986
Unit clerk	Oak	1.0	14.00	29,120

service that is provided. Supply items, such as office supplies, intravenous (IV) solutions, instruments, linens, gloves and other personal protective equipment, medical/surgical supplies, and drugs, are examples of supplies that would vary with a higher volume of patient days. Leases, maintenance contracts, staff education funds for travel to conferences or meetings, and books and subscriptions are all examples of supply items that would not vary with a higher volume of patient days. Dollar amounts are assigned based on historical projections and any known or anticipated adjustments resulting from inflation, contractual increases, or other factors as specified in the organization's budgetary assumptions. The operating budget will also need to include expenses for overhead, depreciation, utilities, telecommunications services, and other related facility expenses.

Revenue budgets are based on a set of calculations that determine expected receipts that will result from charging patients and payers for services. Nursing services are often not viewed as revenue-generating departments; but in many organizations the patient days and related charges are used as a proxy for revenue. Revenue projections are based on volume projections. Factors such as payer mix and contractual rates will affect the overall revenue that is received. Contractual allowances (discounts), bad debt, and indigent care all become reductions of gross revenue and generally are not under the nurse manager's control (Finkler et al., 2007).

TRACKING AND MONITORING OF BUDGETS

The budget process is often viewed as an event that occurs once a year and then ends until the next budget development process begins. Although the budget development process may occur once a year, the budget sets the stage for ongoing monitoring and evaluation of the organization's financial performance related to the budget projection. Regular budget analyses (e.g., quarterly or monthly) are used for monitoring, feedback, and managerial control. The variance (difference) between budgeted and actual revenue and expenses is determined to identify problem areas, enhance control, and ensure timely adjustments. Variances between actual and budgeted (planned) performance need to be analyzed to determine the cause so that nurses can take the appropriate action. Variances can be favorable or unfavorable. Most organizations now use electronic reporting formats that automatically calculate variance rates, but it is important that nurses understand the reasons for the variances. Variances can result from a single cause (e.g., volume of patients; a rate change such as salary, usage, or price) or from a combination of causes.

Nurse executives often require nurse managers to document their analysis of budget variances. Many nurse managers also find it is useful to share variance reports and the reasons for budget variances at unit meetings with their nursing staff. If, for example, the overtime was 4% over the budget rate, staff can engage in discussing the reasons for this expense. It may be that acuity was very high, that there were sick calls that required nurses to "work short," resulting in overtime. This will enhance the nursing staff's awareness of the unit's financial performance. Engaging unit staff in discussions about the unit's financial performance will also provide nursing staff the opportunity to suggest cost-saving strategies to control costs at the unit level.

LEADERSHIP AND MANAGEMENT IMPLICATIONS

Nursing services make up the single largest aggregate expense in most health care organizations because they represent a large personnel component and control a large share of supplies and equipment. This is both a strength and a weakness. It is a strength because nurses clearly manage the organization and system, especially at the operational unit level. With powerful and accurate data and analysis support, unit-level management becomes effective and efficient. However, many organizations simply do not provide a nurse-friendly support structure.

It is a weakness to be the largest aggregate expense because quick, short-term economic gains can be made by ratcheting down resources allocated to nursing services. This often occurs at the expense of long-term gains, staff morale, group cohesion, and sometimes safety. Because health care generally faces strict fiscal constraints, both staff nurses and nurse managers must be knowledgeable and skilled in anticipating financial fluctuations and trends and in making bold decisions based on rapid analysis of information. Staff nurses often will be handling day-to-day budgetary decisions; thus they must be aware of the unit's budget, the financial status of the unit and the organization, and the impact of their decisions about supply and resource (staff) utilization on the financial performance of the unit. Nurse managers are more involved with strategic or long-range financial planning and decision making.

The budgeting process requires a broad range of leadership and management skills. Resources are limited. This fact is difficult for some nurses, especially if they believe they should be able to do everything for every patient under every circumstance. Some professionals think that their job is to provide the maximum quantity and quality of service and that cost consciousness should not be a concern of direct care providers. Nurses are familiar with managing clinical care delivery. These skills can be transferred into the management of money as a necessary component of providing care. However, the management of any scarce resource such as money includes balancing competing interests and making difficult decisions.

Leadership is involved in influencing others to achieve the group's goals within the constraints of scarce resources. Leaders need to be actively involved in setting the vision for how to accomplish goals through budget planning. Ethical considerations, such as fairness and reasonable targets, are part of leadership decision making. Leaders can influence employee morale and organizational culture through role modeling and the decision-making process. Organizational culture can be engaged to diminish negative aspects of budgeting and financial management.

Fiscal Responsibility for Clinical Practice

Continuous change in the health care delivery and reimbursement systems has created a challenge to controlling costs while continually improving the quality of care. One nurse author has advocated that nurses assume fiscal responsibility for their clinical practice (Murray, 2012). Fiscal responsibility is defined as using the resources of the patient to maximize health benefit while simultaneously utilizing the resources of the institution to maximize cost-effectiveness. In trying to improve client care by improving managerial and clinical decisions in nursing, fiscal responsibility is essential. The cost to clients from health care services is a social and professional concern. Cost and quality remain as two major themes for nursing practice. The questions that will be asked are: What is the cost? What if the cost of the intervention is unaffordable but produces superior quality? What will the cost be (to the patient and to the institution and ultimately to society) if the care is not provided or is not of high quality? Cost variables are one consideration to use in decision making.

Being fiscally responsible means that the nurse manager makes responsible resource allocation decisions. Some decisions a nurse manager might need to make include the following:

- Are there sufficient budgeted hours per patient day to provide quality care?
- Making staff assignments: Who is the member of the patient care team who can care for the patient in a cost-effective manner?
- Discharge planning: Is there a process in place to avoid delays in discharges to nursing homes?
- How are the costs of supplies and equipment captured?

There are also multiple opportunities for staff nurse nurses to demonstrate fiscal responsibility. For a client with poor skin integrity, perhaps the most expensive tape should be used because the tape needs to stick and be waterproof. However, in a routine situation, can a lower-cost item be substituted with equal results? Nurses cannot help reduce costs unless they know the per-item cost of the supplies they use and then use this information to evaluate substitutions. Even small cost reductions can be significant if they are applied to high-volume items. Immediately apparent is the costliness of inappropriate use of items (e.g., wiping up spills with a sterile pad; opening a sterile pack to use only one of the instruments; using a manual paper-based system instead of computerized ones). Convenience versus cost trade-off must be considered (e.g., bag baths may be convenient or necessary in a staffing shortage but are an expensive supply cost).

Evaluation of Budget Expenditures

The public is becoming increasingly knowledgeable regarding the quality and safety of health care. Health care consumers and payers expect that money for new initiatives will result in value added in terms of improved quality or safety of care. Business plans must include specific metrics that will be used to measure the impact of the expenditures on clinical outcomes, quality and safety, as well as on cost. Metrics should specify the impact on nurse-sensitive indicators when feasible to further validate the significant role that nurses play in improving the health status of patients.

Costing Out Nursing Services

Accurately determining the costs of providing nursing service is an important budgetary function. Nurses need to know their costs to plan better and negotiate more effectively. Nursing has historically been seen as a cost center but not a revenue generator. One strategy proposed to compensate for nursing's revenue disparity was to cost out nursing services. This idea became popular for awhile but lost attraction as capitated reimbursement systems gained prominence. With a "per member per month" flat payment structure, many felt that efforts to cost out for purposes of charging a fee for service were useless. Therefore costing out nursing services was abandoned by some. However, the unintended consequence was that the value of knowing precisely what it costs to deliver nursing services was lost.

Costing out nursing services is defined as the determination of the costs of the services provided by nurses. By identifying the specific costs related to the delivery of nursing care to each client, nurses have data to identify the actual amount of services received. In reviews of the literature related to costing out nursing services, a variety of variables were examined, such as length of stay, nursing care costs, direct care costs, and diagnosis-related group (DRG) reimbursements. Fundamentally, nurses need to have their own data on actual and specific costs of nursing care. These data are essential to developing an understanding of the relationship between the use of nursing resources and quality outcomes that are sensitive to direct nursing care (Pappas, 2007).

The process of costing out nursing services provides data for productivity comparisons. Activity-based costing (ABC) is one approach to service costing that

may be useful in multiple settings. The key advantage of ABC is that it reflects what it costs to provide services and identifies why costs were incurred. The first step in ABC is to identify all the cost drivers associated with a specific service. For example, if the service is a preschool physical examination provided by a nurse practitioner, here are some examples of the costs associated with the service:

- Nursing assistant (NA): 5 minutes to room the patient, and 5 minutes to clean the room after the visit. The nursing assistant is paid $15 per hour with a 35% benefit rate and works 52 weeks per year, 40 hours per week. The cost of the NA time is $31,200 + $10,920 = $42,120/2080 (number of hours in a year), for an hourly cost of $20.25, or $20.25/60, $0.3375 per minute or $1.69 cost per visit.
- One-half hour of nurse practitioner (NP) time: The nurse is paid $86,000 per year and associated benefits at 35% ($30,100); the NP works 52 weeks (40 hours per week) per year. The cost of the time of the NP is ($116,100/ 2080) = $55.86 cost per hour or $27.91 cost per NP time.
- All other costs are identified in the same manner: equipment, such as stethoscope, tongue depressor, and linens on exam table; cost of electronic health record; costs of a billing clerk.

Once this process is completed, the costs are aggregated, yielding what it costs to provide one unit of one nursing service: providing a preschool physical exam. The next step is to assign activities to cost centers, or service lines or programs. In the previous example, the cost of the service may be placed in a pediatric well-child clinic program.

Another approach to collecting nursing's cost data is using acuity, or patient classification systems. Many of the classification approaches share a similar approach to the determination of the workload based on the required hours of nursing care. This is intuitively attractive because it can be assumed that a ventilator-dependent patient in an intensive care unit will require more care than a patient who has had a total knee replacement. If the nurse manager uses a classification system whereby, for example, type 1 patients receive 2 to 4 hours of nursing care per day and type 2 patients receive 5 to 8 hours per day, these data can be used in constructing a personnel budget when it is linked to the volume indicator of patient days.

If the nurse manager predicts that the unit will provide 800 days of type 1 patients, this information can be used to predict the staffing requirements for that patient group. Multiple commercial patient classifications systems are available for purchase. Most involve entering nurse-collected patient data into a software program. One caveat to this process is that, when used to create staffing ratios, the judgment of an expert nurse clinician must override an empirical system and be based on patients' needs in real time.

Various approaches are used to determine this acuity level and then relate it to staffing needs. Patient classification software is available for purchase. These systems attempt to categorize the levels of nursing care required by patients and then project appropriate nursing and ancillary staff. Some of these may be expensive to purchase and then modify to meet the needs of a specific hospital; they may also be costly to install and maintain. Critics argue that such systems cannot capture the invisible knowledge work of nursing. The systems often inadequately adjust for the experience level and varied expertise of RNs, such as a new graduate versus an experienced senior nurse.

In general, too little effort has been devoted to isolating actual nursing costs and determining the costs of nursing and the provision of care. With actual data, nurses are in a better position to demonstrate the economic value of their service, and nurse managers will have appropriate information with which to accurately manage nursing services. *Acuity* is defined as a measure of the severity of illness of an individual patient or the aggregate patient population on a unit. Any nurse who has engaged in clinical practice in hospitals for 10 or more years can recount how much the acuity of patients has increased in the past decade. Formerly, patients were admitted for diagnostic tests and for additional preparation before surgery. They typically remained in the hospital until they were able to care for themselves, often through a lengthy convalescence. A nurse was able to provide care to larger numbers of these patients because they required less care and assessment. Today, these patients are receiving care in other settings and only very ill patients remain in the hospital. Utilization review experts have stated that the only reason a patient is in the hospital is because they need monitoring and assessment by a registered nurse. If these skills are not needed, patients can probably be safely cared for in a less expensive setting. The increased acuity seen today decreases the number of patients for whom a nurse may safely provide care. This results in what might look like, on paper, a decrease in productivity. Any measure of the productivity of nursing staff that does not consider the acuity level of patients is seriously flawed and would probably result in a gross underestimation of the output.

PRODUCTIVITY

Understanding the concept of productivity and relating it to the management of professional nursing is a leadership skill that will serve nursing in an era of accelerating health care expenditures. Based on this understanding, the nurse manager will be able to determine the costs associated with providing nursing care. Productivity is defined as the relationship between output and the goods and services used to produce them.

MEASURES OF PRODUCTIVITY

Various measures of productivity exist, but all involve relationships between volume of inputs and cost. Nurses' time is the critical input in the production of nursing care. Home health agencies measure their productivity in patient home visits and hours of care; hospitals measure patient days; and clinics measure the number of patient visits. The cost measure is the cost of the nursing time required to produce this care. Table 22-4 provides additional methods of calculating productivity.

The oldest method of measuring nursing productivity is the analysis of hours per patient day (HPPD). The input is the nursing hours worked. The number of hospitalized patient days is the output. This index is imprecise because of the wide variation in client acuity, with the result that the measure of patient days is not equivalent across cases.

A variety of data sources and productivity indices can also be considered. In nursing, productivity has been tightly linked to staffing numbers. For example, staffing, calculated as the total number of hours of a given staff for a given time period, can be compared with client volume or census. Using this method, if

TABLE 22-4 MEASURES OF PRODUCTIVITY

Productivity(P) = Cost per unit of output

$$P = \frac{Input}{Output}$$

$$P = \frac{Cost}{Unit\ of\ output}$$

$$P = \frac{\$}{Work\ hours}$$

$$P = \frac{Nursing\ hours\ worked}{Number\ of\ hospital\ patient\ days}$$

$$P = \frac{Number\ of\ nursing\ staff}{Census\ or\ patient\ days}$$

the output (patient days) increased while staffing remained the same, then the productivity, strictly speaking, would be increased. This typically happens in hospitals, for example, when the influenza season is severe and a large number of geriatric patients are admitted to the hospital. In this short-term staffing crisis, the same numbers of staff are available to care for the high census, and productivity temporarily increases. However, the gains may be short-lived in that the short-staffing situation may result in nurse burnout and resignations.

No one measure of productivity adequately captures the knowledge-based work of nursing. Productivity measurement is complex for several reasons. The causal linkages between nursing interventions and patient outcomes are not well established. There is little research that addresses economic efficiency: that is, what is the least cost combination of inputs required to produce an outcome.

One solution has been to emphasize outcomes measurement. Research on outcomes measurement is accelerating and provides empirical data to support staffing decision making. Nurse researchers (Cho et al., 2003) demonstrated a relationship between staffing and adverse patient outcomes. They found that an increase in 1 hour worked by RNs per patient day was associated with an 8.9% decrease in the odds of patients acquiring pneumonia. These researchers also found that the occurrence of all adverse events (pneumonia, pressure ulcers, and wound

infections) was associated with a prolonged length of hospital stay, increased mortality, and increased hospital costs. This is an example of outcomes research that will aid managers' decision making in the future. Enhancing the productivity of nurses while protecting the quality of patient care will continue to be a major challenge for nurse leaders.

CURRENT ISSUES AND TRENDS

Evaluation of Budget Expenditures

The public is becoming increasingly knowledgeable regarding the quality and safety of health care. Health care consumers and payers expect that money for new initiatives will be well invested and that a significant return on investment will be realized in terms of improved quality or safety of care. Business plans must include specific metrics that will be used to measure the impact of the expenditures on clinical outcomes, quality and safety, as well as on cost. Metrics should specify the impact on nurse-sensitive indicators when feasible to further validate the significant role that nurses play in improving the health status of patients.

Nurses Nearing Retirement

The 2008 National Sample Survey of Registered Nurses reported that RNs over the age of 50 comprised 44.7% of the total RN population in 2008 compared to 33% in 2000 (HRSA, 2010). The American Nurses Association (ANA) reported that "the nursing shortage isn't stopping soon" (ANA, 2012). The U.S. Bureau of Labor statistics projects a 26% growth rate in registered nurses between 2010 and 2020 (Bureau of Labor Statistics, 2012).

Additionally, consider the following:

- The median age of nurses is 46 years. More than 50% of the nursing workforce is close to retirement.
- The population of people over age 65 years in the United States is increasing. The medical and health care needs of this age group will require an expanded health care system.
- The Patient Protection & Affordable Care Act will give increased access to health care to millions of people, further increasing the demand for registered nurses.

These factors, combined with an anticipated strengthening of the economy that may cause large numbers of nurse retirements, will create a renewed critical shortage of nurses (ANA, 2012).

Although nursing educational institutions have attempted to increase the supply of RNs, they have not been entirely successful. *More than 75,000 qualified applications to professional nursing programs were denied admission in 2011,* despite an overall enrollment increase of 5.1% over the previous year (American Association of Colleges of Nursing [AACN], 2011).

These dire statistics point out the need to maximize the productivity of professional nurses. However, this productivity cannot be accomplished at the cost of nursing care quality. Lucero and colleagues conducted a study about patient care activities left undone by registered nurses in 168 hospitals. On average, 41% left developing or updating care plans undone, 12% left preparing patients and families for discharge undone, and 28.5% left patient teaching undone. The authors suggested that learning the consequences of unmet nursing care may influence nurse managers to develop evidence-based resource allocation (Lucero et al., 2009).

It is possible that increased use of technology will be a partial solution to increasing nursing productivity. Computerized documentation and medication administration systems are widespread applications of technology that have resulted in time savings and subsequent increased productivity for nurses. Information technology is another enhancement to nurses' productivity. Medical records are easily accessed from multiple sites, results of diagnostics tests are communicated instantly, and monitoring devices detect deviations from normal limits and communicate these to the nurse as they occur.

Another responsibility of nurse leaders related to productivity is ensuring a future workforce by participating in the recruitment of future nurses. At a recent conference, a speaker reported that as a colleague leaves her home for work each day, she tells her young children, "Mom is going to go to the hospital to save lives today." Although nursing does not *always* offer that level of drama, it certainly speaks of the importance of the work that nurses do. That importance needs to be communicated to the pool of potential nurses.

Integration of Economics into Clinical Practice

The incorporation of economic evaluation into clinical practice is important to productivity because health care resources are limited and choices must, and will, be made. In the years preceding managed care, health care providers acted as if health care resources were infinite, with the result that health care costs spun out of control. Today, providers are faced with difficult decisions about "who gets what." Although rationing health care is inherently unacceptable to most of the U.S. population, it is true that rationing is occurring. Currently, rationing is done on the basis of the ability to pay for health care, with the uninsured receiving less health care. Well-educated nurse leaders who understand economics and finance are in a unique position to bring the values of nursing to decision making about the allocation of health care resources.

Multigenerational Nursing Workforce

For the first time, four generations of nurses are employed at once in the workforce: the veterans (born between 1922 and 1943), the baby boomers (born between 1943 and 1960), the Generation X'ers (born between 1960 and 1980), and the Nexters (born between 1980 and 2000) (Outten, 2012). Each of these generations brings values and attitudes to the workplace. Veterans or traditionalists are described as hard working and being uncomfortable with change. Their core values are law and order, respect for authority, dedication, and sacrifice. Contrast this with Generation X, whose core values focus on thinking globally, balance, technological literacy, independence, and informality (Stanley, 2010). Clearly, different management strategies are needed to enhance the contributions and productivity of each of these groups.

RESEARCH NOTE

Source

Kotecki, S., & Schmidt, R. (2010). Cost and effectiveness analysis using nursing staff–prepared thickened liquids vs. commercially thickened liquids in stroke patients with dysphagia. *Nursing Economic$, 28*(2), 106-113.

Purpose

The purpose of this project was to evaluate the entire cost of two preparations of thickened liquids: (1) staff prepared, and (2) commercially prepared, in an acute care hospital.

Method

The study was implemented on a 37-bed adult care stroke certified neuroscience unit. Three registered nurses (RNs) and three patient care assistants (PCAs) were timed as they prepared both nectar and honey thickened products from water, milk, and orange juice resulting in 36 total products. The average time to create the product was calculated. The average hourly rate of an RN and a PCA including benefits was obtained.

Other costs included cost of water, milk, and orange juice, the thickener (Resource ThickenUp), cups, spoons, and a portable viscometer.

Discussion

Commercially prepared thickeners were 44% to 59% less expensive than the cost of manually creating the thickened liquids. Commercially prepared liquids were also of more consistent viscosity than the manually prepared liquids. Contrary to the outcome that might have been anticipated, this study showed that it is cost-effective to purchase commercially prepared products for patients with dysphagia. Other benefits of the commercial product included maintenance of viscosity over time, readily available products, decreased risk of aspiration, and increased patient satisfaction.

Application to Practice

This study demonstrated using cost analysis as a method of evaluation. It could be applied to many other care processes.

CASE STUDY

Nurse Manager Susan Lange, RN, MS, is responsible for an inpatient orthopedic surgical unit and the associated orthopedic surgical clinic. The inpatient hospital unit cares for an average of 8 patients each week who have had total hip replacement surgery and 12 patients per week who have had total knee replacement surgery. Most of these patients are older than 75 years and depend on either an elderly spouse or other family caregiver for assistance throughout the surgery and recovery. For elective surgery, patients are admitted to the hospital on the morning of surgery. They have had a preoperative physical and laboratory work within 4 days preceding the surgery.

Nurse Lange is aware of the inconsistency of the quality of the preoperative teaching that the patients receive. Some patients are well prepared, know what to expect, and have practiced ambulation techniques before the surgery. Other patients are confused about the plan of care and appear to have had little or no preparation. Nurse Lange has discussed this problem with the RNs who work in the clinic. The RNs acknowledge the problem and report that they "do the best that time allows." A second problem in the care of this patient population is the frequent need for temporary nursing home placement after the surgery. The difficulty in finding this type of post-hospitalization placement often results in delays in discharge of 1 to 3 days.

Nurse Lange has conducted brainstorming sessions with her staff. They have designed a program whereby an RN would function in the dual role of educator/case manager for this group of patients. The person in the new role would be responsible for designing care plans that would begin in the clinic, follow the patient throughout the surgical experience, and even resume in the clinic at post-surgical follow-up. The person would also function as a patient educator. Now, Nurse Lange must "sell" the program to the chief nursing officer and gain funding for the additional position.

1. What data does Nurse Lange need to present to support the request for the new position?
2. What should be the educational requirements of a person in the new position?
3. What should be the experience requirements of the person in the new position?
4. Is any reimbursement possible to offset the costs of the new position? From what source?
5. What outcomes should be measured to demonstrate the impact of the new program?
6. How will the productivity of the person in the position be measured?
7. What other stakeholders in the care of the patient population should be consulted and have input into the program?

CRITICAL THINKING EXERCISE

Mariah Tokyandak, DNP, RN, is a relatively new nurse manager in the medical intensive care unit at a community hospital in a suburban location in the Pacific Northwest. As part of her scholarly project in doctoral study, she examined the research support for use of remote cardiac monitoring for patients in telemetry units. Dr. Tokyandak has a keen interest in this concept, also having heard about it from a colleague at a large academic medical center on the East Coast. The evidence she found demonstrated that the remote cardiac monitors resulted in lower salary expenses for monitor technicians on every telemetry unit, and patients who are monitored via the remote system have significantly improved clinical outcomes and shorter lengths of stay in the hospital.

Dr. Tokyandak is excited by the possibility of introducing this technology in her own hospital. She approached her chief nurse executive (CNE) to share her enthusiasm about this new technology and was told by the CNE that she should develop a formal proposal for the remote monitoring initiative as part of her capital budget development process for the coming fiscal year. The CNE also indicated that Dr. Tokyandak should include the other two monitored intermediate units in her proposal because the technology could then be used consistently across the organization.

Dr. Tokyandak is pleased that her CNE thinks her idea is a good one, but she is unsure about what to do next. Although Dr. Tokyandak completed the capital budget last year and was successful in obtaining a new overhead lift for bariatric patients on her unit, she has never prepared a capital budget proposal of this magnitude. She knows she will need to consider many factors, especially in light of the fact that capital budget requests are due in less than 2 months.

1. What should Dr. Tokyandak do first?
2. What strategies should Dr. Tokyandak use to increase the likelihood of successful approval of her capital budget proposal?
3. The finance director hears about this initiative and claims that he knows that these systems cannot save money. What actions should Dr. Tokyandak take to respond to his comments?
4. A staff nurse on Dr. Tokyandak's unit is concerned about this new initiative because she thinks that "nurses are being replaced by machines." What should Dr. Tokyandak do to address her concerns?

Performance Appraisal

Lynne S. Nemeth

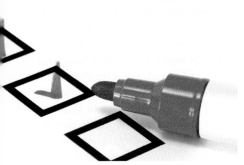

℮volve WEBSITE

http://evolve.elsevier.com/Huber/leadership/

Managing the performance of people is an important organizational strategy designed to exceed expectations of consumers in today's competitive health care environment. Many complex processes and strategies are involved in managing employee behavior. Managers need to clearly define the roles and expectations that are needed in the variety of settings in which individuals provide their efforts in return for compensation. Active engagement by managers in the process of setting standards of performance motivates the staff they employ to achieve goals. By communicating the important issues that affect performance as well as the problem-solving issues that arise with the individual who may experience conflict or difficulty following established procedures, managers can provide a fair appraisal of the individual's abilities, talents, and opportunities for improvement.

DEFINITIONS

Performance is defined as the execution of an action; something accomplished; the fulfillment of a promise, claim, or request (*www.merriam-webster.com*, 2012).

Performance appraisal means evaluating the work of others. It is the process by which a manager examines and

Photo used with permission from Photos.com.

evaluates an employee's work behavior by comparing it with preset standards, documents the results of the comparison and uses the results to provide feedback to the employee to show where improvements are needed and why (*www.businessdictionary.com*, 2012). The employee's work is measured against standards, much like the quality improvement process. Standards, whether explicit or not, are applied to what ought to be or to what is superior, excellent, average, or unacceptable performance.

Peer review in nursing (defined in 1988 by the American Nurses Association and still applicable today) is the process by which nurses systematically evaluate the quality of nursing care provided by peers as measured against professional standards (American Nurses Association, 1988, p. 3).

Self-evaluation is the aspect of performance appraisal whereby employees do self-assessments of their own perceptions about their performance as compared with stated objectives and expectations.

PERFORMANCE APPRAISAL PROCESS

Performance appraisal is a required process in organizations to help ensure that the quality of care is met and to provide a fair human resources management process. Performance appraisals provide staff members

399

with the information necessary to determine whether they are meeting expectations or can improve their performance to the required level.

The process of performance appraisal includes assessing needs and setting goals, establishing objectives and time frames, assessing progress and evaluating performance, and then starting over again (Figure 23-1). At the start of a new job, core competencies (knowledge and skills) of the individual need to be evaluated. During the orientation program, progress should be tracked, and competence needs should be reassessed periodically throughout employment, at least annually.

Performance appraisal is a cyclical process that begins when the employee is hired and ends when the employee leaves. Job analysis identifies competencies required for job performance. The job description lists work standards and the knowledge, skills, and abilities necessary for the job. The performance appraisal specifies employee behaviors and compares job performance with criteria. A variety of measurement methods may be used to ensure that reliable and valid appraisals are conducted. Using the performance appraisal interview, goals are set, corrective action may be taken, or training needs may be identified. Thus meeting established "success criteria" would lead to equitable rewards and recognition that are objectively administered.

The performance appraisal process is both informal and formal. The informal process includes day-by-day supervision or coaching to moderate, modulate, or refine performance. Coaching as a management tool is ongoing, face-to-face collaboration and influence to improve skills and performance. By contrast, the formal performance appraisal should include written documentation and a formal interview with follow-up.

The employee's work is measured against some standard for the purpose of determining the level of quality of the job performance. The guides to evaluation criteria include governmental standards such as Medicare/Medicaid regulations, professional standards published by the American Nurses Association or other specialty organizations, nursing care audits, client feedback in various forms, evidence-based guidelines, and departmentally developed standards. Organizational standards are more prevalent as systems undertake service and operational excellence initiatives to improve customer service, the employee experience, quality, financial performance, and growth. Organizational pillars to "hardwire excellence" provide a platform for all employees to understand and buy into the mission, vision, and values of the organization (Studer, 2003).

Ideally, a performance appraisal measures performance and motivates the person. However, performance appraisal is not the only or major source of motivation for most nurses. Measuring performance is not easy, and motivating someone else is an art. Cultural sensitivity is important to consider as the nursing workforce becomes more diversified (Smith-Trudeau, 2008). The performance appraisal process can create a lot of stress for individuals if it is not managed well by both the manager and the employee (Duncan, 2007). For example, job satisfaction and organizational commitment were found to be positively correlated to satisfaction with the feedback from performance appraisals (Jawahar, 2006). Integral components of a comprehensive performance appraisal system provide an overarching framework for the process. The tools and methods for a comprehensive performance appraisal system involve a clear determination of the abilities required for the position (job description); a match of the key requirements for the position with the individual's capabilities (personnel selection); development of the abilities of the employee (staff development); and use

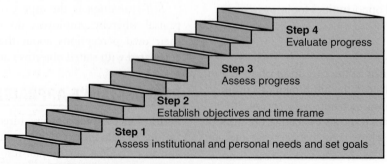

FIGURE 23-1 Four steps of a performance appraisal.

of a motivational reward system to enhance employee performance (reward system). Box 23-1 outlines the key components of the performance appraisal process.

Performance attributes of an individual are determined by two elements: ability and motivation. Ability is made up of a collection of physical and mental capacities that enable a person to exhibit a skill or set of skills. Knowledge, experience, and skill form the ability to successfully complete a task (Hersey et al., 2008). Thus ability is an innate capacity that is molded by experience and training. Motivation is a willingness to work and a desire to achieve.

ORGANIZATIONAL CULTURE AS A CATALYST TO IMPROVING PERFORMANCE

Given the national concerns about patient safety and quality of care, it is important to look at organizational culture as a factor influencing performance appraisal for change and improvement. The change of an error-prone health care system involves leadership and organizational learning, which requires significant strategic commitment and administrative direction. An environment that values and creates a shared vision and purpose can lead to reflection and learning, which then enables and strengthens organizational culture toward creative and effective solutions in health care delivery (Carroll & Edmondson, 2002).

Culture consists of shared norms, behaviors, and values. Schein (1992) defined the culture of a group as "a pattern of shared basic assumptions that the group learned as it solved its problems of external adaptation and internal integration, that has worked well enough to be considered valid and, therefore, to be taught to new members as the correct way to perceive, think, and feel in relation to those problems" (p. 12).

The learning that occurs within the system over time influences organizational culture.

The quality of care and the quality of work life are driven by the culture within a health care organization (Gershon et al., 2004). Culture is reflected in "the way things are done" in an organization (Stetler, 2003), and it surrounds all individuals and influences leadership. Characteristics of the culture are manifested differently in subgroups and by the various stakeholders within the organization, which warrants more in-depth assessment to fully understand.

SUBCULTURES AND STAKEHOLDERS

Socialization of new members into an organization is an important way to learn the rules and norms of a group. New members need to learn the assumptions of the group, which are not always transparent. Group behaviors and perceptions may reveal some elements of the culture, and some of the rituals and processes undertaken within the organization may reflect the assumptions that are held. Groups that are stable and have a history of shared learning are likely to have developed some degree of culture, but groups with significant turnover of members and leaders may lack shared assumptions (Schein, 1992). Organizational culture has been referred to as the *social glue that binds the organization,* in which the deeper meanings of the way things are done in the organization are learned (Cameron & Quinn, 1999; Detert et al., 2000).

Evaluation of organizational culture needs to consider both the larger organization and the smaller unit within which a member belongs. Exploring the microsystem within a health care system reveals the unique disciplinary focus of each department and treatment setting (Donaldson & Mohr, 2000). The performance characteristics of academic departments, clinics, and hospital units and departments highlight the different functions and shared assumptions that members bring to the patient care setting. These varying perspectives enrich the mix of the organization by enabling diverse contributions, attitudes, and skills to be developed.

Members of a larger organizational culture may also belong to subcultures within that organization, whose group learning over time may have generated very different sets of basic assumptions. The behavior and language of organizational members are subject to interpretation through the cultural biases of the subgroup. Conflict may be experienced when members of the subculture do not understand the biases within the larger culture or vice versa. Using an organizational cultural approach to conflict management would enable subcultures to examine the assumptions that underlie the behavior and reinterpret such conflict as the result of diverse experiences. Problem-solving issues that are based on different assumptions, with the intent to evaluate the utility of such differences, demonstrate an effective learning process (Nemeth, 2008).

The criteria for performance appraisals should include measures of key performance indicators that reflect the values of the organizational culture. With these characteristics embedded within appraisal tools, managers can craft the culture within the unit. If there is not an explicit organizational mission, vision, or value statement, managers must translate their vision and values into a clear framework that all can understand. This framework should provide the structure for staff to operationalize the required behaviors for successful performance. The scoring of the performance appraisal tool indicates the weight that these organizational culture characteristics contribute toward performance, which communicates the importance of those to the overall appraisal.

GOALS FOR PERFORMANCE APPRAISAL

The most direct goal of any performance appraisal system is the improvement of performance. Considering the process of performance appraisal systems, the outcome for the system should lead to positive organizational outcomes. Used effectively, the performance appraisal offers the opportunity for numerous organizational goals to be achieved. Box 23-2 provides an overview of the goals of the process of performance appraisal.

Roles and Expectations of Team Members

Numerous stakeholders are represented within the process of performance appraisal of nurses. Most important is the voice of the patient, the end consumer of the care provided. The patient's voice can be obtained from patient satisfaction data that are formally used within the organization. Often, the patient or family member will offer direct verbatim comments that can be used to provide constructive support to individuals or groups. Nurse managers

---

> **BOX 23-2** **GOALS OF PERFORMANCE APPRAISAL**
>
> - Improve performance
> - Improve communication
> - Reinforce positive behavior
> - Communicate about and ultimately correct negative or less-than-optimal behaviors
> - Provide a basis for rewards, which also is a basis for motivation
> - Provide a basis for termination if necessary
> - Identify learning needs and develop personnel

---

should seek out the comments of the patient regarding the patient's experience of care. Through this proactive process, the manager may find that the voice of the patient regarding specific exceptional staff members or those who may need to improve can provide useful input for managing staff behavior.

The peers, who are co-workers in the setting in which the nursing care is delivered, are individuals who have the greatest opportunity to know firsthand how well the individual meets patient care needs and responsibilities as a member of the team. These peers may work on the same shift or alternate shifts or may interact with the individual from the perspective of another unit's function. Experienced with direct communication about the patient's status, they know the specific expectations of care that are required in the individual setting. For example, a nurse may work on a unit that receives patients frequently from the emergency department or the recovery room, and there are bilateral communications and expectations that these staff members have of one another. These are key individuals who interact with the nurse and may be in an excellent position to provide input related to performance.

The interdisciplinary team members who count on the nurse also have expectations for the nurse to communicate and collaborate regarding the plan of care and inform key members of the need to become involved in assisting the patient. For example, social workers or therapists may rely on referrals from the nurse who has made an initial assessment of the patient's needs. If key criteria for referrals are clearly identified but not implemented, then the interdisciplinary care plan for the patient may not be developed as effectively as is needed. Interdisciplinary team members need to work together on behalf of the patient's needs, not just within their own disciplinary silos. Nurse managers need to think about acquiring input from the perspective of the key interdisciplinary team members who provide services within the specific unit or department.

Physicians are valuable sources of feedback in the process for performance appraisal of staff. Effective clinical areas establish a collaborative and inclusive process guided by a strong base of supportive relationships. To develop this level of support requires mutual trust and respect among the physician teams that provide care within the specific area. This would include ongoing communication regarding opportunities for improved performance by staff and physicians alike.

Administrative members have expectations that are more global, but essentially they require that individual staff know the policies and procedures that must be implemented in the care of patients. The commitment of employees to organizational pillars of excellence is important to these stakeholders. With numerous stakeholders, it is important that systematic processes guide the nursing management function of performance appraisals. With data being collected systematically from numerous sources, a more meaningful performance appraisal process can be achieved.

Manager's Role

Leaders who reward positive behavior and punish individuals who behave negatively in the workplace practice transactional leadership. By shifting toward a transformational style of leadership, organizational learning can occur from errors and system issues, and an empowered staff of nurses can work toward the innovations needed in the health care system (Wenberg, 2010).

Managers meet with newly hired employees during a planning stage to discuss the tasks, objectives, competencies, and performance characteristics. Clarity is essential in the performance appraisal process, and the manager has the duty to provide this to all staff members. This process allows the individual to talk specifically about his or her performance goals and to come to agreement with the manager on reasonable performance expectations.

Self-appraisal as an important component in the appraisal process and promotes individual input, personal responsibility, and feedback regarding job performance. Appraisal is a structured process of facilitated self-reflection, which allows individuals to review their professional activities comprehensively and to identify areas of real strength, professional goals, and needs for development (Conlon, 2003).

Managers who create a healthy work environment offer adequate time for feedback and input. Audit and feedback are important mechanisms to provide objective data to the nurse regarding the quality of care provided. To improve clinical practice and motivate nurses to learn, individual self-esteem must be at a level that promotes motivation (Ward, 2003). The imperative for nurse managers is to recognize that the use of feedback in the performance appraisal process may influence an individual's self-esteem, which may affect practice. Providing feedback is a delicate art of nursing management, which should be performed with the goal of encouraging and motivating the individual to improve his or her individual care provision.

Melding Multiple Sources of Input

Incorporating the input of peers in the performance appraisal process also must be handled carefully because the opinions of peers often substantially influence a person's self-esteem (Ward, 2003). This allows managers to determine whether opinions are consistent regarding the employee's job performance. Objectivity can never be presumed in reviewing the input of others; and when perceptions differ, the manager is in the position of determining the final score for the performance appraisal. This process must be used judiciously to avoid creating conflict among staff members and management (Arnold & Pulich, 2003).

Individual self-appraisal, as well as peer and other stakeholder input, provides a mechanism for a 360-degree performance appraisal that enables a wider perspective beyond what the individual manager can provide to the staff member. Organizational cultures that encourage the use of 360-degree feedback do so to provide a learning opportunity for the individual. Financial rewards are not necessarily tied to 360-degree reviews, but development opportunities are to be gained through this method, which is a more important outcome. A key decision in the process of using 360-degree feedback is whether to keep the process as a confidential process or to have it be one in which the person being evaluated knows or selects peers and subordinates to participate in the review.

PERFORMANCE APPRAISAL AND RETENTION

Performance-based career advancement systems provide a means to recognize and reward clinical expertise in direct patient care roles. Differentiated practice models enable employee development and higher performance at a level consistent with individual interest and motivation. For those nurses who seek a higher level of professional contribution, these systems can provide a mechanism for compensation that is based on additional performance and effort. The Vanderbilt Professional Nursing Practice Program is an example of a program that was designed to attract, retain, and reward nurses (Robinson et al., 2003). The concept of Magnet designation offers a framework that attracts and retains registered nurses in work environments that support effective nursing, organizational, and patient outcomes. (Lundmark, 2008). The process for hospitals to meet criteria of the Magnet Recognition Program® from the American Nurses Credentialing Center (ANCC) has led to the development of supportive professional nursing care environments in designated Magnet hospitals.

PERFORMANCE APPRAISAL CRITERIA

It is essential to set expectations regarding job criteria and performance as soon as the nurse begins employment. The organization should have the employee sign the performance tool as a planning stage for the performance criteria that are to be met and should provide a copy for the employee to refer to throughout the year. Armed with clear expectations, the employee should understand how he or she will be rated at the end of the evaluation year.

Managers must maintain objectivity and fairness when conducting performance appraisals. Because of the wide variety of individuals in the workforce and the increased diversity of cultures, there may be instances of personality conflicts with the manager and the employee. Employees may feel that the manager dislikes them and therefore is biased about their performance (Arnold & Pulich, 2003).

RESEARCH NOTE

Source

Meretoja, R., & Koponen, L. (2012). A systematic model to compare nurses' optimal and actual competencies in the clinical setting. *Journal of Advanced Nursing, 68*(2), 414-422.

Purpose

This study addressed a gap in the literature on methods for professional nursing competence assessment and developed a systematic model to compare nurses' optimal and actual competencies in a perioperative clinical setting in Finland.

Discussion

A mixed methods descriptive design used qualitative and quantitative data to address three research questions: What is consensus on optimal competencies required in the research setting? How do nurses and nurse managers assess nurses' actual competencies? How do actual competencies differ from optimal competencies? Twenty-four experts were purposefully selected to represent advanced multidisciplinary expertise in perioperative care. A first qualitative survey was administered, using open-ended questions about the five most important future challenges. Individual experts were then asked to rate the relevance of specific competency items using the Nurse Competence Scale. Group discussions were held to reach consensus on the highest possible agreement of optimal competence items and overall optimal competence levels. A qualitative content analysis and descriptive statistics were used in the analyses. Group consensus was achieved in recognizing challenges, specifying optimal competencies, and identifying educational challenges.

Application to Practice

The study identified future challenges in seven areas: work role, therapeutic interventions, helping role, diagnostic functions, teaching-coaching, ensuring quality, and managing situations. Fifteen important competencies were identified that required delivery at a consistently high level. The highest expectations included the following six competencies: *recognizing early situations posing a threat to life, taking active steps to maintain and improve professional skills, acting appropriately in life-threatening situations, being aware of the limits of one's own resources, analyzing patients well-being from many perspectives,* and *prioritizing activities flexibly according to changing situations.* Differences between optimal and actual competence revealed greatest differences in five areas: *recognizing early situations posing a threat to life, taking active steps to maintain and improve professional skills, promoting flexible team cooperation in rapidly changing situations, coaching others in duties within my responsibility,* and *developing orientation programs for nurses in my area.* This study provided a useful model for the evaluation of competence and performance and could be used to develop a continuous learning culture.

Potential problems may impede a manager from performing a fair evaluation on an employee. Arnold and Pulich (2003) described the following potential problems, called *sources of error*, related to perceptions that may incorrectly influence managerial ratings on performance appraisals:

- *Recent behavior bias:* Occurs when the rater remembers behavior primarily from the most recent period of the employee's performance as opposed to the entire rating period
- *Horn effect:* Occurs when a manager perceives one negative aspect about an employee or his or her performance and generalizes it into an overall poor appraisal rating
- *Halo effect:* Occurs when a manager perceives one positive characteristic about an employee or his or her performance and generalizes it into an overall high rating
- *Similar-to-me effect:* Occurs when a manager rates the employee performance higher when a person is accurately or inaccurately perceived to have the same characteristics as the manager

Developing skill in assessment and interview techniques is a key to effective performance appraisal. Asking questions can elicit important evaluative data. Using a coaching process means studying present behavior and developing planned, purposeful change strategies or intermediate multiple small steps to bring performance closer to what is desired. Coaching uses constant communication and clear consequences. Coaching becomes the management of consequences by praising, reprimanding, and redirecting (Hersey et al., 2008). A process of the employer and employee establishing mutual goals contributes to improved performance.

Distinction can be made between counseling, coaching, and mentoring. *Counseling* addresses problem performers such as employees whose work is consistently substandard, those who regularly miss deadlines, or those who are uncooperative, insubordinate, absent, or tardy. The problem needs to be brought to the employee's attention, the employee should be given time to respond, and specific actions to improve performance should be agreed on. *Coaching* involves all employees in improving their ability to do their job and increase potential. Activities include role modeling, hiring carefully, encouraging growth, creating a positive environment, using praise, and encouraging stretch goals. *Mentoring* is for employees who show promise and is used to shorten learning

curves and increase productivity. Developmental needs demand a greater commitment. The closer the link between the employee's needs and the mentor's competencies, the more likely it is that the mentorship will be productive. Mentoring requires mutual trust and respect (Stone, 1999).

The more explicitly the performance criteria are stated, the less conflict is generally experienced in the scoring. In specific position descriptions, the behaviors that are needed to score a rating of "meets expectations," "exceeds expectations," or "substantially exceeds expectations" can be elaborated. This methodology sets a standard that is institution-wide and provides clarity and consistency among nurse managers on different units.

ALTERNATIVE TYPES OF APPRAISAL

To minimize bias in the performance appraisal, the manager should use multiple methods to fairly evaluate the performance on each employee. The following are some alternative methods:

- *360-Degree evaluation:* The 360-degree evaluation can be obtained by seeking input from approximately four sources: (1) a peer, (2) a physician, (3) a subordinate, and (4) a self-evaluation. Once all the input is obtained, the evaluating manager adds his or her input and merges the feedback to develop the final score. The 360-degree evaluation tends to be more applicable in evaluating advanced practice roles or for management positions because of the diverse interactions that staff in these roles have. For evaluation of the staff nurse role, the 360-degree process may not be as effective because the expectations may be for a more uniform standard of performance.
- *Peer review:* In this process, employees rate the performance of others in the same job classification, using objective criteria that have been established. A peer review committee provides input to the manager. The manager then incorporates the feedback into the person's evaluation along with the manager's comments. The negative aspect of this process is that staff may feel that members of the peer review committee are not fair in their assessment of other staff members' abilities. Peer review is most applicable for evaluating staff positions in which a common set of expectations and performance standards exists, because the staff members

who work with one another are best suited to having the core knowledge about the quality and nature of the work performed by the individual. An effective peer review system may offer the individual honest and specific feedback that allows that person to make specific adjustments in his or her role to better meet objectives and performance standards.

- *Management by objectives:* In this method, the employee and manager establish performance goals for the upcoming appraisal year. This process is difficult for evaluating the entry-level nurse. As the nurse develops and gains more experience, management by objectives may be helpful in defining goals and objectives for the next year and providing the manager with a specific set of goals to follow up with the individual at regular intervals.

RELIABILITY AND VALIDITY IN MEASUREMENT

Reliability and validity are important considerations in any system of measurement. Tools must be constructed so that the score one rater would give would be consistent with another person's rating. If the criteria are developed in a clear, observable manner, they are more likely to lead to increased inter-rater reliability. Inter-rater reliability would be demonstrated if several raters, using the same criteria on the same person, would rate observable performance consistently. If two raters were recording their observations on the same person using the same tool, results should be equivalent. This would indicate a highly reliable tool.

Testing the reliability of a tool involves examining the amount of random error. The characteristics of the tool must be dependable, consistent, accurate, and comparable (Burns & Grove, 2001). Stability of the performance criteria demonstrates consistency with repeated measures of the same tool. Nurse managers who are comfortable with a performance appraisal tool should be able to measure the same person at multiple intervals in a stable and consistent manner. This is referred to as *test-retest reliability.*

Establishing equivalence is a more complex process that involves direct observation of specific processes at the same time by different individuals.

The percentage of agreement is computed to derive inter-rater reliability. Perfect inter-rater reliability would be demonstrated if two individuals rated all performance criteria consistently. The lowest acceptable coefficient for reliability would be 0.80 (Burns & Grove, 2001).

The validity of a tool is the determination of the extent to which the tool is measuring the construct that is under evaluation. Evaluation tools must capture the critical behaviors and outcomes that result from effective nursing care. The term *construct validity* is used to establish that the criteria are appropriate, meaningful, and useful in measuring what they are intending to measure. Perfect validity is not guaranteed, and to define validity in a specific tool often takes many years.

To provide objective measures to ensure that staff members are evaluated fairly, both the reliability and validity of the evaluation tool must be established. Drawing from recent research regarding performance appraisal and variance in measurement, generalizability theory (GT) has been used to describe the variability that is associated with multisource ratings (Greguras et al., 2003). As more employment settings begin to use multiple raters to provide feedback for performance appraisal systems, it is important to understand the nature of the feedback and consider the reliability of its sources. It has been demonstrated that when ratings are used for administrative purposes, the scores have tended to be less reliable than those scores used for development of the person being rated.

Generalizability theory provides a framework for examining the dependability of behavioral measurements of raters. As the information obtained for the performance appraisal is compiled, the final rater must consider the variance due to the person being evaluated, the items being evaluated, and the interaction of the rater with the person being evaluated. For peers and subordinates, amount of variance may be substantial (Greguras et al., 2003).

When compiling the information that is used to complete the performance appraisal, the rater must consider the following factors affecting the reliability and validity of the ratings:

- The way the information is communicated, either verbally or in writing
- How the information is organized

- The potential influence of the relationship the rater has with the person being rated
- The cognitive ability of the rater

LEADERSHIP AND MANAGEMENT IMPLICATIONS

Developing Staff Members Through Performance Appraisal

For managers, the performance appraisal process is an opportunity to gather insight about their staff. This is more than just a piece of paper that is addressed yearly; it is a process in discovering the individual's perception of his or her job. Managers who are leaders consider the performance appraisal an opportunity to identify what motivates their staff members and also to identify their values and interests.

Managers use the performance appraisal process as a way to translate organizational goals into concrete objectives for the individual employee to fulfill. Through a process of communication, coaching, and development, employees are provided with feedback regarding how their performance fits with the expectations for the organization and the manager's vision regarding the culture of the individual microsystem. The manager identifies the strengths and weaknesses of the employee and provides recognition and support of positive behavior, as well as encouragement and specific recommendations regarding opportunities for improvement. The appraisal should show both the employee and the manager what the employee's possibilities for growth and development are. The developmental activities that a manager provides to an individual employee needs to be aimed at helping the individual better utilize his or her skills and improve performance on the current position or develop toward desired future opportunities for advancement. Leaders, supervisors, and managers who model preferred organizational behaviors, identified through the performance appraisal process, inevitably motivate staff to adapt desired outcomes.

The prevailing purpose of performance appraisal is to improve and motivate the staff, which in turn will enhance organizational effectiveness. This clearly identifies the process of performance appraisal as a means to addresses institutional needs, as well as individual staff needs and abilities. The manager who uses the performance appraisal process effectively will become more capable in supporting, coaching, and managing the development of his or her staff members.

CURRENT ISSUES AND TRENDS

The appraisal of performance occurs at multiple levels. At the individual level, performance is measured by a performance appraisal. At the unit level, performance may be estimated using budget or patient safety/quality criteria. At the organizational level, performance is appraised by accreditation review by such entities as the Centers for Medicare and Medicaid Services (CMS), National Committee for Quality Assurance (NCQA), or The Joint Commission (TJC) accreditation. High performance is rewarded with incentive payments for achieving high quality on national quality indicators specific to hospitals and ambulatory care environments. Achievement of patient-centered medical homes certification by NCQA may provide resources from third-party payers that contract with primary care settings for care. Quality indicators published by CMS and the Agency for Healthcare Research and Quality (AHRQ) drive performance improvement. Abundant performance criteria, quality indicators, evidence-based approaches, and incentives for quality outcomes have influenced professional advancement and development of career ladders. New roles and opportunities for nursing continue to develop. Research from evaluations of Magnet and non-Magnet hospitals demonstrated a stronger work environment in Magnet facilities (Kelly et al., 2011), and Magnet reviews emphasize peer evaluation and strong performance appraisal.

With the increased concern for patient safety identified by the Institute of Medicine (IOM) (2000, 2001, 2003, 2004), the drive for a blame-free culture of safety, and current research regarding nursing-sensitive outcomes and nurse staffing (Aiken et al., 2002; IOM, 2004; Needleman et al., 2002), nurse managers and administrators have much to consider regarding how this process can best be crafted. Performance appraisal is one important element.

Considering the multitude of system errors and the current emphasis by regulatory agencies on improvements in system performance and patient safety, nurses are in an extremely visible position at the forefront of health care delivery. The 44,000 to 98,000 deaths per year in American hospitals that were presented as evidence in *To Err Is Human: Building a Safer System* (IOM, 2000) provide the impetus for health care leaders to redesign safer systems of care. Errors occur when planned actions fail or when wrong plans are used, resulting in unintended outcomes. Health care interventions that injure patients are adverse events and are considered preventable (IOM, 2004). Performance appraisal can be fine-tuned to aid in prevention efforts.

Health systems managers and administrators need to consider that to reduce errors that harm patients, a systems approach is needed. Recognition of the fact that human error is to be expected in all organizations (Reason, 2000), combined with diligence to uncover the root causes of events that result in patient harm, is a management responsibility. Multiple factors in health care systems increase the vulnerability of the nurse to errors. The experience and educational background of the nurse, the supervision and feedback that the individual nurse receives daily in the process of care, and the maturity of the nurse to raise issues in the environment that pose a risk to safe patient care are factors to be considered. Nursing performance can be enhanced in an environment in which open and honest feedback to individuals is valued, shared leadership and decision making are encouraged, and errors are discussed or risky situations are analyzed by all participants. Nurse managers and leaders need to develop their staff members as critical "systems thinkers" who explore issues that

negatively affect patient outcomes and/or job satisfaction. Critical systems thinkers can see the bigger context than their individual perspective within the subculture to which they belong. Individual goals and performance should be viewed within the context of how one interacts within a system; but clearly the competencies of the individual, as well as the behaviors that are enacted, must be developed and strengthened for optimal performance. Performance appraisal is one component of a performance management system used by organizations to motivate employees and to address elements of overall system performance risks.

INTERACTIVE GROUP EXERCISE

A useful method to promote creative group interaction and discussion is role-playing. Role-playing allows participation in actual challenging situations. For this exercise, the readers are asked to conduct a mock performance appraisal. One participant will portray the employee and one will portray the manager. In preparation for this exercise, the employee will complete a self-evaluation and the manager will complete an evaluation. Role-playing will provide participants the opportunity to present different employee and management styles in a creative manner. This interaction should occur in a setting that promotes open dialogue regarding the performance appraisal process.

CASE STUDY

Nurse manager Jane Finch, MSN, RN, has prioritized an improvement initiative to implement in her unit after receiving data that showed that her unit had a higher level of catheter-associated urinary tract infections (CAUTIs). Most of the nursing staff members have attended staff meetings that have provided the opportunity to discuss performance on CAUTIs on the unit. A new evidence-based protocol was developed and implemented to reduce CAUTIs. Ms. Finch and an advanced practice nurse consultant led small group sessions on the day and night shifts to introduce the protocol and clarify expectations regarding implementation of the standing order to discontinue/remove catheters at the appropriate time. Emphasis was placed on educating the nurses regarding the research studies and resulting evidence

in order to establish the relative advantage, compatibility, and support of the intervention. The medical staff signed off on the protocol for the nurses to discontinue/remove the catheter, and this was made a unit policy. Communication was ongoing during the initial implementation of the project, with posters and feedback given to the nursing staff on the unit. Additionally, nursing staff members were asked for input during the initial trial to identify any issues that were problematic in the implementation of this protocol. No problems were identified.

Two of the older nurses on the unit have not embraced the protocol, but they also have not spoken up about their concerns with the implementation of this protocol during opportunities when this input was requested. As part of the evaluation of this protocol's implementation, Ms. Finch has audited patients' medical records and learned that there was not consistent adoption of the protocol and standing order. Ms. Finch has to bring this feedback to the individuals who are not acting on behalf of a quality improvement initiative that the unit has undertaken. She has chosen to round on the staff to assess their feedback, perceptions, and goals with regard to this initiative. This provides objective data to use with the annual performance appraisal that is due later in the year. She learns that two of the nurses do not think it is appropriate for them to undertake the discontinuation of catheters as a standing order. By rounding and seeking mid-year feedback, Ms. Finch learns that a more in-depth assessment of nursing staff buy-in is needed to implement change.

CRITICAL THINKING EXERCISE

Mary Gold has completed her first year as a nurse on a general medical-surgical floor. During her first year, she has worked three 12-hour shifts per week, a rotating day-night position, and has begun to assume charge nurse duties. She arrives to work in a timely fashion and completes her tasks. She is quiet and reserved but does not necessarily appreciate some of her co-workers who she perceives are a bit aggressive. Her co-workers described her as quiet and a bit distant.

One day, Mary Gold's nurse manager hands her the self-appraisal form that is part of her performance appraisal and asks her to complete it by the end of her shift. Her nurse manager will be back in the morning to discuss the performance appraisal with her. Two of Mary Gold's co-workers, picked by her manager, have already completed peer evaluations. This is the first time Mary Gold had seen or heard about a performance appraisal. She attempts to finish her evaluation but is unclear about how to complete the form. In the morning, at the end of her shift, her nurse manager asks her to come to her office to discuss her performance appraisal. During their discussion, her manager shares the perception that Mary Gold is distant and unapproachable. The manager continues by telling Mary Gold that immediate improvement is necessary for her to remain in her position. Mary Gold is stunned. She has never had a conversation with her manager regarding job performance before this moment. She signs the appraisal at her manager's request because she does not want to appear difficult. She leaves her unit distraught and confused.

1. What is the problem?
2. Why is it a problem?
3. Whose problem is it?
4. What should Mary Gold do?
5. How should the problem be handled?
6. Describe the management and leadership style of Mary Gold's nurse manager.
7. What parts of the performance appraisal process could be improved? How?

CHAPTER

24

Prevention of Workplace Violence

L. Jean Henry, Gregory O. Ginn

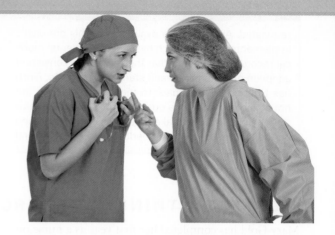

⊖volve WEBSITE

http://evolve.elsevier.com/Huber/leadership/

Nursing is a challenging profession. Recent violent incidents in hospitals and care facilities have pushed the issue of workplace violence into the forefront of concerns among nursing communities and agencies charged with ensuring staff and patient safety. The health care industry is the site of more violence than any other industry, and nurses are victimized twice as often as other health care workers. Although the number of homicides in the health care industry is rather small, 48% of all nonfatal injuries from occupational assaults and violent acts in 2000 occurred in health care and social services (Occupational Safety and Health Administration [OSHA], 2004, p. 5). To add to the gravity of the situation, most researchers agree that violence against nurses is significantly underreported.

Nurses are harmed by workplace violence. A systematic review of the literature on the effects of violence toward nurses reported the predominant responses to be anger, fear or anxiety, posttraumatic stress disorder symptoms, guilt, self-blame, and shame (Hogh & Viitasara, 2005). One researcher reported that physical and psychological aggression experienced by nurses was related to job dissatisfaction, turnover intention, physical symptoms, injuries, and exposure to contagious disease directly and/or indirectly through their emotional strain (irritation, anxiety, and depression) (Needham et al., 2005).

Violence in hospitals is caused by a combination of internal and external factors. External conditions include a society where violence is prevalent and the fact that many health care facilities are located in inner cities where crime rates are higher than average. Internal factors include inadequate staffing levels, larger numbers of dangerous patients, poor security for drugs and money, staff members working alone, poorly lit facilities, and unsecured, continuous access to health care facilities (OSHA, 2004).

Further, the very nature of the jobs that nurses perform places them at high risk for workplace violence, and circumstances inherent in health care work increase workers' susceptibility to homicide or assault. Nurses often deal with people who are in pain, emotionally disturbed, or cognitively impaired; and often their families are experiencing strong emotions brought on by grief, catastrophic injuries, criminal victimization, or severe psychiatric disturbances. Staffs in nursing home/long-term

Photo used with permission from Photos.com.

care facilities, intensive care, psychiatric/behavioral or emergency departments, and geriatric facilities appear to be the most at risk. In addition, nurses are frequently confronted with situations that cause them moral distress. As professionals, nurses are engaged in a moral endeavor and thus confront many challenges in making the right decision and taking the right action. When nurses cannot do what they think is right, they experience moral distress that leaves a moral residue (Corley, 2002). The resultant stress can generate aggressive behaviors. Thus for a number of reasons, violence in the workplace is a particular concern for nurses.

From a public health perspective, it makes sense to approach workplace violence prevention in much the same way as other types of illnesses or injuries. From the perspective of an organization, the connection between workplace violence prevention and the attainment of broader organizational objectives such as financial performance may seem tenuous. However, the organization is uniquely situated to exert a powerful influence over the environment of the workplace, and, because of its position, has far more ability to effectively reduce both the incidence and severity of incidents of workplace violence.

Policies to prevent workplace violence can make a difference. Research has demonstrated that a stronger violence prevention climate (i.e., good prevention practices/response and low tolerance or incentives for unsafe practices) was related to less frequent violence and psychological aggression incidents experienced by nurses (Yang, 2009). Results of multiple regression analyses, controlling for appropriate factors, indicated that the odds of physical assault decreased for having a zero-tolerance policy and having policies regarding types of prohibited violent behaviors (Nachreiner et al., 2005). Reporting must be encouraged and staff asked to contribute to the development of efficient programs, thus leading to a sense of empowerment (Lanza et al., 2011). Therefore the issue is to convince organizations that (1) they can effectively institute a public health objective such as workplace violence prevention, and (2) the attainment of broader organizational objectives such as acceptable operational and financial performance is very much facilitated by successful workplace violence prevention programs (Ginn & Henry, 2002).

DEFINITIONS

Violence is narrowly defined as assault, battery, manslaughter, or homicide; and broadly defined as a range from verbal abuse, threats, and unwanted sexual advances to physical assault and homicide. **Workplace violence** may be conceptualized as a spectrum. One end is aggressive behavior such as verbal abuse, threats, harassment, and menacing behavior that may cause psychological harm. The other end is behavior such as assault, battery, manslaughter, or homicide that causes physical harm. It is important to define workplace violence as a spectrum because people often manifest aggressive psychological behavior as a precursor to violent physical behavior. By using a broad definition of violence, workplace violence prevention policies can respond to the psychological precursors of violence in order to preempt physical violence (Romano et al., 2011)

Sources of violence vary. One source of violence is from criminals with no other connection to the workplace, but who simply intend to commit a crime. A second source is from customers, clients, patients, or students; this is regarded as the most prevalent source of violence against nurses. A third source is from a current or former employee. A fourth source is from someone who is not employed at the workplace but has a personal relationship with an employee, such as a spouse or domestic partner (Rugala & Isaacs, 2004).

Risk factors for violence in health care organizations include working with volatile people, understaffing, long waits, poor environmental design, lack of training, inadequate security, substance abuse, poor lighting, and unrestricted access by the public. Working in hospitals may be dangerous because of the availability of drugs or money in the pharmacy area, the necessity of working evening or night shifts in high-crime areas, and the availability of furniture or medical equipment that could be used as weapons (OSHA, 2004, pp. 6-7).

REGULATORY BACKGROUND

Workplace violence has received increasing attention over the past three decades as a substantial contributor to occupational injury and death. The National Institute for Occupational Safety and Health

(NIOSH) reported that homicide has become the second leading cause of occupational injury and death. Assaults represent a serious safety and health hazard for American workers, and violence against employees continues to increase (NIOSH, 2004).

Acknowledging that workplace violence was a pervasive and growing problem, the Occupational Safety and Health Act of 1970 declared that employers had a general duty to provide safe and healthy working conditions. Through this act, NIOSH was charged with drafting and recommending occupational safety and health standards (OSHA, 2004).

OSHA followed up on the general duty requirement in 1989 with voluntary generic safety and health program management guidelines for all employers to use as a foundation for their safety and health programs. The guidelines were not regulations; however, under the OSHA act, employers face fines if an incident of workplace violence occurs. The agency made it clear that safety and health programs could include workplace violence prevention programs (OSHA, 2004).

In 1998, OSHA built on the 1989 generic workplace safety and health guidelines by announcing guidelines specifically targeted at the health care and social services industry. The new guidelines identify common risk factors and include policy recommendations and practical corrective methods to help prevent and mitigate the effects of workplace violence (OSHA, 2004). Clearly, managers of health care organizations have an ethical obligation to protect the safety of workers. Managers also have a general legal duty to prevent workplace violence. Given the significant economic costs of workplace violence and the potential legal liability, managers have a fiscal responsibility to prevent workplace violence.

NIOSH Recommendations

NIOSH is located within the Centers for Disease Control and Prevention (CDC). NIOSH recognizes that workplace violence is a particular issue in the health care industry and recommends the following violence prevention strategies for employers: environmental designs, administrative controls, and behavior modifications. **Environmental designs** include signaling systems, alarm systems, monitoring systems, security devices, security escorts, lighting, and architectural and furniture modifications

to improve worker safety. **Administrative controls** include (1) adequate staffing patterns to prevent personnel from working alone and to reduce waiting times, (2) controlled access, and (3) development of systems to alert security personnel when violence is threatened. **Behavior modifications** provide all workers with training in recognizing and managing assaults, resolving conflicts, and maintaining hazard awareness (NIOSH, 2002).

OSHA Guidelines

OSHA is an agency in the U.S. Department of Labor. OSHA suggests that all health care organizations have a violence prevention program. Ideally, **violence prevention programs** are available to all employees, track progress in reducing work-related assaults, reduce severity of injuries sustained by employees, decrease the threat to worker safety, and reflect the level and nature of threat faced by employees (OSHA, 2004). The main components in a violence prevention program are (1) a written plan, (2) worksite analysis, (3) hazard prevention and control, (4) safety and health training, and (5) recordkeeping and evaluation of program (Box 24-1 and Figure 24-1). **Violence prevention written plans** demonstrate management commitment by disseminating a policy that all types of violence will not be tolerated, ensures that no reprisals are taken against employees who report or experience workplace violence, encourages prompt reporting of all violent incidents, and establishes a plan for maintaining security in the workplace. **Worksite analysis** is a commonsense look at the workplace to find existing or potential hazards for workplace violence. **Hazard prevention and control** implement work practices to prevent and control identified hazards. **Safety and health training** makes all the staff aware of security hazards and how to protect themselves through established policies, procedures, and training. **Recordkeeping and evaluation of programs** provide the data to track progress in reducing work-related assaults.

LEADERSHIP AND MANAGEMENT

Management Frameworks

Levels of workplace violence may vary depending on how much organizations focus on the root causes of workplace violence, such as individual characteristics

BOX 24-1   ENVIRONMENTAL ANALYSIS

Hazard Prevention and Control

Identify hazards found in the worksite analysis and then provide administrative and work practice controls to make hospitals a safer workplace. For example, the following measures may increase safety:

- Provide better visibility and good lighting, especially in high-risk areas such as the pharmacy or isolated treatment areas.
- Implement safety measures to prevent handgun entry to the facility—for example, use metal detectors.
- Install Plexiglas in the payment window in the pharmacy area.
- Use security devices such as panic buttons, beepers, surveillance cameras, alarm systems, two-way mirrors, card-key access systems, and security guards.
- Place curved mirrors at hallway intersections or concealed areas.
- Control access to work areas.
- Provide training for staff in recognizing and managing hostile and assaultive behavior.
- Provide adequate staffing even during night shifts. Increase staffing in areas in which assaults by patients are likely (e.g., emergency department).
- Increase worker safety during arrival and departure by encouraging car pools and by providing security

escorts and shuttle service to and from parking lots and public transportation.

- Ensure accurate reporting of all violent behavior.
- Make patients aware of zero-tolerance policy for violence.
- Establish liaison with police authorities, and contact them when indicated.
- Obtain previous records of patients to learn of any past violent behaviors.
- Establish a system to chart or track and evaluate possible assaultive behaviors, including a way to pass on information from one shift to another.
- Implement a violence prevention plan to develop strategies to deal with possibly violent patients.

A safer room for a possibly violent patient features the following:

- It has furniture arranged to prevent entrapment of staff; furniture should be minimal, lightweight, without sharp corners, and/or affixed to the floor.
- It is free from clutter, with nothing available on countertops to throw at workers or use as weapons.
- A secondary door is available for escape in case the main door is blocked by patient.
- Every room should be entered with a buddy; do not be alone with patient.

Modified from Occupational Safety and Health Administration [OSHA]. [2004]. *Guidelines for preventing workplace violence for health care and social service workers.* Washington, DC: OSHA, U.S. Department of Labor. Retrieved July 26, 2012 from *http://www.osha.gov/Publications/OSHA3148/osha3148.html.*

and organizational environment factors (Hutchinson et al., 2010; O'Leary-Kelly et al., 1996). The implications for management of the threat of workplace violence vary depending somewhat on the source of violence. With regard to the first source of violence (criminals with no connection to the employer), a risk management approach is appropriate. With the second source of violence (patients), a total quality management approach may be effective. Concerning the third source of violence (current or former workers), good human resource management policies are essential. In dealing with the fourth source of violence (someone who has a personal relationship with an employee), employee assistance programs can be especially useful.

Risk management is an integrated effort across all disciplines and functional areas to protect the financial assets of an organization from loss by focusing on

the prevention of problems that can lead to untoward events and lawsuits. A wide variety of measures are appropriate to prevent violence from criminal activity. Among these measures are posting security guards, restricting access to the general public, adequate lighting, escort services for those coming or going from parking lots, and installing alarm systems and systems to call for emergency assistance. If efforts at prevention fail, insurance is available to cover the specific costs of workplace violence (Law & Pettit, 2007). All of these actions can help prevent or mitigate losses from actions by criminals with no connection to the workplace.

Total quality management (TQM) comprises the general processes of setting standards, collecting information, assessing outcomes, and adjusting policies. TQM and risk management share the goals of eliminating problems, enhancing performance, and

Workplace Violence Checklist

The following items serve merely as an example of what might be used or modified by employers to help identify potential workplace violence problems.

This checklist helps identify present or potential workplace violence problems. Employers also may be aware of other serious hazards not listed here.

Designated competent and responsible observers can readily make periodic inspections to identify and evaluate workplace security hazards and threats of workplace violence. These inspections should be scheduled on a regular basis; when new, previously unidentified security hazards are recognized; when occupational deaths, injuries, or threats of injury occur; when a safety, health and security program is established; and whenever workplace security conditions warrant an inspection.

Periodic inspections for security hazards include identifying and evaluating potential workplace security hazards and changes in employee work practices that may lead to compromising security. Please use the following checklist to identify and evaluate workplace security hazards. **TRUE** notations indicate a potential risk for serious security hazards:

_____ T _____ F   This industry frequently confronts violent behavior and assaults of staff.

_____ T _____ F   Violence has occurred on the premises or in conducting business.

_____ T _____ F   Customers, clients, or coworkers assault, threaten, yell, push, or verbally abuse employees or use racial or sexual remarks.

_____ T _____ F   Employees are **NOT** required to report incidents or threats of violence, regardless of injury or severity, to employer.

_____ T _____ F   Employees have **NOT** been trained by the employer to recognize and handle threatening, aggressive, or violent behavior.

_____ T _____ F   Violence is accepted as "part of the job" by some managers, supervisors, and/or employees.

_____ T _____ F   Access and freedom of movement within the workplace are **NOT** restricted to those persons who have a legitimate reason for being there.

_____ T _____ F   The workplace security system is inadequate—i.e., door locks malfunction, windows are not secure, and there are no physical barriers or containment systems.

_____ T _____ F   Employees or staff members have been assaulted, threatened, or verbally abused by clients and patients.

_____ T _____ F   Medical and counseling services have **NOT** been offered to employees who have been assaulted.

_____ T _____ F   Alarm systems such as panic alarm buttons, silent alarms, or personal electronic alarm systems are **NOT** being used for prompt security assistance.

_____ T _____ F   There is no regular training provided on correct response to alarm sounding.

_____ T _____ F   Alarm systems are **NOT** tested on a monthly basis to ensure correct function.

_____ T _____ F   Security guards are **NOT** employed at the workplace.

_____ T _____ F   Closed circuit cameras and mirrors are **NOT** used to monitor dangerous areas.

_____ T _____ F   Metal detectors are **NOT** available or **NOT** used in the facility.

_____ T _____ F   Employees have **NOT** been trained to recognize and control hostile and escalating aggressive behaviors and to manage assaultive behavior.

_____ T _____ F   Employees **CANNOT** adjust work schedules to use the "Buddy system" for visits to clients in areas where they feel threatened.

_____ T _____ F   Cellular phones or other communication devices are **NOT** made available to field staff to enable them to request aid.

_____ T _____ F   Vehicles are **NOT** maintained on a regular basis to ensure reliability and safety.

_____ T _____ F   Employees work where assistance is **NOT** quickly available.

FIGURE 24-1 Checklist for violence in the workplace. (From Occupational Safety and Health Administration [OSHA]. [2003]. *Guidelines for preventing workplace violence for health care and social service workers* [rev. 2003]. Washington, DC: OSHA, U.S. Department of Labor. Retrieved July 26, 2012, from *http://www.osha.gov/SLTC/etools/hospital/hazards/workplaceviolence/checklist.html*.)

eliciting total organizational commitment. Under TQM, the organization uses all available resources, builds long-term relationships with both employees and patients, and remains open to ways in which processes can be improved to enhance the quality of operations. Teamwork is an integral part of TQM, along with a system for tracking violent incidents (Lanza et al., 2011; Smith, 2001; Wagner et al., 2001). All levels of the organization are expected to be involved in decision-making and employee training. Training topics should impart skills that support the strategic goals of the organization and could include prevalence, incidence, and warning signs of violence; policies and procedures; critical incident response; and availability of services associated with violence in the workplace (OSHA, 2004). Health care organizations can expand the team concept to include strategic partnerships and alliances (OSHA, 2004).

Essential to establishing a safe working environment is developing systems for reporting and documenting incidents of assaults and acts of aggression, as well as taking prompt action when a report is made. The reporting system should include the creation of special forms to report violent incidents, as well as the establishment of a hotline and confidential procedures for employees, to encourage timely and accurate reporting of all forms of violence (OSHA, 2004, pp. 21-24). The principles of TQM are manifested in OSHA's guidelines for violence prevention programs in health care; Henry and Ginn (2002) illustrated and discussed this relationship in more depth.

Human Resource Management Policies

A comprehensive violence prevention policy and procedural manual should be developed to guide organizational violence prevention efforts. Violence prevention occurs on three levels: primary, secondary, and tertiary. *Primary* refers to lowering the risk of occurrence; *secondary* refers to containing or limiting the violence; and *tertiary* refers to retrospective assistance and support to the injured (Hogh & Viitasara, 2005).

A number of management policy recommendations in the literature can be applied to the prevention of workplace violence. Organizations should be particularly careful regarding employees' perceptions of procedural fairness concerning layoffs, performance, and conflict resolution. Explaining to employees how or why certain events, such as layoffs, have occurred

will lessen the likelihood of workplace aggression. Further, organizations can train employees on how to handle situations of unfairness and how to create fair working environments. Organizations can implement a zero-tolerance policy toward aggression to lessen the possibility of work groups encouraging an individual to act aggressively (Beugre, 2005).

In the area of personnel, some suggest that organizations have policies to require thorough screening of applicants to weed out those who may have a propensity for violence. Such procedures may eliminate some violence from co-workers, because a history of violence is the best indicator of future violence (Corbo & Siewers, 2001). One possibility is to include screening for domestic violence in new employee screening (Anderson, 2002). Thorough employee screening and appropriate termination policies will, at the least, contribute to a legal defense that reasonable action to prevent violence has been taken.

In dealing with potential violence from co-workers, threat assessment and threat management are important concepts to consider. **Threat assessment** consists of the evaluation of the threat itself and an evaluation of the threatener. Health care managers must make some effort to determine whether the person making threats was serious about inflicting harm or just verbalizing frustration; however, this is not to diminish the seriousness of verbal assaults. **Threat management** refers to the course of action taken after conducting a threat assessment. Health care managers might want to investigate the person making threats and admonish, reprimand, counsel, or terminate the employee, as well as provide post-incident counseling for the victim of the threats (Rugala & Isaacs, 2004). Still another procedural approach is to circulate generalized information such as typical profiles of workplace killers (violent employees), characteristics of disgruntled employees, motivations for violent actions, and factors that contribute to the problem (Boxes 24-2 and 24-3).

An essential issue for human resource management is accurate reporting of violent incidents. Nurses often fail to report threats or other verbal assaults because institutional policies, or culture, fail to classify them as violence (Harulow, 2000). Nurses frequently encounter acts of intimidation—an implied threat when someone hits a wall, throws an object, or glares at someone in the immediate area—yet do not acknowledge it as violence. Unfortunately, tolerating hostile or threatening behavior can lead to escalation and ultimately physical harm (Romano et al., 2011). Numerous regulatory bodies and agencies (e.g., OSHA, National Health Service [NHS]) advocate for training to meet the needs of different types of staff groups. At a minimum, staff should be trained in basic violence behavior prevention and correct emergency response procedures (Beech & Leather, 2005). Training programs should emphasize the broad definition of violence and the importance of reporting all incidents of violence (Sheehan, 2000).

Human resource management policies are essential for the prevention of violence from current or former workers in health care organizations. Policies on hiring, discipline, counseling, training, threat assessment, threat management, and reporting can prevent or mitigate loss caused by violence from co-workers.

Employee assistance programs (EAPs) provide a range of services to help employees cope with stressors that occur at home and at work. Family counseling might be useful in reducing domestic violence that can spill over into the workplace. Programs that counsel both the victim and the abuser could be instrumental in initiating needed interventions to defuse domestic violence situations that could impact the worksite.

BOX 24-3   THREAT ASSESSMENT: A TRUE-LIFE EXAMPLE—cont'd

His retirement papers contained disturbing comments. For example, recalling a meeting with a human resources staff member, he said, "I started to grab her by the throat and choke her, until the top part of her head popped off. Then I was going to step on her throat and pluck her bozo hairdo bald. Strand by strand."

Some months later, the subject told a former co-worker that he was following a former supervisor and her family. He provided specific information, stating that he knew where some of the targets lived and the types and colors of vehicles they drove. The subject also made comments about the target's family members and stated that he had three guns for each of his former supervisors.

At this point, law enforcement was notified. While the police investigation was under way, the subject made threats against five former female co-workers. A threat assessment was conducted, analyzing letters, voice mails, reports from EAP, and interviews with various individuals. The subject's communications were organized and contained specific threats. For example, he wrote, "Don't let the passage of time fool you, all is not forgotten or forgiven," and "I will in my own time strike again, and it will be unmerciful." The material suggested that he was becoming increasingly fixated on the targets, and his communications articulated an action imperative suggesting that the risk was increasing. After obtaining additional information, the investigators informed the subject of specific limits and consequences that would occur if he continued his threatening behavior and communications.

The subject assured law enforcement agents that his intent was to pursue legal reparations. Four months later, however, he mailed letters to his five targets stating that he wanted to "execute" one of them. The letters indicated that he was close to committing an attack. Based on the foregoing assessment and insight into his thinking and behavior over several months, the threat assessment team, consisting of an investigator and a mental health professional, initiated a conference call with the district attorney. In the conference, the mental health professional provided an assessment of the subject's potential for violence, and the investigator presented evidence regarding the laws violated and law enforcement actions taken to date.

The threat assessment report, along with other evidence, was used by the district attorney in obtaining an arrest warrant and a search warrant. The final recommendation by the team was that the subject should be arrested and held without bond. Six months later, he was found not guilty by reason of insanity.

From Rugala, E.R., & Isaacs, A.R. (Eds.). (2004). Workplace violence: Issues in response. Washington, DC: U.S. Department of Justice, Federal Bureau of Investigation (FBI). Retrieved July 26, 2012 from *http://www.fbi.gov/stats-services/publications/workplace-violence*.

Furthermore, individual counseling can help employees cope with personal stressors that might contribute to unpredictable or violent behaviors. EAPs can be very useful in preventing or mitigating loss caused by domestic violence that extends to the workplace.

Leadership and Management Implications

It is important to establish and maintain a corporate culture that is serious about protecting employees from violence. Similar to safety climate, a perceived violent climate can exist that correlates to both physical and verbal aggression. Depending on the choices that are made, organizations can create a violent or nonviolent climate (Spector et al., 2007). Data from The Joint Commission's Sentinel Event Database indicate that leadership was a causal factor of violence in 62% of reported events—notably policy and procedures development and implementation (The Joint Commission, 2010). The U.S. health care industry is experiencing substantial turbulence as a result of proposed new laws and policies and the development of new forms of inter-organizational relationships. Organizational changes, such as restructuring, mergers, and downsizing, create significant levels of uncertainty and anxiety in employees, which can eventually lead to stress-related consequences, possibly including violence. Employees often perceive the failure of management to prevent violent incidences, or to respond quickly and appropriately when incidents do occur, as lack of organizational commitment and loyalty. Ensuring a nonviolent workplace may require culture change, and alterations in practice may be necessary in such areas as labor relations, injury management, and other human resource procedures (McKoy & Smith, 2001). Consistent with the principles of quality improvement, leadership for such tasks as worksite analysis, threat assessment, and development of organizational policies and procedures should be provided by multidisciplinary teams composed of representatives of all aspects of the organization.

LEGAL IMPLICATIONS

Although the levels of threat vary among the issues (Matchulat, 2007), several *legal issues* surround workplace violence, as follows (Dolan, 2000):

- Employers may be faced with paying higher workers' compensation rates after injuries are sustained from workplace violence.
- Employers may be subject to claims of negligence with regard to the security provided.
- Employers may be subject to claims concerning negligent hiring, retention, and supervision.
- Employers may be subject to claims that they failed to warn subsequent employers about the criminal propensities of former employees.
- Threat management is complicated in that disability discrimination legislation restricts employers from taking action against employees solely because of their psychological disabilities and requires that action be taken only when the employee poses a direct threat.
- Sexual discrimination laws make employers liable in some instance for sexual harassment.
- Employers may be liable for citations, fines, and even criminal penalties.

Legal defense can be based on a variety of proactive actions by management, including conducting a risk assessment to determine what would be reasonable and appropriate action (Egger, 2000). Following OSHA's guidelines for violence prevention, developing written antiviolence policies and procedures is the first step in reducing workplace violence and should address issues related to employees, patients, non-hospital employee providers, and visitors. Policies clearly defining violence, requiring the reporting of violent acts, and specifying appropriate disciplinary actions for committing violence are essential (Ginn & Henry, 2002). The following policies are useful in both preventing workplace violence and providing a legal defense if violence should occur: policies forbidding weapons, alcohol, drug use, bullying, and sexual harassment; and policies requiring pre-employment screening and appropriate termination procedures. Although no program can guarantee violent acts will not occur, the existence of a program can provide evidence in court

that the health care organization has taken appropriate and reasonable action.

If all prevention efforts fail, health care organizations should have a plan for **damage control.** Emergency response teams should be staffed appropriately to be prepared to respond at the times of day when the threat is greatest (Sheehan, 2000). The literature outlines the desired "trained response" to a workplace violence incident as follows (Romano et al., 2011):

- Recall training
- Prepare
- Commit to action

After a violent incident, employers must address the emotions of employees and notify family members. Employers must also take steps to preserve the company image, quash rumors, prepare for ancillary incidents, ward off lawsuits, and return to normal operations (Botting, 2001). Critical incident response teams should be activated to provide immediate debriefing to all persons involved in a violent incident, whereas EAPs can serve as a valuable tool in long-term support of employees after an incident. In combination, these strategies reduce the potential negative impact on both the employees and the organization.

CURRENT ISSUES AND TRENDS

In recent years, violence in the workplace has come to be viewed in the same light as other occupational hazards, allowing some measure of controllability by health and safety professionals. Publicized violent incidents against nurses and evidence in the literature that violence against nurses continues to rise have prompted increased emphasis on prevention of violence, rather than just responding to violent events. The following topics have been determined in the literature to warrant discussion as critical or new perspectives: improving prediction of violence, environmental design, collaboration among organizations and agencies, increasing government oversight, horizontal violence, and post-incident response.

Predicting Violence as a Prevention Strategy

Most research regarding how to prevent workplace violence focuses on issues within the realm of social psychology, such as stress, justice, and social cognition theory. The large legal questions revolve around negligent employment, workplace harassment, and the Americans with Disabilities Act accommodation issues. Thus most of the gaps that exist between legal theory and workplace practices would fall in the realm of psychology. To enable a proactive response to workplace violence, research is needed that would identify people who would likely be aggressive in a way that was a genuine threat to others; establish the effectiveness of anti-harassment policies; and establish the relationships between various mental illnesses and genuine threats to co-workers (Paetzold et al., 2007).

Environmental Design

In addressing workplace violence, it is easy to focus attention strictly on individuals and their behaviors; however, there is growing emphasis on evaluation of the contribution of the physical environment and institutional/organizational factors. Clearly, physical aspects could enable or contribute to the perpetration of violent incidents. NIOSH (2002) presented a variety of suggestions for designing a safe work environment, including the following: emergency signaling alarms and monitoring systems; metal detectors at entrances and security cameras in hallways; appropriate design of waiting areas for patients and families; adequate lighting and security escorts in parking lots; and design of triage and other public areas to minimize risk for assault. In a systems approach, organizational culture is also considered an aspect of environment. A worksite analysis conducted by a threat assessment team or similar taskforce or coordinator is among the recommendations of

---

RESEARCH NOTE

Source

Hutchinson, M., Wilkes, L., Jackson, D., & Vickers, M.H. (2010). Integrating individual, work group and organizational factors: Testing a multidimensional model of bullying in the nursing workplace. *Journal of Nursing Management, 18,* 173-181.

Purpose

A number of studies have documented the frequency and consequences of bullying among nurses, yet few attempts have been made to develop models to increase understanding of contributory factors of the behavior. This study tested a multidimensional model of bullying in the nursing workplace.

Discussion

Nurses are a high-risk occupational group for exposure to workplace violence and aggression. Of particular concern, in recent years, is an apparent increase in bullying among nurses, also known as horizontal or lateral violence. Bullying is noted to be widespread, with estimates suggesting 80% of nurses experience bullying at some point in their careers. The negative consequences of bullying are well-documented, and include both personal, such as psychological trauma, depression, and physical illness; and organizational, such as decreased job satisfaction, and increased absenteeism and sick leave. Most previous research has explored individual or dyadic features of the behavior. Little research has reported on the relationship between bullying and work group or institutional processes. This sequential mixed-methods study of Australian nurses used three stages: in-depth qualitative interviews; developing, testing, and refining a valid set of coherent measures of bullying;

and testing a multidimensional model of bullying. This article reported the results of stage 3—structural equation modeling and confirmatory factor analysis of the proposed model. The results confirmed that organizational characteristics are critical antecedents of bullying, influencing both the occurrence of bullying and the resultant consequences. The identified antecedents were found to be informal organizational alliances; organizational tolerance and reward; and misuse of legitimate authority, processes, and procedures. The model also depicts the negative consequences of bullying: health effects, distress and avoidance at work, and normalization of bullying in work teams; and it confirms the strength of the relationships. The authors suggested that many current policies and procedures are predicated on the assumption that bullying only takes place at the individual level. Effectively addressing bullying in the nursing workplace may, instead, necessitate changes in existing policies, procedures, and organizational culture, based on the understanding that organizational factors may actually be more important in influencing the occurrence of bullying.

Application to Practice

The apparent increase in the prevalence of bullying in nursing underscores the need to explore new understanding of the contributing factors of and approaches to prevention of horizontal violence in the health care environment. The presented model directs nurse administrators to focus on features of the organization, rather than of the individuals. The model may assist nurse managers to better understand features of the work climate that perpetuate bullying, thus providing the basis for developing effective prevention strategies.

OSHA and TQM approaches. Such an effort analyzes records, trends, workplace security, physical characteristics, operating policies, and screening surveys of staff to provide an overview of the work environment. Based on the results of this assessment, direct action should be taken to resolve any identified areas of concern.

Collaboration

Nursing care occurs in many different settings, involves both professionals and laypersons, and exposes nurses to unacceptably high levels of many different types of violence. Thus there is the potential for various organizations and agencies to work together to develop strategies to minimize violence against nurses. McPhaul and Lipscomb (2004) explored the application of three theoretical perspectives in the approach to workplace violence prevention in academic, union, and employer partnerships. Based on their reviews, they advocated that any effective intervention needs to use a collaborative, systemic approach. When necessary, advice and assistance should be sought from resources outside the health care facility, such as threat-assessment psychologists, psychiatrists, and other professionals; social service agencies; and law enforcement agencies. Rugala and Isaacs (2004) offered a number of suggestions for strengthening the relationship between health care organizations and local law enforcement for preventing workplace violence.

Increased Government Oversight

OSHA is the only regulatory agency that directly oversees the safety and health of health care workers, although several health care oversight agencies attempt to provide industry self-regulation of the safety of health care workers. At this time, OSHA's guidelines are voluntary, thus lacking in power of enforcement. The Joint Commission (TJC) (formerly the Joint Commission on Accreditation of Healthcare Organizations [JCAHO]) provides clear standards for support of patient safety but does not offer the same guidance for the safety of health care workers. The American Nurses Association (ANA) supports the establishment of the OSHA recommendations as mandatory requirements.

Horizontal Violence

A major source of violence against nurses is horizontal, or lateral, violence from other nurses. This type of violence is prevalent in female dominated professions such as nursing (Weinand, 2010). The literature is exploding with theories and research around horizontal violence, which consists of antagonistic behaviors that result from historical, geographical, gender-related, and workplace-related issues. The behaviors may include gossip, innuendo (verbal and nonverbal), scapegoating, passive-aggressive behavior, disrespecting privacy, and bullying (Walrafen et al., 2012; Weinand, 2010). Interestingly, nurses are particularly vulnerable to psychological abuse at work, judging by the number of articles and published studies (Miller & Hartung, 2011).

The impact of horizontal violence is in some ways greater than that of other types. In addition to dealing with the violent episode itself, the victim also has to deal with the ramifications of poor working relationships—a situation that affects co-workers, as well. The negative consequences of bullying are well-documented, and include both personal and organizational effects. Examples of the former include psychological trauma, depression, and physical illness; whereas the latter include decreased job satisfaction and increased absenteeism and sick leave. McKenna and colleagues (2003) found the consequences of horizontal violence to include demoralization, feelings of vulnerability, a changed-to-negative attitude to work, loss of confidence, and impaired work performance.

Taking the problem of horizontal violence beyond the direct impact on the individual and the organization, research also indicates that the resultant reduction in nurses' satisfaction with the job will lead to reduced patient satisfaction (Tzeng & Ketefian, 2002). Of even more concern is the effect that the climate and culture created by horizontal violence could have on patient care and safety. The Joint Commission issued a sentinel event alert that called for organizations to address bullying, on the basis that such behaviors "undermine a culture of safety." The Center for American Nurses (2008) issued a position statement noting the effect of horizontal violence on patient safety, quality of care, and the profession's ability to attract and retain nurses. Recommendations for effective resolution of horizontal violence include addressing contributory factors at all levels, including individual, interpersonal, and institutional.

Post-Incident Response

Post-incident response is becoming recognized as a critical element in reducing both the short-term and the long-term impacts of workplace violence. Failure to respond quickly and appropriately to violent incidents is perceived by employees as lack of management commitment and concern for the workforce. In an effort to limit the losses to the profession from nurses leaving due to trauma from workplace violence, researchers studied how nurses adapted cognitively after incidents of workplace violence. They concluded that critical incident debriefing may facilitate a nurse victim's psychological recovery after an episode of workplace violence (Chapman et al., 2010). OSHA (2004) and the Federal Bureau of Investigation (FBI) (Rugala & Isaacs, 2004) have recommended that post-incident response include such measures as prompt medical treatment, psychological evaluation, counseling, support groups, stress debriefing, trauma crisis counseling, and employee assistance programs. The first responsibility of the response team is to ensure the safety and well-being of the victim(s) of violence. Response team members may be called in at any stage of a violent inci-

dent—to defuse an escalating situation, intervene in an event, or respond to the aftermath of a traumatic event. Consequently, response teams should receive special training in evaluation, threat assessment, and conflict resolution, as well as procedures to monitor, document, and respond to situations. Teams should also have plans for dealing with other issues, such as news media and public reaction to a major incident. Post-incident response should involve an integrated system of services and procedures to reduce the potential impact of a violent incident on employees. Incident debriefing should be offered to all employees, not just to those involved in the event (Henry & Ginn, 2002).

Clearly, violence in the workplace has an impact that goes beyond a particular victim. It damages trust, community, and the sense of security that every employee has a right to feel while at work. Employing agencies need to show a commitment to safety for nurses, providing protection against acts of violence in all clinical areas and especially in high-risk settings. Educational institutions and employers need to share responsibility for properly preparing nurses to deal with potentially violent situations.

CASE STUDY

Good Samaritan County Hospital is located in an inner city neighborhood. It is summer, and the emergency department (ED) has been extremely busy at all hours. Nurse Phillip Knotts is the hospital's Nurse Administrator. In the work room, Nurse Knotts has overheard ED nurses talking about how the heat must be affecting people, because patients have been more irritable and impatient, even cursing at and threatening staff. Nurse Knotts also hears rumors that kids have been harassing staff in the parking lot. Nurse Knotts is surprised to hear these stories, because there have only been three incident reports filed in the past 2 months, and the hospital has a violence prevention program that includes a zero-tolerance policy. He decides to investigate what is really happening, determining there are two questions to be answered. What really is the status of violent incidents at the hospital? Is there a difference between actual violent incidents and reported incidents?

Nurse Knotts' first step is to complete OSHA's 2003 Workplace Violence Checklist. In gathering the information to complete the assessment, he determines that, in fact, there have been a number of encounters that were not reported, being deemed "minor" or "insignificant" at the time. The violent incidents (reported and unreported) included some involving criminals with no connection to the hospital (parking lot incidents), but most involved clients, patients, or people accompanying them to the ED. Thus Nurse Knotts concludes that a combined approach, using risk management and TQM strategies, is appropriate. Using the NIOSH recommendations, he devises a plan that incorporates attention to environmental design, administrative controls, and behavior modifications. Among the environmental design strategies are improving lighting in the parking lot, installing additional cameras in the waiting area with signage to inform clients of their presence, and establishing a security officer station prominently in the waiting area of the ED. Strategies in the area of administrative controls include restricting access points to the ED, conducting a work analysis to determine appropriate staffing for each shift,

Continued

CASE STUDY—cont'd

and simplifying and clarifying the incident reporting process. Suggested behavior modification strategies include reviewing, revising, and enhancing the violence prevention module in staff training and new employee orientation, with particular attention focused on clearly defining what constitutes "violence," instructing staff not to walk through parking lots alone, and encouraging staff to immediately report, to a security officer, anyone in the ED who appears to be becoming agitated or does not seem to belong. By completing a thorough assessment, guided by recommendations of OSHA, NIOSH, and The Joint Commission's Sentinel Event Alert, the risk of future violent incidents was reduced, and reporting of violent incidents increased.

CRITICAL THINKING EXERCISE

Nurse Katie Gardner, a first-year nurse new to care of the elderly, works the night shift in a long-term care facility that has experienced a 10% increase in residents in the last 3 months, many in the early stages of dementia and Alzheimer disease. Several times in recent weeks, Nurse Gardner has expressed her frustration with the increasing workload, inadequate staffing of her shift, and not having enough time to assist residents with their needs, including basic activities of daily living (ADLs). This particular night, Nurse Gardner heard Mr. Jones yell, several times, that he needs help getting into his bed clothes, but she has not yet had time to go to his room. As she rushes down the corridor toward the nursing station, she stops briefly at Mr. Jones' room to tell him she will get to him as soon as she can. As she enters the doorway, Mr. Jones curses at her and throws a drinking glass, hitting her on the side of the head.

1. What are the warning signs of a potential problem?
2. Why is each a problem?
3. What is the "source" of violence? Based on the source, which management approach is appropriate? Apply the components of OSHA's Violence Prevention Plan to identify what should be done to ensure that such a situation does not happen again.
4. How could Nurse Gardner have handled the situation differently?

All-Hazards Disaster Preparedness

Elizabeth T. Dugan, Karen Drenkard,
Gene S. Rigotti

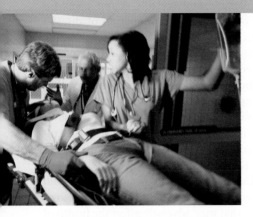

Photo used with permission from Photos.com.

⊝volve WEBSITE

http://evolve.elsevier.com/Huber/leadership/

TRANSITIONING THEORY INTO PRACTICE FOR ALL-HAZARDS PREPAREDNESS

September 11, 2001, was a tragic day that touched everyone's lives and changed Americans' perception of a "safe" world forever. As a result, people of all backgrounds have given thought to preparing themselves, their homes, and their work environments for the eventuality of a disaster. Most people are knowledgeable on how to prepare for potential natural disasters within their local regions; however, many have not had to consider the devastation that can be caused by terrorism. A list of terrorism possibilities is endless: biological exposures, chemical spills, radiological exposures, nuclear blasts, conventional bombings, agricultural contamination, cyber viruses, and other unforeseen cataclysmic events. Thus developing a contingency plan for most types of disasters, including bioterrorism, is most appropriately termed **all-hazards disaster preparedness**.

Since the occurrence of major disasters such as the attack on the World Trade Center, Hurricane Katrina, and the devastating tornado in Joplin, MO,

in 2011, key community stakeholders, such as local government, fire and rescue workers, and hospitals, have been focused on gathering information from a variety of resources, developing collaborative response plans, and preparing for a probable disaster. The Joint Commission (TJC) has advanced hospital efforts through the development of six crucial areas for emergency preparedness: communication, safety and security, resources and assets, staff responsibilities, utilities management, and patient clinical and support activities (The Joint Commission Resources, 2008). These crucial areas create a framework for all-hazards disaster preparedness planning in hospitals. So how does one go about preparing for an event in the workplace, and more specifically, the hospital environment? Traditionally the community hospital is a place of refuge for the sick and wounded. How is all of this impacted in the event of a disaster?

Health care executives across the country understand the need to dedicate resources to support effective all-hazards preparedness. The Health Insurance Portability and Accountability Act (HIPAA) and TJC require all health care facilities to have detailed all-hazard preparedness plans. Nursing leaders are an integral part of the planning process and should have knowledge of the national response plan (NRP) and state and local disaster response plans (Danna et al., 2009). Effective planning skills, for all-hazards preparedness is an essential management competency for nurse executives.

This chapter describes how to orchestrate a multilevel plan for a health care facility. A comprehensive all-hazards preparedness plan will assist in establishing the following: (1) an organized hospital-based plan for both internal and external disasters at the department/unit level, (2) an inter-hospital plan for effectively collaborating with other hospitals within a health care system and within the vicinity, (3) a community plan that will integrate the hospital plan with other external community plans, and (4) a national plan that will guide nurse leaders in accessing financial assistance from federal and state all-hazards preparedness resources.

DEFINITIONS

From a health care perspective, a **disaster** is an unforeseen and often sudden event of sufficient magnitude that causes great destruction, human suffering and most often requires external assistance (World Health Organization, 2005). There are a wide variety of types and causes of disasters. Although often triggered by nature, disasters can be caused by human acts; these can include biological, chemical, radiological, nuclear, cyber, or conventional terrorist events. Wars and civil disturbances that destroy homelands and displace people are included among man-made disasters. Causes of natural disasters include blizzards, wildfires, floods, tsunamis, volcanic eruptions, earthquakes, tornadoes, and hurricanes such as the devastation caused by Hurricane Katrina in 2005 or the earthquake and resulting tsunami in Japan in 2011. Disasters can be *internal,* such as a catastrophic event that occurs within a facility, making it difficult to maintain operations (TJC, 2012); or *external,* a catastrophic event that affects the community, which may or may not affect the facility.

Other disaster-related definitions are as follows:
- *All-hazards:* A general term that is descriptive of all types of natural and/or human terrorist events.
- *All-hazards disaster preparedness:* Multifaceted internal and external disaster preparedness that

establishes flexible and scalable action plans for every type of disaster or combination of disaster events (TJC, 2008).
- *Altered standards of care:* The definition of the term "altered standards" has not reached national consensus but generally is assumed to mean a shift to providing care and allocating scarce equipment, supplies, and personnel in a way that saves the largest number of lives, in contrast to the traditional focus on saving individuals (Agency for Healthcare Research and Quality [AHRQ], 2005a).
- *Biological disaster:* An incident occurring as a result of the deliberate or unintentional release of biological materials that may adversely affect the health of those exposed (U.S. Department of Defense, 2007).
- *Chemical disaster:* An incident occurring as a result of the deliberate or unintentional release of toxic chemical materials that may adversely affect the health of those exposed (U.S. Department of Defense, 2007).
- *Conventional disaster:* A catastrophic event caused by the use of weapons such as guns, bombs, missiles, or grenades.
- *Cyber disaster:* A catastrophic event that results from the use of information technology systems to control or disrupt critical infrastructure systems (U.S. Department of Veterans Affairs, 2005).
- *Hazard Vulnerability Analysis:* An exercise that identifies an organization's potential emergencies, the likelihood of the event occurring, and the impact it would have on the organization (California Hospital Association, 2009).
- *Mass casualty event (MCE):* A catastrophic public health or terrorism-related event that results in the community's health care system being overwhelmed by the needs of victims (AHRQ, 2005a. MCEs can be organized into two categories: (1) immediate or sudden impact; and (2) events resulting in ongoing or sustained impact (AHRQ, 2007).
- *Radiological/nuclear disaster:* A radiological or nuclear emergency that may result from accidents occurring within a facility (e.g., the departments of nuclear medicine and radiation oncology) or from external sources involving vehicles transporting radioactive materials (RAM) or caused by terrorism events (U.S. Department of Defense, 2007).

GETTING STARTED: FIRST STEPS

Starting any complex systems project can be confusing and difficult. Beginning the work of establishing a comprehensive all-hazards preparedness plan is no exception. Historically, most hospitals have had some type of disaster plan in place. Being the leader in the evaluation of the hospital's existing emergency operations plan (EOP), in light of a focus on maintaining a state of constant readiness, can be a complicated process. One of the first steps to gaining participation from appropriate stakeholders and moving the evaluation process forward is the creation of an oversight committee, or an all-hazards preparedness task force (AHPTF, referred to as *Task Force*). The nursing executive, often called the *chief nursing officer (CNO)*, will play a pivotal role in facilitating the initial Task Force.

Creating an All-Hazards Preparedness Task Force

As nurses know, effective projects that create lasting change start with the basic nursing process: assessment, planning, implementation, evaluation, and modification. The AHPTF will similarly follow this process. It is essential to get administrative support regarding the need for an all-hazards preparedness plan. This is best accomplished by establishing a high-level administrative Task Force whose purpose will be oversight of the multilevel all-hazards preparedness plan development. Whether the hospital is part of a larger health care system or is a freestanding, independent hospital, the Task Force will function similarly.

Health care systems with multiple facilities are very familiar with the complexity and intricacies of trying to establish a standardized system-wide approach to care needs. In organizations such as these, system-wide executive administrators need to be part of the Task Force. Having a senior executive administrator of the health care system serve as the chairperson of the Task Force will provide the leadership needed to communicate the importance of all-hazards preparedness as a system priority. A representative CNO and emergency medicine physician, serving as co-chairs with the senior executive administrator, will create a dynamic team that is uniquely prepared to tackle any issues that arise. A project facilitator is helpful in getting the Task Force started and operational. The project facilitator can also serve in a pivotal maintenance role, keeping the all-hazards preparedness plan current and in the forefront of the administration's strategic planning over time.

Establishing the Task Force requires that all departments be committed to the tasks at hand and cognizant of the need for consensus building and standardization of processes. Bidirectional communication is imperative. The standing membership should be composed of stakeholders representing all areas of the organization. Because not all departments can logistically be on the Task Force, the members will have large areas of oversight and communication. The Task Force membership might typically look like that outlined in Table 25-1.

As the team evolves in its work, ad hoc members can be added as needed. Internal ad hoc members might include radiology, facility engineering, telecommunications, volunteer support, chaplain services, physician chairs, social work, case management, and dietary, respiratory, and laboratory services. External ad hoc members might include representatives from the local public health department, government liaison, police, fire and rescue, public school system, representatives from the faith community, community physicians, and even vendor representatives, who can be contracted to provide such things as oxygen, ice, food, cots, and linens in the event of a disaster.

During the start up, the system-wide Task Force will need to meet frequently. To begin, the Task Force should perform a hazard vulnerability analysis (HVA). The HVA will be used as a starting point to create an EOP that addresses potential hazards that are identified specific to the organization (Joint Commission Resources, 2008). For specific details on the HVA process, there are several resources available including the Federal Emergency Management Agency (FEMA) and Joint Commission Resources websites.

TABLE 25-1	ALL-HAZARDS PREPAREDNESS TASK FORCE MEMBERSHIP RESPONSIBILITIES	
RESPONSIBILITY AREA(S)	**POSITION TITLE**	**DETAIL OF AREA COVERED**
Executive owner (chair)	Executive administrator	Leads the all-hazards preparedness task force as chair. If the hospital is part of a health care system, this person will be a system-wide senior administrator. If the hospital is a freestanding, independent facility, this person will be the hospital's chief operating officer.
Clinical operations (co-chair)	Chief nurse officer	Represents all nursing and clinical departments. Co-chairs the Task Force.
Chemical/radiological/ conventional threats (co-chair)	Emergency department/ air care medical director	Represents all aspects of emergency medicine and physician needs related to all-hazards preparedness. This person also will co-chair the Task Force.
Physician liaison(s)	Department chiefs	Serve as spokespersons for physician needs with regard to disaster preparedness. Facilitate communication of timely information should an event occur. Have oversight for physician credentialing in times of a disaster. Assist in approval of medical standards established for various types of disasters.
Chief operating officers (COOs) from health care system facilities	Chief operating officer(s)	Represent the needs of their facilities in establishing an effective all-hazards preparedness plan. Facilitate system-wide collaboration in standardizing practices and communicate essential information to employees.
Security	Safety and security director	Serves as liaison for system-wide safety and security departments in the system. Coordinates and synchronizes efforts of all departments as related to all-hazards preparedness. Responsible for rapid "lockdown" of all entrances and flow of people in the event of a disaster.
Communications	Chief information technology officer	Oversees successful operation of the integrated information system, including telephones, radios, and computers and satellite technology, during times of instability. Creates and maintains redundant systems to ensure an ability to communicate within facilities, outside to other hospitals, and partners with community.
Messages/media	Marketing director	Plays an active role in communicating the "All-Hazards Preparedness" message to all employees, patients, and community. Acts on behalf of the health care system or hospital in speaking with press about impending or actual disaster situations.
Human resources	Human resources director	Serves as the staff's voice in meeting the needs of employees during a disaster. Creates manuals to guide staff in preparing for and responding to a disaster.
Financial reimbursement	Chief financial officer	Leads efforts in monitoring financial expenses related to establishing an effective all-hazards preparedness plan. Seeks out state/federal reimbursement opportunities for planning.

TABLE 25-1	ALL-HAZARDS PREPAREDNESS TASK FORCE MEMBERSHIP RESPONSIBILITIES—cont'd	
RESPONSIBILITY AREA(S)	**POSITION TITLE**	**DETAIL OF AREA COVERED**
Government funding	Government affairs director	Serves as a vital link to local, state, and federal boards representing the system financial and operational needs regarding all-hazards preparedness. Advocates for funding related to all-hazards preparedness.
Biological threats	Infectious disease medical director	Serves as the liaison for all infection control (IC) departments in the system.
Infection control	Infection prevention and control practitioner	Coordinates and synchronizes efforts of all IC departments as related to all-hazards preparedness. Responsible for development, dissemination, and understanding of procedures related to biological events.
Legal	Executive attorney	Advises all-hazards preparedness task force in legal matters related to establishing an effective all-hazards preparedness plan.
Education planning	Education director	Has oversight for planning and implementing educational efforts for staff and patients. As needed, coordinates "just in time" training for any arising incident. Is an integral partner in planning and implementing internal and external disaster drills.
Logistics	Pharmacy director	Serves as the liaison for all system pharmacies. Has oversight for stockpiling medications for use in a disaster. Establishes par levels of drugs for use in "patient surge" situations. Establishes contracts with pharmaceutical vendors to ensure adequate supply of medications in the event of a disaster. Has oversight for any medical supply trucks ready for deployment in times of a disaster (e.g., stocking par level of drugs used in a chemical disaster).
Logistics	Materials management director	Serves as an active participant on the task force. This liaison is the system representative for all materials management departments. Is very involved in setting par levels for supplies and equipment on the units at the time of a disaster. Establishes contracts with materials management vendors to ensure adequate supply of medications in the event of a disaster (e.g., stocking a supplemental supply truck for use in a disaster).
Logistics	Engineering	Directs any operational building redesign needed to prepare hospital for handling a disaster (e.g., decontamination showers).

Courtesy Inova Health System, Falls Church, VA.
NOTE: This assessment tool was developed by Inova Health System based on a bioterrorism preparedness survey created by a committee consisting of representatives from Baylor University's Graduate Program in Healthcare Administration, the U.S. Army Center for Healthcare Education and Studies, and the University of Texas Health Science Center at San Antonio. (For more information, see Drenkard et al., 2002.)

Performing an Effective Gap Analysis

There are many ways to perform an all-hazards preparedness gap analysis and a multitude of online reference websites exist, including, but not limited to, the following examples:

- FEMA: *www.emforum.org/vforum/FEMA/Gap Analysis Program Guidance 03-13-2009.pdf*
- Office of Preparedness and Emergency Operations, U.S. Department of Health and Human Services: *www.hhs.gov* (*http://www.phe.gov/about/opeo/Pages/default.aspx*) American Hospital Association (AHA): *www.aha.org*
- Centers for Disease Control and Prevention (CDC): *www.cdc.gov*
- Agency for Healthcare Research and Quality (AHRQ): *www.ahrq.gov/research/epri*
- CCHC (Clinics and Community Health Centers) Emergency Preparedness Gap Analysis: *http://www.cpca.org/cpca/assets/File/Emergency-Preparedness/Resources/2011-08-11-Gap-Analysis-Tool-Final.pdf*

The guiding principle for creating a hospital-specific all-hazards gap analysis is to "keep it simple!" One example of a simple way to assess the current state is to create an emergency preparedness survey that is easy to read and requires the department directors to answer in simple checklists one of two ways: (1) "Yes, we have it," or (2) "No, we don't have it." Survey questions need to be concise and clear. The goal is to begin by identifying the areas where there are gaps in the facility's preparedness plans. Questions should be addressed to appropriate departments, who then assess the items and determine the current state. A review of the literature and online searches will assist the team in identifying the areas of assessment (Joint Commission Resources, 2008; Mangeri, 2006). Examples of questions to ask in the survey might include those listed in Box 25-1.

Once the survey is created, it should be distributed to all stakeholders. Directors should be challenged to complete and return it in 5 business days so that work can be initiated to address outstanding issues. The Task Force should review the survey results and start an issues list to address deficiencies. Nursing leaders will play key roles in creating aggressive timelines for resolving issues identified. Most resolutions will be modified and enhanced over time as the Task Force gains more knowledge about all-hazards planning.

BOX 25-1   HOSPITAL GAP ANALYSIS SURVEY: SAMPLE QUESTIONS

General
- Has your organization conducted a thorough hazard vulnerability analysis (HVA)?
- Does your organization have an emergency operations plan (EOP) that specifically addresses the four disaster phases?
- Does your EOP identify how to activate an emergency response and who is in charge of the command center in a disaster?
- Are those in charge identified by a vest or have some other sort of physical distinction?
- Does your facility have an operational command center to coordinate the hospital's response to a disaster?
- Does your department staff know the chain of command in an emergency?
- Does your department know their role in a disaster?
- Does your hospital know their role in the community in an emergency situation?
- Are there specific plans for biological, chemical, nuclear, and conventional emergencies? Do all staff in your department know their roles in each type of emergency?
- Is there a bed and staffing plan for surge capacity for 50 patients? 100 patients? 250 patients? Do you have portable cots contracted for use in a surge situation?

Human Resources
- Does your department staff know how to prepare themselves, their significant others, and pets in the event of a disaster?
- Is there a credentialing plan for health care professionals who come to the nearest facility in a disaster to volunteer their services?

Safety and Security
Does your facility have the following:
- A lockdown plan in case of an emergency?
- A plan for allowing staff to get to work and be allowed entry to hospital during an emergency?
- A plan for facility traffic flow during an emergency?
- Multi-language signage to direct people where to go during an emergency?

Communication
- Does your hospital have emergency-powered phones in case of a disaster?
- Does your facility have a backup radio system and volunteer staff to run it?

BOX 25-1   HOSPITAL GAP ANALYSIS SURVEY: SAMPLE QUESTIONS—cont'd

- Does your facility have a tiered paging system that can reach multiple staff simultaneously?
- Does your department know the central command center telephone number (if there is one)?
- Is there an on-call procedure for notifying the administrator on-call and opening the command center in the event of a disaster?
- Are there established linkages to the external community (e.g., other hospitals in the region, fire department, police, emergency medical system, public schools, public health)?
- Do the telephone operators know how to link patients and families both in your facility and in the community should a disaster occur?
- Is there an on-call list for administrative coverage of the command center? If so, do the telephone operators know how to contact the administrator on-call for the command center?
- Is there a plan for contacting essential employees and administrators in a disaster?

Logistics

- Does your facility have:
  - Backup emergency supplies, pharmaceuticals, and equipment?
  - The ability to release and send pharmaceuticals, medical supplies, and equipment such as respirators to the areas in need in the event of a chemical or biological emergency?
  - Prearranged plans with physicians, ambulances, nearby churches, and nursing homes to clear beds in an emergency? (What sites can take patients?)
  - Contracts with vendors to bring in food, ice, oxygen, and other needed supplies?
- Is there an established written psychosocial role for social work, chaplains, psychiatry, employee health, and case management in the event of a disaster?
- Are there contingency plans for 4 to 5 days for no power, no water, no computers, and/or no food?
- Are there contingency plans for staff to report to nearest facility to work?
- Are there contingency plans for childcare during an emergency so that parents can work?
- Is there common nomenclature used during an emergency so that everyone understands what is happening and who has what responsibility?

Clinical Operations

- Does your facility have:
  - Procedures established to maximize staff safety in the event of a disaster?
  - Procedures for fit testing of respiratory masks for staff?
  - Procedures and training for using protective equipment?
  - The ability to track patients until discharge, admission, or death using HIPAA guidelines?
  - Clear established policies and procedures to respond to biological, chemical, nuclear, and conventional emergencies?
  - A decontamination area and detailed step-by-step procedures on how to work in this area?
  - A backup staff to assist with people/patients arriving to the hospital?
- Does your facility have procedures for how to:
  - Track available beds?
  - Track staff working and direct them to a designated area?
  - Track volunteer staff and direct them to a designated area?
  - Track arriving patients and direct them to a designated area?
  - Operate every department of the hospital during an emergency?
  - Track discharged patients and direct them to a designated area?
  - Handle surge capacity situations?
  - Handle OR cases in the event of an emergency?
- Track biological, chemical, or nuclear events and report them to authorities?

Financial

- Is there an established plan to tracking costs during an emergency?
- Is there an established plan for submitting for disaster reimbursement?

Messages/Media

- Is there an established communication plan in case of an emergency?
- Is there an established communication script in the event of an emergency?
- Is there an alternative communication plan if power, telephones, and radios are not working?

Courtesy Inova Health System. From Drenkard, K., & Rigotti, G. (2002, updated 2011). *Inova Health System survey.* Falls Church, VA: Inova Health System.

From the gap analysis, the Task Force should establish high-level, multifaceted standards of practice and system-wide goals for all-hazards preparedness. These standards and goals will be implemented at the facility level and department level as directed by the chief operating officer (COO), CNO, and emergency department medical director. At this point, there is latitude for departments to design and implement the standards and goals based on the unique needs of the populations served. Annual review and evaluation of goals is an effective project management activity, with new goals being created based on the HVA, changing regulatory requirements, and the results of gaps identified during drills. Sustaining attention and focus on disaster preparedness efforts becomes a key role of the nurse executive in ensuring a constant state of organizational readiness. The project facilitator could be very valuable in assisting the nurse executive in researching new initiatives evolving in the discipline of all-hazards preparedness, determining the importance of new trends to the effective operations of the health care organization's all-hazard plan, and implementing relevant enhancements that support the strategic vision for preparedness within the organization.

Keeping the Momentum Going

Once the gap analysis is completed and the issues are identified, development of a comprehensive plan is a critical next step. The work can appear daunting, and it is hard to know where to start. It is at this point that nursing leadership has the opportunity to take charge of the process. Even though the gap analysis may show a multitude of areas for improvement, issues are solvable one step at a time. The CNO and nurse leaders can help focus the Task Force and

---

RESEARCH NOTE

Source

Christian, M.D., Hawryluck, L., Wax, R.S., Cook, T., Lazar, N.M., Herridge, M.S., et al. (2006). Development of a triage protocol for critical care during an influenza pandemic. *Canadian Medical Association Journal, 175*(11), 1377-1381.

Purpose

The development of a protocol for use in determining which patients should receive care is a necessary tool, but this is one that is subject to interpretation in a crisis situation. Planning in advance and creating a method for distributing potentially scarce resources, such as ventilators and antiviral medications, is a key activity that should be carried out by health care organizations. The purpose of this research process was to develop a protocol that could be used to prioritize access to critical care resources.

Discussion

The researchers applied a collaborative process including expert panels, consultation, and ethical principles application to create a triage protocol for prioritizing access to resources that might be needed during a pandemic, including mechanical ventilation and antiviral medications. The triage protocol describes an assessment tool called the *Sequential Organ Failure Assessment (SOFA)* score and has four main components: inclusion criteria, exclusion criteria, minimum qualifications for survival, and a prioritization tool.

Basically, a patient is assessed using clinical parameters and receives a score in each of the key clinical indicators, including respiratory status, hemodynamic status (i.e., blood pressure and shock symptoms), kidney function, end-organ function, and cardiac function. If a patient meets exclusion criteria (e.g., metastatic malignant disease), then he or she is excluded from treatment. Patients arriving at treatment centers would be assigned a SOFA score, which would then guide clinical triage decision making. Training results indicated 36% of staff had received training. Only 3.2% of facilities reported meeting all 10 of the readiness criteria.

Application to Practice

The authors noted that "This protocol is intended to provide guidance for making triage decisions during the initial days to weeks of an influenza pandemic if the systems and resources for providing critical care become overwhelmed. Although the authors designed this protocol for use during an influenza pandemic, the triage protocol would apply to patients both with and without influenza, since all patients must share a single pool of critical care resources." A key practice application will be planning well in advance about how to apply a tool such as the SOFA scale. Once the scale is available for use, a plan needs to be developed to ensure that a process exists for initiating the protocol as well as for identifying key clinical decision makers who have the challenge of putting the protocol into action.

department directors. Focused effort on creating a streamlined, comprehensive internal all-hazards preparedness plan will set the foundation for later steps when the hospital begins to work externally with the community.

Working the Issues List

Over the next phase, the development of an issues list will become the working action plan used to prioritize and organize work to be done. Subgroups made up of members from the Task Force, who are content experts, can be assigned to lead efforts to resolve issues. Issues need to be constantly added and resolved on an ongoing basis as the facility refines the plan. Reports from subgroup progress should be relayed to the Task Force at least monthly, depending on the meeting schedule of the Task Force. The Task Force should have oversight for the subgroups and should strive to "clear the road" for subgroup progress as needed. Hospitals may need to address some common issues such as allocation of resources, including funds to educate staff. Educating the nursing workforce will be critical to promoting an effective disaster response (National Advisory Council on Nurse Education and Practice, 2009.

Establishing a Common Nomenclature, Structure, and Role Definition for Writing All-Hazards Preparedness Plans

When working with the community, recognizable nomenclature becomes especially important for communication in crisis situations. Therefore the National Incident Management System (NIMS) was created by the U.S. Department of Homeland Security Secretary to further standardize and integrate response practices nationally (Emergency Medical Services Authority, 2006):

> NIMS is designed to provide a framework for interoperability and compatibility among the various members of the response community. The end result is a flexible framework that facilitates governmental and nongovernmental agencies working together at all levels during all phases of an incident regardless of size. NIMS also provides standardized organizational structures and requirements for process and procedures. (p. 13).

In the past, the limited focus of the disaster plan on file at a hospital usually related specifically to safety and security preparedness. Today the primary responsibility of the safety and security department, in conjunction with nursing leadership, is to develop or refine the hospital's EOP for incidents based on the HVA. The safety and security department needs to have assigned oversight for facility security, quick lockdown or controlled access, and management of people flowing into and out of the hospital.

Nursing leadership needs to ensure that all facility departments understand their role in a disaster situation. The role of the staff nurse in a disaster must be clearly defined and contain performance standards, including policies that speak to expected hours or refusal to work (Danna et al., 2009). Nurse leaders are the coordinators in synchronizing department plans so that everything fits together to meet the essential needs of the staff, patients, hospital, and community. Once the comprehensive all-hazards preparedness plans are complete, every department should understand their identified written role.

Creating Procedural Annexes to All-Hazards Preparedness Plans

In addition to the overall all-hazards preparedness plans, the hospital will need to define procedures regarding what will be done in any biological, chemical, nuclear/radiological, or conventional disaster, and the surge capacity needs related to any of the events. *Surge capacity* refers to a health care system's ability to rapidly expand or flex up beyond normal capacity to meet an increased demand for qualified personnel, beds, and medical care services in the event of a large-scale emergency or disaster (Adams, 2009; AHRQ, 2005b). These specific procedures are added separately to the plan and are called annexes. The Task Force can assign the creation of each of these procedures to a subgroup. These teams are often led by nursing leadership and the emergency medicine director with appropriate ad hoc participation. For example, the infection prevention and control department, in partnership with public health, can co-lead the biological planning efforts; the radiology department can co-lead the nuclear/radiological efforts, partnering closely with local authorities; and nursing, pharmacy, and emergency medicine can co-lead the conventional, chemical, and surge capacity efforts, partnering closely with police, fire, and rescue. The goal with these procedural annexes is to create easy, step-by-step action plans, fact sheets, and algorithms for identifying, intervening, and notifying the appropriate authorities. As with most all-hazards preparedness literature, the most current references will be online. Some essential websites to assist in writing specific hospital procedures include the CDC, the Department of Homeland Security (DHS), and the U.S. Department of Labor's Occupational Safety and Health Administration (OSHA).

In establishing procedural annexes and the overall all-hazards disaster preparedness plan, the general thought in the literature is to be able to surge beyond daily capacity and plan to manage without external assistance for several days (Kaji, 2007). The Joint Commission's emergency management accreditation standards call for hospitals to sustain disaster operations for at least 96 hours should an external disaster occur that impacts the local area or region (TJC, 2012). Lessons learned from Hurricane Katrina illustrate just how long it can take before assistance is available. Hospital leadership needs to make sure every operating unit and department is prepared. In general, the following are only a few examples of what hospitals will need:

- A conservative stockpile of essential antibiotics for biological threats
- Antidotes for chemical exposures
- Basic food and bottled water surpluses for environmental contamination events
- Preplanned contracts with local supply companies and businesses for ice, oxygen and other gases, and emergency power
- Alternative communication methods and plans, both internally and externally, in case of power outage
- Staff and volunteer credentialing and identification procedures
- Established entrances for staff during lockdowns or controlled access situations
- Patient identification systems for families in search of loved ones
- Downtime procedures for cyber threats (with the ability to function up to 5 days)
- Accommodations for staff to bring in their children for care while they are working

Creating an All-Hazards Planning Subgroup

Even with comprehensive all-hazards preparedness plans and annexes, the unexpected will happen, as in threats and incidents involving anthrax, severe acute respiratory syndrome (SARS), monkeypox, smallpox, and potentially harmful H1N1 influenza. Initially, no one will know whether these are true terrorist threats or isolated spontaneous incidents. At all times, the hospital must be ready to respond. An ongoing all-hazards planning subgroup needs to be formed and chaired by a nurse executive who sits on the Task Force, along with key stakeholder membership (including emergency department, employee health staff, and infection prevention and control). Based on the changing needs of the events, this planning subgroup will enable the facility to respond quickly to the "just in time" educational needs of the staff, allow for rapid procedural planning for community needs, and ensure appropriate authority notification in the event of a disaster. For example, the staff will be expected to recognize the symptoms and presentation of smallpox and respond by critical thinking, as follows:

- Triaging and isolating the patient on admission to the emergency department (ED) and placing the patient in the hospital or facility negative pressure room if available
- Obtaining and having the staff wear appropriate personal protective equipment (PPE)
- Controlling access to the ED and possibly the entire hospital.
- Identifying (name, address, telephone number) all patient contacts, transport services (emergency medical services [EMS]), staff, and patients in the waiting room
- Notifying the infection prevention and control practitioner, hospital/facility infectious disease physician or epidemiologist, public health officials, and police

Developing a Command Center

In the event of a disaster, the hospital would need a dedicated centralized command center where all department directors can report for instructions. The four essential elements of a command center, explained in more detail in later sections, are as follows:

1. Setting up the room
2. Developing processes in the command center

3. Establishing the hospital's role in the community
4. Testing the all-hazards preparedness plans and command center functionality

Setting up the Command Center Room. The location of the incident command center will depend on the organization's physical layout; however, it often is located near the safety and security department. It is commanded by the on-call administrator along with the CNO, the ED medical director, and the safety and security director. The following equipment should be available in the room:

- Multiple telephones/telephone lines with speed dial for frequently called numbers
- Computer access (with both intranet and Internet capabilities)
- Printing capability
- Batch fax and copying capabilities
- Alternative phone options (e.g., 800 MHz radio technology and/or voice over Internet Protocol technology—a phone system that operates over Internet lines with functioning antenna) and people trained to use them
- Tiered paging capability
- Television access
- Office-related supplies such as paper, pens, easels, dry erase boards, work tables, phone books, and reference materials such as the all-hazards preparedness plans for each hospital area

The command center should be available at a moment's notice and fully functional within minutes. A common scenario is that the call comes into the ED; however many internal disasters, such as utility failures, may come from other sources. When an external disaster occurs, nursing leadership staff in the ED, along with medical staff, will determine the gravity of the situation and decide whether the incident can be handled in the ED or whether the hospital administrator needs to be contacted. If it is deemed appropriate to contact the hospital administrator, there will be dialogue among nursing leadership, medical leadership, and the administrator to decide whether the command center should be opened. If the command center is to be opened, the hospital administrator will start the process and call in the additional staff necessary to assist with incident command operations. In the event that the disaster involves the area where the command center is located, the hospital will have to have a predetermined plan to establish a back-up command center in another location. In the

case of a multifacility system, the alternate command center could be at another hospital.

Developing Processes in the Command Center. Because one of the rotating on-call administrators may be called upon to open the command center, the creation of a simple, step-by-step, short document (one to two pages) of how to open, operate, and close down the command center is important. A more extensive manual can also be created, but in times of a disaster, the short "How to Open the Command Center" document is crucial. If the facility does not have an on-call administrator list, one should be established; and staff must know how to reach the on-call person(s). A clear decision matrix should be in place, outlining when to open the command center and who needs to be notified. It may be helpful to create a communication tree identifying the process for notifying administrative team and AHPTF members quickly. Using a group paging function can be helpful for rapid notification of the leadership team.

To facilitate the incident command structure during a disaster, many hospitals have adopted the Hospital Incident Command System (HICS) for their all-hazards preparedness plans, because it allows logical standardization with common nomenclature that is understood both in the hospital environment and in the community setting (U.S. Department of Homeland Security, 2008). In addition, the HICS organizational chart provides a comprehensive structure that is scalable to the size of the event and has standardized role descriptions. Techniques such as using vests to identify people in charge during a disaster with a one-page job action sheet in each vest pocket are essential in a crisis situation. Color-coded vests may also be useful in identifying the role of each leader based on the incident command structure utilized. All hospital and department all-hazards preparedness plans must be on hand and clearly labeled in the command center, along with in-house phone and pager directories.

Testing the All-Hazards Preparedness Plans and Command Center. Having comprehensive all-hazards preparedness plans requires frequent (at least biannual) drills to work through problems and allow for a streamlined preparedness plan that are flexible and sustainable (Mahan et al., 2007). There are many types of drills, including the following:

- *Internal drills* to test specific department and/or hospital responses; examples include setting up and operating the command center, recognizing a biological event both in the emergency department and on the units, locking down the hospital entrances, simulating decontamination processes, operating using downtime procedures during a communications or cyber disaster event, and handling various surge capacity situations

- *External drills* in collaboration with community agencies and departments involving patients (police, fire, and rescue; public health); tabletop drills simulating an unknown biological, nuclear/radiological, or chemical scenario and prioritizing the response by departments; and surge capacity drills, testing a community's ability to respond to overwhelming demand.

All of these drills offer great insight into the merit of the all-hazards preparedness plan and allow facilities the opportunity to modify plans to improve processes.

Establishing the Hospital's Role in the Community. The hospital will play an important role in the community in the case of a disaster. Knowing how the hospital fits into the all-hazards disaster response plan from the perspective of such entities as the police and fire departments, EMS, public health department, and the local school system will be important in coordinating efforts. The Task Force will be instrumental in defining the hospital's role locally in the community, as well as nationally to meet federal government expectations and regulatory compliance.

On a local level, the lead person of the Task Force (often this will be a designated hospital administrator) will partner with public health, local police, fire departments, EMS, community physicians, regional alliances with other health care facilities, and local emergency management agencies/councils. It will be important to define the hospital's and community's role in emergency situations. Testing of plans using local community disaster drills, often biannually, is essential to continually improve processes. The hospital should strive to test its internal all-hazards preparedness plans whenever there is a planned community drill in order to get a full picture of its ability to respond in a disaster in step with the community response.

Nationally, each hospital will play an important role in the political arena by helping local and federal government personnel understand that hospitals, like police and fire departments, are first responders in a disaster. The materials, equipment, and training required for hospitals to prepare adequately for their role in responding to disasters are very expensive. Capital expenditures will be required to create decontamination facilities; purchase PPE; train and educate staff on effective all-hazards preparedness; stockpile emergency equipment, supplies, and pharmaceuticals; ensure adequate isolation rooms; and outfit a hospital command center. Hospitals need financial assistance to do this well, and the AHPTF members can be advocates for federal and state funding. It is helpful to establish a financial subgroup whose mission will be to develop a set plan for capturing costs related to the event as the disaster unfolds. This will enable the hospital to submit immediately for any reimbursement funding that becomes available after the event. In addition, the subgroup can identify potential federal grants or public funding that might be available to support expensive financial expenditures.

Helping Staff Overcome Fear Associated with Disaster and All-Hazards Preparedness

It is important to know that the first rule of disaster preparedness is to keep staff safe. In a disaster, the paradigm of keeping the patient safe first must be modified to focus on helping staff members (and their families) feel as safe as possible. This may be a shift in thinking, but the reality is that if staff members do not feel comfortable coming to work, then the patients' needs cannot be met.

Nursing leadership, in partnership with human resources and the education department, will need to develop educational tools to assist staff in creating personal disaster preparedness plans for themselves and their significant others. Many websites are available to assist in developing educational tools, such as the FEMA and the America Red Cross websites. Tools such as personal disaster preparedness plans should be effectively communicated so that employees know that the facility will "keep staff safe" as their first priority in a disaster. Then when a disaster occurs, the staff will feel as comfortable as possible coming to work. Arrangements will need to be made for 24-hour childcare somewhere close to the hospital or on-site. Employee assistance programs need to be available at all times to help employees cope with fear related to a disaster. It is important that nurse leaders understand the psychological impact of a disaster on the victims as well as the staff (Tillman, 2011).

LEADERSHIP AND MANAGEMENT IMPLICATIONS

Moving into the Future with Confidence

Nursing leaders can effect change and ensure that a fully functional all-hazards preparedness plan for the hospital is developed within 6 to 12 months. The journey toward preparedness is ongoing and constant. Nursing leadership competencies in disaster planning and crisis management are invaluable, and fortunately they have been developed by a collaborative group led by the Department of Veterans Affairs, Office of Nursing Services. These disaster competencies are categorized into four domains: assessment of the disaster scene, technical skills, risk communication, and critical thinking (Coyle et al., 2007).

Clearly, nurse executives are in a position to take a greater role in planning and implementing a disaster response for their organizations. Nurse leaders are called upon to take charge, make decisions, successfully implement protocols, and then modify their action plans based on routine evaluation. Emotional competencies include good interpersonal skills, excellent and clear communication skills, and calm, controlled delegation (Fahlgren & Drenkard, 2002). In addition, being willing to take risks is an important attribute of the nursing leader. Nurse executives are in a unique position to forge new pathways in the arena of disaster preparedness because of their combination of clinical skills, strong organizational ability, networking expertise, and training in clinical crises. If the AHPTF is not diligent in its efforts to keep everyone focused on preparedness, there may even be a sense of complacency about refining all-hazard preparedness plans instead of the necessary awareness that improvements must be ongoing. With strong nursing leadership at the managerial and executive level, the oversight of disaster planning can be proactively addressed, and a constant state of readiness can be achieved.

CURRENT ISSUES AND TRENDS

Current nursing and medical literature is focused on specific departments and how they are establishing their unique roles and responsibilities in a disaster. Nurse leaders can use these benchmark articles to motivate units and departments to move forward in fully assessing and defining their roles in all-hazards preparedness. As the CNO explores the breadth of disaster nursing within his or her facility, care can be enhanced in many ways during a disaster. For instance, making decisions about consolidating care sites may require closing clinics, emergency care centers, and community health programs during a disaster to free up clinical staff to assist in a hospital's surge capacity planning in a disaster, provide staff for vaccination teams in a biological event, or help with decontamination in a chemical exposure event. Allocation of staff may be required to build capacity in outpatient and community arenas depending on the disaster threat. Decisions about alternate care sites should be considered well ahead of an event and often require regional collaboration across many disciplines and agencies.

As we continue in the "new world order," in which all-hazards preparedness is a way of life and knowledge about the level of alertness is an everyday expectation, hospital staff and leadership have begun to settle in at a heightened state of preparedness. In April 2011, the federal government implemented a new alert system, the National Terrorism Advisory System (NTAS), which replaced the colored coded system implemented by the Department of Homeland Security. The new two-level system will alert the American public about an "elevated threat," in the event of a credible terrorist threat; or an "imminent threat," if a credible and specific terrorist threat is about to occur (U.S. Department of Homeland Security, 2012).

One area of all-hazards preparedness that has not been fully developed, yet has great potential in disaster planning, is the role of various community resources such as outpatient centers and even churches. The nurse executive can facilitate the establishment of partnerships between the hospital and the community facilities. Once established, these partnerships can be used to set up communication centers where people can congregate to receive support and obtain information about the disaster situation or family and friends who may have been injured.

To effectively manage large-scale events, networking beyond the hospital will be critical to create partnerships with other facilities, hospitals, community agencies, and local, state, and federal departments. To assist in this process it may be helpful to have a signed agreement or "memorandum of understanding" (MOU) with community organizations and businesses for assistance. A trend is underway, evidenced by a growing alliance between regional hospitals and the community at large throughout the United States, to strategically plan for allocation and sharing of federal and state resources in the event of a disaster. As an example, in Virginia, a Regional Hospital Command Center (RHCC) has been established in which 14 northern Virginia hospitals have been networked to more effectively respond in a disaster. This is accomplished via radio communication and a shared web-based bed availability tracking system, displaying each hospital's ability to take varying levels of patient acuities. These hospitals can directly link with hospitals in Washington, D.C., to coordinate efforts during an event and communicate effectively with fire, police, EMS, public health, the emergency operating center (a local command center for overseeing the event), and the field incident commander in coordinating the disaster response. Cohorts of hospitals, firefighters, EMS, law enforcement, schools, public health, and businesses, similar to the Virginia RHCC just mentioned, are joining together to form regional alliances and collaborations to leverage their capability to respond in a coordinated manner.

Under the direction of NIMS, incident management assistance teams (IMATs) were created to provide rapidly deployable supplemental assistance to the region affected by a disaster. These teams consist of "trained personnel from different departments, organizations, agencies, and jurisdictions within a state or DHS Urban Area Security Initiative region, activated to support incident management at major or complex emergency incidents or special events that extend beyond one operational period" (FEMA, 2010).

Building on the idea of partnering with the community to strengthen preparedness, in 2012, the current Secretary of Homeland Security, Janet Napolitano, commissioned the implementation of a community-based assistance program called FEMA Corps. FEMA Corps will "help communities prepare for, respond to, and recover from disasters by supporting disaster recovery centers; assisting in logistics, community relations, and outreach; and performing other critical functions. We know from experience that quick deployment of trained personnel is critical during a crisis.

The FEMA Corps will provide a pool of trained personnel, and it will also pay long-term dividends by adding depth to our reserves–individuals trained in every aspect of disaster response who augment our full-time FEMA staff" (*http://blog.fema.gov/2012/03/announcing-creation-of-fema-corps.html*). Hospital executives need to stay abreast of these newly emerging resources and explore ways to partner with them. These types of programs will be pivotal in providing extra manpower and support services desperately needed for hospitals to function effectively in times of crisis.

One other emerging issue that challenges care during a disaster is allocation of scarce resources when the system is overwhelmed. This need was directly experienced in the United States during the Hurricane Katrina event, and was also witnessed with the Haiti earthquake, and again with the tsunami in Japan. As a result of these devastating events, both the state and national disaster preparedness leaders are examining planning needs for response requirements when resources are scarce. These efforts include substantial planning efforts to address immediate needs, including ethical considerations and planning assumptions, as well as management issues regarding responder protection, with the health care workforce as a primary concern. In recommendations of the Ethics Subcommittee of the Advisory Committee to the Director, Centers for Disease Control and Prevention (CDC), ethical guidelines were outlined for pandemic planning (CDC, 2007). To maximize the level of national and regional preparedness, these principles included the identification of clear overall goals, principles of transparency in decision making, public engagement and involvement in the process, use of sound scientific evidence for decision making, and thinking in a global context.

The guidelines recommended early planning efforts that balance utilitarian concepts with respect of persons, nonmaleficence, and justice. The recommendations gave examples of distribution criteria that will need to be considered well ahead of the time of an actual event. The development of triage criteria for allocation of scarce resources has been documented in several articles (Hick & O'Laughlin, 2006; Kraus et al., 2007). Also, adopting standards of care under altered conditions has been described and addressed in numerous documents from states and associations seeking to offer guidelines to care providers (American Nurses Association, 2007; New York State Department of Health Task Force on Life and the Law, 2007; Phillips & Knebel, 2007). Each nursing leader and team needs to understand these guidelines and begin the planning process at both a local and a regional level for developing protocols to allocate scarce resources and implementing triage criteria for care in overwhelming events. Implementing periodic tabletop discussions regarding how to allocate resources in a time of scarcity will prove to be a powerful tool in setting the stage for what to do if such an event occurs. Collaborative professional staff and hospital leadership discussions about scarce resource allocation will present ethical dilemmas that need to be thoughtfully considered in

a planning time that is devoid of emotion. Questions to be discussed at the tabletop include (1) Which hospital and/or clinical leader will make the final decision about ventilator allocation and other scarce resource distribution? (2) What are the criteria used to determine which patients receive aggressive treatment and which will receive palliative care, both imminently and long term, as other life-threatening complications ensue? (3) How are prophylactic pharmaceutical dissemination plans going to be activated to protect staff and their families? Knowing the hospital's approach to handling these types of scenarios will be a critical precursor in implementing an effective plan in the event of a disaster that is compounded by a shortage of resources.

CASE STUDY

Day 1 (Wednesday):
A hurricane's projected path takes it north over mountainous regions near your area. It will be a tropical storm by the time it reaches you in 2 days. The winds are forecast to be in the 50 mph range with higher gusts in the 60 to 65 mph range. Conditions are such that tornado watches are predicted. Heavy rains are expected to reach 10 inches, because the weather system is moving slowly. Your community hospital is 50 miles from the nearest health care facility, is not in a direct flood plain (it is located near the commercial area of your town), and has an average daily inpatient occupancy of 120. Your service line includes a small 8-bed pediatric wing; a 12-bed labor, delivery, and postpartum unit; an emergency department; 4 operating rooms; and a 10-bed medical-surgical intensive care unit.

Considerations:
How do you plan for the following areas of potential impact on service given the weather forecast?

Communications	What are your redundant systems? At this point who would you communicate with about preplanning (both in the hospital and with community partners)?
Safety and security	Are there particular safety issues to be concerned about with the approaching storm?
Resources and assets	Do you have adequate supplies, including fuel, food, water and staffing, in the event your transportation avenues are cut off?
Staff responsibilities	Is your staff prepared to come in to work if needed and have their homes and families prepared for the storm? Does your staff understand the "essential personnel" requirements for health care facilities?
Utilities management	What types of redundancy might you expect would be needed in your facility's department functions? Are there any preparations that should take place in the days before this forecasted event?
Patient clinical and support activities	Do you want to consider decreasing the number of inpatients via early discharge? Should you consider canceling elective surgeries at this point?

Day 3 (Friday, 4 PM):
The tropical storm hits, with the predicted high winds and heavy rain. Your ED is receiving an increase in

Continued

motor vehicle accidents, some with severe injuries that potentially need transfer out to a trauma center. No helicopters are flying because of the poor weather. Trees are down and multiple roads in the community are flooding. Staff begins to become concerned about their homes, and incoming evening shift staff is calling stating that roads are blocked and they are attempting to find alternate routes in. Electricity has been flickering off and on for the past hour. The outside temperatures are in the 70s, with relative humidity at 100%.

Considerations:

- Do you set up your incident command center, if not already done?
- Do you have a written incident action plan already in your emergency operations plan, which addresses potential power outages, staffing and supply chain shortages, and facility integrity?
- What is your plan for the next 12 hours? For the next 24 hours?
- Who have you communicated with regarding your plan?
- Do staff, patients, and community partners all know of your situation and your plan?
- What do you have in place for lighting and cooling during the night hours if the power completely fails?

Day 4 (Saturday, 7 AM)

Staff is now unable to get in to or go home from the hospital. You are holding 27 patients in the ED, some of whom have been discharged but have no transportation home. One patient is a trauma patient who needs surgery and blood transfusions, but there is no transport available because of the road conditions. The power failed around 5 AM, and you are running on 100% generator power. Local media are calling in to ask about your plans, and if you have food and power.

Considerations:

- What is your internal surge plan?
- Do you have a plan for managing discharged patients and families who cannot leave?
- How are you staffing your incident command at this point? Which positions are filled, and what are your operational objectives?
- How are you communicating with your staff, patients, and the public?
- How are you feeding everyone? Is there a plan for cold food storage and possible need to prepare

food without power? Is there a plan for conservation of food supplies or for alternate sources because resupply chains are unable to get into town?

- What is your water supply situation?
- Do you have a plan for lighting after it gets dark?
- Where are staff sleeping/resting?
- How are you getting cell phones charged? What about staff's personal phones?

Day 5: (Sunday, 5 PM)

The tropical storm has stalled over the nearby mountains, causing massive flooding. Your hospital has been sheltering patients in place for 2 days, but you are now told that the community water treatment plants have failed, and an advisory to boil water has been issued. The temperatures are in the upper 70s; relative humidity is at 100%. Residents in the community are arriving at the hospital looking for power, food, and clean water. The pharmacy tells you it is low or out of many critical medications needed for treatment of infection and pain control.

Considerations:

- What is your plan for clean, potable water for staff and patient use?
- Is water available to keep the electrical system "chillers" operational?
- Do you have adequate fuel to continue running the generators?
- Where will you get more fuel, because the roads are blocked by high water and/or downed lines and trees?
- How are you handling sanitary systems/waste disposal?
- Are you able to perform surgeries?
- Without air conditioning, is the environment safe for continuing patient care?
- When the sun comes out tomorrow, the temperatures will rise into the 90s. How will you keep patients and staff cool?
- How can food be prepared without power? Do you have enough supplies for feeding staff and patients?
- How do you handle the influx of people who are not patients?
- Who are your community partners who might help in this scenario? Are they overwhelmed as well?
- Where could you get emergency supplies of medications?

CASE STUDY—cont'd

Day 6: (Monday, 8 AM)

A tornado strikes the commercial district next to your facility. You lose many windows, all power is out, and water pressure drops significantly. Injured people are arriving at your ED for care. You decide to begin a systematic evacuation of your facility.

Considerations:

- CAN you evacuate? Are there open routes?
- What do you do about people continuing to arrive at your facility?
- Do you set up an alternate care site for ED patients?
  You find that one transportation route will be open around noon, although it takes approximately twice as long to travel to the nearest hospital taking that route.
- What resources do you have to coordinate with to plan this evacuation?
- How do you prioritize the order in which patients are evacuated?
- How are communications handled with power out?

- How is medical information documented and readied for transfer?
- How do you tag patients being transferred?
- Does your staff go with patients or stay behind?
- Do families get to go with their loved ones being transferred?
- How can you notify families of patients who are evacuated?
- How will you handle media inquiries/presence?
- How will you support critical care patients with all power shut down?
- How do you coordinate patient tracking for reunification purposes once patients are moved?

After Action:

Did your incident command team maintain planning using the six critical areas of preparedness (communications, resources and assets, safety and security, staff responsibilities, utilities management, patient clinical and support activities), which are key to successful responses? Did you document every action over the past 6 days, with time, date, and names?

CRITICAL THINKING EXERCISE

The All-Hazards Preparedness Task Force has been debriefed on an incident involving a chemical exposure from a patient who attempted suicide by ingesting a poisonous chemical. A review of the current literature on chemical exposures to aluminum phosphide is limited; however, it does reveal that severe off-gassing will occur from the gastrointestinal and respiratory tracts. The team decides that a planning session is needed to create a protocol for caring for patients with this type of chemical exposure because it could threaten the safety of the ED staff and patients. Members of the Task Force and the appropriate stakeholders from the ED have gathered to begin planning how your hospital is going to respond should this incident or a similar one occur again.

Planning process: Readiness preparation for chemical exposures in the ED.

Purpose: To prepare and educate staff on how to care for a patient who has been exposed to dangerous chemicals before presenting to the ED and be prepared to protect other ED patients, staff, and the facility from harm.

Background information: You are the chief nurse officer of a 500-bed hospital that serves as the leader of the community for acute care response. You are leading the effort to develop a plan to better respond to chemical exposures from patients who present to the ED after ingesting a chemical that when ingested creates a poisonous gas and a danger to everyone around the patient.

1. What planning framework should you use to develop the plan for addressing a chemical exposure in the ED?
2. What triage considerations need to be included in the plan if you are already aware of the chemical ingestion?
3. What considerations will you include to identify where to care for this type of patient? Is there an adequate negative pressure room?
4. Is there an alternate location such as a decontamination tent that could be used?

5. What is the chain of command in notification of a chemical exposure event that could threaten the staff and ED patients and may require closing your ED?
6. What training needs exist for the staff that can be completed pre-event? What "just in time" training needs are evident? How will this training be delivered during an emerging event?
7. How will the staff be protected from exposure to off-gassing? What PPE should staff wear?
8. What ethical considerations need to be addressed in the planning process? Knowing this is almost always a lethal ingestion and off-gassing presents a danger to caregivers, how aggressive should the treatment be?
9. What should be done to secure the area ED, and how do you keep other patients safe?

Data Management and Clinical Informatics

Jane M. Brokel

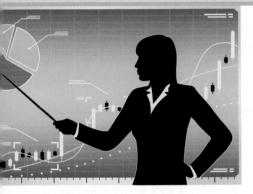

evolve WEBSITE

http://evolve.elsevier.com/Huber/leadership/

The information and knowledge age has pushed decision support toward greater sharing and exchanging of patient and population data. In the past 40 years, society has seen the widespread adoption of wireless personal computers, smart phones with database and digital applications and multi-messaging capabilities, global positioning systems, and satellite and cable networks for real-time broadcasting and contiguous communication. Information can now be transmitted or exchanged across the world, immediately, in a variety of formats. Information technology has changed the way people work, play, learn, manage their personal lives, and view the world. Consequently, information and evidence-based knowledge databases and applications have become a commodity to be bought, sold, and managed.

The business of health care information technologies is evolving rapidly. Management of the health care industry and care delivery relies extensively on the device capture, collection, and analysis of data. Data about the patient, provider, outcomes, and processes of care delivery are collected from many individuals practicing in different specialties and must be

standardized, integrated, coordinated, and managed. Moreover, widespread demand to use these data for performance measurement and reporting to accountable care customers, regulators, and accrediting/certification bodies comes at a time when incentive payments to providers and health care institutions is linked with patient outcome measures (Centers for Medicare & Medicaid Services [CMS], 2011; Petersen et al., 2006). Reimbursement for health care services can be increased, decreased, or denied based on the patient's response to treatment. In 2008, Medicare stopped paying for eight hospital-acquired patient conditions deemed preventable, including objects left in the patient during surgery, urinary tract infections, and pressure ulcers. Redesigned payment for more hospital-acquired complications is proposed (Fuller et al., 2009). Regulatory and governmental agencies require the collection of data to measure performance (e.g., The Joint Commission [TJC]), the organization of these data into specific formats (e.g., Medicare/Medicaid), and adequate protections to ensure the confidentiality of these data (e.g., Health Insurance Portability and Accountability Act [HIPAA]). To meet these demands, administrators need data that can be compared across multiple settings, both geographically and clinically.

DEFINITIONS

Health information technology (HIT) applications in nursing services arise from the intersection of three areas: nursing administration, clinical informatics, and effectiveness research, including research on client outcomes. The technologies are tools for downloading, collecting, organizing, and analyzing vast amounts of complex data; and providing clinical decision support. By having these data in an accessible format, nursing leaders, managers, and administrator are better able to make informed decisions regarding the organization and delivery of patient care. When information cannot be accessed in a timely manner, leaders are forced to make critical decisions without considering key elements or facts.

The domain of technology and informatics combines the sciences of engineering, computers, and information with the cognitive health sciences. **Nursing informatics** is a specialty that integrates nursing science with computer and information sciences to manage and communicate data, information, knowledge, and wisdom in nursing practice. Nursing informatics supports consumers, patients, nurses, and other providers in their decision making in all roles and settings. This support is accomplished through the use of information structures, information processes, and information technology (American Nurses Association [ANA], 2008).

Effectiveness research applies epidemiological methods to large databases to study relationships among health care problems, interventions, outcomes, and costs. These methods can be used to identify alternatives and their effects and reveal associations with different patient characteristics and intervening variables (Ozbolt, 1991).

Health information management (HIM), management information system (MIS), and biomedical technicians provide integrated services to automate and support clinicians' and managers' decision-making processes. These services include downloading, collecting, storing, retrieving, and processing collective sets of data through the use of networking technology and applications to locate and aggregate the data from an integrated data repository. A management information system (MIS) is an integrated system for collecting, storing, retrieving, and processing a collective set of data; the data are queried from repository storage for direct use and application in the process of directing and controlling resources and for measurement, comparison, and evaluation of the achievement of specific management objectives. **Clinical information systems** (CISs) capture clinical data to support more efficient and effective decision making and clinical care delivery (Ward et al., 2006). The **health information exchange** (HIE) is defined as the electronic movement of health-related information among organizations according to nationally recognized standards (U.S. Department of Health and Human Services [USDHHS], 2008, p. 6). The HIE is a process within either a state health information network or a regional health information organization (RHIO), often for a geographic area. Today MIS and HIM departments work with clinical informatics roles (i.e., nurse informaticians) to organize and process information and provide accessible knowledge resource databases (e.g., drug and nursing evidence-based databases) to guide and support decisions during patient care workflow; to monitor patient safety, satisfaction, and quality of care; to manage human resources, physical resources, fiscal resources; and more recently evidence-based knowledge resources (Hannah et al., 2006; Osheroff, 2009; Sewell & Thede, 2013). The 10 characteristics identified by Austin in 1979 for a good MIS are that it is (1) informative, (2) relevant, (3) sensitive, (4) unbiased, (5) comprehensive, (6) timely, (7) action-oriented, (8) uniform, (9) performance-targeted, and (10) cost-effective; these still hold true today. An example of a component of an MIS is a nursing workload management system (NWMS), also called a *patient classification system (PCS)*. These systems automate the collection of patient acuity data to calculate the number of patient care hours needed to provide care to the same group of patients (Hannah et al., 2006). An example of a component of an HIM is a continuity of care document for the health information exchange network. Both departments are capable of extracting nurses' documentation from an electronic health records repository to support reports for analysis and to exchange nursing data with other organizations.

In the current health care industry, the National Institute for Standards and Testing (NIST) raised concerns about the information infrastructure that is needed to allow cross-enterprise document sharing, messaging profiles, medical device communication, a nationwide health information exchange network, patient identification matching, and continuity of care document specifications or semantic interoperability of patient data (NIST, 2011). Automated CISs are used for the device capture (e.g., monitors, ventilators) and electronic documentation of clinical data related to the direct care of clients and managing care processes. CISs organize clinical data and trend clinical parameters and results for display, scan and check medications for interactions and errors before administration, and can provide a summary of the client's story from nursing documentation. Nursing documentation systems include structured entry using drop-down menus, checklists, and computerized ordering/planning for scheduled care interventions. When completed, the documentation is often used within clinical decision support logic to automate actions for communication, add problems or risk diagnoses to the problem list, or elicit intervention reminder messages for evidence-based practice (Brokel et al., 2011). CISs also allow unstructured narrative documentation that is not included in the structured portion of the system (Moss et al., 2007). Integrating these data with other knowledge database systems can facilitate safe medication administration practice and adherence to evidence-based practice protocols (Brokel, 2007). Information collected through the use of CISs is integrated with financial and patient management systems within large data warehouses and queried to evaluate the effectiveness of nursing care and track adverse events.

NURSING'S DATA NEEDS

Nursing's data needs fall into four domains: (1) client care, (2) provider competencies and staffing, (3) administration of care and sustainability of the organization, and (4) knowledge-based research for evidence-based practice. The first three are distinct areas for work-flow processes, whereas research, the fourth domain, interacts with all of the other three. The four areas and the sources for the data are as follows:

1. *Client:* Longitudinal client care/clinical care and its evaluation, clinical findings, and client outcomes. Source: the client's health care record, their personal health record, patient-provider messages, and information from the health information exchange network.

2. *Provider:* Professional data, role responsibilities (i.e., competencies, skills), caregiver outcomes, and decision-maker variables. Source: personnel records, national data banks, and documentation links to client records.

3. *Administrative:* Management and resource oversight, organization statistics, system outcomes, contextual variables, and comparative targets. Source: administrative, fiscal, population, registry, and regulatory performance data.

4. *Research:* Knowledge base development and comparative effectiveness with phenotype data dictionaries (Pathak et al., 2011). Source: existing and newly gathered data, relational databases, and common data elements from emerging exchange networks.

Table 26-1 displays examples of outcomes and variables to be measured in relation to the three distinct domains of nursing's data needs. For example, in the client domain, the cost and continuity of care for the client are important because data are now shared among providers within the HIE to manage care. In the provider domain, professional skills/knowledge and intensity of nursing care are variables that may be measured to monitor variability and control workforce capacity. The quality and type of services is dependent on the competencies of the professional workforce, and nurse administrators need data to prepare a plan for strengthening the quality and capacity of not only the nursing workforce but also other needs, such as for mental health services (Institute of Medicine [IOM], 2006, 2011).

The collection and analysis of data are critical to propel health services research. Data analysis is aimed at cost, safety, quality, and effectiveness outcomes. Collecting and extracting data that describe the processes and outcomes of nursing care electronically has provided evidence for the design of care protocols and delivery models (Horn & Gassaway, 2010). The formal process of using these patient data for providing this evidence is termed *practice-based evidence* (DeJong, 2007). This comparative effectiveness research framework analyzes a comprehensive set of patient, treatment, and outcome variables to identify treatments associated with better outcomes while controlling for patient differences (Horn & Gassaway, 2010). Although both are used to inform the delivery of practice with evidence, in reality, practice-based evidence and evidence-based practice are derived from different

TABLE 26-1	OUTCOMES AND VARIABLES IN THREE DOMAINS OF NURSING DATA NEEDS	
DOMAIN	**OUTCOMES**	**VARIABLES**
Client	Client satisfaction	Attitudes/beliefs
	Achieved care outcomes	Diagnosis, gender, age
	Preferences for personal outcomes	Marital status
	Costs	Support system
	Access to care	Satisfaction
	Continuity of care	Level of dependency
	Access to personal health records	Severity of illness
	Medication reconciliation	Intensity of nursing care
		Nursing patient sensitive outcomes
		Provider-patient messaging
Provider	Job enrichment	Attitudes/beliefs
	Job/work satisfaction	Education level
	Physician/nurse satisfaction	Competency with care interventions
	Job stress	Years of experience
	Intent to leave	Age
	Certification	Work excitement
	Hours work	Position level with electronic health record/ electronic medical record EHR/EMR
	Access to information	Provider-provider messaging
	Skill set/competency with HIT	Health information exchange network
		Clinical decision support automations
Administration	Costs	Agency philosophy/culture
	Productivity	Priorities
	Turnover	Organizational structure
	Income	Fiscal data
	Workforce capacity	Climate data
	Safety culture	Policies and procedures
	Quality performance/benchmarks	Workflow/process data
	Effective communication	Technology capability data
	Health Information exchange	Workforce positions/demand data
	Adherence to best clinical evidence	Patient population—risks & problems
		Community networks/relationships
		Educational institution relations

sources. Deriving evidence for informing practice from research is termed *evidence-based practice*, whereas informing practice from the analysis of patient data collected during the delivery of care is termed *practice-based evidence*. However, this contribution rests on structuring the input logically and providing a level of accuracy and completeness to ensure valid and reliable output. Explicit data definitions, valid linkage between datasets, and well-defined coding of input are essential in securing meaningful and usable output. The aggregation of consistent meaningful information over time and how daily workflow affects the quality of information are especially important to uniform datasets. Using practice-based evidence requires the compilation of clinical data into a *clinical data repository*. This compilation may also be called a *data warehouse* or *data repository*. Data are stored longitudinally over multiple episodes of care. These data are accessed to provide continuity of care to the individual patient, extracted to measure care effectiveness and productivity, queried to provide evidence for care delivery, and analyzed to inform public policy.

NURSING INFORMATICS

Recognized by the American Nurses Association (ANA) as a nursing specialty in 1992, informatics was one of the fastest growing practice areas in health care. As defined by ANA (2008) the practice of nursing informatics views the relationship of data, information, knowledge, and wisdom as a continuum with increasing complexity and interrelations as nurses aggregate and apply them in decision making (Englebardt & Nelson, 2002, p. 12). *Data* are defined as discrete, objective entities, without interpretation; *information* is data that are structured, organized, or interpreted; and *knowledge* is information that is synthesized with identified relationships and meaning. Wisdom is appropriate use of knowledge in managing and solving patient problems, risks, and needs for health enhancement (i.e., nursing diagnoses). Wisdom is knowing when and how to apply the evidence-based knowledge with client information (Englebardt & Nelson, 2002), which nurses exercise through critical thinking and clinical reasoning skills.

Nursing informatics specialists assist practitioners by providing information and evidence-based knowledge to support clinical decision making and delivery of safe patient care. Although these specialists may not be directly involved with care delivery, their effort is integrally related to reengineering workflow for clinical and administrative practice. Nursing informatics specialists participate in analysis, design, and implementation of information and communication systems; effectiveness and informatics research; and education of nurses in informatics and information technology through the Technology and Informatics Guiding Education Reform initiative. More recently, nursing informatics specialists represent nurses at the policy table in building better interoperable frameworks for care coordination and delivery through optimizing processes and technology usability (Sensmeier, 2011).

The first master's degree in nursing informatics was offered by the University of Maryland in 1989. In 1992, that same university followed with the first doctoral program in nursing informatics. Now, programs in nursing informatics can be found throughout the United States. These programs offer a variety of educational options, including master's degrees, post-master's certificates, and doctoral degrees. Nurses prepared at the master's level in nursing informatics are titled *informatics nursing specialists (INSs)* (Hannah et al., 2006). Nurses prepared at the baccalaureate or master's level can obtain certification in nursing informatics from the American Nurses Credentialing Center (ANCC).

ELECTRONIC HEALTH RECORD

In 1965, El Camino Hospital in Mountain View, California, was one of the first to attempt to develop an electronic health record (EHR). Along with Technicon Medical Information Systems and Lockheed Missiles and Space Company, an information system was created that communicated physicians' orders, retrieved laboratory results, and supported the documentation of nursing care (Staggers et al., 2001). The development of early information systems designed to support an EHR were confined to large tertiary care centers and federal agencies such as the U.S. Department of Veterans Affairs (VA) and the National Institutes of Health (NIH). The high cost of these systems provided little incentive for most health care institutions to change. The U.S. Department of Health and Human Services (USDHHS) funded programs that stimulated EHR implementations across eligible providers in ambulatory settings and critical access hospitals through incentives from CMS, regional training curriculums, and regional extension centers staffed with HIT skilled workers (USDHHS, 2010).

The shift from a retrospective fee-for-service and managed care to accountable care organization financial structure for the payment of medical services changes how partners develop informational, technical, financial, and professional capabilities that allow rewarding savings for coordinated longitudinal population-based care (Fisher et al., 2011). Currently, patient data are of interest not only to health care providers and accountable care organizations but also to governmental payers, who want to ensure that specific data and information are present and distributed to patients or public health entities, thus providing incentives when achieving meaningful use indicators (CMS, 2010). These data are also analyzed by health care providers to ensure that patient needs are transpiring in the most efficient and cost-effective manner with these required indicators. An indicator such as the quality of the patient problem list can meet the demands of the final rule, but it needs to also inform the providers using a clinicians' vernacular of patient conditions, co-morbidities, or long-term risks (e.g., hyperlipidemia, diabetes type 2, risk for falls) (Ochylski et al., 2012).

RESEARCH NOTE

Source

Ward, M.M., Vartak, S., Schwichtenberg, T., & Wakefield, D.S. (2011). Nurses' perceptions of how clinical information system implementation affects workflow and patient care. *Computers Informatic Nursing* 29(9), 502-511.

Purpose

Eighty-one percent of acute care nonfederal hospitals plan to achieve meaningful use of EHRs by the end of 2011-2012. This study examined the impact of clinical information system implementation on nurses' perceptions of workflow and patient care throughout the implementation process in a community rural setting.

Discussion

Nurse leaders can expect major changes in nurses' workflow with EHR implementation. The EHR technologies did not decrease provider-patient communications, inter-provider communications, or inter-organizational communications; work life; patient care processes; or quality of care as perceived by nurses. Nurses did identify time spent documenting patient care, recording diagnoses and symptoms, and time directly with patients degraded; whereas four aspects improved. The communication with patients receiving follow-up outpatient care or any readmissions was better. The access to patient information improved the nurses' ability to make good patient care decisions. The timeliness for available patient-related data and the clarity of patient care orders were greatly improved.

Application to Practice

Setting realistic expectations about the implementation of EHRs is important, and the evolution of changes will continue with health information technology. Assessing the nurses' perceptions throughout the implementation process is useful for designing training to meet the needs of the users, because it allows organizations to adapt training and the implementation processes to support nurses who will have concerns.

RESEARCH NOTE

Source

Vogelsmeier, A., Halbesleben, J., & Scott-Cawiezell, J. (2008). Technology implementation and workarounds in the nursing home. *Journal of the American Medical Informatics Association, 15,* 114-119.

Purpose

Medication administration errors can occur at multiple points along the process of preparing, administering, and/or monitoring medications. Technological solutions such as computerized provider order entry, electronic medication administration records, and decision support have the potential to decrease medication error. When the solutions do not fit nursing work processes, nurses work around the technology. The purpose of this study was to explore the relationship of workarounds related to the implementation of an electronic medication administration record and medication safety practices in five Midwestern nursing homes.

Discussion

Nurses developed work-arounds to two types of process blocks—intentional and unintentional technology blocks. Intentional technology blocks were those integrated into the system to specifically prevent an error, and unintentional technology blocks were those impedances to work processes that were not intended by the system design. Working around the system-induced blocks negates the system safeguards provided. These work-arounds can result in an increased number of medication administration errors. Unintentional system blocks can also result in an increased number of medication errors caused by the unintended consequences of system implementation.

Application to Practice

Work-arounds to technology implementation occur because the system design is not congruent with nursing work processes. Before system implementation, practices must be clearly defined and the proposed system customized to adapt to processes. In addition, a thorough understanding of processes will uncover steps that could be improved and redesigned with the implementation of the information system. Analysis of nursing processes must also be conducted before and after implementation to determine what practices are affected and may need to be altered.

Using standards and an interoperability framework for data collection (Office of National Coordinator for Health Information Technology [ONC], 2010), client-protected health information within an EHR can be accessed across health exchange networks, linking clinical and business processes, reducing data replication, and increasing the availability and accessibility of information. Well-designed electronic health records and clinical data repositories can facilitate the collection and exchange of complete and accurate data in a form that is easily accessible to enhance clinical practice (Minthorn & Lunney, 2010; ONC, 2010), support reuse of historical data for current care decisions, analyze patient outcomes over time (Brokel et al., 2011), continuously improve patient safety and quality (Horn & Gassaway, 2010), or manage institutional resources.

The purpose of an EHR is to document patient care in a single repository as a clinical, financial, and legal record. The electronic digital format supports the storage and exchange of the continuity of care document from the record that is accessible and available among health care members regardless of their location. The EHR is a virtual record of retrospective, concurrent, and prospective information to support continuous, efficient, and integrated health care (Häyrinen et al., 2008). It does not originate from one place. It is a compilation of information from a variety of integrated systems through health information exchange networks regionally or via state organizations.

HEALTH INFORMATION EXCHANGES

The health information exchange (HIE) is defined as the electronic movement of health-related information among organizations according to nationally recognized standards (USDHHS, 2008, p. 6). The HIE is a process within either a state health information network or a regional health information organization (RHIO), often for a geographic area. The organizations provide oversight to authorize the locations of health information and the process for secure access and use of the information. In 2010, the Office of National Coordinator provided direction in guiding state-based entities in operational plans to implement HIEs across the nation using Health Information Technology for Economic and Clinical Health (HITECH) funding (USDHHS, 2010). Initial services are a statewide provider directory, secure provider-provider messaging, e-prescribing for ambulatory medications, and exchanging the continuity of care document (e.g., problem lists, medications, plan of care, advance directive, patient instructions), laboratory results, immunization registry, and public health surveillance of contagious diseases (CMS, 2010). Expansion of services would include personal health records and exchanging of other vital diagnostic, outcome, and coordinated care information.

In 2004, President George W. Bush created the position of Office of National Coordinator for HIT within USDHHS. The coordinator's role involved leadership to develop the standards and interoperability framework and establish the infrastructure necessary to harness the use of information technology and exchange of health information nationwide. The goals included improving patient care and reducing health care costs through support of CMS, the Agency for Healthcare Research and Quality (AHRQ), and HIT committees (USDHHS, 2010). The President's mandate was for each American to have an EHR by 2014. In 2009, President Barack Obama furthered this agenda with USDHHS and other federal agencies through funding state and regional programs (USDHHS, 2010). To facilitate the development of interoperable EHR systems across the country, standardized vocabularies such as Systematized Nomenclature of Medicine Clinical Terms (SNOMED CT) have been purchased and made available for download through the National Library of Medicine (USDHHS, 2011).

SNOMED CT is a comprehensive clinical terminology, originally created and compiled by the College of American Pathologists (CAP) using multiple clinical classifications such as evidence-based nursing classifications. In April 2007, the International Health Terminology Standards Development Organization (IHTSDO), a not-for-profit association in Denmark, took over ownership, maintenance, and license distribution. The National Library of Medicine is the U.S. Member of the IHTSDO and distributes SNOMED CT at no cost in accordance with the IHTSDO uniform international license terms, which have been incorporated into the License for Use of the Unified Medical Language System (UMLS) Metathesaurus. This includes both English and Spanish versions as part of the UMLS Metathesaurus, where nurses can find the origins of the biomedical terminologies.

The development of an EHR has been escalated by the public's demand to be partners in decisions about their health care (USDHHS, 2011). This client partnership with providers is necessary to improve continuity and prevent errors among the client's different care providers. This begins by preventing errors by phase of medication process. Kopp and colleagues (2006) reported that lack of drug knowledge was the cause of 10% of errors and that slips and memory lapses were responsible for 40% of errors at the administration phase. Because health care workflow transpires in an interruption-driven environment, it is not surprising that medication administration errors are attributable to omissions. Integrating an EHR with pharmacy, laboratory, and clinical documentation supports the implementation of computerized provider order entry (CPOE), clinical decision support (CDS), and bar code scanning and electronic medication administration records (eMARs) applications designed to reduce errors in health care systems.

Implementing technological solutions such as provider order sets, clinical decision support interventions, evidence-based knowledge database resources, and personal health records in health care are extremely expensive, and it has been difficult to show a return on investment (ROI) for these expenditures. However, an estimated $12.7 to $36 billion could be saved annually from the national implementation of an EHR through the associated reduction in adverse events, unnecessary clinical procedures, and staff time, along with more rapid record retrieval (Staggers et al., 2001). The growing trend is to regard these expenditures as part of the cost of institutional infrastructure and to tie them to the cost savings gained by improving patient outcomes. All eligible providers and health care organizations plan to add CPOE, CDS, and other solutions to achieve stages of meaningful use indictors by 2015 (CMS, 2010).

EFFECTIVENESS

The first person to analyze patient outcomes associated with nursing care delivery was Florence Nightingale in the nineteenth century. Today, health care systems continue to contain costs but need to achieve effective care through accountable care organizations and partnerships (CMS, 2011). Prior measures that focused solely on reduced mortality, length of stay, and hospital costs provided little information about the quality of health care provided. Health information technology and the development of nursing classification systems have made the measurement and evaluation of

nursing-sensitive outcomes feasible (Brokel et al., 2011; Sampaio Santos et al., 2010; Schneider et al., 2008).

Nurses spend approximately 19% of their time in patient care, 7% with assessments, 17% managing medications, 20% coordinating care, and 35% documenting patient information in EHRs (Burnes-Bolton, 2009). Fortunately, more and more data are documented in standardized formats that are now accessible to extract and analyze. The standardized nursing data captured within information tables and well-defined data fields allow the extraction of any standard data object into a report. Nursing informatics specialists work to organize and aggregate these data for real-time decision making in care delivery management and to a degree in the analysis of patient outcomes. These activities require extracting data that can be organized in nursing outcomes databases. Without clinical outcomes databases that reflect nursing care across patient care providers, only data available in current coding and billing systems will provide for generic outcome evaluation. Nursing outcome databases are critical for two reasons: (1) nurses are able to measure and document how nurses influence patient outcomes across care providers for populations of patients, and (2) the study of nursing-sensitive outcomes allows for comparisons among interventional strategies and advancement of the science of nursing care delivery (Furukawa et al., 2011; Minthorn & Lunney, 2010; Muller-Staub, 2009; Scherb et al., 2011).

Formulation of the Nursing Minimum Data Set (NMDS) was an effort to standardize the collection of essential nursing information for comparison of nursing data across patient populations. Three categories of data elements are included in the NMDS: nursing care, demographic, and service. Data elements related to nursing care included nursing diagnosis, intervention, outcome, and intensity of nursing care (Werley & Lang, 1988). Expanding on the use of the NMDS as a guide now helps ensure that data are collected regarding institutional structure (having the right things), process (doing things right), and outcomes (having the right things happen). Linking nursing care data to Donabedian's (1986) quality criteria of structure, process, and outcomes is necessary for the accurate evaluation of efficiency and effectiveness. The NMDS identified the data essential for inclusion in clinical information systems necessary to support decision making in clinical and administrative nursing practice (Brokel, 2007). The challenge has been capturing nursing decisions and care without variation in documentation. Harrington and colleagues (2011) identified where HIT fails nursing usability of EHRs by violating heuristic principles. They found 3 of the 14 principles accounted for most of the concerns with usability. The highest concern was the mismatch between the EHR design and nursing care models, because the design did not match nursing process workflow and nursing documentation of care (Harrington et al, 2011). Another concern was the lack of nursing language in the design, where programmers used financial or medical records coded terms that were not defined in the nurses' vernacular or in evidence-based nursing classifications. The third concern was the lack of the minimalist approach, which caused nurses many more clicks to finish the documentation than necessary (Harrington et al., 2011).

STANDARDIZED CLINICAL TERMINOLOGY

Nurses spend a great deal of their time collecting and documenting information related to patient care delivery. Vast amounts of data are compiled, describing every holistic detail of the patient's encounter, including personal health record messages and calls with the health care system or ambulatory care services. These data are more often encoded and recorded in a standard way that makes them amenable to analysis. When documenting the description of the same surgical incision, five different nurses may use picklist or narration to capture five different entries. They may describe the size of the wound in centimeters or inches, which the HIT can convert and then display both. The wound color could be depicted as pink, slightly reddened, or slightly inflamed. When different terms are used to describe the same observable fact, it is difficult to know that everyone is referring to the same phenomenon. Defined and evidence-based descriptions associated with clinical terminologies provide nurses a method of harmonizing the documentation to foster consistency in accurately describing the wound. The access to reference text definitions and databases to define and identify the context of clinical concepts helps in the quality of documented nursing information.

June Clark and Norma Lang, pioneers in nursing informatics, once wrote, "If we cannot name it, we cannot control it, practice it, research it, teach it, finance it, or put it into public policy" (Clark & Lang, 1992, p. 109). For nearly 40 years, nurses have been developing classification systems that itemize the diagnoses, interventions, and outcomes of the professional domain. More recently this process has been supported by different taxonomic infrastructures for classification. These variations were viewed as disruptive to the profession. However, the result has been a richer, more inclusive representation of "what nurses do" in different practice environments. Currently, the ANA recognizes 13 standardized terminologies. These include terminologies for nursing administration, home health care, perioperative nursing, acute care, and other nursing scopes of practice. The ANA-recognized terminologies for nursing are as follows: NANDA International nursing diagnosis, characteristics, and factors; Nursing Interventions Classification (NIC) interventions with associated activities; Nursing Outcomes Classification (NOC) outcomes with measurable indicators; Nursing Management Minimum Data Set (NMMDS), Clinical Care Classification (CCC); Omaha System; Perioperative Nursing Data Set (PNDS); SNOMED CT; NMDS; International Classification for Nursing Practice (ICNP); ABC codes; Alternate Link; and Logical Observation Identifier Names & Codes (LOINC) (ANA, 2007).

Classification systems are non-combinatorial hierarchical languages designed to categorize objects (Ingenerf, 1995). In health care classification systems, objects classified are generally patient diagnoses, outcomes, and care interventions. Nursing classifications, also referred to as *interface terminologies,* are generally implemented at the point of care to describe and document clinical practice (Coenen et al., 2001).

Concept-oriented or reference terminologies have the potential to provide the necessary basic structure for many classifications, with multiple translations that support documentation in health information systems. Reference/concept-oriented terminologies require the user to combine terms, making them awkward for their direct use as a documentation tool (Hardiker & Rector, 2001). Classification systems help provide the evidence-based terms used in documenting practice, and the reference terminology model provides the structure for organization with other interdisciplinary teams' documentation in the database (Bakken et al., 2001).

The International Standards Organization (ISO) Technical Committee ISO/TC 215 Health Informatics, Working Group 3 Health Concept Representation (ISO/TC 215/WG 3) focused specifically on the conceptual structure required by a nursing reference terminology model (ISO, 2002). Through the use of these terminology models, diagnosis, patient outcomes, and intervention terms contained within existing clinical classification systems can be mapped for harmonization across medical and nursing terminologies.

NURSING MANAGEMENT MINIMUM DATA SET

Awareness of the need for standardized, uniformly collected, retrievable, and comparable service-related management data elements was the impetus for the research to develop and test a Nursing Management Minimum Data Set (NMMDS) (Huber et al., 1992; Huber et al., 1997) (Figure 26-1).

Building on the NMDS, the NMMDS specifically identified variables essential to nurse managers for decision making about nursing care effectiveness. For example, the NMMDS can be linked to the nursing care elements of intensity/staff mix to provide an enhanced assessment of the consumption of health care resources to produce specific client care outcomes for a specific age cohort, racial/ethnic group, or geographical region. Linkage of NMDS and NMMDS elements provide data useful for the financial and clinical management of patient care (Delaney & Huber, 2001). In addition, the NMMDS is being mapped to LOINC for meaningful use (Westra et al., 2010).

The NMMDS has 18 elements potentially critical to evaluating the impact of nursing interventions on client outcomes. The NMMDS work facilitates what to link and augments how other minimum health data sets provide information uniquely important to nursing administrative decisions and thus to the evaluation of nursing services for cost and quality outcomes of care delivery. This contributes to evidenced-based management, as called for by the Institute of Medicine (IOM, 2004).

The NMMDS work clarifies and expands the data points that tap contextual variables, which intervene between provider actions and client outcomes. Nursing will need to extract standardized data sets via queries from data warehouses to facilitate decision making and policy development in such areas as job satisfaction, turnover, cost of nursing services, allocation of nursing personnel, and comparison of nursing care delivery models. Such data sets would foster consistent data collection, retrieval, analysis, and comparison of nursing management outcomes across settings, populations, time intervals, and geographical regions. Using a core set of variables captured by health information systems, data essential to nursing care delivery management can be analyzed and used to meet nursing's goals and objectives. MIS and HIM staff jointly support large database repositories and applications to generate reports and trends for nursing leadership and management. Data warehouses hold more types of data for data analysts to extract nursing variables to answer clinical questions. The reports can be designed to display in real time on portable computers and handheld devices or can be used with expert systems and more advanced decision support and modeling systems. The data analysts need guidance from clinical nurse leaders and nurse informatics specialists to identify the NMDS and NMMDS elements to query for those clinical questions. Data analysts and clinical informatics nurses can design summary reports to display data, CDS logical algorithms to generate messages or automate steps to support decisions in the continuous care of clients, or add to the dashboard display to support administrators and nurse managers in planning patient services and workforce capacity.

LEADERSHIP AND MANAGEMENT IMPLICATIONS

The Institute of Medicine (IOM, 2011) recommended acquiring better data on the health care workforce in their report, *The Future of Nursing: Leading Change, Advancing Health*. The data should include numbers and types of professionals available to meet future needs. Nurse leaders will need to understand the impact of bundled payments, medical homes, accountable care organizations, health information technologies, comparative effectiveness, patient engagement with personal health records, the diversity of the population

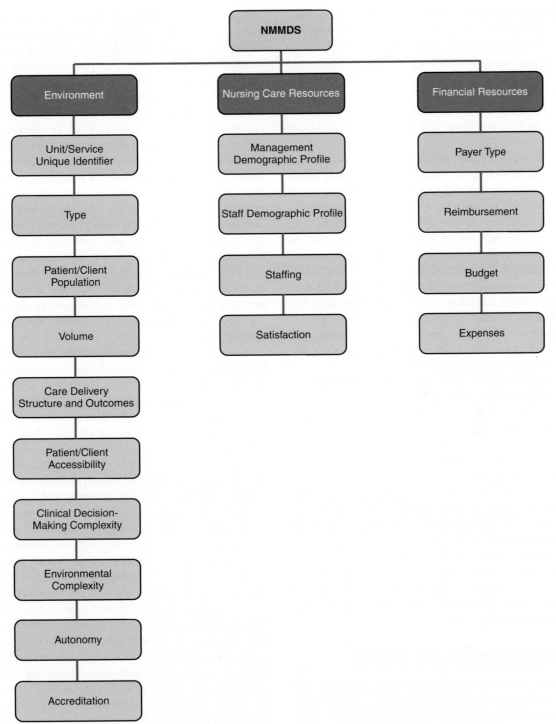

FIGURE 26-1 Nursing Management Minimum Data Set (NMMDS) variables. These elements are at the unit-of-service level. (Copyright © 2008 D. Huber, C. Delaney. All rights reserved. Reprinted with permission.)

and the level of safety. Technological applications have the capability to change system processes to improve delivery. Having nursing data is a necessary step in developing accurate models for projecting workforce capacity (IOM, 2011). Salsberg (2009) provided a model of factors to determine health care workforce demand, which requires elements of the NMMDS on population, health conditions and disease, and utilization rates.

It is implicitly acknowledged that collecting, sharing, and analyzing information will positively affect the quality of care delivered. Nurse leaders are in the position of ensuring that information systems are selected that collect and extract nursing data to support the way nurses work and the decisions to improve workforce capacity for different populations of clients. Implementing and upgrading information systems without the involvement of all user groups often results in work-arounds because the HIT failed to support the clinician's or client's decisions. Successful information systems are those with the ability to accurately measure and analyze the efficiency and effectiveness of care.

Nurse managers are being asked to participate in the selection, design, and implementation of institutional information systems. Managers will need a combination of informatics knowledge and technical skills, quality improvement and project management skills, and organizational skills (Lorenzi & Riley, 2003). During this process, managers and clinical nursing leaders will serve as change agents to overcome resistance. A basic understanding of the dynamics of the change process is essential for successful adoption and cyclical updating and maintenance of these systems (Jones & Moss, 2006). Successful implementation and sustainability of these systems will require nurse managers, nurse informaticians, clinical nurse leaders, and quality experts to have leadership, vision, and commitment.

CURRENT ISSUES AND TRENDS

Nursing and health care organizations are calling for the redesign and reengineering of the existing work environment and patient-centered workflows. Their intent is to improve clinician and client satisfaction, client outcomes and client access to their information, and the sustainability of all health care organizations and services. The American Organization of Nurse Executives (AONE) called for the redesign of work through the use of technology to augment nursing practice (Kennedy, 2003). This goal of nursing work redesign was initially to build systems and safeguards to decrease error and to enhance patient safety. The Institute of Medicine's (IOM, 2004) report, *Keeping Patients Safe: Transforming the Work Environment of Nurses,* emphasized that risks to patient safety are embedded in many work processes. *The Future of Nursing* report (IOM, 2011) established a blueprint to ensure that nurses practice to the full extent of their education and training and that nursing education is improved. Nurses are asked to be partners to redesign and improve care (lead change) and find ways to improve data collection and analysis for workforce planning and policy making. This encourages the full scope of practice for nurses to intervene not only when diagnosing problems and risks, but also when diagnosing needs for health promotion (advance health) and systems change.

Toward this goal, system designers must focus on how to communicate and exchange information for the automation and coordination of health care work. According to Stetson and colleagues (2001), there is no instance in which coordination of care takes place in the absence of communication, and there is no instance in which clinical information exchange occurs in the absence of clinical communication. It is now possible to integrate smart phones, handheld devices, global positioning systems, and bar code scanners with medication administration systems. It is also now possible to integrate health information exchange networks with traditional information systems through secure wireless intranets and internet connections. These technological advances now permit the immediate communication of information to the correct person, at the correct time, in the correct format. For example, it is now possible to link laboratory systems with nursing call systems to alert a patient's nurse when laboratory values fall outside of set limits. It is now possible to connect nursing homes and home care nurses to a web portal with access to the health information exchange network to access client data from multiple providers. It is now possible for clients to have access to their personal health record and to securely send and receive messages from their health care providers.

The integration of these systems can enhance the efficiency of the collection and aggregation of clinical data for use in the management of workload and staffing as recommended by the IOM (2011). Calculating acuity data directly from nursing documentation and treatment plans can more accurately reflect scheduling needs for immediate online retrieval (Kennedy, 2003). This documentation can also be used to determine the quality of care delivered on an institutional, unit, population, or individual level. Efficiency and effectiveness can be compared between units, or the data can be used for an individual nurse's performance evaluation. The possibilities for greater efficiency and effectiveness are boundless.

CASE STUDY

Kim, Mark, and Joyce are chief nursing executives (CNEs) at three different large community hospitals in cities within 100 miles of each other. All three work with the nearby nursing schools to discuss their need for nurses with BSN degrees and nurse practitioners. All three have identified common administrative and clinical questions that must be answered to plan for workforce capacity and to support clinical experiences for students at the nursing schools. Each hospital and community uses standardized nursing classifications to support documentation requirements within the clinical information systems, and they share some of the same client populations. The nurse managers have access to basic object-oriented reports using the data warehouse repositories. The repositories include client medical diagnoses as well as problems, risks and needs for health promotion using nursing diagnoses in the diagnoses and problem list tables. All of the surgery departments use the Perioperative Nursing Data Set to record care for the operating room services. The state and communities have promoted the use of personal health records with the patient populations and clients who are using the hospitals and ambulatory clinics. They have been involved in requesting a set of preferred measurable patient outcomes using a standardized nursing classification (e.g., post-procedure recovery, ambulation/walking, infection severity) at the time of admission and the outcome level achieved at time of departure. The nursing service departments evaluate competencies using a well-defined evidence-based standardized nursing classification for interventions and have asked nurses to document these same interventions when providing care to clients using the standardized documentation terms within their respective electronic health records (EHRs).

Each of the CNEs have asked their unit managers and their nurse informatics specialists to help identify workforce capacity and competencies by extracting data from the EHR data repositories on the frequency of nursing interventions per quarter per unit, numbers of staff in each position, and hours worked by staff position per quarter per unit. The CNEs also question the types of patient populations by medical diagnoses per unit and the types and frequency of nursing diagnoses the nurses must care for per quarter per unit. The CNEs were also interested in what the clients are asking for outcomes within their respective hospitals. The CNEs asked the MIS/HIM data analysts to work with the informatics nurse specialist, two nurse managers, and two clinical nurse leaders to design the various reports to extract the correct data fields from the data warehouse information tables. The EHRs were designed differently so the clinical nurse leaders could help operationally define where the data had been documented by the RNs and other personnel on the units. The data analysts were asked to ensure there was a primary key that would link the nurse provider to not only their educational competencies from orientation, position and nursing education level, but also their frequency of documented interventions, clients, client outcomes preferred, their unit setting, their hospital setting, and the primary medical and nursing diagnoses that nurses cared for.

The data analyst, nurse informatics specialist and CNEs were all aware that these administrative and clinical questions will require many smaller reports that are initially extracted from the repository from base reports and subsequently divided up for each nurse manager or aggregated for the CNE. Once the reports are extracted, the reports provide multiple tables of information that the quality department staff or clinical data analyst, with the help of nurse managers, can use with data analysis tools to find frequencies, averages, ranges, and modes. They can then begin to show distinct similarities or differences and derive comparisons between units and between hospitals on the types of workforce staff used to obtain existing outcomes. Often the comparative analysis will require statistical tools to identify any significant differences. Many of the analytical tools are part of the package of tools hospitals and health systems use to answer questions.

Many of these reports that were generated initially can be programmed to run and extract the data at regular intervals such as weekly, monthly, quarterly, or annually. When the reports are simple to extract basic data elements into a table of information, the query can run efficiently. The simpler reports with primary key variables can be aggregated into a common database for use with analytic tools that allow the linking of multiple tables of information and more robust analysis and comparison. Once the queries are well tested and of proven value, steps can be taken with MIS/HIM departments to add the extraction of data and analysis to monitoring dashboards. Monitoring dashboards display common administrative numbers for the day, such as census, average length of stay of inpatients, number of RNs staffed per unit, number of patients with diagnosed infections (e.g., Catheter-Associated Urinary Tract Infection (CAUTI), Ventilator Associated Pneumonia (VAP), problems on the problem list, and up-to-date plans of care.

CRITICAL THINKING EXERCISE

No nurse wants to make a wrong decision or mistake. However, the nurses on a busy and short-staffed medical-surgical floor of an acute care tertiary-level hospital know the many decisions that need to be made about client diagnoses, assessments, and outcomes as well as the need to monitor the timing of interventions and administered medications. The nurse manager meets with the Nurse Manager Council from time to time to discuss the problem of high rates of missed interventions and medication omissions. The discussion focuses on what questions go unanswered because the data within the EHR repository have not been used to determine the extent and causes of the problem. Short-staffing leaves nurses exhausted from running from task to task. Now the administration has announced that incentive payments will be based on the accuracy and frequency of specific types of interventions. Nurses will need to enter all the data, including patients' preferred outcomes, to ensure this is extracted into the client's personal health record (PHR) for continuity of care at discharge. The nurse managers need information and knowledge about the units' patients, the current staff, competencies, current quality statistics, and what care is omitted.

1. What problem(s) can you identify in this scenario?
2. What makes this (or these) problematic?
3. What should the nurse manager do?
4. What questions are being raised?
5. What factors do the nurses and the nurse manager need to assess and analyze?
6. What data are needed?
7. What can the nurse manager do to form a persuasive data management plan?
8. Who needs to be involved in developing the clinical queries?

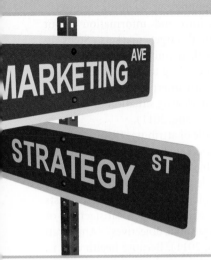

Marketing

Alice R. Boyington,
Jane M. Fusilero

e**volve** WEBSITE

http://evolve.elsevier.com/Huber/leadership/

Marketing is a business function focused on establishing customer relationships and satisfying customer needs and wants. Although definitions of the term marketing vary, most include an exchange process whereby something of value is created and delivered and strong profitable customer relationships are established. The overarching goals of marketing are to "attract new customers by promising superior value and keep and grow current customers by delivering satisfaction" (Kotler & Armstrong, 2011, p. 4). It is easy to accept that organizations and companies that offer tangible products rely on marketing for their success. However, sound marketing is equally as critical to organizations that primarily deliver services instead of more tangible products. Hospitals and other health care organizations fall into this latter group.

Marketing activities within hospitals and other health care organizations occur at the organizational, departmental, and unit levels. Such activities are also classified as internal or external, with each targeting a different audience or market. Target audiences can be patients and families, physicians, payers, and employees. Marketing departments within health care agencies take the lead in organizational level activities and ensure that customer-driven marketing strategies and programs are in alignment with the organization's strategic plan. The primary product that is marketed by hospitals is their care. Nurses deliver most of that product because they spend considerable time with patients and their families. Patient satisfaction is an accepted indicator of product (care) quality, and a high level of satisfaction is imperative to viability in today's competitive marketplace (Wagner & Bear, 2008). Thus nurses and nurse leaders are important marketers.

Not only are nurses at the center of care delivery, but nurse leaders are accountable for the workforce who provides that service. Marketing initiatives that focus on care delivery, customer satisfaction and recruitment and retention of the nursing workforce are not uncommon in hospitals. Nurse leaders who possess marketing acumen within their business skill set are invaluable to the development of high quality services delivered by a competent, experienced nursing workforce.

Previous chapters in this text have addressed the challenges faced by top-level and frontline nurse leaders. Challenges include the delivery of high-quality

Photo used with permission from Photos.com.
The authors of this chapter on Marketing gratefully acknowledge Dana Woods and Nikola Ross for editorial review of this chapter.

patient-centered care; recruitment and retention of a culturally diverse, competent workforce; promotion of a positive and inspiring image of nursing; design of a healthy work environment; and practices to satisfy patients and improve outcomes. Marketing initiatives can be designed and implemented to help meet these challenges.

The purpose of this chapter is to present an introduction to key marketing concepts and definitions, the application of marketing to health care, and implications for nurse leaders and managers. Familiarity with marketing terminology will position a nurse leader to better understand the organization, and possess the tools and techniques to respond to the challenges faced (Woods, 2002). Exposure to more in-depth descriptions of marketing terminology and applications can be expected as the nurse advances in education and career.

DEFINITIONS

Whereas a **market** was once defined as the physical place where buyers and sellers assembled and exchanged goods and wares according to a bartering system, it is defined today as "the set of actual and potential buyers of a product or services" (Kotler & Armstrong, 2011). Actual and potential customers are categorized as external markets, and employees comprise internal markets. Exchange has always been the defining concept underlying marketing. Exchange indicates action whereby a desired product or service is received from someone by offering something in return (Kotler & Armstrong, 2011). Today, exchange relationships take place in person, by phone, by mail, or in a virtual environment such as the Internet.

Marketing is a process that relates to transactions when products (i.e., goods or services) are exchanged in a market. The process begins with understanding what the customer needs and wants, includes the design of programs and services that fulfill these needs and wants, and ends with capturing value from the customers (Kotler & Armstrong, 2011). Marketing ensures a focus on an organization's annual, long-range, and strategic plans. Objectives in the various plans include customer-driven strategies and programs that create customer value and relationships within internal and external target markets (Kotler & Armstrong, 2011).

Market research applies a scientific approach to ascertain insights into and information about customers and potential target markets. Steps in the approach begin with defining the problem and research objectives, proceeding to data collection and analysis, and ending with interpretation of findings relevant to a specific marketing situation or decision making (Kotler & Armstrong, 2011).

A **product** "is a bundle of attributes (features, functions, benefits, and uses) capable of exchange or use; usually a mix of tangible and intangible forms. Thus a product may be an idea, a physical entity (a good), a service, or any combination of the three. It exists for the purpose of exchange in the satisfaction of individual and organizational objectives" (American Marketing Association, 2011). Because health care is, for the most part, a service industry, the use of the term *product* depicts health care service(s) and is often used interchangeably with *service* by health care marketers.

Service is "a form of product that consists of activities, benefits, or satisfactions offered for sale that are essentially intangible and do not result in the ownership of anything" (Kotler & Armstrong, 2011, p. 224). Services are differentiated from products that are goods by four characteristics: (1) intangibility, (2) inseparability, (3) variability, and (4) perishability. A service denotes action, occurs at the time of provider-customer interactions, and varies according to circumstances related to both the provider and customer. Services cannot be saved or stored for later use (American Marketing Association, 2011; Kotler & Armstrong, 2011).

Needs can be biological, psychological, and social. For example, a hospital patient may require special attention to safety concerns, pain management, compassionate care, infection prevention and control measures, and prevention of complications. Nurses, who compose an internal market, seek competitive salaries, continuing education to remain competent, access to evidence to guide practice, and sufficient human resources to meet staffing requirements. These are needs. **Wants** are wishes, desires, or preferences of individuals (American Marketing Association, 2011). A hospital patient's wants may include a quiet and spacious room, high-quality food, and cable television. Nurses may desire uniform allowances, self-scheduling, input in decision making, and flexible work hours. Employers consider the needs and wants of employees, beginning from the time of orientation and continuing throughout their tenure with the organization (Peltier et al., 2008).

BACKGROUND

Marketing is focused on "creating customer value and building profitable customer relationships" (Kotler & Armstrong, 2011, p. xvi). The business goal of a for-profit company is to maximize value so that shareholders will eventually benefit from their financial investment. The business goal of a non-profit or social sector organization, which includes many health care organizations, is to fulfill its mission of meeting consumer needs. Thus marketing is fundamental to creating value for customers that in turn leads to financial viability. Because of its for-profit roots, the term *marketing* often carries a negative connotation when applied to health care. Many question the appropriateness of marketing initiatives that seem focused on net income at the expense of patient care. Because nursing care composes much of the health care product, further questions about the appropriateness of health care marketing have surfaced among nurses.

Profitable may be the word that at first consideration seems foreign to the fabric of nursing and not related to what we do. Nurses are educated and socialized to give care, not to sell care. Although nurses experience the impact of marketing in their daily lives as consumers, they are unlikely to be exposed to it as an essential ingredient of their professional practice. However, when basic marketing concepts and aspects of the marketing process are explored and understood, their importance to not only the health care organization at-large, but also nurses and nurse leaders, becomes clear.

Whether or not they realize it, nurses, as essential providers of the health care product, are engaged in marketing when delivering care. This is in part because interpersonal relationships are a part of the therapeutic "product" of care. A health care organization dedicated to achieving excellence realizes this and works hard to inform all care providers and support staff about meeting customer needs. In excellence-driven organizations, marketing is more than a department; it is at the core of the organizational business framework. The American Organization of Nurse Executives (AONE) has identified "marketing" as a key business skill for nurse leaders in executive practice and for those with a career goal of leadership (American Organization of Nurse Executives, 2011). Nurse leaders and aspiring nurse leaders, who operate within a business framework, benefit from understanding marketing concepts that underlie programs and initiatives in health care organizations.

MARKETING STRATEGY

Strategic planning, a process discussed in previous chapters of this text, sets the overall direction for an organization. Defining the business, determining the mission, and developing long-term objectives form the basis of an organization's strategic plan. Marketing strategies and programs must be aligned and guided by the organization-wide strategic plan (Kotler & Armstrong, 2011). This cannot be done effectively without investing adequate time and resources in evaluating the organization's competitive environment.

A market research approach is used for environmental scanning and is a critical step in both the strategic and marketing planning processes. During the environmental scanning, marketing departments explore and evaluate the internal and external environments to gain an understanding of demographic and societal trends, competition, and potential customers. Also, internal business performance indicators such as financial results, customer and staff satisfaction, and quality indicators are evaluated. To be most effective, compilation, review, and analysis of environmental data should involve every functional area in an organization, including the nursing department. The results of the market research must be shared across business units, and all key stakeholders must participate in the subsequent planning process.

Marketing strategy is based on how target markets are defined. Markets are both broad and narrow. Mass marketing, which is broad, offers a product to an entire external market. Niche marketing is a more narrow view and focuses on capturing a small but important part of the market. Consider the difference between a full-service community hospital and a children's hospital. The former serves a broad market, the latter targets very specific customers—children and their families. Four critical concepts—segmentation, targeting, product differentiation, and positioning—are essential to understanding and becoming fluent in the language of marketing. The following are brief explanations of these concepts. The definitions of these terms, along with an example of each, are in Table 27-1.

Segmentation and targeting are the means of decision making about which customers will be served. Segmentation involves identifying pieces of the total market that contain potential customers with distinguishable characteristics such as age, gender, geographic location, or ethnicity. The essence of segmentation is to break down the mass market into submarkets of individuals with similar needs (Harvard Business School Press, 2006). Targeting takes into account the whole market that can then be considered in terms of attractive smaller market segments. Differentiation and positioning clarify how customers will be served. A product offering's differentiation calls for the creation of superior customer value and is typically what strengthens its position in the market against competitors. Positioning the product such that customers perceive it to be distinctive and desirable is the foundation of the marketing program (Kotler & Armstrong, 2011).

By analyzing information about the competitive market, a hospital can determine key strategies to meet the unmet needs in its service area. A small rural community hospital in a market 200 miles from any other hospital will adopt strategies for defining and serving its market that are very different from the strategies of a large suburban hospital in a market with four other hospitals within a 25-mile radius. The rural hospital would likely position itself as a full-service facility capable of meeting the most frequently occurring needs of their target audience or the local community. For example, its profile of services is likely to include women's services, emergency care, diagnostic care, and general surgery. On the other hand, the large suburban hospital in a highly competitive market might seek to differentiate itself from competitors by creating a specialty center for heart disease or cancer. However, product or service lines are not the only way to differentiate. Differentiation can be based on quality measures and other distinctions that are prevalent today. These include the following:

- The Joint Commission (TJC) accreditation for meeting performance standards
- Malcolm Baldrige National Quality Award for performance excellence
- Beacon Award for Excellence in critical care nursing
- Truven Health Analytics 100 Top Hospitals® award
- American Nurses Credentialing Center's Magnet Recognition Program® for excellence in nursing
- Planetree Designation Program for excellence in patient- and person-centered care

TABLE 27-1 CRITICAL MARKETING CONCEPTS

DEFINITION	EXAMPLE
Segmentation is "the process of dividing a market into distinct groups of buyers who have different needs, characteristics, or behaviors, and who might require separate products or marketing programs" (Kotler & Armstrong, 2011, p. 49).	*Example:* Services are designed according to culture and ethnicity of potential markets and are promoted accordingly.
Targeting is "identifying the buyers sharing common needs or characteristics that the company decides to serve" (Kotler & Armstrong, 2011, p. 201).	*Example:* A skin cancer screening program is designed for migrant farm workers who have regular sun exposure.
Product differentiation is "differentiating the market offering to create superior customer value" (Kotler & Armstrong, 2011, p. 51).	*Example:* A center of excellence for geriatric care is put in place in a large retirement community.
Positioning is "arranging for a product to occupy a clear, distinctive, and desirable place relative to competing products in the minds of target consumers" (Kotler & Armstrong, 2011, p. 49).	*Example:* The primary focus is placed on the advantages of receiving cancer care in a National Cancer Institute Comprehensive Cancer Center in comparison to a community-based center.

Heightened patient and regulatory scrutiny, fueled by more frequent accounts in the media of medical errors, has motivated hospitals to refocus on patient care excellence and seek ways to promote this excellence to the public to gain a competitive advantage. Logos depicting the previously mentioned designations of excellence are displayed on the organization's website home page and are used to promote differentiating distinctions.

Setting marketing strategy is a shared responsibility within a health care organization. This critical activity must be guided by the strategic plan with input from every key stakeholder group—especially nursing—who is engaged in meeting customer needs during many and varied exchanges. Likewise, the organization's marketing team is engaged at the start when new services are planned. With multiple perspectives represented at the planning table, an organization will respond more effectively to the needs and challenges of its markets.

THE MARKETING PROCESS: FOCUS ON MARKETING MIX

Previous sections of this chapter have focused on marketing at the organizational level to external markets. Familiarity with the marketing terminology and concepts that have been presented are imperative to building business skills and to applying the marketing mix. There are many complex marketing models that depict steps in the marketing process. Most begin with an appraisal and understanding of the environment and potential customers, include the design and delivery of a customer-driven marketing strategy, and end with customer loyalty and equity. A more in-depth understanding of such models will be required with career advancement. At this point, understanding basic aspects of the marketing process are more meaningful. The marketing mix is the set of tactical tools used in the marketing process. The marketing mix was introduced almost 50 years ago (McCarthy, 1964), but remains a useful organizing framework for successful marketing programs. Nurse leaders at all levels can apply this framework in programs and initiatives designed to meet everyday challenges.

The specific tools in the mix are custom-designed to influence the buyer's decision to purchase the product or service and to be the basis for operational marketing activities. From the seller's point of view, the marketing mix emerges as a unique combination of the four P's of (1) product, (2) price, (3) place, and (4) promotion. From the customer's point of view, the marketing mix emerges from the four C's of (1) customer needs and wants, (2) cost to customer, (3) convenience to buy, and (4) communication (Kotler, 2006; Lauterborn, 1990). Because the four P's framework is streamlined and robust, it can be used to guide important aspects of marketing initiatives. Brief descriptions of the four P's as they pertain to the marketing mix follow.

A *product* is the basis of any business and is the focus of exchange between the provider and customer. It is whatever is offered to satisfy a target market's need, desire, or preference. Products generally include objects, services, and ideas. Goods and services may also be combined into a product (Kotler & Armstrong, 2011). The primary hospital product is the "care" delivered by nurses.

The *place* refers not only to the location of the product exchange, but also to activities that make the product available to the customer. Examples of obvious places for health care delivery are hospitals, which are composed of individual departments and units, practitioner offices in ambulatory settings, and outpatient surgical centers. Less obvious factors to consider are *hours of* and *access to* the service. The place nursing care is delivered is well prescribed—a hospital, home, clinic, or other health care setting.

In a narrow sense, *price* is described as the amount of money customers pay to obtain the product. Customers consider the cost in terms of reasonableness. However, in a broader sense, cost is more than the money that is exchanged. Customers place value on products and services not only according to financial issues, but also according to psychosocial and emotional concerns. For example, delayed services that result in an excessive time commitment by the customer, may be a "greater price" than they are willing to pay. The "price" that is perceived by the customer may be very subjective.

Promotion is composed of communications with target markets about the product offered to meet needs, desires, or preferences. It is inclusive of publicity and advertising that seeks to persuade target markets that a given health care organization can deliver on their promise, meaning they provide a high quality product. Promotion often initiates relationships with customers.

In addition to emphasizing the important aspects of a marketing initiative to expand health care services, the marketing mix can be used as an organizing framework for developing and disseminating innovations related to patient care, nursing, and the practice environment. For example, one hospital used the marketing mix to design an educational campaign to educate and engage nurses in evidence-based practice (Boyington et al., 2010). Table 27-2 displays the marketing mix applied to this campaign. To further delineate a product that could be promoted to the internal market (nurses), a theme that reflected the overall goal of the campaign was selected. The goal was to identify outdated practices and consider them in light of current, relevant evidence. Thus a slogan that guided nurses to stop **C**linging **R**igidly to **O**utdated **C**are, with an accompanying logo, was developed (Figure 27-1). Buttons and other promotional materials used the CROC® theme and logo to call attention to the product.

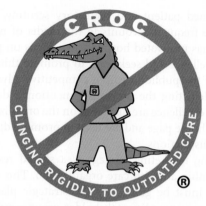

FIGURE 27-1 Product brand: CROC®. (Used with permission from the H. Lee Moffitt Cancer Center & Research Institute, Tampa, FL.)

LEADERSHIP AND MANAGEMENT IMPLICATIONS

At a glance, nurses may consider that nursing and marketing go together like oil and water. However, nurses (and nursing) are critical components to health care marketing. This is because marketing is about building relationships with customers so needs and wants are satisfied and value is created. Marketing goals are incorporated into the organizational strategic plan. These goals focus on satisfying and creating value with respect to customers. They also may be focused on attracting new customers or increasing volume to enhance financial viability. Nursing is impacted by such strategies and also can have an impact on goal achievement.

An understanding of basic marketing concepts and their application within the organization's strategic plan allows nurse leaders and managers to be knowledgeable contributors at the table where high-level goals are established and decisions about meeting goals are made. They are prepared to design or redesign nursing services according to markets identified in segmenting and targeting strategies and are best prepared to identify the resources required to further position customary services or establish new ones.

Nurse leaders and managers can describe the value nursing brings to the organizational marketing mix and thus to financial viability. Nurses deliver high quality care (product) across varied settings (place) and in a timely and efficient manner (price).

TABLE 27-2	**MARKETING MIX APPLIED TO EDUCATIONAL CAMPAIGN FOR NURSES**
MARKETING MIX ELEMENTS	**EDUCATIONAL CAMPAIGN**
Product	Evidence-based practice workshop
	Evidence-based practice tool kit
Place	Intranet
	Classroom
	Clinical area
	E-mail
Price	Staff time
	Staff effort
Promotion	Available 24/7
	Workshop invitations
	Branding of materials
	Management support

Adapted from Boyington, A.R., Ferrall, S.M., & Sylvanus, T. (2010). Marketing evidence-based practice: What a CROC®! *Clinical Journal of Oncology Nursing, 14*(5), 653-655.

Advertising messages (promotion) about nurses and nursing care communicated to internal and external markets can reinforce a positive image of nursing to internal and external markets. One opportunity for promotion of nursing to all markets is to have a nursing focus on the hospital website. Nurse leaders should ensure the presence of nursing on websites to communicate the importance of nursing, nursing practice, or nursing care to potential target markets (Boyington et al., 2006; Finkler et al., 2007).

There is no question that marketing is an important mind-set in organizations (Kumar, 2008). All employees should focus on establishing and maintaining satisfactory customer relationships. In hospitals and other health care organizations, frontline nurses are critical to creating value for customers. Nurse managers can turn to the reported work of the Nursing Executive Center (NEC) (Berkow et al., 2012) for a framework to engage frontline nurses in achieving goals concerning patient care and in understanding where the organization is headed. Underlying the NEC framework is the need to foster frontline nurse accountability such that key organizational goals and performance targets are met. Table 27-3 displays three ways to strengthen accountability in order to align with strategies for successful marketing initiatives at the organizational, departmental, and unit levels.

Another marketing application for nurse leaders and managers relates to workforce characteristics. Nurses who are employed make up an internal market, and the pool of nurses who are potential new hires make up an external market. In these instances, nurses are the customers. Nurse leaders can use marketing to increase "customer" retention and attraction. When considering nurse retention and recruitment, leaders consider what (product) the nursing department or unit offers to nurses. Highlighting department or unit characteristics deemed important, such as shared governance, professional development opportunities, and workplace fun (Karl et al., 2010) provide details about the product. Leaders can give attention

TABLE 27-3   FRONTLINE NURSE ENGAGEMENT IN ORGANIZATIONAL GOALS TO BUILD CUSTOMER RELATIONSHIPS

MARKETING PERSPECTIVE	NURSING EXECUTIVE CENTER STRATEGIES*	INTEGRATION INTO NURSING PRACTICE
Employees from all levels are involved in setting marketing goals in strategic plans.	Establish a greater line of sight for frontline staff (i.e., recognize the connection between what they do on a daily basis and the institution's larger priorities).	Nurses at all levels • Participate in strategic planning. • Value and engage in activities linked to unit and organizational patient-centered goals.
Employees with direct customer contact and in supportive roles are responsible for creating and maintaining a culture of customer-orientation.	Create a culture of shared responsibility to all patients and outcomes across the unit or institution as a whole.	Nurses at all levels • Form collaborative partnerships across units to promote patient-centered care and patient satisfaction. • Hold peers accountable for optimizing patient throughput.
Employees are cognizant that their performance and attitude play important roles in service delivery to customers.	Provide an appropriate level of external motivation through formal and informal approaches.	Nurse leaders • Reflect unit and organizational priorities in the performance appraisal process and clinical ladder advancement program. • Link reward and recognition events to achievement of best practice benchmarks and performance indicators.

*Data from Berkow, S., Workman, J., & Aronson, S. (2012). Strengthening frontline nurse investment in organizational goals. *Journal of Nursing Administration, 42*(3), 165-169.

to the unit (place) where nurses provide service. Consideration of the physical layout and whether the unit design is conducive to an efficient and effective work flow is important (Woods & Cardin, 2002). Nurse leaders can ensure that nurse salaries are competitive and that nurses do not feel underpaid and undervalued. Market research in collaboration with the human resources department can analyze salaries (price) in the external market and adjust salaries accordingly. Nurse leaders and managers are responsible for promoting the merits of nursing service internally and externally. The presence of nursing on the hospital's website will promote nursing to current staff and to prospective new hires (Boyington et al., 2006).

CURRENT ISSUES AND TRENDS

Accountable payment models are shifting costs from payer to provider and mandate that organizations improve performance and quality, and thus customer satisfaction with the patient care experience. These models do not unbundle nursing care from room and board, therefore adjustments for nursing intensity in billing mechanisms are not possible. Recommendations for incorporating a nursing intensity adjustment to existing inpatient billing could lead to determination of the economic value of that care. Marketing mix could more closely reflect the "price" of nursing care, which would contribute to the effort in establishing a value-based purchasing system for hospitals (Welton & Dismuke, 2008; Welton et al., 2006). Moss and Saba (2011) have demonstrated the feasibility of observing nurses carrying out common nursing interventions and of applying a costing method to develop the cost of routine care. Because of the need to deliver and market cost-effective and efficient care, there will be continued efforts and initiatives to address costs of nursing care and subsequent reimbursement decisions. Nurses must also discuss evolving accountable payment models to create care delivery systems that prevent negative outcomes for which reimbursement will be withheld.

A focus on patient-centered care began in the 1970s, but how to implement it remains an issue for many health care organizations. Varied patient-centered models and frameworks exist. Attributes in patient-centeredness are patient satisfaction, the patient experience of care, patient engagement, and shared decision making. Evidence supports that patient-centered care improves patient outcomes and is a solution for addressing racial, ethnic, and socioeconomic disparities in health care and health care outcomes (Epstein et al., 2010). The dialogue surrounding patient-centered care can sound complex. However, Planetree is a designation that differentiates a hospital on the basis of excellence in patient- and person-centered care. The Planetree philosophy reveals a simple view of what it means to be patient-centered. "Care should be organized first and foremost around the needs of patients" (Planetree, n.d.). Components of the Planetree model that move an organization toward a culture of patient-centeredness can be found on their website. It is easy to determine the importance of patient-centeredness to marketing goals and ultimately to patient satisfaction. Models for delivery of patient-centered care will continue to evolve (Millenson & Macri, 2012).

Though there is a debate regarding whether the nursing shortage is over, there is sufficient evidence to support that nurses who are baby boomers are on the cusp of retirement and that the baby boomer population as a whole will increase the demand for health care services over the next 20 years (Buerhaus, 2008). In fact, a large prolonged shortage of nurses is predicted in the United States (Buerhaus et al., 2009). This trend calls for internal marketing initiatives that address nurse turnover, job satisfaction, and occupational and organizational commitment. External marketing challenges will be encountered by hospitals seeking a more qualified nurse workforce (i.e., those with baccalaureate [BSN] degrees). This standard is supported by the Institute of Medicine (Committee on the Robert Wood Johnson Foundation Initiative on the Future of Nursing, at the Institute of Medicine, 2011) and the American Nurses Credentialing Center's Magnet Recognition Program® (American Nurses Credentialing Center, 2012), and calls for competitive marketing strategies to recruit successfully from the target market of BSN prepared nurses. Clearly, nurses, as essential providers of the health care product, are engaged in marketing. Frontline nurses are critical to creating value for customers.

RESEARCH NOTE

Source

Press Ganey Associates, Inc. (2011). 2011 hospital pulse report: Patient perspectives on American health care. South Bend, IN: Author.

Purpose

The purpose of this study was to examine the experiences and perceptions of hospital inpatients treated in 2010.

Discussion

Press Ganey is a leader in health care performance improvement in organizations throughout the United States and is an approved vendor for a government-sponsored public report of hospital performance titled *Hospital Consumer Assessment of Healthcare Providers and Systems* (HCAHPS). They focus on care delivery, and clinical and business outcomes. Specifically, they guide health care organizations to improve quality, increase market share, operate efficiently, and optimize reimbursement. Press Ganey emphasizes the value of patients' perspectives in their data collection and analyses, and thus their reports have relevance to a marketing orientation. For many years, Press Ganey has published the *Pulse Report* about patients' perspectives of their health care experiences. Although their 2011 report included varied indicators of clinical and business outcomes, patient satisfaction remained a focus area. Satisfaction data are based on the responses of 2,854,198 patients, from 2067 hospitals, received from January 1, 2010, to December 31, 2010. The inpatient priority index is based on survey items of subjective experiences of hospital patients. The 2011 report revealed the following as *very important* to hospital patients:

- Response to concerns and complaints made during the hospital stay
- Degree to which hospital staff addressed emotional stress associated with the hospital stay
- Staff effort to include patients in treatment decisions
- Promptness in responding to the call button
- How well the nurses kept patients informed

A 5-year trend supports an increase in inpatient satisfaction across 2006-2010. Increases are due in part to changes in employee annual performance appraisals that reflect quality and behavioral expectations and to employee reward and recognition programs that reinforce quality and patient satisfaction. The Press Ganey Consulting Group recommends that "the standards of behavior in health care organizations must establish clear expectations for how to treat others–being responsive, looking people in the eyes and speaking directly to them, building relationships, and including patients in decisions."

Application to Practice

The inpatient satisfaction survey allows customers to rate a recent hospital experience according to their perspectives of care received—or not received. Reports to the public about health care agency performance are becoming the norm for the industry. Regardless of where they work, nurses must be familiar with patient satisfaction survey results and interpretation of findings. The top five items on the inpatient priority index in the Press Ganey *2011 Hospital Pulse Report* are evidence that nurses have a prominent role in patient satisfaction with the health care product and thus are contributors to a hospital's ability to be competitive in the marketplace.

CASE STUDY

As the nurse manager in the emergency department of Stockbridge Regional Medical Center (SRMC), Alexander Robbins has been appointed to serve on a committee to develop a marketing plan for the department. SRMC, a 500-bed hospital in an area with an estimated population of 200,000, has competition from four smaller hospitals in surrounding communities. SRMC has a reputation for being a very good acute care hospital with an emergency department (Level II trauma center) that has over 150,000 visits per year. Because SRMC has the only full-service emergency room in the area, they have experienced minimal competition from the smaller organizations.

Although quarterly patient satisfaction surveys have revealed concerns with wait time, length of stay, and "door-to-doc" times, hospital administration has been satisfied with the patient volume. Nurses are frustrated with perceived slow turnaround times for lab and radiology services. A marketing strategy was unnecessary for their competitive advantage in the external market, and the concerns of employees (internal market) were not addressed.

One of the smaller hospitals in a surrounding community entered into a partnership with an academic medical center (AMC) located 100 miles away. A center of excellence in the immediate care of stroke

Continued

patients was created. Virtual communication technology was implemented to allow their emergency room physicians to have around-the-clock access to neurologists at the AMC. The stroke center quickly gained an excellent reputation in the area. Plans are underway to expand the partnership to include other specialties over time.

SRMC noted a decrease in their emergency room patient volume and particularly a decline in stroke patient visits. A marketing committee has been formed to investigate their loss in market share and to move forward with strategic and marketing planning processes to reverse the trend.

From a marketing point of view, what should the committee consider about the product, place, price, and promotion of care delivered in the emergency room? Discuss how frontline nurses can be involved. What are the implications from the customer's perspective? What is the value of having nurse manager Alexander on the marketing committee?

CRITICAL THINKING EXERCISE

Sarah Glenn has been a critical care nurse in a community hospital for 10 years and has been the assistant manager of the adult critical care unit (CCU) for the past 3 years. Sarah was recently promoted and is now the CCU manager. The CCU is described as progressive, with a highly qualified nursing staff dedicated to continuing their education and to achieving critical care national certification. Over the past 2 months, there has been little response to routine advertising strategies employed by the human resources department in effort to fill three vacant staff nurse positions in the CCU. Sarah faces additional recruitment challenges with the opening of a new 12-bed expansion in 6 months. Sarah is aware of recruitment challenges because the target market is specialty nurses who may need or want attractive incentives.

1. What is the problem?
2. With whom should Sarah discuss the problem?
3. How can Sarah apply the marketing mix framework to approach the problem?
4. Who are the key stakeholder groups that should be involved in a recruitment campaign?

REFERENCES

Chapter 1

Alvesson, M., & Sveningsson, S. (2003). Managers doing leadership: The extra-ordinarization of the mundane. *Human Relations, 56*(12), 1435–1459.

American Nurses Association (ANA). (2009). *Nursing administration scope and standards of practice.* (3rd ed.). Washington, DC: Author.

American Nurses Credentialing Center (ANCC). (2008a). Modifying the Magnet™ model: The shape of things to come. *American Nurse Today, 3*(10), 52.

American Nurses Credentialing Center (ANCC). (2008b). *Overview of ANCC Magnet Recognition Program® new model.* Silver Spring, MD: Author.

American Organization of Nurse Executives (AONE). (2005a). AONE nurse executive competencies. *Nurse Leader, 3*(1), 15–21.

Bass, B. (1985). *Leadership and performance beyond expectations.* New York: The Free Press.

Bass, B., & Avolio, B. (1990). *Transformational leadership development: Manual for the Multifactor Leadership Questionnaire.* Palo Alto, CA: Consulting Psychologists Press.

Bennis, W. G. (1994). *On becoming a leader.* Reading, MA: Addison-Wesley.

Bennis, W. G. (2004). The seven ages of the leader. *Harvard Business Review, 82*(1), 46–53.

Bennis, W. G., & Nanus, B. (1985a). *Leaders: The strategies for taking charge.* New York: Harper & Row.

Bennis, W. G., & Thomas, R. J. (2002). Crucibles of leadership. *Harvard Business Review, 80*(9), 39–45.

Blake, R., & Mouton, J. (1964a). *The managerial grid.* Houston: Gulf Publishing.

Blake, R. R., & McCanse, A. A. (1991). *Leadership dilemmas—Grid solutions.* Houston: Gulf Publishing.

Brakey, M. (1991). Are you a good follower? *Nursing, 21*(12), 78–81.

Bureau of Health Professions (BHPr). (2010a). *The Registered Nurse population: Findings from the 2008 National Sample Survey of Registered Nurses.* Washington, DC: Author. Retrieved October 22, 2012, from http://bhpr.hrsa.gov/healthworkforce/rnsurveys/rnsurveyfinal.pdf.

Burns, J. (1978a). *Leadership.* New York: Harper & Row.

Cartwright, D., & Zander, A. (Eds.), (1960). *Group dynamics: Research and theory.* (2nd ed.). Evanston, IL: Row, Peterson.

Castle, N. G., & Decker, F. H. (2011). Top management leadership style and quality of care in nursing homes. *The Gerontologist, 51*(5), 630–642.

Chaleff, I. (2003). *The courageous follower: Standing up to and for our leaders* (2nd ed.). San Francisco: Berrett-Koehler.

Clancy, T. R. (2003). Courage and today's nurse leader. *Nursing Administration Quarterly, 27*(2), 128–132.

Curtin, L. L. (2000a). The first ten principles for the ethical administration of nursing services. *Nursing Administration Quarterly, 25*(1), 7–13.

Drucker, P. F. (1988). The coming of the new organization. *Harvard Business Review, 68*(1), 45–53.

Drucker, P. F. (1996). Foreword. In F. Hesselbein, M. Goldsmith, & R. Beckhard (Eds.), *The leader of the future: New visions, strategies, and practices for the next era.* San Francisco: Jossey-Bass.

Drucker, P. F. (2004). What makes an effective executive. *Harvard Business Review, 82*(6), 58–63.

Dunham, J., & Klafehn, K. (1990). Transformational leadership and the nurse executive. *Journal of Nursing Administration, 20*(4), 28–34.

Fayol, H. (1949). *General and industrial management.* London: Pitman & Sons.

Fiedler, F. (1967). *A theory of leadership effectiveness.* New York: McGraw-Hill.

Fiedler, F., & Chemers, M. (1984). *Improving leadership effectiveness: The leader match concept* (2nd ed.). New York: John Wiley & Sons.

Fiedler, F., & Garcia, J. (1987). *New approaches to effective leadership: Cognitive resources and organizational performance.* New York: John Wiley & Sons.

Foust, J. (1994). Creating a future for nursing through interactive planning at the bedside. *Image, 26*(2), 129–131.

Gittell, J. H. (2009). *High performance healthcare: Using the power of relationships to achieve quality, efficiency and resilience.* New York: McGraw-Hill.

Goleman, D. (2007). *Social intelligence: The new science of social relationships.* New York: Bantam Dell Publishing Group.

Gosling, J., & Mintzberg, H. (2003). The five minds of a manager. *Harvard Business Review, 81*(11), 54–63.

Grant, A. (1994). *The professional nurse: Issues and actions.* Springhouse, PA: Springhouse.

Greenleaf, R. K. (2002). *Servant leadership: A journey into the nature of legitimate power and greatness* (25th anniversary ed.). Mahwah, NJ: Paulist Press.

Hayes-Roth, B., & Hayes-Roth, F. (1979). A cognitive model of planning. *Cognitive Science, 3*, 275–310.

Helgeson, S. (1995a). *The web of inclusion: A new architecture for building organizations.* New York: Doubleday.

Helgeson, S. (1995b). *The female advantage: Women's ways of leadership* (2nd ed.). New York: Doubleday.

Hersey, P. H., Blanchard, K. H., & Johnson, D. E. (2013a). *Management of organizational behavior: Leading human resources* (10th ed.). Upper Saddle River, NJ: Pearson Education.

Huber, D. L., & Watson, C. A. (2001). *Effective leadership in health care organizations.* Indianapolis: The College Network.

Huber, D. L., Maas, M., McCloskey, J., Scherb, C. A., Goode, C. J., & Watson, C. (2000). Evaluating nursing administration instruments. *Journal of Nursing Administration, 30*(5), 251–272.

Institute of Medicine (IOM). (2004a). *Keeping patients safe: Transforming the work environment of nurses.* Washington, DC: National Academies Press.

Institute of Medicine (IOM) (2011a). *The future of nursing: Leading change, advancing health.* Retrieved October 1, 2012, from http://www.iom.edu/Reports/2010/The-Future-of-Nursing-Leading-Change-Advancing-Health.aspx/.

Jennings, B. M., Scalzi, C. C., Rodgers, J. D., III, & Keane, A. (2007). Differentiating nursing leadership and management competencies. *Nursing Outlook, 55*, 169–175.

Kanter, R. M. (1989). The new managerial work. *Harvard Business Review, 69*(6), 85–92.

Kellerman, B. (2008). *Followership: How followers are creating change and changing leaders.* Boston: Harvard Business Press.

Kelley, R. (1988). In praise of followers. *Harvard Business Review, 66*, 142–148.

Kelley, R. E. (1992). *The power of followership: How to create leaders people want to follow and followers who lead themselves.* New York: Doubleday.

Kison, C. (1989). Leadership: How, who and what? *Nursing Management, 20*(11), 72–74.

Kleinman, C. (2004a). The relationship between managerial leadership behaviors and staff nurse retention. *Hospital Topics, 82*(4), 2–9.

Knickman, J. R., & Snell, E. K. (2002). The 2030 problem: Caring for aging baby boomers. *Health Services Research, 37*(4), 849–884.

Koontz, H. (1961). The management theory jungle. *Academy of Management Journal,* (December) 174–188.

Kotter, J. (2001). What leaders really do. *Harvard Business Review, 79*(11), 85–96.

Kouzes, J., & Posner, B. (1988). *The leadership practices inventory.* San Diego: Pfeiffer & Company.

Kouzes, J., & Posner, B. (1995). *The leadership challenge: How to keep getting extraordinary things done in organizations.* San Francisco: Jossey-Bass.

Lewin, K. (1947a). Frontiers in group dynamics: Concept, method, and reality in social science; social equilibria and social change. *Human Relations, 1*(1), 5–41.

Lorenz, E. N. (1993). *The essence of chaos.* Seattle: University of Washington Press.

Malloch, K. (2002). Trusting organizations: Describing and measuring employee-to-employee relationships. *Nursing Administration Quarterly, 26*(3), 12–19.

Marchionni, C., & Ritchie, J. (2008). Organizational factors that support the implementation of a nursing Best Practice Guideline. *Journal of Nursing Management, 16*(3), 266–274.

Mathena, K. A. (2002). Nursing manager leadership skills. *Journal of Nursing Administration, 32*(3), 136–142.

McCauley, G. (2005). *Leadership in a quantum age.* Ottawa, Ontario, Canada: WEL-Systems Institute. Retrieved October 21, 2012, from www.partnersinrenewal.com/articles/Leadership.htm.

McClure, M. (1991a). Introduction. In I. Goertzen (Ed.), *Differentiating nursing practice: Into the twenty-first century* (pp. 1–11). Kansas City, MO: American Academy of Nursing.

McDaniel, C., & Wolf, G. (1992). Transformational leadership in nursing service: A test of theory. *Journal of Nursing Administration, 22*(2), 60–65.

McNamara, C. (1999a). *Skills and practices in organizational management.* Minneapolis, MN: Authenticity Consulting, LLC. Retrieved October 22, 2012, from http://208.42.83.77/mgmnt/skills.htm.

McNamara, C. (1999b). *Basic guidelines for successful planning process.* Minneapolis, MN: Authenticity Consulting, LLC. Retrieved October 22, 2012, from http://208.42.83.77/plan_dec/gen_plan/gen_plan.htm.

McNamara, C. (1999c). *Management function of organizing: Overview of methods.* Minneapolis, MN: Authenticity Consulting, LLC. Retrieved October 22, 2012, from http://208.42.83.77/orgnzing/orgnzing.htm#anchor121585.

McNamara, C. (1999d). *Management function of coordinating/controlling: Overview of basic methods.* Minneapolis, MN: Authenticity Consulting, LLC. Retrieved October 22, 2012, from http://managementhelp.org/managementcontrol/index.htm.

McNamara, C. (1999e). *Introduction to management.* Minneapolis, MN: Authenticity Consulting, LLC.

Retrieved October 22, 2012, from http://208.42.83.77/mng_thry/mng_thry.htm.

McNamara, C. (1999f). *New paradigm in management.* Minneapolis, MN: Authenticity Consulting, LLC. Retrieved October 22, 2012, from http://managementhelp.org/management/paradigms.htm.

McNamara, C. (1999g). *Historical and contemporary theories of management.* Minneapolis, MN: Authenticity Consulting, LLC. Retrieved October 22, 2012, from http://managementhelp.org/management/theories.htm.

Metts, L. (2008). The emotionally intelligent case manager. *Case In Point*, (April/May), 11–13.

Mintzberg, H. (1973). *The nature of managerial work.* New York: Harper & Row.

Mintzberg, H. (1975). The manager's job: Folklore and fact. In M. Matteson & J. Ivancevich (Eds.), *Management classics.* (3rd ed., (pp. 63–85). Plano, TX: Business Publications.

Mintzberg, H. (1994). Managing as blended care. *Journal of Nursing Administration*, 24(9), 29–36.

Mintzberg, H. (1998). Covert leadership: Notes on managing professionals. *Harvard Business Review*, 76(6), 140–147.

O'Connor, M. (2008). The dimensions of leadership: A foundation for caring competency. *Nursing Administration Quarterly*, 32(1), 21–26.

O'Neil, E., Morjikian, R. L., Cherner, D., Hirschkorn, C., & West, T. (2008). Developing nursing leaders: An overview of trends and programs. *Journal of Nursing Administration*, 38(4), 178–183.

Pagonis, W. (1992). The work of the leader. *Harvard Business Review*, 70(6), 118–126.

Patrick, A., Laschinger, H. K. S., Wong, C., & Finegan, J. (2011). Developing and testing a new measure of staff nurse clinical leadership: The clinical leadership survey. *Journal of Nursing Management*, 19, 499–460.

Pediani, R. (1996). Chaos and evolution in nursing research. *Journal of Advanced Nursing*, 23(4), 645–646.

Pipe, T. B. (2008). Illuminating the inner leadership journey by engaging intention and mindfulness as guided by caring theory. *Nursing Administration Quarterly*, 32(2), 117–125.

Porter-O'Grady, T. (2003a). A different age for leadership, Part 1. *Journal of Nursing Administration*, 33(2), 105–110.

Rosenhead, J. (1998). Complexity theory and management practice. *The Human Daily Review*. Retrieved October 24, 2012, from http://human-nature.com/science-as-culture/rosenhead.html.

Shirey, M. R. (2006). Building authentic leadership and enhancing entrepreneurial performance. *Clinical Nurse Specialist*, 20(6), 280–282.

Shirey, M. R. (2007a). Leadership and organizational strategies to increase innovative thinking. *Clinical Nurse Specialist*, 21(4), 191–194.

Smola, B. (1988). Refinement and validation of a tool measuring leadership characteristics of baccalaureate nursing students. In O. Strickland & C. Waltz (Eds.), *Measurement of nursing outcomes* (Vol. 2, pp. 314–366). New York: Springer.

Stodgill, R. (1963). *Manual for the Leader Behavior Description Questionnaire—Form XII: An experimental revision.* Columbus, OH: Ohio State University.

Sull, D. N. (2003). Managing by commitments. *Harvard Business Review*, 81(6), 82–91.

Tannenbaum, R. & Schmidt, W. H. (1973). How to choose a leadership pattern. *Harvard Business Review*, 51(3), 162–180.

Tornabeni, J. (2001). The competency game: My take on what it really takes to lead. *Nursing Administration Quarterly*, 25(4), 1–13.

U.S. Census Bureau. (2012). *Profile America: Facts for features.* Washington, DC: Author. Retrieved October 22, 2012, from http://www.census.gov/newsroom/releases/archives/facts_for_features_special_editions/cb12-ff07.html.

Upenieks, V. (2003a). Nurse leaders' perceptions of what compromises successful leadership in today's acute inpatient environment. *Nursing Administration Quarterly*, 27(2), 140–152.

Upenieks, V. (2003b). What constitutes effective leadership? *Journal of Nursing Administration*, 33(9), 456–467.

Waldrop, M. M. (1992). *Complexity: The emerging science at the edge of order and chaos.* New York: Simon & Schuster Paperbacks.

Walsh, M. (2000). Chaos, complexity and nursing. *Nursing Standard*, 14(3), 39–42.

Wheatley, M. J. (1992). *Leadership and the new science: Learning about organization from an orderly universe.* San Francisco: Berrett-Koehler.

Wheatley, M. J. (1999a). *Leadership and the new science: Discovering order in a chaotic world* (2nd ed.). San Francisco: Berrett-Koehler.

Wolf, G. A., Triolo, P., & Ponte, P. R. (2008a). Magnet Recognition Program: The next generation. *Journal of Nursing Administration*, 38(4), 200–204.

Chapter 2

Agency for Healthcare Research and Quality (AHRQ). (2012). *AHRQ Health Care Innovations Exchange.* Retrieved from: www.innovations.ahrq.gov/innovations_qualitytools.aspx.

Alas, R. (2007). Organizational change from learning perspective. *Problems and Perspectives in Management*, 5(2), 43–50.

American Organization of Nurse Executives (AONE). (2005b). AONE nurse executive competencies. *Nurse Leader, 3*(1), 15–21.

Anderson, L. A., & Anderson, D. (2009). *Awake at the wheel: Moving beyond change management to Conscious Change Leadership.* Retrieved from www.BeingFirst.com.

Aranda, D. A., & Molina-Fernandez, L. M. (2002). Determinants of innovation through a knowledge-based theory lens. *Industrial Management and Data Systems, 102,* 289–296.

Balfour, M., & Clarke, C. (2001). Searching for sustainable change. *Journal of Clinical Nursing, 10,* 44–50.

Balogun, J. (2006). Managing change: Steering a course between intended strategies and unanticipated outcomes. *Long Range Planning, 39,* 29–49.

Bartunek, J. M., Rousseau, D. M., Rudolph, J., & DePalma, J. A. (2006). On the receiving end: Sensemaking, emotion, and assessments of an organizational change initiated by others. *Journal of Applied Behavioral Science, 42,* 182–206.

Bennis, W., Benne, K., Chin, R., & Corey, K. (1976). *The planning of change.* New York: Holt, Rinehart & Winston.

Bennis, W. G., Benne, K. D., & Chin, R. (Eds.). (1961). *The planning of change: Readings in the applied behavioral sciences.* New York: Holt, Rinehart & Winston.

Bola, H. S. (1994). The CLER model: Thinking through change. *Nursing Management, 25*(5), 59–63.

Bowditch, J. L., & Buono, A. F. (2001). *A primer on organizational behavior* (5th ed.). New York: John Wiley.

Burns, J. (1978b). *Leadership.* New York: Harper & Row.

Burnes, B. (2004). Kurt Lewin and complexity theories: Back to the future? *Journal of Change Management, 4*(4), 309–325.

Cartwright, D., & Zander, A. (Eds.). (1960). *Group dynamics: Research and theory.* (2nd ed.). Evanston, IL: Row, Peterson.

Christensen, C. M., Bohmer, R., & Kenagy, J. (2000). Will disruptive innovations cure health care? *Harvard Business Review, 78*(5), 102–112.

Copnell, B., & Bruni, N. (2006). Breaking the silence: Nurses' understandings of change in clinical practice. *Journal of Advanced Nursing, 55*(3), 301–309. http://dx.doi:10.1111/j.1365-2648.2006.03911.x.

Drucker, P. (1992). *Managing for the future: The 1990s and beyond.* New York: Truman Talley Books/Plume.

Falk-Rafael, A. R. (2000). Nurses' orientations to change: Debunking the "resistant to change" myth. *Journal of Professional Nursing, 16*(6), 336–344.

Gilmartin, M. J. (1999). Creativity: The fuel of innovation. *Nursing Administration Quarterly, 23*(2), 1–8.

Grant, B., Colello, S., Reihle, M., & Dende, D. (2010). *Journal of Nursing Management, 18,* 326–331. http://dx.doi:10.1111/j1365-2834.2010.01076.x.

Havelock, R. (1973). *The change agent's guide to innovation in education.* Englewood Cliffs, NJ: Educational Technology Publications.

Hersey, P., Blanchard, K. H., & Johnson, D. E. (2008a). *Management of organizational behavior: Leading human resources* (9th ed.). Upper Saddle River, NJ: Pearson Education.

Hughes, F. (2006). Nurses at the forefront of innovation. *International Nursing Review, 53,* 94–101.

Institute of Medicine (IOM) (2011b). *The future of nursing: Leading change, advancing health.* Washington, DC: The National Academies Press.

Issel, L. M., & Anderson, R. A. (1996). Take charge: Managing six transformations in healthcare delivery. *Nursing Economic$, 14*(2), 78–85.

Jones, J. E., & Bearley, W. L. (1996). *Organizational change-readiness scale.* Amherst, MA: HRD Press.

Kanter, R. M. (1983). *The change masters: Innovation and entrepreneurship in the American corporation.* New York: Simon & Schuster.

Kerfoot, K. (1998). Leading change is leading creativity. *Nursing Economic$, 16*(2), 98–99.

Leeman, J., Baernholdt, M., & Sandelowski, M. (2007). Developing a theory-based taxonomy of methods for implementing change in practice. *Journal of Advanced Nursing, 58*(2), 191–200. http://dx.doi:10.1111/j.1365-2648.2006.04207.x.

Lewin, K. (1947b). Frontiers in group dynamics: Concept, method, and reality in social science; social equilibrium and social change. *Human Relations, 1*(1), 5–41.

Lewin, K. (1951). *Field theory in social science: Selected theoretical papers.* New York: Harper & Row.

Lippitt, G. (1973). *Visualizing change: Model building and the change process.* La Jolla, CA: University Associates.

Porter-O'Grady, T. & Malloch, K (2011a). *Quantum leadership: Advancing innovation, transforming health care* (3rd ed.) Sudbury, MA: Jones and Bartlett.

Robbins, B., & Davidhizar, R. (2007). Transformational leadership in healthcare today. *The Health Care Manager, 26*(3), 234–239.

Robert Wood Johnson Foundation (RWJF). (2008). *The transforming care at the bedside (TCAB) toolkit.* Princeton, NJ: Robert Wood Johnson Foundation. Retrieved June 7, 2012, from www.rwjf.org/healthpolicy/product.jsp?id=30051.

Rogers, E. M. (2003a). *Diffusion of innovations* (5th ed.). New York: Free Press.

Rost, J. C. (1994). Leadership: A new conception. *Holistic Nursing Practice, 9*(2), 1–8.

Romano, C. (1990). Diffusion of technology innovation. *Advances in Nursing Science, 13*(2), 11–21.

Savcik, P. O., Tvedt, S. T., Nytro, K., Andersen, G. R., Andersen, T. K., Buvik, M., et al. (2007). Developing criteria for healthy organizational change. *Work & Stress, 21*(3), 243–263.

Senge, P. M. (1990). *The fifth discipline: The art and practice of the learning organization.* New York: Doubleday.

Senge, P. M., Kleiner, A., Roberts, C., Ross, R. B., & Smith, B. J. (1994). *The fifth discipline fieldbook.* New York: Doubleday.

Shanley, C. (2007). Management of change for nurses: Lessons from the discipline of organizational studies. *Journal of Nursing Management, 15*, 538–546.

Shirey, M. R. (2007b). Leadership and organizational strategies to increase innovative thinking. *Clinical Nurse Specialist, 21*(4), 191–194.

Tiffany, C. R., & Lutjens, L. R. J. (1998). *Planned change theories for nursing: Review, analysis, and implications.* Thousand Oaks, CA: Sage.

Valente, S. (2011). Rapid cycle change projects improve quality of care. *Journal of Nursing Care Quality, 26*(1), 54–60.

Van Woerkum, C., Aarts, N., Van Herzele, A. (2011). Changed planning for planned and unplanned change. *Planning Theory, 10*, 144–161. http://dx. doi:10.1177/1473095210389651.

Watzlawick, P., Weakland, J. H., & Fisch, R. (1974). *Change: Principles of problem formation and problem resolution.* New York, NY: Norton.

Weimer, B. J., Amick, H., & Lee, S. D. (2008). Conceptualization and measurement of organizational readiness for change: A review of the literature in health services research and other fields. *Medical Care Research and Review, 65*(4), 379–436.

Wheatley, M. J. (2007). *Finding our way: Leadership for an uncertain time.* San Francisco, CA: Berrett-Koehler.

Workman, R., & Kenney, M. (1988). The change experience. In S. Pinkerton, & P. Schroeder (Eds.), *Commitment to excellence: Developing a professional nursing staff* (pp. 17–25). Rockville, MD: Aspen.

Chapter 3

Agency for Healthcare Research and Quality. (2002). *National healthcare quality report: update.* Fact Sheet. AHRQ Publication No. 02-P028. Rockville, MD: Author.

Aiken, L. H., Clarke, S. P., Sloane, D. M., Lake, E. T., & Cheney, T. (2008). Effects of hospital care environments on patient mortality and nurse outcomes. *Journal of Nursing Administration, 38*(5), 223–229.

Aiken, L. H., Clarke, S. P., Sloane, D. M., Sochalski, J. A., Busse, R., Clarke, H., et al. (2001a). Nurses' reports on hospital care in five countries. *Health Affairs, 20*(3), 43–53.

Aiken, L. H., & Fagin, C. M. (1997). Evaluating the consequences of hospital restructuring. *Medical Care, 35*(10), OS1–OS4.

Aiken, L. H., Lake, E. T., Sochalski, J., & Sloane, D. M. (1997a). Design of an outcomes study of the organization of hospital AIDS care. *Research in the Sociology of Health Care, 14*, 3–26.

Aiken, L. H., Sochalski, J., & Lake, E. T. (1997b). Studying outcomes of organizational change in health services. *Medical Care, 35*(11), NS6–NS18.

Aiken, L. H., Smith, H. L., & Lake, E. T. (1994). Lower Medicare mortality among a set of hospitals known for good nursing care. *Medical Care, 32*, 771–785.

Alderfer, C. P. (1980). *Consulting to under bounded systems.* (Vol. 2) New York: Wiley.

American Nurses Association (ANA). (1997). *Implementing nursing's report card: A study of RN staffing, length of stay and patient outcomes.* Washington, DC: American Nurses Publishing.

American Nurses Credentialing Center (ANCC). (2004). *Magnet Recognition Program®, Forces of Magnetism.* Silver Spring, MD: Author. Retrieved February 22, 2008, from http://www.nursecredentialing.org/Magnet/ ProgramOverview/HistoryoftheMagnetProgram/ ForcesofMagnetism.

American Nurses Credentialing Center (ANCC). (2008c). *Magnet Recognition Program®.* Silver Spring, MD: Author. Retrieved July 30, 2008, from http:// nursecredentialing.org/Magnet.aspx.

Anthony, M. K., Standing, T. S., Glick, J., Duffy, M., Paschall, F., Sauer, M., et al. (2005). Leadership and nurse retention: The pivotal role of nurse managers. *Journal of Nursing Administration, 35*, 146–155.

Bellot, J. (2011). Defining and assessing organizational culture. *Nursing Forum, 46*(1), 29–37.

Blegen, M. A., Pepper, G. A., & Rosse, J. (2005). *Safety climate on hospital units: A new measure.* Retrieved February 1, 2008, from http://ahrq.gov/downloads/pub/ advances/vol4/Blegen.pdf.

Boyle, D. K., Bott, M. J., Hansen, H. E., Woods, C. Q., & Taunton, R. L. (1999). Managers' leadership and critical care nurses' intent to stay. *American Journal of Critical Care, 8*, 361–371.

Boyle, S. M. (2004). Nursing unit characteristics and patient outcomes. *Nursing Economic$, 22*, 111–119.

Brennan, P. F., & Anthony, M. K. (2000). Measuring nursing practice models using multiattribute utility theory. *Research in Nursing and Health, 23*, 372–382.

Clarke, S., Rockett, J., Sloane, D., & Aiken, L. (2002a). Organizational climate, staffing, and safety equipment as predictors of needlestick injuries and near-misses in hospital nurses. *American Journal of Infection Control, 30*(4), 207–216.

Clarke, S., Sloane, D., & Aiken, L. (2002b). Effects of hospital staffing and organizational climate on needlestick injuries to nurses. *American Journal of Public Health, 92*(7), 1115–1119.

Coeling, H., & Simms, L. (1993). Facilitating innovation at the nursing unit level through cultural assessment. Part 1. *Journal of Nursing Administration, 23*, 46–52.

Connor, M., Duncombe, D., Barclay, E., Bartel, S., Borden, C., Gross, E., et al. (2007). Creating a fair and just culture: One institution's path toward organizational change. *The Joint Commission Journal on Quality and Patient Safety, 33*, 617–624.

Daft, R. L. (2001). *Organizational theory and design* (7th ed.). New York: West Publishing.

DeJoy, D. M., Schaffer, B. S., Wilson, M. G., Vandenbert, R. J., & Butts, M. M. (2004). Creating safer workplaces: Assessing the determinants and role of safety climate. *Journal of Safety Research, 35*, 81–90.

Duchscher, J. E., & Cowin, L. (2004). Multigenerational nurses in the workplace. *Journal of Nursing Administration, 34*, 493–501.

Friese, C., Lake, E., Aiken, L., Silber, J., & Sochalski, J. (2008). Hospital nurse practice environments and outcomes for surgical oncology patients. *Health Services Research, 43*(4), 1145–1163.

Hart, K., & Moore, M. (1989). The relationship among organizational climate variables and nurse stability in critical care units. *Journal of Professional Nursing, 5*(3), 124–131.

Hemingway, M., & Smith, C. (1999). Organizational climate and occupational stressors as predictors of withdrawal behaviors and injuries among nurses. *Journal of Occupational and Organizational Psychology, 72*, 285–299.

Hinshaw, A. S. (2008). Navigating the perfect storm: Balancing a culture of safety with workforce challenges. *Nursing Research, 57*, S4–S10.

Institute of Medicine (IOM). (2001a). *Crossing the quality chasm*. Washington, DC: National Academies Press.

Kimball, B., & O'Neill, E. (2002). *Health care's human crisis: The American nursing shortage*. Princeton, NJ: Robert Wood Johnson Foundation. Available: www.rwjf.org/news/special/nursing_report.pdf.

Koerner, J. G. (1996). Congruency between nurses' values and job requirements: A call for integrity. *Holistic Nursing Practice, 10*, 69–77.

Kohn, L. T., Corrigan, J. M., & Donaldson, M. S. (Eds.). (2000a). *To err is human: Building a safer health system*. Washington, DC: National Academies Press.

Kramer, M., & Hafner, L. P. (1989a). Shared values: Impact on staff nurse job satisfaction and perceived productivity. *Nursing Research, 38*, 172–177.

Litwin, G., & Stringer, R. (1968). *Motivation and organizational climate*. Boston: Division of Research, Graduate School of Business Administration, Harvard University.

Lustbader, W. (2001). The Pioneer Challenge: A radical change in the culture of nursing homes. In L. S. Noelker, & Z. Harel (Eds.), *Linking quality of long-term care and quality of life* (pp. 185–203). New York: Springer.

Manojlovich, M. (2005). The effect of nursing leadership on hospital nurses' professional practice behavior. *Journal of Nursing Administration, 35*, 366–374.

Mark, B. A. (1996). Organizational culture. In J. J. Fitzpatrick, & J. Norbeck (Eds.), *Annual review of nursing research* (Vol. 14, pp. 145–163). New York: Springer.

Mark, B. A., Hughes, L. C., Belyea, M., Chang, Y., Hoffman, D., Jones, C. B., et al. (2007a). Does safety climate moderate the influence of staffing adequacy and work condition on nurse injuries? *Journal of Safety Research, 38*, 431–446.

Marx, D. (2001). *Patient safety and the "Just Culture": A primer for health care executives*. New York: Columbia University.

Mitchell, P. H., & Shortell, S. M. (1997). Adverse outcomes and variations in organization of care delivery. *Medical Care, 35*, NS19–NS32.

Needleman, J., Buerhaus, P. I., Mattke, S., Stewart, M., & Zelevinsky, K. (2001a). *Nurse staffing and patient outcomes in hospitals*. (Contract No. 230-99-0021). Boston: Health Resources Services Administration.

Peters, T., & Waterman, R. H. (1982). *In search of excellence*. New York: Warner Communications.

Omnibus Budget Reconciliation Act of 1987. http://www.ncmust.com/doclib/OBRA87summary.pdf.

QSEN (2002). *Quality and safety education for nurses*. Retrieved March 25, 2012 from www.qsen.org/.

Schein, E. H. (1996). Culture: The missing concept in organization studies. *Administrative Science Quarterly, 41*(2), 220–240.

Schmalenberg, C., & Kramer, M. (2008). Essentials of a productive work environment. *Nursing Research, 57*, 2–13.

Scott, T., Mannion, R., Davies, H., & Marshall, M. (2003). The quantitative measurement of organizational culture in health care: A review of the available instruments. *Health Services Research, 38*, 923–945.

Seago, J. A. (2001). Nurse staffing, models of care delivery, and interventions. In K. G. Shojania, B. W. Duncan, K. M. McDonald, & R. M. Wachter (Eds.), *Making health care safer: A critical analysis of patient safety practices* (Vol. 43, pp. 427–450). Rockville, MD: Agency for Healthcare Research and Quality.

Shields, S. (2004). Pioneering approaches to long term care. In *Symposium,* May 2004: Springfield, IL.

Sleutel, M. R. (2000). Climate, culture, context, or work environment? Organizational factors that influence nursing practice. *Journal of Nursing Administration, 30*, 53–58.

Snow, J. (2002). Enhancing work climate to improve performance and retain valued employees. *Journal of Nursing Administration, 33*(2), 111–117.

Sochalski, J., Estabrooks, C. A., & Humphrey, C. K. (1999). Nurse staffing and patient outcomes: Evolution of an international study. *Canadian Journal of Nursing Research, 31*, 69–88.

Sorrentino, E., Nalli, B., & Schriesheim, C. (1992). The effect of head nurse behaviors on nurse job satisfaction and performance. *Hospital and Health Services Administration, 37*, 103–113.

Sovie, M. D., & Jawad, A. F. (2001). Hospital restructuring and its impact on outcomes. *Journal of Nursing Administration, 31*, 588–600.

Stock, R., Mahoney, E., Reece, D., & Cesario, L. (2008). Developing a senior healthcare practice using the chronic care model: Effect on physical function and health-related quality of life. *Journal of the American Geriatrics Society, 56*(7), 1342–1348.

Stone, P. W., Harrison, M. I., Feldman, P., Linzer, M., Peng, T., Roblin, D., et al. (2005). *Organizational climate of staff working conditions and safety: An integrative model.* Retrieved February 1, 2008, from http://www.ncbi.nlm.nih.gov/books/NBK20497/.

Stone, P. W., Larson, E. L., Mooney-Kane, C., Smolowitz, J., Lin, S. X., & Dick, A. W. (2006). Organizational climate and intensive care nurses' intention to leave. *Critical Care Medicine, 34*, 1907–1912.

Taunton, R. L., Boyle, D. K., Woods, C. Q., Hansen, H. E., & Bott, M. J. (1997). Manager leadership and retention of hospital staff nurses. *Western Journal of Nursing Research, 19*, 205–226.

Upenieks, V. (2003c). What constitutes effective leadership? Perceptions of Magnet and non-Magnet nurse leaders. *Journal of Nursing Administration, 33*, 456–467.

U.S. Department of Health and Human Services: Health Resources and Services Administration. (2010, September). *The registered nurse population: Findings from the 2008 National Sample Survey of Registered Nurses.* Retrieved March 25, 2012, from http://bhpr.hrsa.gov/healthworkforce/rnsurveys/rnsurveyfinal.pdf.

Uttal, B. (1983, October). The corporate culture vultures. *Fortune Magazine, 108*(8), 66. (October).

Wolf, G. (2006). A road map for creating a magnet work environment. *Journal of Nursing Administration, 36*, 458–462.

Wooten, L. P., & Crane, P. (2003). Nurses as implementers of organizational culture. *Nursing Economic$, 21*, 275–279.

Chapter 4

Albarran, J. W. (2004). Creativity: An essential element of critical care nursing practice. *Nursing in Critical Care, 9*(2), 47–49.

Alfaro-LeFevre, R. (2009). *Critical thinking and clinical judgment: A practical approach to outcome-focused thinking* (4th ed.). St. Louis: Saunders Elsevier.

American Association of Colleges of Nursing. (2008). *Essentials of baccalaureate education for professional nursing practice.* Retrieved May 1, 2012 www.aacn.nche.edu/education-resources/BaccEssentials08.pdf.

American Nurses Association. (2009). *Nursing administration scope and standards.* Silver Springs, MD: Author.

Benham-Hutchins, M., & Clancy, T. R. (2010). Social networks as embedded complex adaptive systems. *Journal of Nursing Administration, 40*(9), 352–356.

Benner, P. (1984). *From novice to expert: Excellence and power in clinical practice.* Menlo Park, CA: Addison-Wesley.

Benner, P. (2003). Beware of technological imperatives and commercial interests that prevent best practices! *American Journal of Critical Care, 12*(5), 469–471.

Burke, D. S., Epstein, J. M., Cummings, D. A. T., Parker, J. I., Cline, K. C., Singa, R. M., et al. (2006). Individual computational modeling of smallpox epidemic control strategies. *Academic Emergency Medicine, 13*(11), 1142–1149.

Campbell, E. M., Sittig, D. F., Ash, J. S., Guappone, K. P., & Dykstra, R. H. (2006). Types of unintended consequences related to computerized provider order entry. *Journal of the American Medical Informatics Association, 13*(5), 547–556.

Cannon, S., Boswell, C., & Robinson, M. (2007). Making research come alive at the bedside. *Nursing Management, 38*(10), 16–17.

Castaldo, J. (2010). Getting drowned out by the brainstorm. *Canadian Business, 83*(10), 91.

Chambers, C. C. (2009). *Creative nursing leadership and management.* Sudbury, MA: Jones & Bartlett.

Choo, C. W. (2006). *The knowing organization* (2nd ed.). New York: Oxford University Press.

Chu, D., Strand, R., & Fjelland, R. (2003). Theories of complexity. *Complexity, 8*(3), 19–30.

Clancy, T. R., & Delaney, C. W. (2005). Complex nursing systems. *Journal of Nursing Management, 13*, 192–201.

Cohen, S. (2002). Don't overlook creative thinking. *Nursing Management, 33*(8), 9–10.

Committee on the Robert Wood Johnson Foundation Initiative on the Future of Nursing, at the Institute of Medicine; Institute of Medicine (IOM). (2011). *The future of nursing: Leading change, advancing health.* Retrieved June 15, 2011 from www.nap.edu.

Cornell, P., Riordan, M., Townsend-Gervis, M., & Mobley, R. (2011). Barriers to critical thinking: Workflow interruptions and task switching among nurses. *Journal of Nursing Administration, 41*(10), 407–414.

Coyle, G. A., Sapnas, K. G., & Ward-Presson, K. (2007a). Dealing with disaster. *Nursing Management, 38*(7), 24–29.

Currie, K., Tolson, D., & Booth, J. (2007). Helping or hindering: The role of nurse managers in the transfer of practice development learning. *Journal of Nursing Management, 15*, 585–594.

De Bleser, L., DePreitere, R., De Waele, K., Vanhaecht, K., Vlayen, J., & Sermeus, W. (2006). Defining pathways. *Journal of Nursing Management, 14*(7), 553–563.

del Bueno, D. (2005). A crisis in critical thinking. *Nursing Education Perspectives, 26*(5), 278–282.

Dexter, F., Wachtel, R. E. & Epstein, R. H. (2011). Event-based knowledge elicitation of operating room management decision-making using scenarios adapted from information systems data. *BMC Medical Informatics and Decision Making, 11*(1), 1–13.

Drummond, H. (2001). *The art of decision making.* Chichester, England: John Wiley & Sons.

Dunbar, B., Park, B., Berger-Wesley, M., Cameron, T., Lorenz, B. T., Mayes, D., et al. (2007). Shared governance: Making the transition in practice and perception. *Journal of Nursing Administration, 37*(4), 177–183.

Effken, J. A., Verran, J. A., Logue, M. D., & Hsu, Y. C. (2010). Nurse managers' decisions: Fast and favoring remediation. *Journal of Nursing Administration, 40*(4), 188–195.

Elder, L., & Paul, R. (n.d.). *Becoming a critic of your thinking.* Retrieved May 9, 2012, from http://www.criticalthinking.org/pages/becoming-a-critic-of-your-thinking/478.

Ellermann, C. R., Katoka-Yahiro, M. R., & Wong, L. C. (2006). Logic models to enhance critical thinking. *Journal of Nursing Education, 45*(6), 220–227.

Etheridge, S. A. (2007). Learning to think like a nurse: Stories from new nurse graduates. *Journal of Continuing Education in Nursing, 38*(1), 24–30.

Etzioni, A. (1986). Mixed scanning revisited. *Public Administration Review, 46*(1), 8–14.

Etzioni, A. (1989). Humble decision making. *Harvard Business Review, 67*(4), 122–126.

Facione, P. (2007). *2007 Update—Critical thinking: What it is and why it counts.* Retrieved May 11, 2008, from www.insightassessment.com/pdf_files/what&why2007.pdf.

Fero, L. J., Witsberger, C. M., Wesmiller, S. W., Zullo, T. G., & Hoffman, L. A. (2008). Critical thinking ability of new graduate and experienced nurses. *Journal of Advanced Nursing, 65*(1), 139–148.

Fioratou, E., Pauley, K., & Fin, R. (2011). Critical thinking in the operating theatre. *Theoretical Issues in Ergonomics Science, 12*(3), 241–255.

Ford, R. (2009). Complex leadership competency in health care: Towards framing a theory of practice. *Health Services Management Research, 22*(3), 101–114.

Forneris, S. G., & Peden-McAlpine, C. (2009). Creating context for critical thinking in practice: The role of the preceptor. *Journal of Advanced Nursing, 65*(8), 1715–1724.

Frings, G. W., & Grant, L. (2005). Who moved my Sigma: Effective implementation of the Six Sigma methodology to hospitals. *Quality and Reliability Engineering International, 21*(3), 311–328.

Gromley, D. K. (2011). Are we on the same page? Staff nurse and manager perceptions of work environment, quality of care and anticipated nurse turnover. *Journal of Nursing Management, 19*(1), 33–40.

Guo, K. L. (2008). DECIDE: A decision-making model for more effective decision making by health care managers. *The Health Care Manager, 27*(2), 118–127.

Hammond, J. S., Keeney, R. L., & Raiffa, H. (1998). The hidden traps in decision making. *Harvard Business Review, 76*(5), 47–58.

Hammond, J. S., Keeney, R. L., & Raiffa, H. (2006). The hidden traps in decision making. *Harvard Business Review, 84*(1), 118–126.

Hammond, J. S., Keeney, R. L., & Raiffa, H. (1999). *Smart choices: A practical guide to making better decisions.* Boston: Harvard Business School Press.

Hart, M. A. (2012). Accountable care organizations: The future of care delivery? *American Journal of Nursing, 112*(2), 23–26.

Hawkins, A., Carter, K., & Nugent, M. (2009). Nurse manager orientation. *AACN Advanced Critical Care, 20*(1), 55–70.

HFMA P & P Board (2012). Medicare incentive payments for meaningful use of electronic health records: Accounting and reporting developments. *Healthcare Financial Management, 66*(2), 90–93.

Holden, L. M. (2005). Complex adaptive systems: Concept Analysis. *Journal of Advanced Nursing, 52*(6), 651–657.

Ignatavicius, D. D. (2008). *Critical thinking skills in the clinical setting.* Message posted to Nursing Educators Discussion List, archived at https://lists.uvic.ca/mailman/private/nrsinged/.

Insight Assessment. (2008a). *California critical thinking skills test—Form 2000.* Milbrae, CA Insight Assessment/California Academic Press. Retrieved May 18, 2008, from www.insightassessment.com/test-cctst.html.

Insight Assessment. (2008b). *The health sciences reasoning test manual.* Retrieved May 18, 2008, from http://www.insightassessment. com/Products/Critical-Thinking-Skills-Tests/ Health-Sciences-Reasoning-Test-HSRT.

Institute of Medicine (IOM). (2001b). *Crossing the quality chasm: A new health system for the 21st century.* Washington, DC: National Academies Press.

Institute of Medicine (IOM). (2003a). *Health professions education: A bridge to quality.* Washington, DC: National Academies Press. Retrieved August 4, 2008, from http://books.nap.edu/openbook. php?record_id=10681&page=4.

Interprofessional Education Collaborative Expert Panel. (2011). *Core competencies for interprofessional collaborative practice: Report of an expert panel.* Washington, D.C.: Interprofessional Education Collaborative. Retrieved May 20, 2011 from: www.aacn. nche.edu/education-resources/IPECReport.pdf.

Junttila, K., Meretoja, R., Seppala, A., Tolppanen, E., Ala-Nikkola, T., & Silvennoinen, L. (2007). Data warehouse approach to nursing management. *Journal of Nursing Management, 15,* 155–161.

Kahneman, D., Lovallo, D., & Sibony, O. (2011). Before you make that decision. *Harvard Business Review, 89*(6), 51–60.

Kane, R. L., Shamliyan, T. A., Mueller, C., Duval, S., & Wilt, T. J. (2007a). The association of registered nurse staffing levels and patient outcomes: Systematic review and meta-analysis. *Medical Care, 45*(12), 1195–1204.

Kerfoot, K. (2006). Reliability between nurse managers: The key to the high-reliability organization. *Nursing Economic$, 24*(5), 274–275.

Keynes, M. (2008). Making good decisions, Part 1. *Nursing Management-UK, 14*(9), 32–34.

Kohn, N. W., & Smith, S. M. (2011). Collaborative fixation: Effects of others' ideas on brainstorming. *Applied Cognitive Psychology, 25*(3), 359–371.

Kramer, M., Schmalenberg, C., & Maguire, P. (2010). Nine structures and leadership practices essential for a magnetic (healthy) work environment. *Nursing Administration Quarterly, 34*(1), 4–17.

Kuraitis, V. (2007). Disease management and the medical home model. *Disease Management and Health Outcomes, 15*(3), 135–140.

Lamont, J. (2010). Data drives decision-making in healthcare. *Healthcare, 19*(3), 12–14.

Layman, E. J. (2011). Decision making for health care managers and supervisors. *The Health Care Manager, 30*(4), 287–300.

Leigh, G. (2011). The simulation revolution: What are the implications for nurses in staff development? *Journal for Nurses in Staff Development, 27*(2), 54–57.

MacPhee, M., Wardrop, A., & Campbell, C. (2010). Transforming work place relationships through shared decision making. *Journal of Nursing Management, 18*(8), 1016–1026.

Mayer, N. J. (2009). Transporting telemetry patients: An algorithm enables safe patient transport without an RN or monitoring. *American Journal of Nursing, 109*(11), [Supplement], 35–37.

McCannon, C. J., Hackbarth, A. D., & Griffin, F. A. (2007). Miles to go: An introduction to the 5 Million Lives Campaign. *The Joint Commission Journal on Quality and Patient Safety, 33*(8), 477–484. Retrieved April 30, 2012 from http://www.ihi.org/knowledge/Pages/Publications/ MilestoGoIntro5MillionLivesCampaign.aspx.

Mick, J. (2011). Data-driven decision making. *Journal of Nursing Administration, 41*(10), 391–393.

Minas, H. (2005). Leadership for change in complex systems. *Australasian Psychiatry, 13*(1), 33–39.

Morgan, S. P., & Cooper, C. (2004). Shoulder work intensity with Six Sigma. *Nursing Management, 35*(3), 29–32.

Pew Health Professions Commission. (1998). *Twenty-one competencies for the twenty-first century.* San Francisco: Center for the Health Professions.

Pidgeon, N., & Gregory, R. (2004). Judgment, decision making, and public policy. In D. J. Koehler & N. Harvey (Eds.), *Blackwell handbook of judgment and decision making* (pp. 604–623). Malden, MA: Blackwell.

Porter-O'Grady, T. (2011). Leadership at all levels. *Nursing Management, 42*(5), 32–37.

Porter-O'Grady, T., Clark, J. S., & Wiggins, M. S. (2010). The case for clinical nurse leaders: Guiding nursing practice into the 21st century. *Nurse Leader, 8*(1), 37–41.

Pulman, A., Scammell, J., & Martin, M. (2009). Enabling interprofessional education: The role of technology to enhance learning. *Nurse Education Today, 29*(2), 232–239.

Robert Wood Johnson Foundation. (2008). *The transforming care at the bedside (TCAB) toolkit.* Retrieved May 9, 2012 from www.rwjf.org/ qualityequality/product.jsp?id=30051.

Rotter, T., Kinsman, L., James, E. L., Machotta, A., Gothe, H., Willis, J., Snow, P, & Kugler, J. (2010). Clinical pathways: Effects on professional practice, patient outcomes, length of stay and hospital costs (review). Retrieved May 3, 2012 from http://www.ncbi.nlm.nih.gov/ pubmed/20238347.

Rubenfeld, M. G., & Scheffer, B. K. (2006). *Critical thinking tactics for nurses.* Sudbury, MA: Jones & Bartlett.

Scheffer, B. K., & Rubenfeld, M. G. (2000). A consensus statement on critical thinking in nursing. *Journal of Nursing Education, 39*(8), 352–359.

Sharma, S., & Ivancevic, V. G. (2010). Nonlinear dynamical characteristics of situation awareness. *Theoretical Issues in Ergonomic Science, 11*(5), 448–460.

Sherman, R. O., Bishop, M., Eggenberger, T., & Karden, R. (2007). Development of a leadership competency model. *Journal of Nursing Administration, 37*(2), 85–94.

Shirey, M. R. (2007c). Competencies and tips for effective leadership: From novice to expert. *Journal of Nursing Administration, 37*(4), 167–170.

Shoemaker, L. K., Kazley, A. S., & White, A. (2010). Making the case for evidence-based design in healthcare: A descriptive case study of organizational decision making. *Health Environments Research & Design Journal, 4*(1), 56–88.

Shoemaker, P. (2011). What value-based purchasing means to your hospital. *Healthcare Financial Management, 60*(8), 60–68.

Sitterding, M. C., Broome, M. E., Everett, L. Q., & Ebright, P. (2012). Understanding situation awareness in nursing work: A hybrid concept analysis. *Advances in Nursing Science, 35*(1), 77–92.

Snowden, D. J., & Boone, M. E. (2007). A leader's framework for decision making. *Harvard Business Review, 85*(11), 68–76.

Sullivan-Mann, J., Perron, C. A., & Fellner, A. N. (2009). The effects of simulation on nursing students' critical thinking scores: A quantitative study. *Newborn and Infant Nursing Reviews, 9*(2), 111–116.

Swinny, B. (2010). Assessing and developing critical-thinking skills in the intensive care unit. *Critical Care Nursing Quarterly, 33*(1), 2–9.

Tan, J., Wen, H. J., & Awad, N. (2005). Health care and services delivery systems as complex adaptive systems: Examining chaos theory in action. *Communications of the ACM, 48*(5), 36–44.

Tanner, C. A. (2000). Critical thinking: Beyond nursing process. *Journal of Nursing Education, 39*(8), 338–339.

Tanner, C. A. (2006). Thinking like a nurse: A research-based model of clinical judgment in nursing. *Journal of Nursing Education, 45*(6), 204–211.

The Critical Thinking Community. (2008). *A brief history of the idea of critical thinking.* Retrieved May 12, 2008, from http://www.criticalthinking.org/pages/a-brief-history-of-the-idea-of-critical-thinking/408.

Thomas, J., & Herrin, D. (2008). Executive master of science in nursing program: Incorporating the 14 Forces of Magnetism. *Journal of Nursing Administration, 38*(2), 64–67.

Toofany, S. (2008). Critical thinking among nurses. *Nursing Management-UK, 14*(9), 28–31.

Toren, O., & Wagner, N. (2010). Applying ethical decision-making tool to a nurse management dilemma. *Nursing Ethics, 17*(3), 393–402.

Vroom, V., & Yetton, P. (1973). *Leadership and decision making.* Pittsburgh: University of Pittsburgh Press.

Watson, G. B., & Glaser, E. M. (1994). *Watson-Glaser critical thinking appraisal form S manual.* San Antonio, TX: Harcourt Brace.

Wheatley, M. (1999). *Leadership and the new science.* San Francisco: Berrett-Koehler.

Wilson, D. S., Talsma, A., & Martyn, K. (2011). Mindful staffing: A qualitative description of charge nurses' decision-making behaviors. *Western Journal of Nursing Research, 33*(6), 805–824.

Zori, S., & Morrison, B. (2009). Critical thinking in nurse managers. *Nursing Economic$, 27*(2), 75–79, 98.

Zori, S., Nosek, L. J., & Musil, C. M. (2010). Critical thinking of nurse managers related to staff RNs' perceptions of the practice environment. *Journal of Nursing Scholarship, 42*(3), 305–313.

Chapter 5

American Association of Critical-Care Nurses. (2005). *AACN standards for establishing and sustaining healthy work environments: A journey to excellence.* Aliso Viejo, CA: AACN.

American Association of Critical Care Nurses (AACN). (2004). *The 4A's to rise above moral distress.* Retrieved June 10, 2012, from www.aacn.org/WD/Practice/Docs/4As_to_Rise_Above_Moral_Distress.pdf.

American Association of Critical Care Nurses (AACN) (2008). *Moral distress position paper.* Retrieved June 10, 2012, from www.aacn.org/WD/Practice/Docs/Moral_Distress.pdf.

American Bankruptcy Institute. (2011). *Annual business and non-business filings by year (1980–2011).* Retrieved June 10, 2012, from www.abiworld.org/AM/AMTemplate.cfm?Section=Home&CONTENTID=65139&TEMPLATE=/CM/ContentDisplay.cfm.

American Psychological Association. (2012). *Stress in America: Our health at risk.* Retrieved June 10, 2012, from www.apa.org/news/press/releases/stress/2011/final-2011.pdf.

Atwood, D., & Uttley, R. (2011). Help! Strategies for preventing information overload. *Nursing Management, 42*(7), 50–52.

Auerbach, D. I., Buerhaus, P. I., & Staiger, D. O. (2011a). Registered nurse supply grows faster than projected amid surge in new entrants ages 23–26. *Health Affairs, 30*(12), 2286–2292.

Benson, H., & Klipper, M. Z. (1976). *The relaxation response.* New York: HarperTorch.

Bureau of Labor Statistics. (2012a). *Labor force statistics from the current population survey: Data bases, tables & calculators by subject*. Retrieved from http://data.bls.gov/timeseries/LNS14000000.

Cummings, G. G., Macgregor, T., Davey, M., Lee, H., Wong, C. A., Lo, E., et al. (2010). Leadership styles and outcome patterns for the nursing workforce and work environment: A systematic review. *International Journal of Nursing Studies, 47*, 363–385.

Curtin, L. (1994). Restructuring: What works and what does not! *Nursing Management, 25*, 7–8.

Fairchild, R. M. (2010). Practical ethical theory for nurses responding to complexity in care. *Nursing Ethics, 17*, 353–362.

Fischer, J., & Keenan, N. (2010). *Prioritizing self-care: The key to stress management*. Retrieved June 10, 2012, from http://ezinearticles.com/?Prioritizing-Self-Care:-The-Key-to-Stress-Management&id=5499316.

Gionta, D. (2009). *Setting boundaries at work: Steps to making them a reality*. Retrieved June 10, 2012, from www.psychologytoday.com/blog/occupational-hazards/200901/setting-boundaries-work-steps-making-them-reality.

Han, K., Trinkoff, A. M., Storr, C. L., & Geiger-Brown, J. (2011). Job stress and work schedules in relation to nurse obesity. *Journal of Nursing Administration, 41*, 488–495.

Hoolahan, S. E., Greenhouse, P. K., Hoffmann, R. L., & Lehman, L. A. (2012). Energy capacity model for nurses: The impact of relaxation and restoration. *The Journal of Nursing Administration, 42*(2), 103–109.

Institute of Medicine. (2010). *The future of nursing: Leading change, advancing health*. Washington, DC: National Academies Press.

Kanter, R. M. (1977). *Work and family in the United States: A critical review and agenda for research and policy*. New York: Sage.

Kath, L. M., Stichler, J. F., & Ehrhart, M. G. (2012). Moderators of the negative outcomes of nurse manager stress. *Journal of Nursing Management, 42*, 215–221.

Katherine, A. (2000). *Where to draw the line: How to set healthy boundaries every day*. New York: Touchstone.

Langner, B. E. (1995). Health care reform: A missed opportunity. *The Kansas Nurse, 70*, 1.

Levitin, A. J., & Wachter, S. M. (2011). *Explaining the housing bubble*. University of Pennsylvania Institute for Law & Economics Research Paper No. 10–15; Georgetown Public Law Research Paper No. 10–60; Georgetown Law and Economics Research Paper No. 10–16. Available at SSRN: http://ssrn.com/abstract=1669401.

Lewis, P. S., & Malecha, A. (2011). The impact of workplace incivility on the work environment, manager skill, and productivity. *Journal of Nursing Administration, 41*, 41–47.

Lindy, C., & Schaefer, F. (2010). Negative workplace behaviours: An ethical dilemma for nurse managers. *Journal of Nursing Management, 18*, 285–292.

McCarthy, J., & Deady, R. (2011). Moral distress reconsidered. *Nursing Ethics, 15*(2), 254–262.

McNeely, E. (2005). The consequences of job stress for nurses' health: Time for a check-up. *Nursing Outlook, 53*(6), 291–299.

Mind Tools. (2010). *The mind tools e-book*. (7th ed.). Mind Tools Limited. Retrieved June 10, 2012, from http://www.mindtools.com/cgi-bin/sgx2/shop.cgi?page=orderform_mindtools.htm.

The New York Times. (2010, June 10). Credit crisis – Bailout plan (TARP). *The New York Times*. Retrieved June 10, 2012, from http://topics.nytimes.com/top/reference/timestopics/subjects/c/credit_crisis/bailout_plan/index.html.

O'Driscoll, M. P. (1996). The interface between job and off-job roles: Enhancement and conflict. *International Review of Industrial and Organizational Psychology, 11*, 279–306.

O'Driscoll, M., Brough, P., & Kalliath, T. (2006). Work-family conflict and facilitation. In F. Jones, R. J. Burke, & M. Westman (Eds.), *Managing the work-home interface* (pp. 117–142). Hove, Sussex, UK: Psychology Press.

Office of Press Secretary. (2002). *President hosts conference on minority homeownership*. Retrieved June 10, 2012, from http://georgewbush-whitehouse.archives.gov/news/releases/2002/10/20021015.html.

Randel, J. (2010). *The skinny on time management: How to maximize your 24-hour gift*. Westport, CT: Rand Media.

Redman, B. K., & Fry, S. T. (2000). Nurses' ethical conflicts: What is really known about them? *Nursing Ethics, 7*, 360–366.

Rego, A., & Pina e Cunha, M. (2008). Workplace spirituality and organizational commitment: An empirical study. *Journal of Organizational Change Management, 21*, 53–75.

Richmond, P. A., Book, K., Hicks, M., Pimpinella, A., & Jenner, C. A. (2009). C.O.M.E. be a nurse manager. *Nursing Management, 40*(2), 52–54.

Robert Wood Johnson Foundation. (2011). *Action coalitions*. Retrieved June 10, 2012, from http://www.thefutureofnursing.org/content/action-coalitions.

Rosenthal, M. S. (2002). *50 ways to prevent and manage stress*. New York: McGraw-Hill.

Rushton, C. H. (2006). Defining and addressing moral distress. *AACN Advanced Critical Care, 17*(2), 161–168.

Shirey, M. R., McDaniel, A. M., Ebright, P. R., Fisher, M. L., & Doebbeling, B. N. (2010). Understanding nurse manager stress and work complexity. *Journal of Nursing Administration, 40*, 82–91.

Small, S. A., & Riley, D. (1990). Towards a multidimensional assessment of work spillover into family life. *Journal of Marriage and the Family, 52*(1), 51–61.

Tracy, B. (2007). *Eat that frog!: 21 great ways to stop procrastinating and get more done in less time*. San Francisco, CA: Berrett-Koehler.

Weberg, D. (2010). Transformational leadership and staff retention: An evidence review with implications for healthcare systems. *Nursing Administration Quarterly, 34*, 246–258.

Chapter 6

Agency for Healthcare Research and Quality (AHRQ). (2004). *Hospital nurse staffing and quality of care. Research in Action Issue #4*. Washington, DC: U.S. Department of Health and Human Services. Retrieved January 2, 2012, from http://www.ahrq.gov/research/findings/factsheets/services/nursestaffing/index.html.

Aiken, L. H., Clarke, S. P., Sloane, D. M., Sochalski, J., & Silber, J. H. (2002a). Hospital nurse staffing and patient mortality, nurse burnout, and job dissatisfaction. *Journal of the American Medical Association, 288*(16), 1987–1993.

Aiken, T. D. (2004). *Legal, ethical, and political issues in nursing* (2nd ed.). Philadelphia: F.A. Davis.

American Hospital Association (AHA). (2002). *In our hands: How hospital leaders can build a thriving workforce*. Chicago: Author.

American Medical Association (AMA). (2000). *Organizational ethics in health care*. Chicago: Author.

American Medical Association. (2012–2013). *Code of Medical Ethics of the American Medical Association*. Retrieved from http://www.ama-assn.org/ama/pub/physician-resources/medical-ethics/code-medical-ethics/code-medical-ethics.page? ISBN#:978-1-60359-209-3.

American Nurses Association (ANA). (2001). *Code of ethics for nurses: With interpretive statements*. Washington, DC: Author. Retrieved December 1, 2007, from nursingworld.org/ethics/code/protected_nwcoe813.htm.

American Nurses Association (ANA). (2010a). *Nursing's social policy statement: The essence of the profession*. Kansas City, MO: Author.

Andrews, D. R. (2004). Fostering ethical competency: An ongoing staff development process that encourages professional growth and staff satisfaction. *The Journal of Continuing Education in Nursing, 35*(1), 27–33.

Auerbach, D. I., Buerhaus, P. I., & Staiger, D. O. (2011b). Registered nurse supply grows faster than projected amid surge in new entrants ages 23–26. *Health Affairs, 30*(12), 2286–2292.

Austin, S. (2011). Stay out of court with proper documentation. *Nursing, 41*(4), 24–29.

Austin, W. (2007). The ethics of everyday practice: Healthcare environments as moral communities. *Advances in Nursing Science, 30*(1), 81–88.

Bailey, M. L., & Aulisio, M. P. (2011). The nurse administrator on the ethics committee: A collaborative approach. *Nursing Management, 42*(12), 52–54. http://dx.doi:10.1097/01.NUMA.0000406574.81214.9e.

Beauchamp, T., & Childress, J. (2001). *Principles of biomedical ethics* (5th ed.). New York: Oxford University Press.

Bell, J., & Breslin, J. M. (2008). Healthcare provider moral distress as a leadership challenge. *JONA'S Healthcare Law, Ethics, and Regulation, 10*(4), 94–97.

Brothers, D. (2005). *A practical guide to legal issues: Skills for nurse managers*. Marblehead, MA: HCPro, Inc.

Buerhaus, P. I., Donelan, K., Ulrich, B. T., DesRoches, C., & Dittus, R. (2007a). Trends in the experiences of hospital-employed registered nurses: Results from three national surveys. *Nursing Economic$, 25*(2), 69–80.

Buerhaus, P. I., Donelan, K., Ulrich, B. T., Norman, L., & Dittus, R. (2006). State of the registered nurse workforce in the United States. *Nursing Economic$, 24*(1), 6–12.

Buerhaus, P. I., Donelan, K., Ulrich, B. T., Norman, L., Williams, M., & Dittus, R. (2005a). Hospital RNs' and CNOs' perceptions of the impact of the nursing shortage on the quality of care. *Nursing Economic$, 23*(5), 214–221.

Cooper, R. W., Frank, G. L., Gouty, C. A., & Hansen, M. C. (2002). Key ethical issues encountered in health care organizations: Perceptions of nurse executives. *Journal of Nursing Administration, 32*(6), 331–337.

Cooper, R. W., Frank, G. L., Gouty, C. A., & Hansen, M. C. (2003). Ethical helps and challenges faced by nurse leaders in the health care industry. *Journal of Nursing Administration, 33*(1), 17–23.

Cooper, R. W., Frank, G. L., Hansen, M. M., & Gouty, C. A. (2004). Key ethical issues encountered in health care organizations: The perceptions of staff nurses and nurse leaders. *Journal of Nursing Administration, 34*(3), 149–156.

Cotter, B. M., & Vaszar, L. T. (2008). Hospital ethics case consultation: An overview. *PCCSU*, .01.01.08. Retrieved from http://www.chestnet.org/accp/pccsu/hospital-ethics-case-consultation-overview?page=0,3.

Croke, E. M. (2003). Nurses, negligence, and malpractice. *American Journal of Nursing, 103*(9), 54–63. Retrieved December 3, 2007, from www.nursingcenter.com/library/journalarticle.asp?article_id=423284.

Curtin, L. L. (2000b). The first ten principles for the ethical administration of nursing services. *Nursing Administration Quarterly, 25*(1), 7–13.

Douglas, M. R. (2007). Encourage corporate compliance and disclosure. *Nursing Management, 38*(1), 16–17.

Edmonson, C. (2010). Moral courage and the nurse leader. *OJIN: The Online Journal of Issues in Nursing, 15*(3), Manuscript 5.

Epstein, E. G., & Delgado, S. (2010). Understanding and addressing moral distress. *OJIN: The Online Journal of Issues in Nursing, 15*(3), Manuscript 1.

Epstein, E. G., & Hamric, A. B. (2009). Moral distress, moral residue, and the crescendo effect. *Journal of Clinical Ethics, 20*(4), 330–342.

Frank-Stromborg, M., & Christensen, A. (2001a). Nurse documentation: Not done or worse, done the wrong way—Part I. *Oncology Nursing Forum, 28*(4), 697–702.

Frank-Stromborg, M., & Christensen, A. (2001b). Nurse documentation: Not done or worse, done the wrong way—Part II. *Oncology Nursing Forum, 28*(5), 841–846.

Gaudine, A., LeFort, S., Lamb, M., & Thorne, L. (2011). Ethical conflicts with hospitals: The perspective of nurses and physicians. *Nursing Ethics, 18*(6), 756–766.

Gordon, S. (2005). *Nursing against the odds: How health care cost-cutting, media stereotypes, and medical hubris undermine nursing and patient care.* Ithaca, NY: Cornell University Press.

Guido, G. W. (2010). *Legal and ethical issues in nursing* (5th ed.). Upper Saddle River, NJ: Pearson Prentice-Hall.

Hassmiller, S. B., & Cozine, M. (2006). Addressing the nurse shortage to improve the quality of patient care. *Health Affairs, 25*(1), 268–274.

Johnson, R. (2005). Shifting patterns of practice: Nurse practitioners in a managed care environment. *Research and Theory for Nursing Practice: An International Journal, 19*(4), 323–340.

Lachman, V. D. (2007a). Moral courage: A virtue in need of development? *Medsurg Nursing, 16*(2), 131–133.

Lachman, V. D. (2007b). Moral courage in action: Case studies. *Medsurg Nursing, 16*(4), 275–277.

Lachman, V. D. (2010, September 30). Strategies necessary for moral courage. *OJIN: The Online Journal of Issues in Nursing, 15*(3), Manuscript 3 http://dx.doi:10.3912/OJIN.Vol15No03Man03.

LaSala, C. A., & Bjarnason, D. (2010). Creating workplace environments that support moral courage. *OJIN: The Online Journal of Issues in Nursing, 15*(3), Manuscript 4.

Miller, J. (2006). Opportunities and obstacles for good work in nursing. *Nursing Ethics, 13*(5), 471–487.

Miller, J., & Glusko, J. (2003). Standing up to the scrutiny of medical malpractice. *Nursing Management, 34*(10), 20.

Needleman, J., Buerhaus, P., Pankratz, S., Leibson, C. L., Stevens, S. R., & Harris, M. (2011a). Nurse staffing and inpatient mortality. *The New England Journal of Medicine, 364*(11), 1037–1045.

Nelson, W. A. (2011). Ethics: A foundation for quality. *Healthcare Executive, 26*(6), 46, 48–49.

Nurses Service Organization (NSO). (2012). *Commonly asked questions about medical malpractice insurance.* Hatboro, PA: Author. Retrieved January 2, 2012, from www.nso.com/professional-liability-insurance/need-coverage.jsp.

O'Neil, E., & Seago, J. A. (2002). Meeting the challenge of nursing and the nation's health. *Journal of the American Medical Association, 288*(16), 2040–2041.

O'Neill, O. (2001). Practical principles and practical judgment. *Hastings Center Report, 31*(4), 15–23.

Pavlish, C., Brown-Saltzman, K., Hersh, M., Shirk, M., & Nudelman, O. (2011a). Early indicators and risk factors for ethical issues in clinical practice. *Journal of Nursing Scholarship, 43*(1), 13–21.

Pavlish, C., Brown-Saltzman, K., Hersh, M., Shirk, M., & Rounkle, A. (2011b). Nursing priorities, actions, and regrets for ethical situations in clinical practice. *Journal of Nursing Scholarship, 43*(4), 385–395.

Porter-O'Grady, T. (2003b). A different age for leadership, Part 2. *Journal of Nursing Administration, 33*(3), 173–178.

Schluter, J., Winch, S., Holzhauser, K., & Henderson, A. (2008). Nurses' moral sensitivity and hospital ethical climate: A literature review. *Nursing Ethics, 15*(3), 304–321.

Schyve, P. M. (2009). *Leadership in healthcare organizations: A guide to Joint Commission leadership standards.* San Diego: The Governance Institute.

Shirey, M. R. (2005). Ethical climate in nursing practice: The leader's role. *JONA'S Healthcare Law, Ethics, and Regulation, 7*(2), 59–67.

Silverman, H. (2000). Organizational ethics in health care organizations: Proactively managing the ethical climate to ensure organizational integrity. *Hospital Ethics Committee Forum, 12*, 202–215.

Ulrich, C. M., Taylor, C., Soeken, K., O'Donnell, P., Farrar, A., Danis, M., et al. (2010). Everyday ethics: Ethical issues and stress in nursing practice. *Journal of Advanced Nursing, 66*(11), 2510–2519.

Upenieks, V. (2003d). Nurse leaders' perceptions of what compromises successful leadership in today's acute care inpatient environment. *Nursing Administration Quarterly, 27*(2), 140–152.

Weld, K., & Bibb, S. (2009). Concept analysis: Malpractice and modern-day nursing practice. *Nursing Forum, 44*(1), 2–10.

Wetter, D. (2007). *The best defense is a good documentation offense (Online course).* Wilmington, DE: Corexcel.

Retrieved December 3, 2007, from www.corexcel.com/html/body.documentation.title.ceus.htm.

Zuzelo, P. R. (2007). Exploring the moral distress of registered nurses. *Nursing Ethics, 14*(3), 344–359.

Chapter 7

Aiken, L. H., Clarke, S. P., Sloane, D. M., Sochalski, J. A., Busse, R., Clarke, H., et al. (2001b). Nurses' reports on hospital care in five countries. *Health Affairs, 20*(3), 43–53.

Anthony, M. K., & Preuss, G. (2002). Models of care: The influence of nurse communication on patient safety. *Nursing Economic$, 20*(5), 209–215, 248.

Apker, J., & Fox, D. H. (2002). Communication: Improving RNs' organizational and professional identification in managed care hospitals. *Journal of Nursing Administration, 32*(2), 106–114.

Argenti, P. A. (2002). *Corporate communication* (3rd ed.). Burr Ridge, IL: Richard D. Irwin.

Baldacchino, D. R. (2006). Nursing competencies for spiritual care. *Journal of Clinical Nursing, 15*(7), 885–896.

Battey, B. W. (2006). *Spiritual assessment in health care: Guidelines for providing the third dimension of holistic health care (a workshop for nursing staff and other health care providers)*. Antioch, CA: Author.

Battey, B. W. (2007). *The practice of faith community (parish) nursing: A computer assisted instructional program with instructor's manual and student handbook*. Antioch, CA: Author. Computer assisted instructional tools are available from A.S.K. Data Systems, Inc. www.askdatasystems.com.

Bavelas, A. (1953). Communication patterns in task-oriented groups. In D. Cartwright & A. Zander (Eds.), *Group dynamics: Research and theory*. Evanston, IL: Row, Peterson.

Bettinghaus, E. P. (1968). *Persuasive communication*. New York: Holt, Rinehart & Winston.

Boyle, D. K., & Kochinda, C. (2004). Enhancing collaborative communication of nurse and physician leadership in two intensive care units. *Journal of Nursing Administration, 34*(2), 60–70.

Brann, M., & Mattson, M. (2004). Toward a typology of confidentiality breaches in health care communication: An ethic of care analysis of provider practices and patient perceptions. *Health Communications, 16*(2), 231–251.

Buerhaus, P. I., Donelan, K., Norman, L., & Dittus, R. (2005b). Nursing student's perceptions of a career in nursing and impact of a national campaign designed to attract people into the nursing profession. *Journal of Professional Nursing, 21*(2), 75–83.

Buerhaus, P. I., Donelan, K., Ulrich, B. T., Norman, L., DesRoches, C., & Dittus, R. (2007b). Impact of the nurse shortage on hospital patient care: Comparative perspectives. *Health Affairs, 26*(3), 853–862.

Childers, L. (2004). Bullybusters: Nurses in hostile work environments must take action against abusive colleagues. *Nurse Week*, April 19; 11(9): 12–13.

Clancy, T. R. (2007a). Organizing: New ways to harness complexity. *Journal of Nursing Administration, 37*(12), 534–536.

DeMarco, R., Roberts, S. J., Norris, A. E., & McCurry, M. (2007). Refinement of the silencing the self scale: Work for registered nurses. *Journal of Nursing Scholarship, 39*(4), 375–378.

de Shazer, S. (1985). *Keys to solution in brief therapy*. New York: W.W. Norton.

Duddle, M., & Boughton, M. (2007). Intraprofessional relations in nursing. *Journal of Advanced Nursing, 59*(1), 29–37.

Duldt, B. W. (2008). *Nursing communication observation tool (NCOT) instruction manual*. Springfield, VA: Duldt & Associates. (Battey, B. W.; Revised & reprinted, 2008, and available from the author.)

Duldt, B. W. (1989). *Nursing communication observation tool (NCOT) instruction manual*. Springfield, VA: Duldt & Associates, Inc. (Battey, B. W.; Revised & reprinted, 2008, and available from the author.)

Duldt, B. W., & Giffin, K. (1985). *Theoretical perspectives for nursing*. Boston: Little Brown.

Farley, M. (1989). Assessing communication in organizations. *Journal of Nursing Administration, 19*(12), 27–31.

Gardner, M. (2008, January 28). Happiness is a warm "thank you": Seven things that workers want. *Christian Science Monitor*, Monday, 13, 16. Retrieved October 30, 2012, from www.csmonitor.com/Business/2008/0128/p13s03-wmgn.html.

Harvey, K. (1990). The power of positive questioning. *Nursing Management, 21*(5), 94–96.

Hersey, P. H., Blanchard, K. H., & Johnson, D. E. (2013b). *Management of organizational behavior: Leading human resources* (10th ed.). Upper Saddle River, NJ: Pearson Education.

Institute for Safe Medication Practices (ISMP). (2004, March 25). *Intimidation: Mapping a plan for cultural change in healthcare (Part II)*. Huntingdon Valley, PA. Retrieved October 26, 2012, from https://ismp.org/Newsletters/acutecare/articles/20040325.asp.

Johnson, J. (2000). The nursing shortage: A difficult conversation. *Journal of Nursing Administration, 30*(9), 401–402.

Keefe, S. (2007). Bullying among nurses. *Advance for Nursing, 9*(16), 34–36.

Kramer, M., & Schmalenberg, C. (2003). Securing "good" nurse/physician relationships. *Nursing Management, 34*(7), 34–38.

Kraus, P. D., & Holmes, W. D. (2007). *Pastoral care: A computer assisted instruction program.* St. Louis: A.S.K. Data Systems.

Lindeke, L. L., & Sieckert, A. M. (2005). Nurse-physician workplace collaboration. American Nurses Association. *Online Journal of Issues in Nursing, 10*(1). Retrieved October 26, 2012, from www.nursingworld. org/MainMenuCategories/ANAMarketplace/ ANAPeriodicals/OJIN/TableofContents/Volume102005/ No1Jan05/tpc26_416011.aspx.

McClung, E., Grossoehme, D. H., & Jacobson, A. F. (2006). Collaborating with chaplains to meet spiritual needs. *Medsurg Nursing, 15*(3), 147–156.

Moss, J., & Xiao, Y. (2004). Improving operating room coordination: Communication pattern assessment. *Journal of Nursing Administration, 34*(2), 93–100.

Namie, R., & Namie, G. (2008). *The Workplace Bullying Institute, WBI.* Retrieved January 27, 2008, from www. bullyinginstitute.org/.

Patterson, K., Grenny, J., McMillan, R., & Switzler, A. (2002). *Crucial conversations: Tools for talking when stakes are high.* New York: McGraw-Hill.

Patton, B. R., & Giffin, K. (1977). *Interpersonal communication in action.* New York: Harper & Row.

Patton, B. R., & Giffin, K. (1981). *Interpersonal communication in action: Basic text and readings.* New York: Harper & Row.

Pincus, J. (1986). Communication: Key contributor to effectiveness—The research. *Journal of Nursing Administration, 16*(9), 19–25.

Power, J. (2006). Spiritual assessment: Developing an assessment tool. *Nursing Older People, 18*(2), 16–18.

Sanford, F. H. (1950). *Authoritarianism and leadership.* Philadelphia: Institute for Research in Human Relations.

Sherer, J. (1994). Resolving conflict (the right way). *Hospitals and Health Networks, 68*(8), 52–55.

Smetzer, J. L., & Cohen, M. R. (2005). Intimidation: Practitioners speak up about this unresolved problem. *Joint Commission Journal on Quality and Patient Safety, 31*, 594–599.

The Joint Commission (TJC). (2008). *Comprehensive accreditation manual for hospitals.* Oakbrook Terrace, IL: Author.

Troupin, B. (2001, July 11). *16th WONCA World Conference of Family Doctors Conference Summary.* June 2001. Retrieved October 26, 2012, from www.medscape.com/ viewarticle/407928.

Ulrich, B. (2004). Fear factor: Management must stay on top of hostile behavior for nurses'—and patients'— sake. *California NurseWeek: A Nursing Spectrum Publication, 17*(9), 4.

U.S. Department of Labor, Bureau of Labor Statistics. (2012a). *Occupational outlook handbook: Registered nurses.* Retrieved October 26, 2012, from http://www. bls.gov/ooh/healthcare/registered-nurses.htm.

Chapter 8

Adams, A., & Bond, S. (2003). Staffing in acute hospital wards, II: Relationships between grade mix, staff stability and features of ward organizational environment. *Journal of Nursing Management, 11*(5), 293–298.

Aguayo, R. (1990). *Dr. Deming: The American who taught the Japanese about quality.* New York: Carol Publishing Group.

Book, C., & Galvin, K. (1975). *Instruction in and about small group discussion.* Falls Church, VA: Speech Communication Association.

Cherniss, C., & Goleman, D. (2001). *The emotionally intelligent workplace: How to select for, measure, and improve emotional intelligence in individuals, groups, and organizations.* San Francisco: Jossey-Bass.

Dabney, D. (1995). Workplace deviance among nurses: The influence of work group norms on drug diversion and/or use. *Journal of Nursing Administration, 25*(3), 48–55.

Darr, K. (1989). Applying the Deming method in hospitals, Part 1. *Hospital Topics, 67*(6), 4–5.

DiMeglio, K., Padula, C., Piatek, C., Korber, S., Barrett, A., Ducharme, M., et al. (2005). Group cohesion and nurse satisfaction: Examination of a team-building approach. *Journal of Nursing Administration, 35*(3), 110–120.

Farley, M., & Stoner, M. (1989). The nurse executive and interdisciplinary team building. *Nursing Administration Quarterly, 13*(2), 24–30.

Goldratt, E. M., & Cox, J. (2004). *The goal.* Great Barrington, MA: North River Press.

Hersey, P., Blanchard, K. H., & Johnson, D. E. (2008b). *Management of organizational behavior: Leading human resources* (9th ed.). Upper Saddle River, NJ: Pearson Education.

Jacobs, B., & Rosenthal, T. (1984). Managing effective meetings. *Nursing Economic$, 2*(2), 137–141.

Jay, A. (1982). How to run a meeting. *Journal of Nursing Administration, 12*(1), 22–28.

Kalisch, B., Begeny, S., & Anderson, C. (2008). The effect of consistent nursing shifts on teamwork and continuity of care. *Journal of Nursing Administration, 38*(3), 132–137.

Kalisch, B., & Begeny, S. (2005). Improving nursing unit teamwork. *Journal of Nursing Administration, 35*(12), 550–556.

Kalisch, B., & Lee, K. H. (2010). The impact of teamwork on missed nursing care. *Nursing Outlook, 58,* 233–241.

Katzenbach, J., & Smith, D. (1993). *The wisdom of teams: Creating the high-performance organization.* New York: Harper Collins.

Kohn, L. T., Corrigan, J. M., & Donaldson, M. S. (Eds.). (2000b). *To err is human: Building a safer health system.* Washington, DC: National Academies Press.

Lancaster, J. (1981). Making the most of meetings. *Journal of Nursing Administration, 11*(10), 15–19.

Laramee, A. (1999). The building blocks of successful relationships. *The Journal of Care Management, 5*(4), 40, 42, 44–45.

Lencioni, P. (2002). *The five dysfunctions of a team.* San Francisco: Jossey-Bass.

Lencioni, P. (2004). *Death by meeting.* San Francisco: Jossey-Bass.

Lencioni, P. (2006). *Silos, politics and turf wars.* San Francisco: Jossey-Bass.

Leppa, C. J. (1996). Nurse relationships and work group disruption. *Journal of Nursing Administration, 26*(10), 23–27.

Manion, J. (2004). Strengthening organizational commitment: Understanding the concept as a basis for creating effective workforce retention strategies. *The Health Care Manager, 23*(2), 167–176.

Manion, J. (2009). *The engaged workforce: Proven strategies to build a positive healthcare workplace.* Chicago: AHA Press.

Manion, J. (2011). *From management to leadership: Strategies for transforming health care.* San Francisco: Jossey-Bass.

Manion, J., & Bartholomew, K. (2003). Community in the workplace: A proven retention strategy. *Journal of Nursing Administration, 34*(1), 46–53.

Manion, J., Lorimer, W., & Leander, W. J. (1996). *Team-based health care organizations: Blueprint for success.* Gaithersburg, MD: Aspen.

Sorrells-Jones, J. (1997). The challenge of making it real: Interdisciplinary practice in a "seamless" organization. *Nursing Administration Quarterly, 21*(2), 20–30.

Sorrells-Jones, J., & Weaver, D. (1999). Knowledge workers and knowledge-intense organizations. I. A promising framework for nursing and healthcare. *Journal of Nursing Administration, 29*(7/8), 12–18.

Veninga, R. (1982). *The human side of health administration: A guide for hospital, nursing, and public health administrators.* Englewood Cliffs, NJ: Prentice-Hall.

Weaver, T. (2008). Enhancing multiple disciplinary teamwork. *Nursing Outlook, 56*(3), 108–114.

Chapter 9

American Association of Critical-Care Nurses (AACN). (2004). *AACN delegation handbook.* (2nd ed.). Aliso Viejo, CA: Author.

American Journal of Nursing (AJN). (1996a). $3 Million suit exposes "de-skilling". *American Journal of Nursing, 96*(11), 70.

American Journal of Nursing (AJN). (1996b). Pennsylvania lawmakers probe RN cuts, grill hospitals on UAP use. *American Journal of Nursing, 96*(11), 71–72.

American Nephrology Nurses' Association (ANNA). (2010). *The role of unlicensed assistive personnel in dialysis therapy.* Retrieved October 24, 2012, from www.annanurse.org/download/reference/health/position/unlicPersonnel.pdf.

American Nurses Association (ANA). (1992). *Joint statement on maintaining professional and legal standards during a shortage of nursing personnel.* Washington, DC: Author.

American Nurses Association (ANA). (2005a). *Utilization guide for the ANA principles for nurse staffing.* Silver Spring, MD: Author.

Anthony, M. K., Standing, T., & Hertz, J. E. (2000). Factors influencing outcomes after delegation to unlicensed assistive personnel. *Journal of Nursing Administration, 30*(10), 474–480.

Barter, M., & Furmidge, M. (1994). Unlicensed assistive personnel: Issues relating to delegation and supervision. *Journal of Nursing Administration, 24*(4), 36–40.

Fisher, M. (2000). Do you have delegation savvy? *Nursing, 30*(12), 58–59.

Gravlin, G., & Bittner, N. P. (2010). Nurses' and nursing assistants' reports of missed care and delegation. *Journal of Nursing Administration, 40*(7/8), 329–335.

Hansten, R., & Jackson, M. (2009). *Clinical delegation skills* (4th ed.). Sudbury, MA: Jones & Bartlett.

Hodge, M. B., Romano, P. S., Harvey, D., & Samuels, S. J. (2004). Licensed caregiver characteristics and staffing in California acute care hospital units. *Journal of Nursing Administration, 34*(3), 125–133.

Hudspeth, R. (2007). Understanding delegation is a critical competency for nurses in the new millennium. *Journal of Nursing Administration Quarterly, 32*(2), 183–184.

Institute for Healthcare Improvement (IHI). (2008). *Failure modes and effects analysis (FMEA) tool (IHI tool).* Boston, MA. Retrieved October 24, 2012, from www.ihi.org/knowledge/Pages/Tools/FailureModesandEffectsAnalysisTool.aspx.

Lightfoot, R. J., II (2011). Nurse delegation in LTC and assisted living. *Long-Term Living,* November 8, 1–2. Retrieved October 24, 2012, from www.ltlmagazine.com/article/nurse-delegation-ltc-and-assisted-living.

Marthaler, M. (2003). Delegation of nursing care. In P. Kelly-Heidenthal (Ed.), *Nursing leadership and management* (pp. 266–279). Clifton Park, NY: Delmar.

Martin, J., & Cain, S. K. (2003). Legal aspects of patient care. In P. Kelly-Heidenthal (Ed.), *Nursing leadership and management* (pp. 266–279). Clifton Park, NY: Delmar.

McIntosh, J. (2003). Questions we should ask about community nursing practice. *Primary Health Care Research and Development, 4,* 137–145.

National Council of State Boards of Nursing (NCSBN) (1995). *Delegation: Concepts and decision-making process.* Chicago: Author.

National Council of State Boards of Nursing (NCSBN). (2005). *Working with others: A position paper.* Chicago: Author.

National Council of State Boards of Nursing (NCSBN) and the American Nurses Association (ANA). (2006). *Joint statement on delegation.* Retrieved October 24, 2012, from www.ncsbn.org/Joint_statement.pdf.

National Council of State Boards of Nursing (NCSBN). (2012). *Boards of nursing.* Chicago: Author. Retrieved October 24, 2012, from www.ncsbn.org/boards.htm.

Nelson, R. (1994). *Empowering employees through delegation.* Burr Ridge, IL: Richard D. Irwin.

Nightingale, F. (1859). *Notes on nursing: What it is and what it is not.* London: Harrison & Sons.

Niven, C., & Scott, P. (2003). The need for accurate perception and informed judgment in determining the appropriate use of the nursing resource: Hear the patient's voice. *Nursing Philosophy, 4,* 201–210.

Poteet, G. (1989). Nursing administrators and delegation. *Nursing Administration Quarterly, 13*(3), 23–32.

Potter, P., & Grant, E. (2004). Understanding RN and unlicensed assistive personnel working relationships in designing care delivery strategies. *Journal of Nursing Administration, 34*(1), 19–25.

Richards, A., Carley, J., Jenkins-Clarke, S., & Richards, D. (2000). Skill mix between nurses and doctors working in primary care-delegation or allocation: A review of the literature. *International Journal of Nursing Studies, 37,* 185–197.

Rushton, H. C. (2007). Respect in critical care: A foundational ethical principle. *AACN Advanced Critical Care, 18*(2), 149–156.

Saccomano, S. J., & Pinto-Zipp, G. (2011). Registered nurse leadership style and confidence in delegation. *Journal of Nursing Management, 19,* 522–533.

The Joint Commission (TJC). (2007). *National patient safety goals.* Oakbrook Terrace, IL: Author.

The Joint Commission (TJC). (2012a). *Hospital: 2013 national patient safety goals.* Retrieved October 24, 2012, from www.jointcommission.org/standards_information/npsgs.aspx.

Weydt, A. (2010). Developing delegation skills. *Online Journal of Issues in Nursing, 15*(2), Manuscript 1. Retrieved October 25, 2012 from www.nursingworld.org/MainMenuCategories/ANAMarketplace/ANAPeriodicals/OJIN/TableofContents/Vol152010/No2May2010/Delegation-Skills.html.

Zolnierek, C. (2011). RN delegation rules under review in 2011. *Texas Nursing,* Summer, 6–7.

Chapter 10

Abood, S. (2007). Influencing health care in the legislative arena. *Online Journal of Issues in Nursing, 12*(1). Retrieved October 1, 2012, from http://www.nursingworld.org/MainMenuCategories/ANAMarketplace/ANAPeriodicals/OJIN/TableofContents/Volume122007/No1Jan07/tpc32_216091.html.

Almost, J. (2005). Conflict within nursing work environments: Concept analysis. *Journal of Advanced Nursing, 53*(4), 444–453.

Amason, A. (1996). Distinguishing effects of functional and dysfunctional conflict on strategic decision making: Resolving a paradox for top management teams. *Academy of Management Journal, 39,* 123–148.

Amason, A., & Sapienza, H. (1997). The effects of top management team size and interaction norms on cognitive and affective conflict. *Journal of Management, 23,* 496–516.

American Nurses Association (2011). *Fact sheet: Registered nurses in the U.S. nursing by the numbers.* Silver Spring, MD: Author.

Bacharach, S. B., & Lawler, E. J. (1980). *Power and politics in organizations.* San Francisco: Jossey-Bass.

Barden, A. M., Quinn Griffin, M. T., Donahue, M., & Fitzpatrick, J. J. (2011a). Governance and empowerment in registered nurses working in a hospital setting. *Nursing Administration Quarterly, 35*(3), 212–218.

Barki, H., & Hartwick, J. (2001). Interpersonal conflict and its management in information system development. *MIS Quarterly, 25,* 195–228.

Barki, H., & Hartwick, J. (2004). Conceptualizing the construct of interpersonal conflict. *International Journal of Conflict Management, 15*(3), 216–244.

Bartol, G., Parrish, R. S., & McSweeney, M. (2001). Effective conflict management begins with knowing your style. *Journal of Nursing Staff Development, 17*(1), 34–40.

Barton, A. (1991). Conflict resolution by nurse managers. *Nursing Management, 22*(5), 83–86.

Bennis, W., & Nanus, B. (1985b). *Leaders: The strategies for taking charge.* New York: Harper & Row.

Blake, R., & Mouton, J. S. (1964b). *The managerial grid.* Houston, TX: Gulf Publishing.

Blau, P. M. (1964). *Exchange and power in social life*. New York: Wiley.

Boswell, C., Cannon, S., & Miller, J. (2005). Nurses' political involvement: Responsibility versus privilege. *Journal of Professional Nursing, 21*(1), 5–8.

Brown, L. D. (1983). *Managing conflict at organizational interfaces*. Reading, MA: Addison-Wesley.

Centers for Medicare & Medicaid Services (CMS). (2011a). *Health Disparities and Inequalities Report – United States, 2011*. Retrieved October 1, 2012, from www.cdc.gov/minorityhealth/reports/CHDIR11/ExecutiveSummary.pdf.

Centers for Disease Control and Prevention (CDC). (2011, January 14). CDC Health Disparities & Inequalities Report – United States, 2011. *Morbidity & Mortality Weekly Report (MMWR) Supplement, 60*, 1–116. Retrieved October 1, 2012, from www.cdc.gov/mmwr/pdf/other/su6001.pdf.

Classen, D., Resar, R., Grifin, F., Federico, F., Frankel, T., Kimmel, N., et al. (2011). Global trigger tool shows that adverse events in hospitals may be ten times greater than previously measured. *Health Affairs, 30*(4), 581–588.

Conrad, C. (1990). *Strategic organizational communication: An integrated perspective* (2nd ed.). Fort Worth, TX: Holt, Rinehart & Winston.

Coser, L. A. (1956). *The functions of social conflict*. Glencoe, IL: Free Press.

Cox, K. B. (2004). The intragroup conflict scale: Development and psychometric properties. *Journal of Nursing Measurement, 12*(2), 133–146.

Daft, R. L. (2013). *Organization theory and design* (11th ed.). Mason, OH: South-Western Cengage Learning.

Dahl, R. A. (1957). The concept of power. *Behavioral Science, 2*, 202–210.

DeDreu, C. K. W., & Weingart, L. R. (2003). Task versus relationship conflict, team performance, and team member satisfaction: A meta-analysis. *Journal of Applied Psychology, 88*(4), 741–750.

Deutsch, M. (1973). *The resolution of conflict: Constructive and destructive processes*. New Haven, CT: Yale University Press.

Dumont, C., Meisinger, S., Whitacre, M. J., & Corbin, G. (2012). Nursing 2012 horizontal violence survey report. *Nursing, 42*(1), 44–49.

Einarsen, S., Raknes, B. I., & Matthiesen, S. M. (1994). Bullying and harassment at work and their relationships to work environment quality: An exploratory study. *European Work and Organizational Psychologist, 4*, 381–401.

Emerson, R. M. (1957). Power-dependence relations. *American Sociological Review, 27*(1), 31–40.

Esperat, M. C. R., Hanson-Turton, T., Richardson, M., Debisette, A. T., & Rupinta, C. (2012). Nurse-managed health centers: Safety-net care through advanced nursing practice. *Journal of the American Academy of Nurse Practitioners, 24*(1), 24–31.

Faulkner, J., & Laschinger, H. (2008). The effects of structural and psychological empowerment on perceived respect in acute care nurses. *Journal of Nursing Management, 16*(2), 214–221.

Filley, A. C. (1975). *Interpersonal conflict resolution*. Glenview, IL: Scott Foresman.

Fisher, R., Ury, W., & Patton, B. (1992). *Getting to yes: Negotiating agreement without giving in* (2nd ed.). New York: Penguin Books.

Folger, J. P., Poole, M. S., & Stutman, R. K. (1997). *Working through conflict: Strategies for relationships, groups, and organizations*. New York: Longman.

French, J., & Raven, B. (1959). The bases of social power. In D. Cartwright (Ed.), *Studies in social power* (pp. 150–167). Ann Arbor, MI: University of Michigan, Institute for Social Research.

Gardner, D. L. (1992). Conflict and retention of new graduate nurses. *Western Journal of Nursing Research, 14*, 76–85.

Gerardi, D. (2004). Using mediation techniques to manage conflict and create healthy work environments. *AACN Clinical Issues, 15*(2), 182–195.

Glaser, J., & Latimer, G. (2011, July 28). Nursing in the new era of accountability. *Hospitals and Health Networks*. Retrieved October 1, 2012, from www.hhnmag.com/hhnmag/HHNDaily/HHNDailyDisplay.dhtml?id=5990002017.

Green, A. (2012). Accountable care organizations: A new approach to care delivery. *Nursing Spectrum, 22*(9), 160–165.

Hampton, D. R., Summer, C. E., & Webber, R. A. (1987). *Organization behavior and the practice of management*. Glenview, IL: Scott Foresman.

Hardy, C., & Leiba-O'Sullivan, S. (1998). The power behind empowerment: Implications for research and practice. *Human Relations, 51*(4), 451–483.

Hassmiller, S. (2010). Nursing's role in healthcare reform. *American Nurse Today, 5*(9). Retrieved October 1, 2012, from www.americannursetoday.com/article.aspx?id=7086&fid=6850.

Hersey, P., Blanchard, K. H., & Johnson, D. E. (2008c). *Management of organizational behavior: Leading human resources* (9th ed.). Upper Saddle River, NJ: Pearson Education.

Hersey, P., Blanchard, K. H., & Natemeyer, W. E. (1979). Situational leadership, perception, and the impact of power. *Group and Organization Studies, 4*, 418–428.

Hickson, D. J., Hinings, C. R., Lee, C. A., Schneck, R. E., & Pennings, J. M. (1971). A strategic contingencies theory of intraorganizational power. *Administrative Science Quarterly, 16*, 216–229.

Institute of Medicine (IOM) (2010). *The future of nursing: Leading change, advancing health.* Retrieved October 1, 2012, from www.iom.edu/Reports/2010/The-Future-of-Nursing-Leading-Change-Advancing-Health.aspx/.

Jehn, K. A. (1995). A multimethod examination of the benefits and detriments of intragroup conflict. *Administrative Science Quarterly, 40,* 256–282.

Jehn, K. A. (1997). A qualitative analysis of conflict types and dimensions in organizational groups. *Administrative Science Quarterly, 42,* 530–557.

Jehn, K. A., Northcraft, G., & Neale, M. (1999). Why differences make a difference: A field study of diversity, conflict, and performance in workgroups. *Administrative Science Quarterly, 44,* 741–763.

Kane, R. L., Shamliyan, T., Mueller, C., Duvai, S., & Wilt, T. (2007b). *Nursing staffing and quality of patient care. Evidence report/technology Assessment No. 151* (prepared by the Minnesota Evidence-based Practice Center under Contract No. 290-0009). AHRQ Publication No. 07-E005. Rockville, MD: Agency for Healthcare Research and Quality.

Kanter, R. M. (1977b). *Men and women of the corporation.* New York: Basic Books.

Kaplan, A. (1964). Power in perspective. In R. L. Kahn & E. Boulding (Eds.), *Power and conflict in organizations* (pp. 11–32). London: Tavistock.

Kelly, J. (2006). An overview of conflict. *Dimensions of Critical Care Nursing, 25*(1), 22–28.

King, I. M. (1981). *A theory for nursing: Systems, concepts, process.* New York: Wiley & Sons.

Kipnis, D., Schmidt, S. M., Swaffin-Smith, C., & Wilkinson, I. (1984). Patterns of managerial influence: Shotgun managers, tacticians, and bystanders. *Organizational Dynamics, 12*(3), 58–67.

Kipnis, D., Schmidt, S. M., & Wilkinson, I. (1980). Intraorganizational influence tactics: Explorations in getting one's way. *Journal of Applied Psychology, 65*(4), 440–452.

Kotter, J. P. (1979). *Power in management: How to understand, acquire, and use it.* New York: AMACOM.

Kouzes, J., & Posner, B. (1987). *The leadership challenge: How to get extraordinary things done in organizations.* San Francisco: Jossey-Bass.

Kramer, M., & Schmalenberg, C. (1990). Fundamental lessons in leadership. In E. Simendinger, T. Moore, & M. Kramer (Eds.), *The successful nurse executive: A guide for every nurse manager* (pp. 5–21). Ann Arbor, MI: Health Administration Press.

Lämås, K., Willman, A., Lindholm, L., & Jacobsson, C. (2009). Economic evaluation of nursing practices: A review of literature. *International Nursing Review, 56*(1), 13–20.

Laschinger, H. K., Finegan, J., & Shamian, J. (2001a). The impact of workplace empowerment, organizational trust on staff nurses' work satisfaction and organizational commitment. *Health Care Management Review, 26*(3), 7–23.

Laschinger, H. K., Finegan, J., Shamian, J., & Casier, S. (2000). Organizational trust and empowerment in restructured healthcare settings: Effects on staff nurse commitment. *Journal of Nursing Administration, 30*(9), 413–425.

Laschinger, H. K., Finegan, J., Shamian, J., & Wilk, P. (2001b). Impact of structural and psychological empowerment on job strain in nursing work settings: Expanding Kanter's model. *Journal of Nursing Administration, 31*(5), 260–272.

Laschinger, H. K., & Havens, D. S. (1997). The effect of workplace empowerment on staff nurses' occupational mental health and work effectiveness. *Journal of Nursing Administration, 27*(6), 4–50.

Laschinger, H. K., Purdy, N., & Almost, J. (2007). The impact of leader-member exchange quality, empowerment, and core self-evaluation on nurse manager's job satisfaction. *Journal of Nursing Administration, 37*(5), 221–229.

Laschinger, H. K., Sabiston, J. A., & Kutszcher, L. (1997). Empowerment and staff nurse decision involvement in nursing work environments: Testing Kanter's theory of structural power in organizations. *Research in Nursing and Health, 20,* 341–352.

Leymann, H. (1996). The content and development of mobbing at work. *European Journal of Work and Organizational Psychology, 5,* 165–184.

Liberatore, P., Brown-Williams, R., Brucker, J., Dukes, N., Kimmey, L., McCarthy, K., et al. (1989). A group approach to problem-solving. *Nursing Management, 20*(9), 68–72.

Manojlovich, M. (2007). Power and empowerment in nursing: Looking back to inform the future. *The Online Journal of Issues in Nursing, 12*(1). Retrieved October 1, 2012, from www.nursingworld.org/MainMenuCategories/ANAMarketplace/ANAPeriodicals/OJIN/TableofContents/Volume122007/No1Jan07/LookingBackwardtoInformtheFuture.aspx.

Marshall, P. (2006, May). *Conflict resolution: what nurses need to know.* Retrieved October 1, 2012, from http://mediatecalm.ca/pdfs/what%20nurses%20need%20to%20know.pdf.

Mason, D. (2010). Health care reform: What's in it for nursing? *American Journal of Nursing, 110*(7), 24–26.

Matthiesen, S. B., Aasen, G. H., Wie, K., & Einarsen, S. (2003). The escalation of conflict: A case study of bullying at work. *International Journal of Management and Decision Making, 4*(1), 96–112.

McBride, A. (2011). Taking leadership seriously. *American Journal of Nursing, 11*(3), 11.

Mullinix, C. (2011). Making nurses full partners in redesigning health care in North Carolina. *North Carolina Medical Journal, 70*(4), 314–316.

National Nursing Centers Consortium (2012). *About nurse-managed care.* Retrieved October 1, 2012, from www.nncc.us/site/index.php/about-nurse-managed-care.

Oetzel, J. G., & Ting-Toomey, S. (2003). Face concerns in interpersonal conflict: A cross-cultural empirical test of the face negotiation theory. *Communication Research, 30*(6), 599–624.

Oetzel, J. G., Ting-Toomey, S., Masumoto, T., Yokochi, Y., Pan, X., Takai, J., et al. (2001). Face and facework in conflict: A cross-cultural comparison of China, Germany, Japan, and the United States. *Communication Monographs, 68*, 235–258.

Pfeffer, J. (1981). *Power in organizations.* Boston: Pitman Books.

Pinkley, R. (1990). Dimensions of the conflict frame: Disputant interpretations of conflict. *Journal of Applied Psychology, 75*(2), 117–128.

Pondy, L. R. (1967). Organizational conflict: Concepts and models. *Administrative Science Quarterly, 12*, 296–320.

Ponte, P. R., Glazer, G., Dann, E., McCollum, K., Gross, A., Tyrrell, R., et al. (2007). The power of professional nursing practice: An essential element of patient and family centered care. *The Online Journal of Issues in Nursing, 12*(1). Retrieved October 1, 2012, from www.nursingworld.org/MainMenuCategories/ANAMarketplace/ANAPeriodicals/OJIN/TableofContents/Volume122007/No1Jan07/tpc32_316092.aspx.

Putnam, L. L., & Poole, M. S. (1987). Conflict and negotiation. In F. M. Jablin, L. L. Putnam, K. Roberts, & L. W. Porter (Eds.), *Handbook of organizational communication* (pp. 549–599). Newbury Park, CA: Sage.

Rahim, M. A. (1983a). A measure of styles of handling interpersonal conflict. *Academy of Management Journal, 26*, 368–376.

Rahim, M. A. (1983b). Measurement of organizational conflict. *The Journal of General Psychology, 109*, 189–199.

Rahim, M. A. (1983c). *Rahim organizational conflict inventories: Experimental edition: Professional manual.* Palo Alto, CA: Consulting Psychologists Press.

Rahim, M. A. (2001). *Managing conflict in organizations* (3rd ed.). Westport, CT: Quorum.

Rahim, M. A., & Bonoma, T. V. (1979). Managing organizational conflict: A model for diagnosis and intervention. *Psychological Reports, 44*, 1323–1344.

Raven, B., & Kruglanski, W. (1975). Conflict and power. In P. Swingle (Ed.), *The structure of conflict* (pp. 177–219). New York: Academic Press.

Robbins, S. P. (2003). *Organizational behavior* (10th ed.). Englewood Cliffs, NJ: Prentice Hall.

Robbins, S. P., & Judge, T. A. (2011). *Organizational behavior* (14th ed.). Upper Saddle River, NJ: Pearson Prentice Hall.

Rosenstein, A. (2002). The impact of nurse-physician relationships on nurse satisfaction and retention. *American Journal of Nursing, 102*(6), 26–34.

Sabiston, J. A., & Laschinger, H. K. (1995). Staff nurse empowerment and perceived autonomy: Testing Kanter's theory of structural power in organizations. *Journal of Nursing Administration, 25*(9), 42–50.

Schira, M. (2004). Reflections on "About power in nursing". *Nephrology Nursing Journal, 31*(5), 583.

Sieloff, C. L. (2003). Measuring nursing power within organizations. *Journal of Nursing Scholarship, 32*, 183–187.

Sportsman, S., & Hamilton, P. (2007). Conflict management styles in the health professions. *Journal of Professional Nursing, 23*(3), 157–166.

Spreitzer, G. M. (1995). An empirical test of a comprehensive model of intrapersonal empowerment in the workplace. *American Journal of Community Psychology, 23*(5), 601–629.

The Joint Commission Online. (2011, November 9). *The term "disruptive behavior" is changed in the standards.* Retrieved October 1, 2012, from http://www.jointcommission.org/assets/1/18/jconline_Nov_9_11.pdf.

Thomas, K. W. (1976). Conflict and conflict management. In M. D. Dunnette (Ed.), *The handbook of industrial and organizational psychology* (pp. 889–935). Chicago: Rand McNally.

Thomas, K. W. (1992). Conflict and negotiation processes in organizations. In M. D. Dunnette, & L. M. Hough (Eds.), *The handbook of industrial and organizational psychology* (2nd ed., Vol. 3, pp. 651–717). Palo Alto, CA: Consulting Psychologists Press.

Thomas, K. W., & Kilmann, R. H. (1974). *Thomas-Kilmann conflict mode instrument.* Tuxedo, NY: Xicom.

Ting-Toomey, S. (1988). Intercultural conflict styles: A face negotiation theory. In Y. Y. Kim & W. Gudykunst (Eds.), *Theories in intercultural communication* (pp. 213–235). Newbury Park, CA: Sage.

Ting-Toomey, S., & Kurogi, A. (1998). Facework competence in intercultural conflict: An updated face-negotiation theory. *International Journal of Intercultural Relations, 22*, 187–225.

U.S. Department of Health and Human Services, Assistant Secretary for Planning and Evaluation Office of Health Policy. Issue Brief. *Overview of the Uninsured in the United States: Summary of the 2011 Current Population Survey*. Retrieved October 1, 2012, from http://aspe.hhs.gov/health/reports/2011/CPSHealthIns2011/ib.pdf.

Wall, J. A., & Callister, R. R. (1995). Conflict and its management. *Journal of Management, 21*, 515–558.

Walton, R. E. (1966). Theory of conflict in lateral organizational relationships. In J. R. Lawrence (Ed.), *Operational research and the social sciences* (pp. 409–426). London: Tavistock Publications.

Weber, M. (1947). *The theory of social and economic organization* (A. M. Henderson, & T. Parsons, Trans.). New York: Oxford University Press (Original work published 1923).

Yukl, G., & Falbe, C. M. (1991). Importance of different power sources in downward and lateral relations. *Journal of Applied Psychology, 76*(3), 416–423.

Yukl, G., Falbe, C., & Joo, Y. Y. (1993). Patterns of influence behavior for managers. *Group and Organization Management, 18*(1), 5–28.

Yukl, G., Lepsinger, R., & Lucia, T. (1992). Preliminary report on development and validation of the Influence Behavior Questionnaire. In K. E. Clar, M. B. Cla, & D. P. Campbell (Eds.), *The impact of leadership* (pp. 417–427). Greensboro, NC: Center for Creative Leadership.

Chapter 11

American Association of Colleges of Nursing (AACN). (2011a). *Enhancing diversity in the nursing workforce. Fact sheet*. Washington, DC: Author. Retrieved August 6, 2012, from www.aacn.nche.edu/media-relations/fact-sheets/enhancing-diversity.

Brett, J., Behfar, K., & Kern, M. C. (2006). Managing multicultural teams. *Harvard Business Review, 84*(11), 84–91.

Halford, G. S., Baker, R., McCredden, J. E., & Bain, J. D. (2005). How many variables can humans process? *Psychological Science, 16*(1), 70–76.

Hall, E. T., & Hall, M. R. (1990). *Understanding cultural differences*. Yarmouth, ME: Intercultural Press.

Henry, P. (2012, August 1). The Catholic church's ritual unites us more than beliefs. *The National Catholic Reporter*. Retrieved August 11, 2012, from http://ncronline.org/news/spirituality/catholic-churchs-ritual-unites-us-more-beliefs.

Hilton, A. (2007). *The different religions' views on abortion*. Retrieved August 6, 2012, from www.helium.com/items/716202-the-different-religions-views-on-abortion.

Merriam-Webster. (2012). *Definition of ethnocentric*. Retrieved August 6, 2012, from www.merriam-webster.com/dictionary/ethnocentrism.

National Coalition Building Institute (NCBI) (2012). *About NCBI*. Washington, DC: NCBI. Retrieved August 6, 2012, from http://www.ncbi.nlm.nih.gov/About/index.html.

Obama, B. (2006). *The audacity of hope*. New York, NY: Random House, Inc.

Office of Minority Health. (2007). *National standards on culturally and linguistically appropriate services (CLAS)*. Rockville, MD: Author, U.S. Department of Health and Human Services. Retrieved August 6, 2012, from http://minorityhealth.hhs.gov/templates/browse.aspx?lvl=2&lvlID=15.

Reuters. (2011). *Most Catholic women use birth control banned by church*. Retrieved August 6, 2012, from www.reuters.com/article/2011/04/13/us-contraceptives-religion-idUSTRE73C7W020110413.

Schyve, P. (2007). Language differences as a barrier to quality and safety in health care: The Joint Commission perspective. *Journal of General Internal Medicine, 22*(Suppl. 2), 360–361. Retrieved August 6, 2012, from www.ncbi.nlm.nih.gov/pmc/articles/PMC2078554/.

The Henry J. Kaiser Family Foundation. (2011). *The uninsured, a primer*. Retrieved August 6, 2012, from www.kff.org/uninsured/upload/7451-07.pdf.

U.S. Census Bureau. (2008). *An older and more diverse nation by midcentury*. Retrieved August 6, 2012, from www.census.gov/newsroom/releases/archives/population/cb08-123.html.

U.S. Census Bureau. (n.d.a). *Census of population and housing. 1930 Census*. Retrieved August 6, 2012 from http://www.census.gov/prod/www/decennial.html.

U.S. Census Bureau. (n.d.b). *1990 Census*. Retrieved August 6, 2012, from www.census.gov/main/www/cen1990.html.

U.S. Census Bureau. (2011a). *2010 Census shows America's diversity*. Retrieved August 6, 2012, from www.census.gov/prod/cen2010/briefs/c2010br-02.pdf.

U.S. Census Bureau. (2011b). *The 2012 statistical abstract. The national data book*. Retrieved August 6, 2012, from www.census.gov/compendia/statab/cats/population/religion.html.

U.S. Census Bureau. (1996). *Population projections of the United States by age, sex, race, and Hispanic origin: 1995 to 2050*. (Current Population Reports, Series

P25–1130). Washington, DC: Author, U.S. Department of Commerce.

U.S. Department of Commerce and Vice President Al Gore's National Partnership for Reinventing Government Benchmarking Study. (1999). *Best practices in achieving workforce diversity*. Retrieved August 6, 2012, from http://govinfo.library.unt.edu/npr/library/workforce-diversity.pdf.

U.S. Department of Health and Human Services. (1998). *Council on graduate medical education twelfth report—Minorities in medicine*. Retrieved August 6, 2012, from www.ask.hrsa.gov/detail_materials.cfm?ProdID=2833&ReferringID=1898.

U.S. Department of Health and Human Services. (2003). *Developing cultural competence in disaster mental health programs*. Retrieved August 6, 2012, from www.hhs.gov/od/documents/CulturalCompetence-FINALwithcovers.pdf.

U.S. Department of Labor, Bureau of Labor Statistics. (2012b). *Occupational outlook handbook*. Retrieved August 6, 2012, from www.bls.gov/ooh/healthcare/registered-nurses.htm.

U.S. Supreme Court. (2012). *In the Supreme Court of the United States*. Retrieved August 6, 2012, from http://civilrightsdocs.info/pdf/healthcare/11-398-tsac-NAAC-legal-defense-educational-fund-et-al.pdf.

Weech-Maldonado, R., Dreachslin, J. L., Brown, J., Pradhan, R., Rubin, K. L., Schiller, C., et al. (2012). Cultural competency assessment tool for hospitals: Evaluating hospitals' adherence to the culturally and linguistically appropriate services standards. *Health Care Management Review, 37*(1), 54–66.

Wendover, R. W. (2002). *The corrosion of character*. Aurora, CO: The Center for Generational Studies.

Chapter 12

Agency for Healthcare Research and Quality (AHRQ). (2007). *Closing the quality gap: A critical analysis of quality improvement strategies Volume 7-Care coordination*. Technical Review 9. (AHRQ Publication No. 04(07)-0051-7). Rockville, MD: Author.

Agency for Healthcare Research and Quality (AHRQ). (2011a). *Care coordination measures atlas*. Retrieved October 28, 2012, from www.ahrq.gov/qual/careatlas/careatlas.pdf.

Agency for Healthcare Research and Quality (AHRQ). (2011b). *Transition of care for acute stroke and myocardial infarction patients: From hospitalization to rehabilitation, recovery, and secondary prevention*. Retrieved October 28, 2012, from http://effectivehealthcare.ahrq.gov/ehc/products/306/821/EvidReport-Transitions_20111031.pdf.

Aikman, P., Andress, I., Goodfellow, C., LaBelle, N., & Porter-O'Grady, T. (1998). System integration: A necessity. *Journal of Nursing Administration, 28*(2), 28–34.

Allen, J. K., Blumenthal, R. S., Margolis, S., Young, D. R., Miller, E. R., III, & Kelly, K. (2002). Nurse case management of hypercholesterolemia in patients with coronary heart disease: Results of a randomized clinical trial. *American Heart Journal, 144*(4), 678–686.

Aliotta, S. (1999). Patient adherence outcome indicators and measurement in case management and health care. *Journal of Care Management, 5*(4), 24, 26, 29–31, 81–82.

Aliotta, S. L. (1996). Components of a successful case management program. *Managed Care Quarterly, 4*(2), 38–45.

American Nurses Association (ANA). (1988a). *Nursing case management*. (Publication No. NS-32). Kansas City, MO: Author.

American Nurses Association (ANA). (2012a). *Care coordination and registered nurses' essential role*. Silver Spring, MD: Author.

Anderson, M. A., & Helms, L. B. (1998). Comparison of continuing care communication. *Image, 30*(3), 255–260.

Anderson, M. A., & Tredway, C. A. (1999). Communication: An outcome of case management. *Nursing Case Management, 4*(3), 104–111.

Aubert, R. E., Herman, W. H., Waters, J., Moore, W., Sutton, D., Peterson, B. L., et al. (1998). Nurse case management to improve glycemic control in diabetic patients in a health maintenance organization: A randomized, controlled trial. *Annals of Internal Medicine, 129*(8), 605–612.

Aurora Health Care. (2004). *Aurora's continuum of care*. Milwaukee, WI: Author. Retrieved October 29, 2012, from www.aurorahealthcare.org/aboutus/continuum/index.asp.

Birmingham, J. (1996). How to apply CMSA's standards of practice for case management in a capitated environment. *Journal of Care Management, 2*(5), 9–10, 12, 14, 16–18, 20, 22.

Birmingham, J. (2007). Case management: Two regulations with coexisting functions. *Professional Case Management, 12*(1), 16–24.

Bower, K. A. (2004a). Patient care management as a global nursing concern. *Nursing Administration Quarterly, 28*(1), 39–43.

Braden, C. J. (2002). *State of the science paper #2: Involvement/participation, empowerment and knowledge outcome indicators of case management*. Little Rock, AR: Case Management Society of America.

Burgess, C. S. (1999). Managed care: The driving force for case management. In E. L. Cohen, & V. DeBack (Eds.),

The outcomes mandate: Case management in health care today (pp. 13–19). St. Louis: Mosby.

Care Continuum Alliance (CCA). (2012a). *Definition of disease management.* Washington, DC: Author. Retrieved October 29, 2012, from www.carecontinuumalliance.org/dm_definition.asp.

Care Continuum Alliance (CCA). (2012b). *Advancing the population health improvement model.* Washington, DC: Author. Retrieved October 30, 2012, from www.carecontinuumalliance.org/phi_definition.asp.

Carroll, P. L. (2004). *Community health nursing: A practical guide.* Clifton Park, NY: Thomson Delmar Learning.

Case Management Society of America (CMSA). (2010). *Standards of practice for case management.* Little Rock, AR: Author.

Case Management Society of America (CMSA). (2012a). *What is a case manager? Definition of case management.* Little Rock, AR: Author. Retrieved September 8, 2012, from www.cmsa.org/Home/CMSA/WhatisaCaseManager/tabid/224/Default.aspx.

Case Management Society of America (CMSA). (2012b). *Our history.* Little Rock, AR: Author. Retrieved October 30, 2012, from www.cmsa.org/Home/CMSA/OurHistory/tabid/225/Default.aspx.

Centers for Disease Control and Prevention (CDC). (2012). *Chronic disease prevention and health promotion.* Atlanta, GA: Author. Retrieved October 29, 2012, from www.cdc.gov/chronicdisease/index.htm.

Centers for Medicare & Medicaid Services (CMS). (2003). Medicare program; Demonstration: Capitated disease management for beneficiaries with chronic illnesses. *Federal Register, 68*(40), 9673–9680.

Cesta, T. G., & Tahan, H. A. (2003). *The case manager's survival guide: Winning strategies for clinical practice* (2nd ed.). St. Louis: Mosby.

Clark, K. A. (1996). Alternate case management models. In D. L. Flarey & S. S. Blancett (Eds.), *Handbook of nursing case management* (pp. 295–304). Gaithersburg, MD: Aspen.

Cline, B. G. (1990). Case management: Organizational models and administrative methods. *Caring: National Association for Home Care Magazine, 9*(7), 14–18.

Coggeshall Press. (2008). *Care for the total population.* Coralville, IA: Author.

Cole, L., & Houston, S. (1999a). Structured care methodologies: Evolution and use in patient care delivery. *Outcomes Management for Nursing Practice, 3*(2), 53–59.

Coleman, J. R. (1999). Integrated case management: The 21st century challenge for HMO case managers, Part 1. *The Case Manager, 10*(5), 28–34.

Commission for Case Manager Certification (CCMC). (2012). *Certification guide to the CCM® examination.* Mount Laurel, NJ: Author.

Cousins, M. S., & Liu, Y. (2003). Cost savings for a preferred provider organization population with multicondition disease management: Evaluating program impact using predictive modeling with a control group. *Disease Management, 6*(4), 207–217.

Dzyacky, S. C. (1998). An acute care case management model for nurses and social workers. *Nursing Case Management, 3*(5), 208–215.

Falk, C., & Bower, K. (1994). Managing care across department, organization, and setting boundaries. *Series on Nursing Administration, 6,* 161–176.

Fitzgerald, J. F., Smith, D. M., Martin, D. K., Freedman, J. A., & Katz, B. P. (1994). A case manager intervention to reduce readmissions. *Archives of Internal Medicine, 154*(15), 1721–1729.

Forbes, M. A. (1999). The practice of professional nurse case management. *Nursing Case Management, 4*(1), 28–33.

Gillespie, J. L. (2002). The value of disease management. Part 3. Balancing cost and quality in the treatment of asthma. *Disease Management, 5*(4), 225–232.

Goldstein, R. (1998). The disease management approach to cost containment. *Nursing Case Management, 3*(3), 99–103.

Goodwin, D. R. (1994). Nursing case management activities: How they differ between employment settings. *Journal of Nursing Administration, 24*(2), 29–34.

Goodwin, J. S., Satish, S., Anderson, E. T., Nattinger, A. B., & Freeman, J. L. (2003). Effect of nurse case management on the treatment of older women with breast cancer. *Journal of the American Geriatrics Society, 51*(9), 1252–1259.

Grimaldi, P. L. (1996a). A glossary of managed care terms. *Nursing Management, 27*(10, Spec. Suppl.), 5–7.

Hall, P. J. (1998). Planning an integrated population-based program. *Journal of Nursing Administration, 28*(10), 40–47.

Hawkins, J. W., Veeder, N. W., & Pearce, C. W. (1998). *Nurse–social worker collaboration in managed care.* New York: Springer.

Hinitz-Satterfield, P., Miller, E., & Hagan, E. (1993). Managed care and new roles for nursing: Utilization and case management in a health maintenance organization. *Series on Nursing Administration, 5,* 83–99.

Ho, S. (2003). The emerging role for health plans: "Info-Mediary". *Disease Management, 6*(Suppl. 1), 4–10.

Huber, D. L. (2005a). The diversity of service delivery models. In D. Huber (Ed.). *Disease management: A guide for case managers.* Philadelphia: Saunders.

Huber, D. L. (2005b). Overview of disease management. In D. L. Huber (Ed.), *Disease management: A guide for case managers.* Philadelphia: Saunders.

Huston, C. J. (2001). The role of the case manager in a disease management program. *Lippincott's Case Management, 6*(5), 222–227.

Improving Chronic Illness Care. (2012). *The chronic care model.* Retrieved October 28, 2012, from www.improvingchroniccare.org/index. php?p=Model_Elements&s=18.

Institute of Medicine (IOM). (2001c). *Crossing the quality chasm: A new health system for the 21st century.* Washington, DC: National Academies Press.

Institute of Medicine (IOM). (2004b). *Crossing the quality chasm: The IOM health care quality initiative.* Washington, DC: National Academies Press.

Javors, J. R., Laws, D., & Bramble, J. E. (2003). Uncontrolled chronic disease: Patient non-compliance or clinical mismanagement? *Disease Management, 6*(3), 169–178.

Johnson, A. (2003, October 15). Why we can't wait to implement disease management. *Business and Health Archive, 21.*

Kramer, M. S. (2004, January 10). Predictive models make smart purchasers. *Business and Health Archive,* 1–4.

Laramee, A. S., Levinsky, S. K., Sargent, J., Ross, R., & Callas, P. (2003). Case management in a heterogeneous congestive heart failure population: A randomized controlled trial. *Archives of Internal Medicine, 163*(7), 809–817.

Levitt, D. A., Starz, T. W., & Higgins, R. (1998). Disease state case management in an academic medical center utilizing osteoarthritis-of-the-knee model. *Journal of Care Management, 4*(5), 45, 48, 51–52, 54, 56.

Lewis, A. (2004). Savings opportunities through Medicaid disease management. *Disease Management, 7*(1), 35–46.

Lipold, A. G. (2002, June 19). Disease management comes of age, not a moment too soon. *Business and Health Archive, 7.*

Lu, C. Y., Ross-Degnan, D., Soumerai, S. B., & Pearson, S. (2008). Interventions designed to improve the quality and efficiency of medication use in managed care: A critical review of the literature—2001–2007. *BMC Health Services Research, 8,* 1–12.

Mark, B. (1992a). Characteristics of nursing practice models. *Journal of Nursing Administration, 22*(11), 57–63.

Martin, D. C., Berger, M. L., Anstatt, D. T., Wofford, J., Warfel, D., Turpin, R. S., et al. (2004). A randomized controlled open trial of population-based disease and case management in a Medicare Plus Choice health maintenance organization. *Preventing Chronic Disease, 1*(4). Retrieved October 29, 2012, from www.cdc.gov/pcd/issues/2004/oct/04_0015.htm.

McClure, M. (1991b). Introduction. In I. E. Goertzen (Ed.), *Differentiating nursing practice: Into the twenty-first century* (pp. 1–11). Kansas City, MO: American Academy of Nursing.

MediLexicon. (2012). *Medical dictionary—Critical pathway.* Retrieved October 28, 2012, from www.medilexicon. com/medicaldictionary.php.

Mikulencak, M. (1993a). Public health stands as a proven model for future delivery systems. *The American Nurse, 25*(6), 18.

Nobel, J. J., & Norman, G. K. (2003). Emerging information management technologies and the future of disease management. *Disease Management, 6*(4), 219–231.

Norris, S. L., Nichols, P. J., Caspersen, C. J., Glasgow, R. E., Engelgau, M. M., Jack, L., Jr., et al. (2002). The effectiveness of disease and case management for people with diabetes: A systematic review. *American Journal of Preventive Medicine, 22*(Suppl. 4), 1–25.

Mike Holt Enterprises, Inc. (2008). *Pareto's Law.* Retrieved October 29, 2012, from www.mikeholt. com/mojonewsarchive/BM-HTML/HTML/ ParetosLaw~20031013.htm.

Park, E. J., Huber, D. L., & Tahan, H. A. (2009). The evidence base for case management practice. *Western Journal of Nursing Research, 6,* 693–714. First published on April 6, 2009 as http://dx. doi:10.1177/0193945909332912.

Patel, P. H., Welsh, C., & Foggs, M. B. (2004). Improved asthma outcomes using a coordinated care approach in a large medical group. *Disease Management, 7*(2), 102–111.

Qudah, F. J., & Brannon, M. (1996). Population-based case management. *Quality Management in Health Care, 5*(1), 29–41.

Raiff, N. R., & Shore, B. K. (1993). *Advanced case management: New strategies for the nineties.* Newbury Park, CA: Sage.

Renholm, M., Leino-Kilpi, H., & Suominen, T. (2002). Critical pathways: A systematic review. *Journal of Nursing Administration, 32*(4), 196–202.

Rheaume, A., Frisch, S., Smith, A., & Kennedy, C. (1994). Case management and nursing practice. *Journal of Nursing Administration, 24*(3), 30–36.

Ridgely, M. S., & Willenbring, M. C. (1992). Application of case management to drug abuse treatment: Overview of models and research issues. *NIDA Monograph, 127,* 12–33.

Riegel, B., Carlson, B., Kopp, Z., LePetri, B., Glaser, B., & Unger, A. (2002). Effect of a standardized nurse case management telephone intervention on resource use in patients with chronic heart failure. *Archives of Internal Medicine, 162*(6), 705–712.

Schuster, G. F., & Goeppinger, J. (1996). Community as client: Using the nursing process to promote health. In M. Stanhope, & J. Lancaster (Eds.), *Community health nursing: Promoting health of aggregates, families, and individuals* (4th ed., pp. 289–314). St. Louis: Mosby.

Sesperez, J., Wilson, S., Jalaludin, B., Seger, M., & Sugrue, M. (2001). Trauma case management and clinical pathways: Prospective evaluation of their effect on selected patient outcomes in five key trauma conditions. *The Journal of Trauma, 50*(4), 643–649.

Shortell, S. M., Anderson, D. A., Gilles, R. R., Mitchell, J. B., & Morgan, K. L. (1993). The holographic organization. *Healthcare Forum Journal, 36*(2), 20–26.

Siefker, J. M., Garrett, M. B., Van Genderen, A., & Weis, M. J. (1998). *Fundamentals of case management: Guidelines for practicing case managers.* St. Louis: Mosby.

Simpson, R. (1993). Case-managed care in tomorrow's information network. *Nursing Management, 24*(7), 14–16.

Tahan, H. A. (1996). A ten-step process to develop case management plans. *Nursing Case Management, 1*(3), 112–121.

Tahan, H. A. (1998). Case management: A heritage more than a century old. *Nursing Case Management, 3*(2), 55–60.

Todd, W. E., & Nash, D. (Eds.). (1997). *Disease management: A systems approach to improving patient outcomes.* Chicago: American Hospital Publishing.

Wagner, E. H., Austin, B. T., Davis, C., Hindmarsh, M., Schaefer, J., & Bonomi, A. (2001a). Improving chronic illness care: Translating evidence into action. *Health Affairs, 20*(6), 64–78.

Ward, M. D., & Rieve, J. A. (1997). The role of case management in disease management. In W. E. Todd, & D. Nash (Eds.), *Disease management: A systems approach to improving patient outcomes* (pp. 235–259). Chicago: American Hospital Publishing.

Weil, M., & Karls, J. M. (1985). *Case management in human service practice: A systematic approach to mobilizing resources for clients.* San Francisco: Jossey-Bass.

Weiman, M. G. (1995). Case management. A means to improve quality and control the costs of cure in children with acute myelogenous leukemia. *Journal of Pediatric Hematology and Oncology, 17*(3), 248–253.

Welch, W. P., Bergsten, C., Cutler, C., Bocchino, C., & Smith, R. I. (2002). Disease management practices of health plans. *The American Journal of Managed Care, 8*(4), 353–361.

Williams, C. A. (1996). Community-based population focused practice: The foundation of specialization in public health nursing. In M. Stanhope, & J. Lancaster (Eds.), *Community health nursing: Promoting health of aggregates, families, and individuals.* (4th ed., pp. 21–33). St. Louis: Mosby.

Wilson, T., & MacDowell, M. (2003). Framework for assessing causality in disease management programs: Principles. *Disease Management, 6*(3), 143–158.

Zander, K. (1990a). Case management: A golden opportunity for whom? In J. McCloskey, & H. Grace (Eds.), *Current Issues in Nursing.* (3rd ed., pp. 199–204). St. Louis: Mosby.

Zander, K. (1991). Case management in acute care: Making the connections. *The Case Manager, 2*(1), 39–43.

Zander, K. (1992a). Nursing care delivery methods and quality. *Series on Nursing Administration, 3,* 86–104.

Zander, K. (2002). Nursing case management in the 21st century: Intervening where margin meets mission. *Nursing Administration Quarterly, 26*(5), 58–67.

Ziguras, S. J., & Stuart, G. W. (2000). A meta-analysis of the effectiveness of mental health case management over 20 years. *Psychiatric Services, 51,* 1410–1421.

Zitter, M. (1997). A new paradigm in health care delivery: Disease management. In W. E. Todd & D. Nash (Eds.), *Disease management: A systems approach to improving patient outcomes* (pp. 1–25). Chicago: American Hospital Publishing.

Chapter 13

Alidina, S., & Funke-Furber, J. (1988). First line nurse managers: Optimizing the span of control. *Journal of Nursing Administration, 18*(5), 34–39.

Altaffer, A. (1998). First-line managers: Measuring their span of control. *Nursing Management, 29*(7), 36–39.

Blau, P. M. (1968). The hierarchy of authority in organizations. *American Journal of Sociology, 73*(4), 453–467.

Blau, P. M. (1970). A formal theory of differentiation in organizations. *American Sociological Review, 35*(2), 201–218.

Carter, N. M., & Cullen, J. B. (1984). A comparison of centralization/decentralization of decision making concepts and measures. *Journal of Management, 10*(2), 259–268.

Champy, J. (2010). *Reengineering health care: A manifesto for radically rethinking health care delivery.* Upper Saddle River, NJ: FT Press.

Charnes, M., & Tewksbury, L. (1993). The continuum of organization structures. In *Collaborative management in health care: Implementing the integrative organization.* (pp. 20–43). San Francisco: Jossey-Bass.

Clegg, S. R. (1990). *Modern organizations: Organization studies in the postmodern world.* London: Sage Publications.

Clegg, S. R., & Hardy, C. (Eds.). (1999). *Studying organization: Theory and method.* (1st ed.). London: Sage Publications.

Curtin, L. (1994b). Restructuring: What works and what does not! *Nursing Management, 25*(10), 7–8.

Donaldson, L. (1996). The normal science of structural contingency theory. In S. R. Clegg & C. Hardy (Eds.), *Studying organization: Theory and method* (pp. 51–70). London: Sage Publications.

Doran, D., McCutcheon, A. S., Evans, M. G., MacMillan, D., McGillis Hall, L., Pringle, D., et al. (2004). *Impact of the manager's span of control on leadership and performance.* Ottawa, ON: Canadian Health Services Research Foundation.

Duffield, C., & Franks, H. (2001). The role and preparation of first-line nurse managers in Australia: Where are we going and how do we get there? *Journal of Nursing Management, 9,* 87–91.

Eisenstein, H. (1995). The Australian femocratic experiment: A feminist case for bureaucracy. In M. M. Ferree & P. Y. Martin (Eds.), *Feminist organizations: Harvest of the new women's movement* (pp. 69–83). Philadelphia: Temple University Press.

Farmer, D. J. (1997). The postmodern turn and the Socratic gadfly. In H. T. Miller & C. J. Fox (Eds.), *Postmodernism "reality" and public administration* (pp. 105–117). Burke, VA: Chatelaine Press.

Feldman, M. S., & Pentland, B. T. (2003). Reconceptualizing organizational routines as a source of change and flexibility. *Administrative Science Quarterly, 48,* 94–118.

Filerman, G. (2003). Closing the management competence gap. *Human Resources for Health, 1*(7), 1–3.

Galbraith, J. R. (1974). Organization design: An information processing view. *Interfaces, 4*(3), 28–36.

Galbraith, J., Downey, D., & Kates, A. (2002). How networks undergird the lateral capability of an organization: Where the work gets done. *Journal of Organizational Excellence, 21*(2), 67–78.

Gittell, J. H. (2002). Coordinating mechanisms in care provider groups: Relational coordination as a mediator and input uncertainty as a moderator of performance effects. *Management Science, 48*(11), 1408–1426.

Gittell, J. H. (2003). A theory of relational coordination. In K. S. Cameron, J. E. Dutton, & R. E. Quinn (Eds.), *Positive organizational scholarship: Foundations of a new discipline* (pp. 279–435). San Francisco: Berrett-Koehler.

Gittell, J. H. (2004). Achieving focus in hospital care: The role of relational coordination. In R. E. Herzlinger (Ed.), *Consumer-driven health care: Implications for providers, payers, and policymakers* (pp. 683–695). San Francisco: Jossey-Bass.

Gittell, J. H., & Weiss, L. (2004). Coordination networks within and across organizations: A multi-level framework. *Journal of Management Studies, 41*(1), 127–153.

Gulick, L. (1937). Notes on the theory of organization. In L. Gulick & L. Urwick (Eds.), *Papers on the science of administration* (pp. 1–46). New York: Institute of Public Administration, University of Columbia.

Hatch, M. J., & Cunliffe, A. L. (2006). *Organization theory: Modern, symbolic, and postmodern perspectives* (2nd ed.). New York: Oxford University Press.

Hoffman, C., Beard, P., Greenall, J. U. D., & White, J. (2006). *Canadian Root Cause Analysis Framework: A tool for identifying and addressing the root causes of critical incidents in health care.* Edmonton, AB: Canadian Patient Safety Institute.

Institute of Medicine of the National Academies. (2004). *Keeping patients safe: Transforming the work environment of nurses.* Washington, DC: National Academies Press.

Jaques, E. (1990). In praise of hierarchy. *Harvard Business Review, 68*(1), 127–133.

Kanter, R. M. (1977c). *Men and women of the corporation.* New York: Basic Books.

Katz, D., & Kahn, R. L. (1978). *The social psychology of organizations* (2nd ed.). New York: John Wiley and Sons.

Kimberly, J. R. (1976). Organizational size and the structuralist perspective: A review, critique, and proposal. *Administrative Science Quarterly, 21*(4), 571–597.

Kirkley, D., Johnson, A. P., & Anderson, M. A. (2004). Technology support of nursing excellence: The magnet connection. *Nursing Economics, 22*(2), 94–98.

Kramer, M., Maguire, P., Schmalenberg, C., Brewe, B., Burke, R., Chmielewski, L., et al. (2007). Nurse manager support: What is it? Structures and practices that promote it. *Nursing Administration Quarterly, 31*(4), 325–340.

Laschinger, H. K. S. (1996). A theoretical approach to studying work empowerment in nursing: A review of studies testing Kanter's theory of structural power in organizations. *Nursing Administration Quarterly, 20*(2), 25–41.

Laschinger, H. K. S., & Finegan, J. (2005). Using empowerment to build trust and respect in the workplace: A strategy for addressing the nursing shortage. *Nursing Economic$, 23*(1), 6–13.

Leape, L. L., & Berwick, D. M. (2005a). Five years after To Err Is Human: What have we learned? *JAMA, 293*(19), 2384–2390.

Leatt, P., Lemieux-Charles, L., & Aird, C. (1994). Program management: Introduction and overview. In L. Lemieux-Charles, P. Leatt, & C. Aird (Eds.), *Program management and beyond: Management innovations in Ontario hospitals* (pp. 1–10). Ottawa, ON: Canadian College of Health Service Executives.

Little, L., & Buchan, J. (2007). *Nursing self sufficiency/sustainability in the global context*. Geneva: International Centre on Nurse Migration.

Lorenz, H. L. (2008). Service line leadership. *Nurse Leader, 6*(1), 42–43.

Mahon, A., & Young, R. (2006). Health care managers as a critical component of the health care workforce. In C. Dubois, M. McKee, & E. Nolte (Eds.), *Human resources for health in Europe* (pp. 116–139). Berkshire, UK: Open University Press.

March, J. G., & Simon, H. A. (1958). *Organization*. New York: John Wiley & Sons.

Mark, B. A., Sayler, J., & Smith, C. S. (1996). A theoretical model for nursing systems outcomes research. *Nursing Administration Quarterly, 20*(4), 12–27.

Matthews, S., Laschinger, H. K. S., & Johnstone, L. (2006). Staff nurse empowerment in line and staff organizational structures for chief nurse executives. *Journal of Nursing Administration, 6*(11), 526–533.

McCutcheon, A. S. (2004). *Relationships between leadership style, span of control and outcomes*. Unpublished doctoral dissertation, Toronto, ON: University of Toronto.

Meier, K. J., & Bohte, J. (2003). Span of control and public organizations: Implementing Luther Gulick's research design. *Public Administration Review, 63*(1), 61–70.

Meyer, R. M. (2008). Span of management: Concept analysis. *Journal of Advanced Nursing, 63*(1), 104–112.

Meyer, R. M., & O'Brien-Pallas, L. (2010). Nursing Services Delivery Theory: An open system approach. *Journal of Advanced Nursing, 66*(12), 2828–2838.

Meyer, R. M., O'Brien-Pallas, L., Doran, D., Streiner, D., Ferguson-Paré, M., & Duffield, C. (2011). Front-line managers as boundary spanners: Effects of span and time on nurse supervision satisfaction. *Journal of Nursing Management, 19*(5), 611–622.

Mintzberg, H. (1983). *Structure in fives: Designing effective organizations*. Englewood Cliffs, NJ: Prentice-Hall.

Morash, R., Brintnell, J., & Rodger, G. L. (2005). A span of control tool for clinical managers. *Canadian Journal of Nursing Leadership, 18*(3), 83–93.

Nedd, N. (2006a). Perceptions of empowerment and intent to stay. *Nursing Economic$, 24*(1), 13–19.

O'Connor, E. S. (1999). The politics of management thought: A case study of the Harvard Business School and the Human Relations School. *Academy of Management Review, 24*(1), 117–131.

Pabst, M. K. (1993). Span of control on nursing inpatient units. *Nursing Economic$, 11*(2), 87–90.

Porter-O'Grady, T. (2003c). A different age for leadership, Part 1. *Journal of Nursing Administration, 33*(2), 105–110.

Porter-O'Grady, T. (2007). The CNE as entrepreneur: Innovation leadership for a new age. *Nurse Leader, 5*(1), 44–47.

Prins, G. (2000). *Testing theories on structure and strategy: An assessment of organizational knowledge*. Delft, The Netherlands: Eburon.

Redman, R. W., & Jones, K. R. (1998). Effects of implementing patient centered care models on nurse and non-nurse managers. *Journal of Nursing Administration, 28*(11), 46–53.

Reed, M. I. (1992). *The sociology of organizations: Themes, perspectives and prospects*. New York: Harvester Wheatsheaf.

Registered Nurses' Association of Ontario (RNAO). (2006). *Developing and sustaining nursing leadership*. Toronto, ON: Author.

Scott, W. R. (1992). *Organizations: Rational, natural, and open systems* (3rd ed.). Englewood Cliffs, NJ: Prentice-Hall.

Taylor, F. W. (2003). Scientific management. In K. Thompson (Ed.), *Early sociology of management and organizations* (Vol. 1). New York: Taylor & Francis. (Online). Retrieved July 3, 2012, from http://blogs.cas.suffolk.edu/govt521/files/2010/09/taylor.pdf.

Taylor, M. (2008). Working through the frustrations of clinical integration. *H&HN: Hospitals & Health Networks, 82*(1), 34–40.

Tichy, N. M., Tushman, M. L., & Fombrun, C. (1979). Social network analysis for organizations. *Academy of Management Review, 4*(4), 507–519.

Van de Ven, A. H., Delbecq, A. L., & Koenig, R. (1976). Determinants of coordination modes within organizations. *American Sociological Review, 41*(3), 322–338.

Venkatraman, N. (1994). IT-enabled business transformation: From automation to business scope redefinition. *Sloan Management Review, 35*(2), 73–87.

Weber, M. (1978). *Economy and society: An outline of interpretive sociology* (E. Fischoff, H. Gerth, A. M. Henderson, F. Kolegar, C. W. Mills, T. Parsons, M. Rheinstein, G. Roth, E. Shils, & C. Wittich, Trans., Vol. 2). Berkeley, CA: University of California Press.

Wenger, E. (2008). *Communities of practice: A brief introduction*. Retrieved July 3, 2012, from www.ewenger.com/theory/communities_of_practice_intro_WRD.doc.

West, E., & Barron, D. N. (2005). Social and geographical boundaries around senior nurse and physician leaders: An application of social network analysis. *Canadian Journal of Nursing Research, 37*(3), 132–148.

Willem, A., Buelens, M., & De Jonghe, I. (2007). Impact of organizational structure on nurses' job satisfaction: A questionnaire survey. *International Journal of Nursing Studies, 44*, 1011–1020.

Young, G. J., Charnes, M. P., & Heeren, T. C. (2004). Product line management in professional organizations: An empirical test of competing theoretical perspectives. *Academy of Management Journal, 47*(5), 723–734.

Young-Ritchie, C., Laschinger, H. K. S., & Wong, C. (2007). The effects of emotionally intelligent leadership behaviour on emergency staff nurses' workplace empowerment and organizational commitment. *Nursing Outlook, 30*(2), 24.

Chapter 14

Adler, P., Hecksher, C., & Prusak, L. (2011). Building a collaborative enterprise. *Harvard Business Review, 89*(7/8), 94–101.

American Nurses Credentialing Center. (2012). *History of the Magnet Program*. Retrieved on March 28, 2012 from www.nursecredentialing.org/Magnet/ProgramOverview/HistoryoftheMagnetProgram.aspx.

Anderson, E. F. (2011). A case for measuring governance. *Nursing Administration Quarterly, 35*(3), 197–203.

Anthony, M. K. (2004). Shared governance models: The theory, practice, and evidence. *Online Journal of Issues in Nursing, 9*(1), 138–153.

Ballard, N. (2010). Factors associated with success and breakdown of shared governance. *Journal of Nursing Administration, 40*(10), 411–416.

Bamford-Wade, A., & Moss, C. (2010). Transformational leadership and shared governance: An action study. *Journal of Nursing Management, 18*(7), 815–821.

Barden, A. M., Griffin, M. T. Q., Donahue, M., & Fitzpatrick, J. J. (2011b). Shared governance and empowerment in registered nurses working in a hospital setting. *Nursing Administration Quarterly, 35*(3), 212–218.

Bednarski, D. (2009). Shared governance: Enhancing nursing practice. *Nephrology Nursing Journal, 36*(6), 585.

Beglinger, J. E., Hauge, B., Krause, S., & Ziebarth, L. (2011). Shaping future nurse leaders through shared governance. *Nursing Clinics of North America, 46*(1), 129–135.

Brody, A. A., Barnes, K., Ruble, C., & Sakowski, J. (2012). Evidence-based practice councils: Potential path to staff nurse empowerment and leadership growth. *Journal of Nursing Administration, 42*(1), 28–33.

Brooks, B. A. (2004). Measuring the impact of shared governance. *Online Journal of Issues in Nursing, 9*(1), Manuscript 1a. Retrieved March 28, 2012 from www.nursingworld.org/MainMenuCategories/ANAMarketplace/ANAPeriodicals/OJIN/TableofContents/Volume92004/No1Jan04/MeasuringtheImpact.aspx.

Drenkard, K. (2010). The business case for Magnet. *Journal of Nursing Administration, 40*(6), 263–271.

Frith, K., & Montgomery, M. (2006). Perceptions, knowledge, and commitment of clinical staff to shared governance. *Nursing Administration Quarterly, 30*(3), 273–284.

Golanowski, M., Beaudry, D., Kurz, L., Laffey, W. J., & Hook, M. L. (2007). Interprofessional shared decision-making: Taking shared governance to the next level. *Nursing Administration Quarterly, 31*(4), 341–353.

Hess, R. (1994). Shared governance: Innovation or imitation? *Nursing Economic$, 12*(1), 28–34.

Hess, R. (2004). From bedside to boardroom: Nursing shared governance. *Online Journal of Issues in Nursing, 9*(1), Manuscript 1. Retrieved March 28, 2012 from www.nursingworld.org/MainMenuCategories/ANAMarketplace/ANAPeriodicals/OJIN/TableofContents/Volume92004/No1Jan04/FromBedsidetoBoardroom.aspx.

Hess, R. (2011). Slicing and dicing shared governance: In and around the numbers. *Nursing Administration Quarterly, 35*(3), 235–241.

Hoying, C., & Allen, S. (2011). Enhancing shared governance for interprofessional practice. *Nursing Administration Quarterly, 35*(3), 252–259.

Institute of Medicine (IOM). (2011c). *The future of nursing: Leading change, advancing health*. Washington, DC: National Academies Press.

Kain, E. (2012). 4.5 Million people signed Google's anti-SOPA petition. *Forbes*. Retrieved March 28, 2012 from www.forbes.com/sites/erikkain/2012/01/19/4-5-million-people-signed-googles-anti-sopa-petition/.

Kanter, R. (1993). *Men and women of the corporation* (2nd ed.). New York: Basic Books.

Kelly, L. A., McHugh, M. D., & Aiken, L. H. (2011a). Nurse outcomes in Magnet and non-magnet hospitals. *Journal of Nursing Administration, 41*(10), 428–433.

Kops, B. (2011). Summer session organizational models at Canadian universities. *Canadian Journal of University Continuing Education, 36*(2), 1–13.

McGuire, E., & Kennerly, S. (2006). Nurse managers as transformational and transactional leaders. *Nursing Economic$, 24*(4), 179–185.

Moore, S. C., & Hutchison, S. A. (2007). Developing leaders at every level: Accountability and empowerment actualized through shared governance. *Journal of Nursing Administration, 37*(12), 564–568.

Newman, K. (2011). Transforming organizational culture through nursing shared governance. *Nursing Clinics of North America, 46*, 45–58.

Orchard, C. (2010). Persistent isolationist or collaborator? The nurse's role in interprofessional collaborative practice. *Journal of Nursing Management, 18,* 248–257.

Poe, M. T. (2011). *A history of communications: Media and society from the evolution of speech to the internet.* New York: Cambridge University Press.

Porter-O'Grady, T. (2009). *Interprofessional shared governance: Integrating practice, transforming health care* (2nd ed.). Sudbury, MA: Jones & Bartlett.

Porter-O'Grady, T., Hawkins, M. A., & Parker, M. L. (1997). *Whole-systems shared governance: Architecture for integration.* Gaithersburg, MD: Aspen.

Porter-O'Grady, T., & Malloch, K. (2011b). *Quantum leadership: Advancing innovation, transforming health care* (3rd ed.). Sudbury, MA: Jones & Bartlett.

Rheingans, J. I. (2012). The alchemy of shared governance: Turning steel (and sweat) into gold. *Nurse Leader, 10*(1), 40–42.

Scherb, C. A., Specht, J. K. P., Loes, J. L., & Reed, D. (2011a). Decisional involvement: Staff nurse and nurse manager perceptions. *Western Journal of Nursing Research, 33*(2), 161–179.

Straub, J. T., & Attner, R. F. (1994). *Introduction to business* (5th ed.). Belmont, CA: Wadsworth.

Tassi, P. (2012). Internet blackout causes 18 senators to flee from PIPA. *Forbes.* Retrieved March 28, 2012 from www.forbes.com/sites/insertcoin/2012/01/19/internet-blackout-causes-18-senators-to-flee-from-pipa/.

Tomey, A. M. (2009). *Guide to nursing management and leadership* (8th ed.). St. Louis: Mosby Elsevier.

Tourangeau, L. A., Cranley, L. A., & Jeffs, L. (2006). Impact of nursing on hospital patient mortality: A focused review and related policy implications. *Quality and Safety in Health Care, 15,* 4–8.

Chapter 15

Abts, D., Hofer, M., & Leafgreen, P. (1994). Redefining care delivery: A modular system. *Nursing Management, 25*(2), 40–46.

Adams, D. (2004). *The pillars of planning: Mission values, vision.* Washington, DC: National Endowment for the Arts. Retrieved October 20, 2012, from http://arts.endow.gov/resources/lessons/adams.html.

Aiken, L. H., Clarke, S. P., Sloane, D. M., Sochalski, J., & Silber, J. H. (2002b). Hospital nurse staffing and patient mortality, nurse burnout, and job dissatisfaction. *Journal of the American Medical Association, 288*(16), 1987–1993.

American Association of Critical Care Nurses. (2005). AACN standards for establishing and sustaining healthy work environments: A journey to excellence. *American Journal of Critical Care, 14*(3), 187–197.

American Nurses Association (ANA). (1988b). *Nursing case management.* (Publication No. NS-32) Kansas City, MO: Author.

American Organization of Nurse Executives (AONE). (2012). *AONE guiding principles for the role of the nurse in future care delivery toolkit.* Washington, DC: Author. Retrieved October 20, 2012, from www.aone.org/resources/leadership%20tools/guidprinciples.shtml.

Anderson, C., & Hughes, E. (1993). Implementing modular nursing in a long-term care facility. *Journal of Nursing Administration, 23*(6), 29–35.

Arford, P. H., & Zone-Smith, L. (2005). Organizational commitment to professional practice models. *Journal of Nursing Administration, 35*(10), 467–472.

Bower, K. A. (2004b). Patient care management as a global nursing concern. *Nursing Administration Quarterly, 28*(1), 39–43.

Bylone, M. (2011). Healthy work environment 101. *AACN Advanced Critical Care, 22*(1), 19–21.

Case Management Society of America (CMSA). (2012a). *What is a case manager?* Little Rock, AR: Author. Retrieved September 8, 2012, from www.cmsa.org/Home/CMSA/WhatisaCaseManager/tabid/224/Default.aspx.

Cohen, E. L., & Cesta, T. G. (2005). *Nursing case management: From essentials to advanced practice applications* (4th ed.). St. Louis: Mosby.

Cole, L., & Houston, S. (1999b). Structured care methodologies: Evolution and use in patient care delivery. *Outcomes Management for Nursing Practice, 3*(2), 53–59.

Comack, M., Paech, G., & Porter-O'Grady, T. (1999). From structure to culture: A journey of transformation. In S. P. Smith & D. L. Flarey (Eds.), *Process-centered health care organizations* (pp. 45–67). Gaithersburg, MD: Aspen.

Deutschendorf, A. L. (2003). From past paradigms to future frontiers: Unique care delivery models to facilitate nursing work and quality outcomes. *Journal of Nursing Administration, 33*(1), 52–59.

Drenkard, K. N. (2001). Creating a future worth experiencing: Nursing strategic planning in an integrated healthcare delivery system. *Journal of Nursing Administration, 31*(7/8), 364–376.

Drucker, P. (1973). *Management: Tasks, responsibilities, practices.* New York: Harper & Row.

Duffy, J. R., Baldwin, J., & Mastorovich, M. J. (2007). Using the Quality-Caring Model to organize patient care delivery. *Journal of Nursing Administration, 37*(12), 546–551.

Eastaugh, S. R., & Regan-Donovan, M. (1990). Nurse extenders offer a way to trim staff expenses. *Healthcare Financial Management, 44*(4), 58–60, 62.

Erickson, J. I., & Ditomassi, M. (2011). Professional practice model: Strategies for translating models into practice. *Nursing Clinics of North America, 46*, 35–44.

Fuzard, R. T., Fox, D. H., & Wells, P. J. (1999). Performance of first-line management functions on productivity of hospital unit personnel. *Journal of Nursing Administration, 29*(9), 12–18.

Gardner, K. (1991). A summary of findings of a five-year comparison study of primary and team nursing. *Nursing Research, 40*(2), 113–117.

Gittell, J. H., Fairfield, K. M., Bierbaum, B., Head, W., Jackson, R., Kelly, M., et al. (2000). Impact of relational coordination on quality of care, postoperative pain and functioning, and length of stay: A nine-hospital study of surgical patients. *Medical Care, 38*(8), 807–819.

Glandon, G., Colbert, K., & Thomasma, M. (1989). Nursing delivery models and RN mix: Cost implications. *Nursing Management, 20*(5), 30–33.

Grimaldi, P. L. (1996b). A glossary of managed care terms. *Nursing Management, 24*(10, Spec Suppl.), 5–7.

Guild, S., Ledwin, R., Sanford, D., & Winter, T. (1994). Development of an innovative nursing care delivery system. *Journal of Nursing Administration, 24*(3), 23–29.

Haase-Herrick, K. S., & Herrin, D. M. (2007). The American Organization of Nurse Executives' guiding principles and American Association of Colleges of Nursing's Clinical Nurse Leader: A lesson in synergy. *Journal of Nursing Administration, 37*(2), 55–60.

Hall, L. M. (1997). Staff mix models: Complementary or substitution roles for nurses. *Nursing Administration Quarterly, 21*(2), 31–39.

Hardin, S. R., & Kaplow, R. (2005a). *Synergy for clinical excellence: The AACN synergy model for patient care.* Sudbury, MA: Jones & Bartlett.

Hoffart, N., & Woods, C. Q. (1996). Elements of a nursing professional practice model. *Journal of Professional Nursing, 12*(6), 354–364.

Institute of Medicine (IOM) (2001d). *Crossing the quality chasm: A new health system for the 21st century.* Washington, DC: National Academies Press.

Jennings, B. M. (2008). Care models. In R. G. Hughes (Ed.), *Patient safety and quality: An evidence-based handbook for nurses.* (Prepared with support from the Robert Wood Johnson Foundation.) AHRQ Publication No. 08–0043. Rockville, MD: Agency for Healthcare Research and Quality.

Jones-Schenk, J., & Hartley, P. (1993). Organization for communication and integration. *Journal of Nursing Administration, 23*(10), 30–33.

Kane, R. L., Shamliyan, T. A., Mueller, C., Duval, S., & Wilt, T. J. (2007c). The association of registered nurse staffing levels and patient outcomes: Systematic review and meta-analysis. *Medical Care, 45*(12), 1195–1204.

Katz, R. E., & Frank, R. G. (2010). A vision for the future: New care delivery models can play a vital role in building tomorrow's eldercare workforce. *Generations: Journal of the American Society on Aging, 34*(4), 82–88.

Kimball, B., Joynt, J., Cherner, D., & O'Neil, E. (2007). The quest for new innovative care delivery models. *Journal of Nursing Administration, 37*(9), 392–398.

Kohn, L. T., Corrigan, J., & Donaldson, M. S. (2000c). *To err is human: Building a safer health system.* Washington, DC: National Academies Press.

Koloroutis, M. (Ed.). (2004a). *Relationship-based care: A model for transforming practice.* Minneapolis: Creative Health Care Management.

Kramer, M., & Schmalenberg, C. (1988a). Magnet hospitals: Institutions of excellence: Part 1. *Journal of Nursing Administration, 18*(1), 13–24.

Kramer, M., & Schmalenberg, C. (1988b). Magnet hospitals: Institutions of excellence: Part 2. *Journal of Nursing Administration, 18*(2), 11–19.

Leape, L. L., & Berwick, D. M. (2005b). Five years after *To Err Is Human*: What have we learned? *Journal of the American Medical Association, 293*(19), 2384–2390.

Lee, J. (1993). A history of care models in nursing. *Series on Nursing Administration, 5*, 20–38.

Lengacher, C., Mabe, P., Bowling, C., Heinemann, D., Kent, K., & Cott, M. (1993). Redesigning nursing practice: The partners in patient care model. *Journal of Nursing Administration, 23*(12), 31–37.

Lookinland, S., Tiedeman, M. E., & Crosson, A. E. (2005). Nontraditional models of care delivery: Have they solved the problems? *Journal of Nursing Administration, 35*(2), 74–80.

Lyon, J. (1993). Models of nursing care delivery and case management: Clarification of terms. *Nursing Economic$, 11*(3), 163–169.

Maehling, J. A. S. (1995). Process reengineering: Strategies for analysis and redesign. In S. S. Blancett & D. L. Flarey (Eds.), *Reengineering nursing and health care: The handbook for organizational transformation* (pp. 61–74). Gaithersburg, MD: Aspen.

Magargal, P. (1987). Modular nursing: Nurses rediscover nursing. *Nursing Management, 18*(11), 98–104.

Manthey, M. (1991). Delivery systems and practice models: A dynamic balance. *Nursing Management, 22*(1), 28–30.

Mark, B. (1992b). Characteristics of nursing practice models. *Journal of Nursing Administration, 22*(11), 57–63.

McCloskey, J. (1991). Creating an environment for success with fun, hope, and trouble. *Journal of Nursing Administration, 21*(4), 5–6.

McCloskey, J., Blegen, M., & Gardner, D. (1991). Who helps you with your work? *American Journal of Nursing*, *91*(4), 43–46.

McNamara, C. (2008). *Basics of developing mission, vision and values statements*. St. Paul, MN: Free Management Library: Authenticity Consulting, LLC. Retrieved October 20, 2012, from http://208.42.83.77/plan_dec/str_plan/stmnts.htm#anchor519441.

Mikulencak, M. (1993b). Public health stands as a proven model for future delivery systems. *The American Nurse*, *25*(6), 18.

Minnick, A. F., Mion, L. C., Johnson, M. E., & Catrambone, C. (2007). How unit level nursing responsibilities are structured in U.S. hospitals. *Journal of Nursing Administration*, *37*(10), 452–458.

Morjikian, R. L., Kimball, B., & Joynt, J. (2007). Leading change: The nurse executive's role in implementing new care delivery models. *Journal of Nursing Administration*, *37*(9), 399–404.

National Transitions of Care Coalition (NTOCC) (2010). *Improving transitions of care: Findings and considerations of the "vision of the national transitions of care coalition"*. Retrieved May 30, 2012, from www.ntocc.org/Portals/0/PDF/Resources/NTOCCIssueBriefs.pdf.

Naylor, M. D., Aiken, L. H., Kurtzman, E. T., Olds, D. M., & Hirschman, K. B. (2011a). The importance of transitional care in achieving health reform. *Health Affairs*, *30*(4), 746–754.

Needleman, J., Buerhaus, P. I., Mattke, S., Stewart, M., & Zelevinsky, K. (2001b). *Nurse staffing and patient outcomes in hospitals*. (Contract No. 230–99–0021). U.S. Department of Health and Human Resources, Health Resources and Services Administration.

Person, C. (2004a). Patient care delivery. In M. Koloroutis (Ed.), *Relationship-based care: A model for transforming practice*. Minneapolis Creative Health Care Management.

Planetree, Inc. (2008). *Patient-centered care improvement guide*. Derby, CT: Author. Retrieved October 20, 2012, from http://planetree.org/wp-content/uploads/2012/01/Patient-Centered-Care-Improvement-Guide-10-28-09-Final.pdf.

Poteet, G., & Hill, A. (1988). Identifying the components of a nursing service philosophy. *Journal of Nursing Administration*, *18*(10), 29–33.

Reverby, S. (1987). *Ordered to care: The dilemma of American nursing, 1850–1945*. Cambridge, MA: Cambridge University Press.

Rust, G., Strothers, H., Miller, W. J., McLaren, S., Moore, B., & Sambamoorthi, U. (2011). Economic impact of a Medicaid population health management program. *Population Health Management*, *14*(5), 215–222.

Shirey, M. R. (2008). Nursing practice models for acute and critical care: Overview of care delivery models. *Critical Care Nursing Clinics of North America*, *20*, 365–373.

Smith, D. S., & Dabbs, M. T. (2007). Transforming the care delivery model in preparation for the clinical nurse leader. *Journal of Nursing Administration*, *37*(4), 157–160.

Tiedeman, M. E., & Lookinland, S. (2004). Traditional models of care delivery: What have we learned? *Journal of Nursing Administration*, *34*(6), 291–297.

Unruh, L. (2003a). Licensed nurse staffing and adverse events in hospitals. *Medical Care*, *41*(1), 142–152.

Unruh, L. (2008a). Nurse staffing and patient, nurse, and financial outcomes. *American Journal of Nursing*, *108*(1), 62–71.

Vlasses, F. R., & Smeltzer, C. H. (2007). Toward a new future for healthcare and nursing practice. *Journal of Nursing Administration*, *37*(9), 375–380.

Watson, J., & Foster, R. (2003). The attending nurse caring model: Integrating theory, evidence and advanced caring-healing therapeutics for transforming professional practice. *Journal of Clinical Nursing*, *12*(3), 360–365.

Wiggins, M. S. (2006). The Partnership Care Delivery Model. *Journal of Nursing Administration*, *36*(7–8), 341–345.

Wolf, G., Boland, S., & Aukerman, M. (1994). A transformational model for the practice of professional nursing. Part 2. Implementation of the model. *Journal of Nursing Administration*, *24*(5), 38–46.

Wolf, G. A., & Greenhouse, P. K. (2007). Blueprint for design: Creating models that direct change. *Journal of Nursing Administration*, *37*(9), 381–387.

Wolf, G. A., Triolo, P., & Ponte, P. R. (2008b). Magnet Recognition Program: The next generation. *Journal of Nursing Administration*, *38*(4), 200–204.

Zander, K. (1990b). Case management: A golden opportunity for whom? In J. McCloskey & H. Grace (Eds.), *Current issues in nursing*. (3rd ed., pp. 199–204). St. Louis: Mosby.

Zander, K. (1992b). Nursing care delivery methods and quality. *Series on Nursing Administration*, *3*, 86–104.

Zander, K., & Warren, C. (2005). Converting case managers from MD/service to unit-based assignments: A before and after comparison. *Lippincott's Case Management*, *10*(4), 180–184.

Chapter 16

Aarons, G. A. (2006). Transformation and transactional leadership: Association with attitudes toward evidence-based practice. *Psychiatric Services*, *57*(8).

Agency for Healthcare Research and Quality (AHRQ). (2002). *Evaluating the impact of value-based purchasing: A guide for purchasers.* Rockville, MD: Agency for Healthcare Research and Quality.AHRQ Publication No. 02-0029. Retrieved from www.ahrq.gov/qual/valuebased/.

Agency for Healthcare Research and Quality (AHRQ). (2011). *What is comparativeness effectiveness research.* Retrieved March 30, 2012, from www.effectivehealthcare.ahrq.gov/index.cfm/what-is-comparative-effectiveness-research1/.

Agency for Healthcare Research and Quality (AHRQ). (2012). *U.S. Preventive Services Task Force (USPSTF).* Retrieved March 31, 2012, from www.ahrq.gov/clinic/uspstfix.htm.

Avorn, J., & Soumerai, S. B. (1983). Improving drug-therapy decisions through educational outreach. A randomized controlled trial of academically based "detailing". *The New England Journal of Medicine, 318*(24), 1457–1463.

Block, J., Lilienthal, M., Cullen, L., & White, A. (2012). Evidence-based thermoregulation for adult trauma patients. *Critical Care Nursing Quarterly, 35*(1), 50–63.

Bloom, B. (2005). Effects of continuing medical education on improving physician clinical care and patient health: A review of systematic reviews. *International Journal of Technology Assessment in Health Care, 21*(3), 380–385.

Boström, A. M., Wallin, L., & Nordström, G. (2007). Evidence-based practice and determinants of research use in elderly care in Sweden. *Journal of Evaluation in Clinical Practice, 13*, 665–673.

Bowman, A., Greiner, J., Doerschug, K., Little, S., Bombei, C., & Comried, L. (2005). Implementaton of an evidence-based feeding protocol and aspiration risk reduction algorithm. *Critical Care Nursing Quarterly, 28*(4), 324–333.

Boyer, D. R., Steltzer, N., & Larrabee, J. H. (2006). Implementation of an evidence-based bladder scanner protocol. *Journal of Nursing Care Quality, 24*(1), 10–16.

Brewer, B., Brewer, M., & Schultz, A. (2009). A collaborative approach to building the capacity for research and evidence-based practice in community hospitals. *Nursing Clinics of North America, 44*(1), 11–25. http://dx.doi:10.1016/j.cnur.2008.10.003.

Brouwers, M., Kho, M. E., Browmna, G. P., Burgers, J. S., Cluzeau, F., Feder, G., et al. (2010). AGREE II: Advancing guideline development, reporting and evaluation in healthcare. *Canadian Medical Association Journal, 182*, E839–E842. http://dx.doi:10.1503/090449.

Bullock-Palmer, R. P., Weiss, S., & Hyman, C. (2008). Innovative approaches to increase deep vein thrombosis prophylaxis rate resulting in a decrease in hospital-acquired deep vein thrombosis at a tertiary-care teaching hospital. *Journal of Hospital Medicine, 3*(2), 148–155.

Burns, S. (2012). Adherence to sedation withdrawal protocols and guidelines in ventilated patients. *Clinical Nurse Specialist, 26*(1), 22–28.

Centers for Disease Control and Prevention. (2012a). *Overweight and obesity.* Retrieved May 21, 2013, from http://www.cdc.gov/obesity/data/index.html.

Centers for Disease Control and Prevention. (2012b). *High blood pressure.* Retrieved May 21, 2013, from www.cdc.gov/bloodpressure/.

Centers for Medicare & Medicaid Services (CMS). (2011). Medicare program: Hospital inpatient value-based purchasing program. Final rule. *Federal Registry, 76*(88), 26490–26547.

Centers for Medicare & Medicaid Services (CMS). (2010). *CMS final rule on meaningful use.* Retrieved March 30, 2012, from http://edocket.access.gpo.gov/2010/pdf/2010-17207.pdf.

Conway, J. (2008). Getting boards on board: Engaging governing boards in quality and safety. *Joint Commission Journal on Quality and Patient Safety, 34*(4), 214–220.

Cullen, L., & Adams, S. (2012). Planning for implementation of evidence-based practice. *Journal of Nursing Administration, 42*(4), 222–230.

Cullen, L., Greiner, J., Greiner, J., Bombei, C., & Comried, L. (2005). Excellence in evidence-based practice: An organizational and MICU exemplar. *Critical Care Nursing Clinics of North America, 17*(2), 127–142.

Cullen, L., & Titler, M. G. (2004). Promoting evidence-based practice: An internship for staff nurses. *Worldviews on Evidence-Based Nursing, 1*(4), 215–223.

Cullen, L., Titler, M. G., & Rempel, G. (2010). An advanced educational program promoting evidence-based practice. *Western Journal of Nursing Research, 33*(3), 345–364.

Cullen, L., Tucker, S., Hanrahan, K., Rempel, G., & Jordan, K. (2012). *Evidence-based practice building blocks: Comprehensive strategies, tools, and tips* (1st ed.). Iowa City: Department of Nursing Services and Patient Care, University of Iowa Hospitals and Clinics.

Cummings, G. G., Estabrooks, C. A., Midodzi, W. K., Wallin, L., & Hayduk, L. (2007). Influence of organizational characteristics and context on research utilization. *Nursing Research, 56*(4S), S24–S39.

Davies, B., Edwards, N., Ploeg, J., Virani, T., Skelly, J., & Dobbins, M. (2006). *Determinants of the sustained use of research evidence in nursing.* Canadian Health Services Research Foundation; Canadian Institutes of Health Research; Government of Ontario, Ministry of Health and Long-Term Care; Registered Nurses' Association on Ontario. www.chsrf.ca/final_research/ogc/pdf/davies_final_e.pdf.

Davies, D. A., Thomson, M. A., Oxman, A. D., & Haynes, R. B. (1995). Changing physician performance: A systematic review of the effect of continuing medical education strategies. *Journal of the American Medical Association*, *274*(9), 700–705.

Debourgh, G. A. (2012). Synergy for patient safety and quality: Academic and service partnerships to promote effective nurse education and clinical practice. *Journal of Professional Nursing*, *28*(1), 48–61.

Department of Health and Human Services (DHHS). (2009). Breach notification for unsecured protected health information. *Federal Registry*, *74*(162), 42740.

Dobbins, M, Ciliska, D., Cockerill, R., Barnsley, J., & DiCenso, A. (2002). A framework for the dissemination and utilization of research for health-care policy and practice. *Online Journal of Knowledge Synthesis for Nursing*, November 18; 9: 7.

Dogherty, E. J., Harrison, M. B., Baker, C., & Graham, I. D. (2012). Following a natural experiment of guideline adaptation and early implementation: a mixed-methods study of facilitation. *Implementation Science*, *7*(1), 9.

Dole, N., & Griffin, E. (2009). *Accurate blood pressure measurement of the obese arm: A staff nurse case example of evidence-based practice*. Paper presented at the 34th Annual Conference for the American Academy of Ambulatory Care Nursing, March 2009. Philadelphia, PA.

Dolezal, N., Cullen, L., Harp, J., & Mueller, T. (2011). Implementing preoperative screening of undiagnosed obstructive sleep apnea. *Journal of PeriAnesthesia Nursing*, *26*(5), 338–342.

Doumit, G., Gattellari, M., Grimshaw, J., & O'Brien, M. A. (2007). *Local opinion leaders: Effects on professional practice and health care outcomes*. Cochrane Database Systematic Review. January 24. (1) Art. No.:CD000125. Retrieved from. http://dx.doi:10.1002/14651858. CD000125.pub3.

Durieux, P., Trinquart, L., Colombet, I., Niès, J., Walton, R. T., Rajeswaran, A., et al. (2008). Computerized advice on drug dosage to improve prescribing practice. *Cochrane Database of Systematic Reviews*, *2008*(3), Art. No.:CD002894. http://dx.doi:002810.001002/14651858. CD14002894.pub14651852.

Eccles, M. P., & Mittman, B. S. (2006). Welcome to Implementation Science. *Implementation Science*, *1*(1), 1–3. http://dx.doi:10.1186/1748-5908-1-1.

Estabrooks, C. A., Midodzi, W. K., Cummings, G. G., & Wallin, L. (2007). Predicting research use in nursing organizations. *Nursing Research*, *56*(4S), S7–S23.

Farmer, A. P., Légaré, F., Turcot, L., Grimshaw, J., Harvey, E., McGowan, J. L., et al. (2008). Printed educational materials: Effects on professional practice and health care outcomes. *Cochrane Database of Systematic Reviews*, *3*, Art No.:CD004398. http://dx.doi:004310.001002/14651858.CD14004398. pub14651852.

Farrington, M., Lang, S., Cullen, L., & Stewart, S. (2009). Nasogastric tube placement in pediatric and neonatal patients. *Pediatric Nursing*, *3*(1), 17–25.

Fleuren, M., Wiefferink, K., & Paulussen, T. (2004). Determinants of innovation within health care organizations. *International Journal for Quality in Health Care*, *16*(2), 107–123.

Forsetlund, L., Bjørndal, A., Rashidian, A., Jamtvedt, G., O'Brien, M. A., Wolf, F., et al. (2009). Continuing education meetings and workshops: Effects on professional practice and health care outcomes. *Cochrane Database of Systematic Reviews*, *2*, CD003030.

Gawlinski, A., & Rutledge, D. (2008). Selecting a model for evidence-based practice changes: A practical approach. *AACN Advanced Critical Care*, *19*(3), 291–300.

Gerrish, K., McDonnell, A., Nolan, M., Guillaume, L., Kirshbaum, M., & Tod, A. (2011). The role of advanced practice nurses in knowledge brokering as a means of promoting evidence-based practice among clinical nurses. *Journal of Advanced Nursing*, *67*(9), 2004–2014.

Gerrish, K., Nolan, M., McDonnell, A., Tod, A., Kirshbaum, M., & Guillaume, L. (2012). Factors influencing advanced practice nurses' ability to promote evidence-based practice among frontline nurses. *Worldviews on Evidence-Based Nursing*, *9*(1), 30–39. http://dx.doi:10.1111/j.1741-6787.2011.00230.x.

Gifford, W., Davies, B., Edwards, N., Griffith, P., & Lybanon, V. (2007). Managerial leadership for nurses' use of research evidence: An integrative review of the literature. *Worldviews on Evidence-Based Nursing*, *4*(3), 126–145.

Gifford, W., Davies, B., Tourangeau, A., & Lefebre, N. (2011). Developing team leadership to facilitate guide utilization: Planning and evaluating a 3-month intervention strategy. *Journal of Nursing Management*, *19*(1), 121–132.

Gifford, W. A., Davies, B., Graham, I. D., & Lefebre, N. (2009). *Interview guide: Leadership/diabetic foot ulcer study*. Ottawa: University of Ottawa.

Goeschel, C. A., Wachter, R. M., & Pronovost, P. J. (2010). Responsibility for quality improvement and patient safety: Hospital board and medical staff leadership challenges. *Chest*, *138*(1), 171–178.

Goode, C. J., Fink, R. M., Krugman, M., Oman, K. S., & Traditi, L. K. (2011). The Colorado Patient-Centered Interprofessional Evidence-Based Practice Model: A framework for transformation. *Worldviews on Evidence-Based Nursing*, *8*(2), 96–105. http://dx.doi:10.1111/j.1741-6787.2010.00208.x.

GRADE. (2012). *GRADE working group*. Retrieved March 31, 2012, from www.gradeworkinggroup.org/.

Granger, B. B., Prvu-Bettger, J., Aucoin, J., Fuchs, M. A., Mitchell, P. H., Holditch-Davis, D., et al. (2012). An academic-health service partnership in nursing: Lessons from the field. *Journal of Nursing Scholarship, 44*(1), 71–79. http://dx.doi:10.1111/j.1547-5069.2011.01432.x.

Greenhalgh, T., Robert, G., Bate, P., Macfarlane, F., & Kyriakidou, O. (2005). *Diffusion of innovations in health service organizations*. Malden, MA: Blackwell Publishing.

Hart, P., Eaton, L., Buckner, M., Morrow, B. N., Barrett, D. T., Fraser, D. D., et al. (2008). Effectiveness of a computer-based educational program on nurses' knowledge, attitude, and skill level related to evidence-based practice. *Worldviews on Evidence-Based Nursing, 5*(2), 75–84.

Harvard Business Essentials. (2004). *Managing projects large and small*. Boston: Harvard Business School Press.

Haynes, A. B., Weiser, T. G., Berry, W. R., Lipsitz, S. R., Breizat, A. H., Dellinger, E. P., et al. (2009). A surgical safety checklist to reduce morbidity and mortality in a global population. *New England Journal of Medicine, 360*(5), 491–499.

Hogan, D. L., & Logan, J. (2004). The Ottawa model of research use: A guide to clinical innovation in the NICU. *Clinical Nursing Specialist, 18*(5), 255–261.

Hudak, M., & Bond-Domb, A. (1996). Postoperative head and neck cancer with artificial airways: The effect of saline lavage on tracheal mucus evacuation and oxygen saturation. *ORL-Head and Neck Nursing, 14*(1), 17–21.

Hughes, L. C., Chang, Y., & Mark, B. A. (2009). Quality and strength of patient safety climate on medical-surgical units. *Health Care Management Review, 34*(1), 19–28.

Institute for Healthcare Improvement (2012). *How-to guide: Governance leadership (get boards on boards)*. Retrieved March 14, 2012, from www.ihi.org/knowledge/pages/tools/howtoguidegovernanceleadership.aspx.

Institute of Medicine (2008). *Knowing what works in health care: A roadmap for the nation*. Washington, DC: The National Academies Press.

Institute of Medicine (2010b). *The future of nursing: Leading change, advancing health*. Washington, DC: The National Academies Press.

Institute of Medicine (2011a). *Clinical practice guidelines we can trust*. Washington, DC: The National Academies Press.

Institute of Medicine (2011b). *Finding what works in health care: Standards for systematic reviews*. Washington, DC: Institute of Medicine.

Jablonski, A., & Ersek, M. (2009). Nursing home staff adherence to evidence-based pain management practices. *Journal of Gerontological Nursing, 35*(7), 28–34. quiz 36–37. http://dx.doi:10.3928/00989134-20090428-03.

Kirchhoff, K. (2004). State of the science of translation research: From demonstration projects to intervention testing. *Worldviews on Evidence-Based Nursing, 1*(Suppl. 1), S6–S12.

Kitson, A. L., Rycroft-Malone, J., Harvey, G., McCormack, B., Seerse, K., & Titchen, A. (2008). Evaluating the successful implementation of evidence into practice using the PARiHS framework: Theoretical and practical challenges. *Implementation Science, 3*, 1.

Logan, J., Harrison, M. B., Graham, I. D., Dunn, K., & Bissonnette, J. (1999). Evidence-based pressure-ulcer practice: The Ottawa model of research use. *Canadian Journal of Nursing Research, 31*(1), 37–52.

Luther, K., & Savitz, L. A. (2012). Leaders challenged to reduce cost, deliver more: Targeted improvements are critical for creating a culture dedicated to efficiency and quality. *Healthcare Executive, 27*(1), 80–81.

Madsen, D., Sebolt, T., Cullen, L., Folkdahl, B., Mueller, T., Richardson, C., et al. (2005). Listening to bowel sounds: An evidence-based practice project. *American Journal of Nursing, 105*(12), 40–50.

Majumdar, R., Tsuyuki, F., & McAlister, F. A. (2007). Impact of opinion leader-endorsed evidence summaries on the quality of prescribing for patients with cardiovascular disease: A randomized controlled trial. *American Heart Journal, 153*(1), 22.

Mallidou, A., Cummings, G., Ginsburg, L., Chuang, Y., Kang, S., Norton, P. G., et al. (2011). Staff, space, and time as dimensions of organizational slack: A psychometric assessment. *Health Care Management Review, 36*(3), 252–264. http://dx.doi:10.1097/HMR.0b013e318208ccf8.

Manning, D. M., Kuchirka, C., & Kaminski, J. (1983). Miscuffing: Inappropriate blood pressure cuff application. *Circulation, 68*(4), 763–766.

Missal, B., Schafer, B., Halm, M., & Schaffer, M. (2010). A university and health care organization partnership to prepare nurses for evidence-based practice. *Journal of Nursing Education, 49*(8), 456–461. http://dx.doi:10.3928/01484834-20100430-06.

Newhouse, R. (2007). Creating infrastructure supportive of evidence-based nursing practice: Leadership strategies. *Worldviews on Evidence-Based Nursing, 4*(1), 21–29.

Nicol, P., Watkins, R., Donovan, R., Wynaden, D., & Cadwallader, H. (2009). The power of vivid experience in hand hygiene compliance. *Journal of Hospital Infection, 72*(1), 36–42. http://dx.doi:10.1016/j.jhin.2009.01.021.

O'Brien, M. A., Rogers, S., Jamtvedt, G., Oxman, A. D., Odgaard-Jensen, J., Kristoffersen, D. T., et al. (2007). Educational outreach visits: Effects on professional practice and health care outcomes. *Cochrane Database of Systematic Reviews, 4*, Art. No.: CD000409. http://dx.doi:10.1002/14651858.CD000409.pub2.

Oxman, A. D., Thomson, M. A., Davis, D. A., & Haynes, R. B. (1995). No magic bullets: A systematic review of 102 trials of interventions to improve professional practice. *Canadian Medical Association Journal, 153*(10), 1423–1431.

Pappas, S. H. (2008). The cost of nurse-sensitive adverse events. *Journal of Nursing Administration, 38*(5), 230–236.

Pepler, C. J., Edgar, L., Frisch, S., Rennick, J., Swidzinski, M., White, C., et al. (2006). Strategies to increase research-based practice. *Clinical Nursing Specialist, 20*(1), 23–31.

Pickering, T. G., Hall, J. E., Appel, L., Falkner, B. E., Graves, J., Hill, M. N., et al. (2005). Recommendations for blood pressure measurement in humans and experimental animals: Part 1: Blood pressure measurement in humans: A statement for professionals from the Subcommittee of Professional and Public Education of the American Heart Association Council on High Blood Pressure Research. *Circulation, 111*(5), 697–716.

Pipe, T., Timm, J., Harris, M., Frusti, D., Tucker, S., Attlesey-Pries, J., et al. (2009). Implementing a health system-wide evidence-based practice educational program to reach nurses with various levels of experience and educational preparation. *Nursing Clinics of North America, 44*(1), 43–55.

Ploeg, J., Skelly, J., Rowan, M., Edwards, N., Davies, B., Grinspun, D., et al. (2010). The role of nursing best practice champions in diffusing practice guidelines: A mixed methods study. *Worldviews on Evidence-Based Nursing, 7*(4), 238–251.

Prior, M., Guerin, M., & Grimmer-Somers, K. (2008). The effectiveness of clinical guideline implementation strategies—A synthesis of systematic review findings. *Journal of Evaluation in Clinical Practice, 14*(5), 888–897.

QSEN. (2012). *Quality and Safety Education for Nurses.* Retrieved April 1, 2012, from http://qsen.org/about-qsen/project-overview/.

Randall, J., Arthur, A., & Vaughan, N. (2010). Twenty-four-hour observational study of hospital hand hygiene compliance. *Journal of Hospital Infection, 76*(3), 252–255. http://dx.doi:10.1016/j.jhin.2010.06.027.

Rauen, C. A., Chulay, M., Bridges, E., Vollman, K. M., & Arbour, R. (2008). Seven evidence-based practice habits: Putting some sacred cows out to pasture. *Critical Care Nurse, 28*(2), 98–124.

Revello, K., & Fields, W. (2012). A performance improvement project to increase nursing compliance with skin assessments in a rehabilitation unit.

Rehabilitation Nursing, 37(1), 37–42. http://dx.doi:10.1002/RNJ.00006.

Rogers, E. (2003b). *Diffusion of innovations* (5th ed.). New York: The Free Press.

Rosamond, W., Flegal, K., Friday, G., Furie, K., Go, A., Greenlund, K., et al. (2007). Heart disease and stroke statistics—2007 update: A report from the American Heart Association Statistics Committee and Stroke Statistics Subcommittee. *Circulation, 115*(5), e69–e171.

Rubenstein, L. V., & Pugh, J. A. (2006). Strategies for promoting organizational and practice change by advancing implementation research. *Journal of General Internal Medicine, 21*, S58–64.

Rushing, J. (2004). Taking blood pressure accurately. *Nursing, 34*(11), 26.

Russo, C., Steiner, C., & Spector, W. (2008). *Hospitalizations related to pressure ulcers among adults 18 years and older, 2006: statistical brief # 64.* Rockville, MD: Healthcare Cost and Utilization Project (HCUP) Statistical Briefs. Agency for Health Care Policy and Research.

Rycroft-Malone, J., & Bucknall, T. (2010). *Models and frameworks for implementing evidence-based practice: linking evidence to action.* Hoboken, NJ: Wiley-Blackwell.

Rycroft-Malone, J., Harvey, G., Kitson, A., McCormack, B., & Titchen, A. (2002). Getting evidence into practice: Ingredients for change. *Nursing Standard, 16*(37), 38–43.

Sackett, D. L., Strauss, S. E., Richardson, W. S., Rosenberg, W., & Haynes, R. B. (2000). *Evidence-based medicine: How to practice and teach EBM.* London: Churchill Livingstone.

Sandström, B., Borglin, G., Nilsson, R., & Willman, A. (2011). Promoting the implementation of evidence-based practice: A literature review focusing on the role of nursing leadership. *Worldviews on Evidence-Based Nursing, 8*(4), 212–223.

Scales, D., Dainty, K., Hales, B., Pinto, R., Fowler, R., Adhikari, N., et al. (2011). A multifaceted intervention for quality improvement in a network of intensive care units: A cluster randomized trial. *Journal of the American Medical Association, 305*(4), 363–372. http://dx.doi:10.1001/jama.2010.2000.

Schell, K. A., Morse, K., & Waterhouse, J. K. (2010). Forearm and upper-arm oscillometric blood pressure comparison in acutely ill adults. *Western Journal of Nursing Research, 32*(3), 322–340.

Schell, K. A., Richards, J. G., & Farquhar, W. B. (2007). The effects of anatomical structures on adult forearm and upper arm noninvasive blood pressures. *Blood Pressure Monitoring, 12*(1), 17–22.

Schimizu, Y., & Shimanouchi, S. (2006). Effective components of staff and organizational development for client outcomes by implementation of action plans in home care. *International Medical Journal, 13*(3), 175–183.

Schmaltz, S. P., Williams, S. C., Chassin, M. R., Loeb, J. M., & Watcher, R. M. (2011). Hospital performance trends on national quality measures and the association with Joint Commission accreditation. *Journal of Hospital Medicine, 6*(8), 454–461. http://dx.doi:10.1002/jhm.905.

Sigma Theta Tau International Research and Scholarship Advisory Committee (2008). Sigma Theta Tau International position statement on evidence-based practice, February 2007 summary. *Worldviews on Evidence-Based Nursing, 5*(2), 57–59.

Slessor, S. R., Crandall, J. B., & Nielsen, G. A. (2008). Case study: Getting boards on board at Allen Memorial Hospital, Iowa Health System. *Joint Commission Journal on Quality and Patient Safety, 34*(4), 221–227.

Sohn, W., Ismail, A., & Tellez, M. (2004). Efficacy of educational interventions targeting primary care providers practice behaviors: An overview of published systematic reviews. *Journal of Public Health Dentistry, 64*(3), 164–172.

Soumerai, S. B., & Avorn, J. (1990). Principles of educational outreach ("academic detailing") to improve clinical decision making. *Journal of the American Medical Association, 263*(4), 549–556.

Spyridonidis, D., & Calnan, M. (2011). Opening the black box: A study of the process of NICE guidelines implementation. *Health Policy, 102*(2–3), 117–125.

Stenger, K., Montgomery, L. A., & Briesemeister, E. (2007). Creating a culture of change through implementation of a safe patient handling program. *Critical Care Nursing Clinics of North America, 19*(2), 213–222.

Stetler, C. (2001). Updating the Stetler Model of Research Utilization to facilitate evidence-based practice. *Nursing Outlook, 49*(6), 272–279.

Stetler, C. B., Ritchie, J. A., Rycroft-Malone, J., Schultz, A. A., & Charns, M. P. (2009). Institutionalizing evidence-based practice: An organizational case study using a model of strategic change. *Implementation Science, 4*, 78. http://dx.doi:10.1186/1748-5908-4-78.

Stevens, K. R. (2004). *ACE Star Model of EBP: Knowledge transformation*. Academic Center for Evidence-Based Practice. The University of Texas Health Science Center at San Antonio.

The Joint Commission (2011). *National patient safety goals*. Retrieved January 16, 2011, from www.jointcommission.org/patientsafety/Nationalpatientsafetygoals/.

Thiel, L., & Ghosh, Y. (2008). Determining registered nurses' readiness for evidence-based practice. *Worldviews on Evidence-Based Nursing, 5*(4), 182–192.

Titler, M. (2004). Methods in translation science. *Worldviews on Evidence-Based Nursing, 1*(March), 38–48.

Titler, M. (2007). *Moving nursing's agenda forward into the 21st century: Sigma Theta Tau International's position on translation research*. Paper presented at the Sigma Theta Tau, International 39th Biennial Convention. Baltimore, MD.

Titler, M. G. (2008). The evidence for evidence-based practice implementation. In R. Hughes (Ed.), *Patient safety & quality: An evidence-based handbook for nurses*. Rockville, MD: Agency for Healthcare Research and Quality. www.ahrq.gov/qual/nurseshdbk/.

Titler, M. G. (2010). Translation science and context. *Research and Theory for Nursing Practice, 24*(1), 35–55.

Titler, M., Cullen, L., & Ardery, G. (2002). Evidence-based practice: An administrative perspective. *Reflect Nurs Leadersh, 2002; 28*(2):26–27, 46, 45.

Titler, M., & Everett, L. Q. (2001). Translating research into practice: Considerations for critical care investigators. *Critical Care Nursing Clinics of North America, 13*(4), 587–604.

Titler, M. G., & Moore, J. (2010). Evidence-based practice: A civilian perspective. *Nursing Research, 59*(Suppl. 1), S2–S6. http://dx.doi:10.1097/NNR.0b013e3181c94ec000006199-201001001-00002 [pii].

Titler, M., Kleiber, C., Steelman, V., Rakel, B. A., Budreau, G., Everett, L. Q., et al. (2001). The Iowa model of evidence-based practice to promote quality care. *Critical Care Nursing Clinics of North America, 13*, 497–509.

Turner, M., Burns, S. M., Chaney, C., Conaway, M., Dame, M., Parks, C., et al. (2008). Measuring blood pressure accurately in an ambulatory cardiology clinic setting: Do patient position and timing really matter? *Medsurg Nursing, 17*(2), 93–98.

Van Den Bos, J., Rustagi, K., Gray, T., Halford, M., Ziemkiewicz, E., & Shreve, J. (2011). The $17.1 billion problem: The annual cost of measurable medical errors. *Health Affairs, 30*(4), 596–603.

van Klei, W. A., Hoff, R. B., van Aarnhem, E. E., Simmermacher, R. K., Regli, L. P., Kappen, T. H., et al. (2012). Effects of the introduction of the WHO "Surgical Safety Checklist" on in-hospital mortality: A cohort study. *Annals of Surgery, 255*(1), 44–49.

VanDeusen, L. C., Engle, R. L., Holmes, S. K., Parker, V. A., Petzel, R. A., Nealon, S. M., et al. (2010). Strengthening organizations to implement evidence-based clinical practices. *Health Care Management Review, 35*(3), 235–245.

Vaughn, T. E., McCoy, K. D., BootsMiller, B. J., Woolson, R. F., Sorofman, B., Tripp-Reimer, T., et al. (2002). Organizational predictors of adherence to ambulatory care screening guidelines. *Medical Care, 40*(12), 1172–1185.

Wallin, L., Ewald, U., Wikblad, K., Scott-Findlay, S., & Arnetz, B. B. (2006). Understanding work context factors: A short-cut to evidence-based practice? *Worldviews on Evidence-Based Nursing, 3*(4), 153–164.

Wallin, L., Rudberg, A., & Gunningberg, L. (2005). Staff experiences in implementing guidelines for Kangaroo Mother Care—A qualitative study. *International Journal of Nursing Studies, 42*, 61–73.

Weeks, S., Moore, P., & Allender, M. (2011). A regional evidence-based practice fellowship: Collaborating competitors. *Journal of Nursing Administration, 41*(1), 10–14. http://dx.doi:10.1097/NNA.0b013e318200282c.

Weiss, C. H., Moazed, F., McEvoy, C. A., Singer, B. D., Szleifer, I., Amaral, L. A., et al. (2011). Prompting physicians to address a daily checklist and process of care and clinical outcomes: A single-site study. *American Journal of Respiratory and Critical Care Medicine, 184*(6), 680–686.

Wells, N., Free, M., & Adams, R. (2007). Nursing research internship: Enhancing evidence-based practice among staff nurses. *Journal of Nursing Administration, 37*(3), 135–143.

Williams, S. C., Schmaltz, S. P., Morton, D. J., Koss, R. G., & Loeb, J. M. (2005). Quality of care in U.S. hospitals and reflects by standardized measures, 2002–2004. *New England Journal of Medicine, 353*(3), 255–264.

Woolf, S. H., & Atkins, D. (2001). The evolving role of prevention in health care. Contributions of the U.S. Preventive Services Task Force. *American Journal of Preventive Medicine, 20*(3, Suppl. 1), 13–20.

World Health Organization. (2007). *Practical guidance for scaling up health service innovations.* Switzerland: World Health Organization.

Zdrojewski, T., Kozicka-Kaol, K., Chwojnicki, K., Szpakowski, P., Konarski, R., & Wyrzykowski, B. (2005). Arm circumference in adults in Poland as an important factor influencing the accuracy of blood pressure readings. *Blood Pressure Monitoring, 10*(2), 73–77.

Zhan, C., Friedman, B., Mosso, A., & Pronovost, P. (2006). Medicare payment for selected adverse events: Building the business case for investing in patient safety. *Health Affair, 25*(5), 1386–1393.

Zohar, D., Livine, Y., Tenne-Gazit, O., Admi, H., & Donchin, Y. (2007). Healthcare climate: A framework for measuring and improving patient safety. *Critical Care Medicine, 35*(5), 1312–1317.

Chapter 17

Agency for Healthcare Research and Quality (AHRQ). (n.d.). *TeamSTEPPS®: National implementation.* Retrieved March 31, 2012, from http://teamstepps.ahrq.gov/.

American Nurses Association (ANA). (2012b). *Guidelines for data collection on the American Nurses Association's national quality forum endorsed measures: Nursing care hours per patient day, skill mix, falls, falls with injury.* Retrieved March 30, 2012, from http://www.odh.ohio.gov/~/media/ODH/ASSETS/Files/dspc/health20care20service/nursestaffingmaterials8-2-2010.ashx.

American Nurses Association (ANA). (2010b). *Position statement: Just culture.* Retrieved March 20, 2012, from http://nursingworld.org/psjustculture.

American Nurses Credentialing Center (ANCC). (2012). *ANCC Magnet Recognition Program®.* Retrieved March 24, 2012, from www.nursecredentialing.org/Magnet.aspx.

American Society for Quality (ASQ). (2007). *Quality glossary - C.* Retrieved March 4, 2012, from www.asq.org/glossary/c.html.

American Society for Quality (ASQ). (2013). *Quality glossary-t.* Retrieved from http://asq.org/glossary/t.html.

American Society for Healthcare Risk Management. (2006). *Enterprise risk management. Part one: Defining the concept, recognizing its value.* Retrieved March 21, 2012, from www.ashrm.org/ashrm/education/development/monographs/ERMmonograph.pdf.

Berwick, D. M., Godfrey, A. B., & Roessner, J. (1990). *Curing health care: New strategies for quality improvement.* San Francisco: Jossey-Bass.

Berwick, D. M., Nolan, T. W., & Whittington, J. (2008). The triple aim: Care, health and cost. *Health Affairs, 27*(3), 759–769.

California Patient Safety Action Coalition (CAPSAC). (2008). *What is CAPSAC.* Retrieved March 22, 2012, from www.capsac.org/.

Carroll, R. (2003). *Risk management handbook for health care organizations* (4th ed.). San Francisco: Jossey-Bass.

Center for Advancing Health. (2010). *A new definition of patient engagement: What is engagement and why is it important?* Washington, DC: Author.

Centers for Medicare & Medicaid Services. (2012). *Hospital quality initiatives: Overview.* Retrieved March 21, 2012, from https://www.cms.gov/HospitalQualityInits/.

Chassin, M. R. (1997). Assessing strategies for quality improvement. *Health Affairs, 16*(3), 151–161.

Cibulka, N., Fischer, H., & Fischer, A. (2012). Improving communication with low-income women using today's technology. *OJIN: The Online Journal of Issues in Nursing, 17*(2). Retrieved July 16, 2012, from http://nursingworld.org/MainMenuCategories/ANAMarketplace/ANAPeriodicals/OJIN/TableofContents/Vol-17-2012/No2-May-2012/Articles-Previous-Topics/Communication-With-Low-Income-Women-and-Technology.html.

Committee on Enhancing Federal Healthcare Quality Programs (CEFHQP) (2002). In J. M. Corrigan, J. Eden, & B. M. Smith (Eds.). *Leadership by example: Coordinating government roles in improving health care quality*. Washington, DC: The National Academies Press.

Corrigan, J. M., Eden, J., & Smith, B. M. (Eds.). (2002). *Leadership by Example: Coordinating Government Roles in Improving Health Care Quality*. Washington, DC: National Academies Press.

Deming, W. E. (2000a). *The new economics for industry, government, education*. Cambridge, MA: MIT Center for Advanced Engineering Studies.

Deming, W. E. (2000b). *Out of the crisis*. Cambridge, MA: MIT Center for Advanced Engineering Studies.

Donabedian, A. (1980). *Explorations in quality assessment and monitoring: The definition of quality and approaches to its assessment* (Vol. 1). Ann Arbor, MI: Health Administration Press.

Donaldson, M. S., & Mohr, J. J. (Eds.). (2000a). *Exploring innovation and quality improvement in health care micro-systems*. Washington, DC: The National Academies Press.

Foster, D. A., & Chenoweth, J. (2011). *Comparison of Baldrige award applicants and recipients with peer hospitals on a national balanced scorecard*. Retrieved March 27, 2012, from www.nist.gov/baldrige/upload/baldrige-hospital-research-paper.pdf.

Fowler, M. D. M. (2008). *Guide to the code of ethics for nurses: Interpretation and application*. Silver Spring, MD: American Nurses Association.

Frost, R. (2005). *New, improved ISO 9000 guidelines for health sector*. Retrieved March 21, 2012, from http://www.iso.org/iso/home/news_index/news_archive/news.htm?refid=Ref977.

Glascow, R. (2002, September). *Technology and chronic care*. Paper presented at the Congress on Improving Chronic Care: Innovations in Research and Practice. Seattle, WA.

Harmon, F. G. (1997). Future present. In F. Hesselbein, M. Goldsmith, & R. Beckhard (Eds.), *The organization of the future* (pp. 239–247). San Francisco: Jossey-Bass.

Harry, M., & Schroeder, R. (2000). *Six Sigma: The breakthrough strategy revolutionizing the world's top corporations*. New York: Currency/Doubleday.

Hesselbein, F., & Johnston, R. (2002). *A leader-to-leader guide: On high-performance organizations*. San Francisco: Jossey Bass.

His Holiness the Dalai Lama, & Cutler, H. C. (1998). *The art of happiness*. New York: Riverhead Books.

Hughes, R. G. (Ed.). (2008). *Patient safety and quality: An evidence-based handbook for nurses*. (AHRQ Publication No. 08-0043). Retrieved March 30, 2012, from www.ahrq.gov/qual/nurseshdbk/.

Hussey, P. S., Mattke, S., Morse, L., & Ridgely, M. S. (2007). *Evaluation of the use of AHRQ and other quality indicators: Final contract report*. (Contract No. WR-426 HS to RAND Health) (AHRQ Publication No. 08-M012-EF) Rockville, MD: Agency for Healthcare Research and Quality.

Hyde, P. S., Falls, K., Morris, J. A., & Schoenwald, S. A. (2003). *Turning knowledge into practice: A manual for behavioral health administrators and practitioners about understanding and implementing evidence-based practices*. Boston: The Technical Assistance Collaborative.

Institute for Healthcare Improvement (IHI). (2004). *About IHI*. Retrieved March 31, 2012, from www.ihi.org/about/Pages/default.aspx.

Institute for Healthcare Improvement (IHI). (2012). *Overview: What is the open school?* Retrieved March 30, 2012, from www.ihi.org/offerings/IHIOpenSchool/overview/Pages/default.aspx.

Institute of Medicine (IOM), Committee on Enhancing Federal Health Care Quality Programs. (2002). *Enhancing federal health care quality programs: Activity description*. Retrieved March 21, 2012, from http://iom.edu/Activities/Quality/FedHCQuality.aspx.

Institute of Medicine (IOM) Committee on the National Quality Report on Health Care Delivery. (2001). *Envisioning the national health care quality report*. Washington, DC: National Academies Press.

Institute of Medicine (IOM), Committee on Quality of Health Care in America (CQHCA). (2001). *Crossing the quality chasm: A new health system for the 21st century*. Washington, DC: National Academies Press.

Institute of Medicine (IOM), Committee on the Robert Wood Johnson Foundation Initiative on the Future of Nursing. (2011). *The future of nursing: Leading change, advancing health*. Washington, DC: National Academies Press.

International Organization for Standardization (ISO). (2011). *Standards*. Retrieved May 21, 2013, from http://www.iso.org/iso/home/standards.htm.

Jones, D., & Womack, J. (2003). *Lean thinking: Banish waste and create wealth in your corporation, revised and updated*. New York: Free Press.

Juran, J. M. (1989). *Juran on leadership for quality: An executive handbook*. New York: The Free Press.

Juran Institute (2009). *Product store*. Retrieved March 31, 2012, from http://www.juran.com/product-store/.

Katz, J. M., & Green, E. (1997). *Managing quality: A guide to system-wide performance management in healthcare* (2nd ed.). St. Louis: Mosby.

Kelly, L. A., McHugh, M. D., & Aiken, L. H. (2011b). Nurse outcomes in Magnet and non-Magnet hospitals. *Journal of Nursing Administration, 41*(10), 428–433. http://dx.doi:10.1097/NNA.0b013e31822eddbc.

Kohn, L. T., Corrigan, J. M., & Donaldson, M. S. (Eds.). (2000d). *To err is human: Building a safer health care system.* Washington, DC: National Academies Press.

Lohr, K. (Ed.). (1990). *Medicare: A strategy for quality assurance* (Vol. 2). Washington, DC: National Academies Press.

Maas, M. L., & Kerr, P. (1999). Risk adjustment in nursing effectiveness research. *Outcomes Management for Nursing Practice, 3*(2), 50–52.

Marcus, L. J., Dorn, B. C., Kritek, P. B., Miller, V. G., & Wyatt, J. B. (1995). *Renegotiating health care: Resolving conflict to build collaboration.* San Francisco: Jossey Bass.

Marx, D. (2007). *Just culture community.* Retrieved March 30, 2012, from www.justculture.org/.

Mayo Foundation for Medical Research and Education. (2012). *Mayo Clinic mission and values.* Retrieved March 30, 2012, from www.mayoclinic.org/about/missionvalues.html.

National Institute of Standards and Technology. (2007). *Presidential award for excellence honors five U.S. organizations: Two nonprofits recognized in first year of category.* Retrieved March 21, 2012, from www.nist.gov/public_affairs/releases/2007baldrigerecipients.cfm.

National Quality Forum (NQF). (2004). *National voluntary consensus standards for nursing-sensitive care: An initial performance measure set.* Washington, DC: National Quality Forum.

National Quality Forum (NQF). (2011). *Measure evaluation criteria.* Retrieved July 16, 2012, from www.qualityforum.org/docs/measure_evaluation_criteria.aspx.

National Quality Forum. (2012). *Nursing-sensitive care: Initial measures.* Retrieved July 16, 2012, from www.qualityforum.org/Projects/n-r/Nursing-Sensitive_Care_Initial_Measures/Nursing_Sensitive_Care__Initial_Measures.aspx.

Nightingale, D. (2009, October). *A lean enterprise systems approach to healthcare transformation.* MIT Conference on Systems Thinking for Contemporary Challenges, Massachusetts Institute of Technology. Retrieved March 28, 2012, from http://sdm.mit.edu/conf09/presentations/deborah_nightingale.pdf.

Nursing Alliance for Quality Care (NAQC). (2010). *Strategic policy and advocacy roadmap.* Retrieved March 21, 2012, from www.gwumc.edu/healthsci/departments/nursing/naqc/documents/Roadmap.pdf.

Omenn, G. (2002). *Public briefing: Opening statement—Leadership by example: Coordinating government roles in improving health care quality.* Washington, DC: Institute of Medicine.

O'Neil, E. H., The Pew Health Professions Commission (PHPC). (1998). *Recreating health professional practice for a new century: The fourth report of the Pew Health Professions Commission.* San Francisco: PHPC.

Palmer, S., & Torgerson, D. J. (1999). Definition of efficiency. *British Medical Journal, 318,* 1136.

Pelletier, L. R. (1998). Guest editorial: Standardization. *Journal of Nursing Care Quality, 13*(1), vii.

Pelletier, L. R. (1999a). On strategic planning [Editorial]. *Journal for Healthcare Quality, 21*(3), 2, 17.

Pelletier, L. R. (1999b). On values and achievements [Editorial]. *Journal for Healthcare Quality, 21*(6), 2, 10–11.

Pelletier, L. R. (2000). On error-free health care: Mission possible! [Editorial]. *Journal for Healthcare Quality, 22*(3), 2, 9.

Pelletier, L. R., & Hoffman, J. A. (2002). A framework for selecting performance measures for opioid treatment programs. *Journal for Healthcare Quality, 24*(3), 24–35.

Plsek, P., & Omnias, A. (1989). *Juran Institute quality improvement tools: Problem solving/glossary.* Wilton, CT: Juran Institute.

PricewaterhouseCoopers' Health Economics Institute. (2008). *The price of excess: Identifying waste in healthcare spending.* Retrieved March 28, 2012, from www.pwc.com/extweb/pwcpublications.nsf/docid/73272CB152086C6385257425006BA2FC.

Quality Interagency Coordination (QuIC). Task Force. (2000). *Doing what counts for patient safety: Federal actions to reduce medical errors and their impact.* Retrieved March 21, 2012, from http://archive.ahrq.gov/quic/report/mederr2.htm.

Quality & Safety Education for Nurses (QSEN). (2012). *About QSEN.* Retrieved March 30, 2012, from www.qsen.org/.

Sackett, D. L., Rosenberg, W. M. C., Gray, J. A. M., Haynes, R. B., & Richardson, W. S. (1996). Evidence-based medicine: What it is and what it isn't. *British Medical Journal, 312*(7023), 71.

Sharp HealthCare. (2012). *Mission, vision, and values.* Retrieved March 21, 2012, from www.sharp.com/choose-sharp/mission-vision-values.cfm.

Shojania, K. G., Duncan, B. W., McDonald, K. M., & Wachter, R. M. (Eds.). (2001). *Making health care safer:*

A critical analysis of patient safety practices. (Evidence Report/Technology Assessment No. 43, AHRQ Publication No. 01-E058). Retrieved July 17, 2012, from http://somaaccess.net/ptsafety.pdf.

Shojania, K. G., McDonald, K. M., Wachter, R. M., & Owens, D. K. (2004). *Closing the quality gap: A critical analysis of quality improvement strategies. Vol. 1: Series overview and methodology.* (Technical Review 9, AHRQ Publication No. 04–0051–1). Rockville, MD: Agency for Healthcare Research and Quality.

Sower, V. E., Duffy, J. A., & Kohers, G. (2008). *Benchmarking for hospitals: Achieving best-in-class performance without having to reinvent the wheel.* Milwaukee, WI: American Society for Quality.

The Commonwealth Fund. (2004). *First report and recommendations of The Commonwealth Fund's International Working Group on Quality Indicators.* Retrieved March 21, 2012, from www.commonwealthfund.org/Publications/Fund-Reports/2004/Jun/First-Report-and-Recommendations-of-the-Commonwealth-Funds-International-Working-Group-on-Quality-In.aspx.

The Commonwealth Fund Commission on a High Performance Health System. (2009). *The path to a high performance U.S. health system: A 2020 vision and the policies to pave the way.* Retrieved March 23, 2012, from www.commonwealthfund.org/Publications/Fund-Reports/2009/Feb/The-Path-to-a-High-Performance-US-Health-System.aspx?page=all.

The Joint Commission (TJC). (2012b). *Core measure sets.* Retrieved March 21, 2012, from www.jointcommission.org/core_measure_sets.aspx.

The Joint Commission (TJC). (2012c). *Specifications manual for national hospital inpatient quality measures.* Retrieved March 21, 2012, from www.jointcommission.org/specifications_manual_for_national_hospital_inpatient_quality_measures.aspx.

The Joint Commission (TJC). (2012d). *Sentinel event.* Retrieved March 21, 2012, from www.jointcommission.org/sentinel_event.aspx.

The Joint Commission (TJC). (2012e). *E-dition: Hospital: Accreditation requirements: Leadership.* Retrieved March 21, 2012, from https://e-dition.jcrinc.com/.

The Joint Commission (TJC). (2011a). *Specifications manual for Joint Commission national quality measures (v2012A): Appendix C: General glossary of terms.* Retrieved March 21, 2012, from https://manual.jointcommission.org/releases/TJC2013A/AppendixCTJC.html.

The Joint Commission (TJC). (2011b). *Sentinel event policies and procedures (hospitals).* Retrieved March 21, 2012, from www.jointcommission.org/assets/1/6/2011_CAMH_SE.pdf.

The Joint Commission (TJC). (2011c). *Facts about ORYX vendors performance measurement systems.* Retrieved March 21, 2012, from http://www.jointcommission.org/facts_about_oryx_performance_measurement_systems/.

U.S. Department of Health and Human Services. (2010). *Official Hospital Compare data.* Retrieved March 21, 2012, from https://data.medicare.gov/data/hospital-compare.

U.S. Department of Veterans Affairs. (2004). *The VA National Center for Patient Safety.* Retrieved March 21, 2012, from www.patientsafety.gov/.

Visiting Nursing Service of New York (VNSNY). (2012). *Vision and mission.* Retrieved March 30, 2012, from www.vnsny.org/about-us/vision-mission/.

Ward, B. (2004). *The five key facets of high performance leadership.* Edmonton, Alberta, Canada: Affinity Consulting. Retrieved March 21, 2012, from www.affinitymc.com/what-makes-a-good-leader/.

Chapter 18

Agency for Healthcare Research and Quality (AHRQ). (n.d.). *Desirable attributes of a quality measure.* Retrieved July 17, 2012, from www.qualitymeasures.ahrq.gov/tutorial/attributes.aspx.

Albanese, M. P., Evans, D. A., Schantz, C. A., Bowen, M., Moffa, J. S., Piesieski, P., et al. (2010). Engaging clinical nurses in quality and performance improvement activities. *Nursing Administration Quarterly, 34*(3), 226–245.

American Nurses Association (ANA). (1996). *Nursing quality indicators: Definitions and implications.* Washington, DC: American Nurses Publishing.

Clancy, C. (2007). The performance of performance measurement. *Health Services Research, 42*(5), 1797–1801.

Clarke, S. P., & Donaldson, N. E. (2008). Nurse staffing and patient care quality and safety. In R. G. Hughes (Ed.), *Patient safety and quality: An evidence-based handbook for nurses.* (AHRQ Publication No. 08-0043). Rockville, MD: Agency for Healthcare Research and Quality. Retrieved July 17, 2012, from www.ahrq.gov/qual/nurseshdbk/.

Clarke, S. P., Raphael, C., & Disch, J. (2008). Challenges and directions for nursing in the pay-for-performance movement. *Policy, Politics and Nursing Practice, 9*(2), 127–134.

Donabedian, A. (1985). *The methods and findings of quality assessment and monitoring: An illustrated analysis.* (Vol. 3). Ann Arbor, MI: Health Administration Press.

Donabedian, A. (2005). Evaluating the quality of medical care. 1966. *Milbank Quarterly, 83*(4), 691–729.

Donaldson, N., & Shapiro, S. (2010). Impact of California mandated acute care hospital nurse staffing ratios: A literature synthesis. *Policy, Politics and Nursing Practice, 11*(3), 184–201.

Donaldson, N., Brown, D. S., Aydin, C. E., Bolton, M. L. B., & Rutledge, D. N. (2005). Leveraging nurse-related dashboard benchmarks to expedite performance improvement and document evidence. *Journal of Nursing Administration, 35*(4), 163–172.

Doran, D., Mildon, B., & Clarke, S. (2011). Towards a national report card in nursing: A knowledge synthesis. *Nursing Leadership, 24*(2), 38–57.

Ellwood, P. M. (1988). Shattuck lecture—Outcomes management: A technology of patient experience. *The New England Journal of Medicine, 318*(23), 1549–1556.

Epstein, A. M. (2009). Revisiting readmissions: Changing the incentives for shared accountability. *New England Journal of Medicine, 360*(14), 1457–1459.

Frith, K. H., Anderson, F., & Sewell, J. P. (2010a). Assessing and selecting data for a nursing services dashboard. *Journal of Nursing Administration, 40*(1), 10–16.

Gallagher, R. M., & Rowell, P. A. (2003). Claiming the future of nursing through nursing-sensitive quality indicators. *Nursing Administration Quarterly, 27*(4), 273–284.

Huber, D., & Oermann, M. (1998). The evolution of outcomes management. In D. L. Flarey & S. S. Blancett (Eds.), *Cardiovascular outcomes: Collaborative, path-based approaches* (pp. 3–12). Gaithersburg, MD: Aspen.

Iezzoni, L. I. (Ed.). (2003). *Risk adjustment for measuring health care outcomes* (3rd ed.). Chicago: Health Administration Press.

Jeffs, L., MacMillan, K., McKey, C., & Ferris, E. (2009). Nursing leaders' accountability to narrow the safety chasm: Insights and implications from the collective evidence base on health care safety. *Canadian Journal of Nursing Leadership, 22*(1), 73–85.

Jeffs, L., Merkley, J., McAllister, M., Richardson, S., & Eli, J. (2011). Using a nursing balanced scorecard approach to measure and optimize nursing performance. *Nursing Leadership, 24*(1), 47–58.

Jennings, B. M., Staggers, N., & Brosch, L. R. (1999). A classification scheme for outcome indicators. *Image— the Journal of Nursing Scholarship, 31*(4), 381–388.

Jha, A. K., Joynt, K. E., Orav, E. J., & Epstein, A. M. (2012). The long-term effect of premier pay for performance on patient outcomes. *New England Journal of Medicine, 366*(17), 1601–1615. http://dx.doi:10.1056/NEJMsa1112351.

Kane, R. L. (2006). Introduction: An outcomes approach. In R. L. Kane (Ed.), *Understanding health care outcomes research* (2nd ed.), (pp. 3–22). Boston: Jones & Bartlett.

Kane, R. L., Shamliyan, T., Mueller, C., Duval, S., & Wilt, T. (2007). *Nursing staffing and quality of patient care.* Evidence report/technology assessment No. 151. (Prepared by the Minnesota Evidence-based Practice Center under Contract No. 290–02–0009) (No. 07-E005). Rockville, MD: Agency for Healthcare Research and Quality.

Klassen, A., Miller, A., Anderson, N., Shen, J., Schiarti, V., & O'Donnell, M. (2010). Performance measurement and improvement frameworks in health, education and social services systems: A systematic review. *International Journal for Quality in Health Care, 22*(1), 44–69.

Kohlbrenner, J., Whitelaw, G., & Cannaday, D. (2011). Nurses critical to quality, safety, and now financial performance. *Journal of Nursing Administration, 41*(3), 122–128.

Lamb, G., & Donaldson, N. (2011). Performance measurement—A strategic imperative and a call to action. *Nursing Outlook, 59*(6), 336–338.

Loan, L. A., Patrician, P. A., & McCarthy, M. (2011). Participation in a national nursing outcomes database: Monitoring outcomes over time. *Nursing Administration Quarterly, 35*(1), 72–81.

McGillis-Hall, L. (2002). Report cards: Relevance for nursing and patient care safety. *International Nursing Review, 49*(3), 168–177.

Mitchell, P. H., Ferketich, S., & Jennings, B. M. (1998). Quality health outcomes model. American Academy of Nursing Expert Panel on Quality Health Care. *Image— The Journal of Nursing Scholarship, 30*(1), 43–46.

Naranjo-Gil, D. (2009). Strategic performance in hospitals: The use of the balanced scorecard by nurse managers. *Health Care Management Review, 34*(2), 161–170.

National Database of Nursing Quality Indicators (NDNQI) by the American Nurses Association. (n.d.). *FAQs.* Retrieved July 17, 2012, from http://www.nursingquality.org/FAQs.

National Quality Forum. (2004). *National voluntary consensus standards for nursing-sensitive care: An initial performance measure set—A consensus report (No. NQFCR-08–04).* Washington, DC: Author.

National Quality Forum. (2009). *Nursing-sensitive care: Measure maintenance.* Retrieved July 17, 2012, from www.qualityforum.org/Projects/n-r/Nursing-Sensitive_Care_Measure_Maintenance/Nursing_Sensitive_Care_-_Measure_Maintenance.aspx.

Naylor, M. (2012). Advancing high value transitional care. The central role of nursing and its leadership. *Nursing Administration Quarterly, 36*(2), 115–126.

Naylor, M. D. (2007). Advancing the science in the measurement of health care quality influenced by nurses. *Medical Care Research & Review, 64*(Suppl. 2), S144–S169.

Naylor, M. D., Aiken, L. H., Kurtzman, E. T., Olds, D. M., & Hirschman, K. B. (2011). The importance of transitional care in achieving health reform. *Health Affairs, 30*(4), 746–754.

Oermann, M. H., & Huber, D. (1997). New horizons. *Outcomes Management for Nursing Practice, 1*(1), 1–2.

Oermann, M. H., & Huber, D. (1999). Patient outcomes: A measure of nursing's value. *American Journal of Nursing, 99*(9), 40–47.

Park, E. J., & Huber, D. L. (2007). Balanced scorecards for performance management. *Journal of Nursing Administration, 37*(1), 14–20.

Patrician, P. A., Loan, L., McCarthy, M., Fridman, M., Donaldson, N., Bingham, M., et al. (2011). The association of shift-level nurse staffing with adverse patient events. *Journal of Nursing Administration, 41*(2), 64–70.

Peters, D. A. (1995). Outcomes: The mainstay of a framework for quality of care. *Journal of Nursing Care Quality, 10*(1), 61–69.

Smith, A. P. (2007). Nursing sensitive care measures: A platform for value and vision. *Nursing Economics, 25*(1), 43–46.

van Walraven, C., Bennett, C., Jennings, A., Austin, P. C., & Forster, A. J. (2011). Proportion of hospital readmissions deemed avoidable: A systematic review. *Canadian Medical Association Journal, 183*(7), E391–E402.

Zrelak, P. A., Utter, G. H., Sadeghi, B., Cuny, J., Baron, R., & Romano, P. S. (2012). Using the agency for healthcare research and quality patient safety indicators for targeting nursing quality improvement. *Journal of Nursing Care Quality, 27*(2), 99–108.

Chapter 19

American Nurses Credentialing Center (ANCC). (2008). *Magnet Recognition Program® manual: Recognizing nursing excellence.* Silver Spring, MD: nursesbooks.org. Retrieved from http://nursesbooks.org/Main-Menu/ Magnet/Magnet-Recognition-Program-Manual-- Recognizing-Nursing-Excellence-.aspx.

Benner, P., Sutphen, M., Leonard, V., & Day, L. (2010). *Educating nurses: A call for radical transformation.* San Francisco: Jossey Bass.

Collins, J. C., & Porràs, J. I. (2004). *Built to last: Successful habits of visionary companies.* New York: HarperCollins.

Collins, J. C., & Hansen, M. T. (2011). *Great by choice: Uncertainty, chaos, and luck: Why some thrive despite them all.* New York: HarperBusiness.

Conway-Morana, P. L. (2009). Nursing strategy: What's your plan? *Nursing Management, 40*(3), 25–29.

Coulter, M. (2009). *Strategic management in action* (5th ed.). Upper Saddle River, NJ: Prentice Hall.

Dess, G. G., Eisner, A., Lumpkin, G. T., & McNamara, G. (2011). *Strategic management: Creating competitive advantages* (6th ed.). New York: McGraw-Hill/Irwin.

Fine, L. (2011). *The SWOT analysis [Kindle edition].* Seattle: Amazon Digital Services.

Institute for Safe Medical Practices (ISMP). (2008). *ISMP issues recommendations on resolving conflicts when safety questions arise.* Huntingdon Valley, PA: Author. Retrieved from www.ismp.org/pressroom/ PR20080319.pdf.

Institute of Medicine. (2011c). *The future of nursing: Leading change, advancing health.* Washington, DC: National Academies Press. Retrieved from www.iom. edu/Reports/2010/The-Future-of-Nursing-Leading-Change-Advancing-Health.aspx.

Oermann, M. H. (2002). Developing a professional portfolio in nursing. *Orthopaedic Nursing, 21*(2), 73–78.

Pearce, J. A., & Robinson, R. (2012). *Strategic management* (13th ed.). New York: McGraw-Hill/Irwin.

Peters, T. J., & Waterman, R. H. (2004). *In search of excellence: Lessons from America's best-run companies.* New York: HarperBusiness.

Sare, M. V., & Ogilvie, L. (2009). *Strategic planning for nurses: Change management in health care.* Sudbury, MA: Jones & Bartlett.

Sigma Theta Tau International. (2011). *The power of ten: Nurse leaders address the profession's ten most pressing issues.* Indianapolis: Author.

Studer, Q. (2003). *Hardwiring excellence.* Gulf Breeze, FL: Fire Starter Publishing.

Chapter 20

Acree, C. M. (2006). The relationship between nurse leadership practices and hospital nursing retention. *Newborn and Infant Nursing Reviews, 6*(1), 34–40.

Aiken, L. H. (2008). Economics of Nursing. *Policy, Politics, & Nursing Practice, 9*(2), 73–79.

Aiken, L. H., Clarke, S. P., Sloane, D. M., Sochalski, J., & Silber, J. H. (2002). Hospital nurse staffing and patient mortality, nurse burnout, and job dissatisfaction. *Journal of the American Medical Association, 288*(16), 1987–1993.

American Association of Colleges of Nursing (AACN). (2007a). *2007 Survey on faculty vacancies.* Washington, DC: Author.

American Association of Colleges of Nursing (AACN). (2008). *Nursing shortage fact sheets.* Washington, DC: Author.

American Association of Colleges of Nursing (AACN). (2011b). *2011 Survey overview: Percentage change in enrollments in entry-level baccalaureate nursing programs: 1994–2011*. Washington, DC: Author. Retrieved October 6, 2012, from www.aacn.nche.edu/ Media-Relations/EnrollChanges.pdf.

American Association of Colleges of Nursing (AACN). (2011–2012d). *Enrollment and graduations in baccalaureate & graduate programs in nursing.* Washington, DC: Author.

American Association of Colleges of Nursing (AACN). (2012a). *New AACN data show an enrollment surge in baccalaureate and graduate programs amid calls for more highly educated nurses.* Washington, DC: Author. Retrieved October 6, 2012, from www.aacn.nche.edu/ news/articles/2012/enrollment-data.

American Association of Colleges of Nursing (AACN). (2012b). *AACN report on 2010–2011 salaries of instructional and administrative nursing faculty in baccalaureate and graduate programs in nursing.* Washington, DC: Author. Retrieved October 6, 2012, from www.aacn.nche.edu/media-relations/fact-sheets/ nursing-faculty-shortage.

American Health Care Association (AHCA). (2008). *Report of findings 2007 AHCA survey: Nursing staff vacancy and turnover in nursing facilities.* Retrieved October 6, 2012, from www.ahcancal.org/research_ data/staffing/Documents/Vacancy_Turnover_ Survey2007.pdf.

American Hospital Association (AHA), Commission on Workforce for Hospitals and Health Systems. (2002). *In our hands: How hospital leaders can build a thriving workforce.* (AHA Product No. 210101). Chicago: Author.

American Nurses Association (ANA). (2002). *Nursing's agenda for the future: A call to the nation.* Silver Spring, MD: Author.

American Nurses Association (ANA). (2011). *Fact sheet: Registered nurses in the U.S. Nursing by the numbers.* Silver Spring, MD: Author.

American Organization of Nurse Executives (AONE). (2002). *Acute care hospital survey of RN vacancy and turnover rates in 2000.* Chicago: Author.

American Organization of Nurse Executives. (2010). *Guiding principles for the newly licensed nurse's transition into practice.* Retrieved from October 6, 2012, www.aone.org/resources/PDFs/AONE_GP_Newly_ Licensed_Nurses.pdf.

Apker, J., Zabava Ford, W., & Fox, D. (2003). Predicting nurses' organizational and professional identification: The effect of nursing roles, professional autonomy, and supportive communication. *Nursing Economic$, 21*(5), 226–233.

Atencio, B. L., Cohen, J., & Gorenberg, B. (2003). Nurse retention: Is it worth it? *Nurs Econ. 21*(6):262–268, 299, 259.

Auerbach, D. I., Buerhaus, P. I., & Staiger, D. O. (2007). Better late than never: Workforce supply implications of later entry into nursing. *Health Affairs, 26*(1), 178–185.

Auerbach, D. I., Buerhaus, P. I., & Staiger, D. O. (2011c). Registered nurse supply grows faster than projected amid surge in new entrants ages 23–26. *Health Affairs, 30*(12), 2286–2292.

Bass, B. (1998). *Transformational leadership: Industrial, military, and educational impact.* Mahwah, NJ: Lawrence Erlbaum Associates.

Blythe, J., & Baumann, A. (2009). Internationally educated nurses: Profiling workforce diversity. *International Nursing Review, 56*, 191–197.

Buerhaus, P. I. (2008a). Current and future state of the US nursing workforce. *Journal of the American Medical Association, 300*(20), 2422–2424.

Buerhaus, P. I., Auerbach, D. I., & Staiger, D. O. (2009a). The recent surge in nurse employment: Causes and implications. *Health Affairs, 28*(4), w657–w668.

Buerhaus, P. I., DesRoches, C., Donelan, K., & Hess, R. (2009b). Still making progress to improve the hospital workplace environment? Results from the 2008 national survey of registered nurses. *Nursing Economic$, 27*(5), 289–301.

Buerhaus, P. I., Donelan, K., Ulrich, B. T., Norman, L., & Dittus, R. (2005c). Is the shortage of hospital registered nurses getting better or worse? Findings from two recent national surveys of RNs. *Nursing Economic$, 2*(2), 61–71, 96.

Buerhaus, P. I., Staiger, D., & Auerbach, D. (2000). Implications of an aging registered nurse workforce. *Journal of the American Medical Association, 283*(22), 2948–2954.

Buerhaus, P. I., Staiger, D., & Auerbach, D. (2009c). *The future of the nursing workforce in the United States: Data, trends and implications.* Burlington, MA: Jones & Bartlett Learning.

Bureau of Health Professions (BHPr). (2002). *Projected supply, demand, and shortages of Registered Nurses: 2000–2020.* Rockville, MD: U.S. Department of Health and Human Services, Bureau of Health Professions, Health Resources and Services Administration, National Center for Health Workforce Analysis.

Bureau of Health Professions (BHPr). (2004). *What is behind the Health Resources and Services Administration's projected supply, demand, and shortage of registered nurses?* Rockville, MD: U.S. Department of Health and Human Services, Bureau of Health Professions, Health Resources and Services Administration.

Bureau of Health Professions (BHPr). (2006). *The registered nurse population: Findings from the March 2004 National Sample Survey of Registered Nurses.* Rockville, MD: U.S. Department of Health and Human Services, Bureau of Health Professions, Health Resources and Services Administration. Retrieved October 5, 2012, from http://bhpr.hrsa.gov/healthworkforce/rnsurveys/rnsurvey2004.pdf.

Bureau of Health Professions (BHPr). (2010b). *The registered nurse population: Findings from the 2008 National Sample Survey of Registered Nurses.* Rockville, MD: U.S. Department of Health and Human Services, Bureau of Health Professions, Health Resources and Services Administration. Retrieved October 5, 2012, from http://bhpr.hrsa.gov/healthworkforce/allreports.html and http://bhpr.hrsa.gov/healthworkforce/rnsurveys/rnsurveyfinal.pdf.

Bureau of Labor Statistics (BLS). (2007). Employment outlook: 2006–16. Occupational employment projections into 2016. In *Monthly Labor Review.* Washington, DC: U.S. Bureau of Labor Statistics. Retrieved October 5, 2012, from www.bls.gov/opub/mlr/2007/11/art5full.pdf.

Carlson, S. M., Cowart, M. E., & Speaker, D. L. (1992). Perspectives of nursing personnel in the 1980s. In M. E. Cowart & W. J. Serow (Eds.), *Nurses in the workplace* (pp. 1–27). Newbury Park, CA: Sage.

Curran, C. R. (2003). Nurse recruitment: A waste of postage, paper, and people. *Nursing Economic$, 21*(1), 5–32.

Daniel, P., Chamberlain, A., & Gordon, F. (2000). Expectations and experiences of newly recruited Filipino nurses. *British Journal of Nursing, 10*(4), 256–265.

Davidhizar, R. (2005). Joining the ranks: Nurses as role models. *Caring: National Association for Home Care Magazine, 24*(1), 50–51.

Donelan, K., Buerhaus, P. I., DesRoches, C., & Burke, S. P. (2010). Health policy thoughtleaders' views of the health workforce in an era of health reform. *Nursing Outlook, 58*(4), 175–180. http://dx.doi:10.1016/j.outlook.2010.06.003.

Duchscher, J. B. (2009). Transition shock: The initial stage of role adaptation for newly graduated registered nurses. *Journal of Advanced Nursing, 65,* 1103–1113.

Duffield, C., Roche, M., O'Brien-Pallas, L., Diers, D., Aisbett, C., King, M., et al. (2007). *Glueing it together: Nurses, their work environment and patient safety.* Australia: University of Technology Sydney, Centre for Health Services Management.

Dumpel, H. (2005). Contemporary issues facing international nurses: Adopting a CAN/NNOC code of practice for international nursing recruitment. *California Nurse,* November, 18–22.

Erickson, J. I., Holm, L. J., & Chelminiak, L. (2004). Keeping the nursing shortage from becoming a nursing crisis. *Journal of Nursing Administration, 34*(2), 83–87.

Grando, V. T. (1998). Making do with fewer nurses in the United States, 1945–1965. *Image, 30*(2), 147–149.

Halfer, D. (2007). A magnetic strategy for new graduate nurses. *Nursing Economic$, 25*(1), 6–11.

Hall, L. M., Lalonde, M., Dales, L., Peterson, J., & Cripps, L. (2011). Strategies for retaining midcareer nurses. *Journal of Nursing Administration, 41*(12), 531–537.

Hart, S. M. (2006). Generational diversity: Impact on recruitment and retention of registered nurses. *Journal of Nursing Administration, 36*(1), 10–12.

Hayhurst, A., Saylor, C., & Stuenkel, D. (2005). Work environmental factors and retention of nurses. *Journal of Nursing Care Quality, 20*(3), 283–288.

Henriksen, C., Page, N. E., Williams, R. I. I., & Worral, P. S. (2003). Responding to nursing's agenda for the future: Where do we stand on recruitment and retention? *Nursing Leadership Forum, 8*(2), 78–84.

Hunt, S. T. (2009). *Nursing turnover; Costs, causes, & solutions.* SuccessFactors, Inc. Retrieved October 6, 2012, from www.uexcel.com/resources/articles/NursingTurnover.pdf.

Institute of Medicine (IOM). (2001c). *Crossing the quality chasm: A new health care system for the 21st century.* Washington, DC: National Academies Press.

Institute of Medicine (IOM). (2011d). *The future of nursing: Leading change, advancing health.* Retrieved October 1, 2012, from www.iom.edu/Reports/2010/The-Future-of-Nursing-Leading-Change-Advancing-Health.aspx/.

International Council of Nurses (ICN). (2007a). *Nurse retention and migration.* Geneva: Author. Retrieved October 5, 2012, from www.icn.ch/images/stories/documents/publications/position_statements/C06_Nurse_Retention_Migration.pdf.

International Council of Nurses (ICN). (2007b). *Ethical nurse recruitment: Position statement.* Geneva: Author. Retrieved October 5, 2012, from www.icn.ch/images/stories/documents/publications/position_statements/C03_Ethical_Nurse_Recruitment.pdf.

Jenkins, J., & Jarrett-Pulliam, C. (2012). A comparative of Magnet organizations and accountable care organizations. *JONA's Healthcare Law, Ethics, and Regulation, 14*(2), 55–63.

Johnson & Johnson (J&J). (2012). *The campaign for nursing's future.* Retrieved October 6, 2012, from www.discovernursing.com/.

Jones, C. B. (2004a). The costs of nurse turnover. Part 1. An economic perspective. *Journal of Nursing Administration, 34*(12), 562–570.

Jones, C. B. (2004b). The costs of nurse turnover. Part 2. Application of the nursing turnover cost calculation methodology. *Journal of Nursing Administration, 35*(1), 41–49.

Jose, M. M. (2011). Lived experiences of internationally educated nurses in hospitals in the United States of America. *International Nursing Review, 58*, 123–129.

Juraschek, S. P., Zhang, X., Ranganathan, V., & Lin, V. W. (2012). United States registered nurse workforce report card and shortage forecast. *American Journal of Medical Quality, 27*(3), 241–249.

Kane, R., Shamliyan, T., Mueller, C., Duval, S., & Wilt, T. (2007e). *Nurse staffing and quality of patient care.* Report No. 151 prepared for U.S. Department of Health and Human Services, Agency for Healthcare Research and Quality. Retrieved October 5, 2012, from www.ncbi.nlm.nih.gov/books/NBK38315/.

Kawi, J., & Xu, Y. (2009). Facilitators and barriers to adjustment of international nurse: An integrative review. *International Nursing Review, 56*, 174–183.

King, M. G. (1989). Nursing shortage, circa 1915. *Image, 21*(3), 124–127.

Kleinman, C. S. (2004b). Leadership: A key strategy in staff nurse retention. *The Journal of Continuing Education in Nursing, 35*(3), 128–132.

Kovner, C. T., Brewer, C., Fairchild, S., Poornima, S., Kim, H., & Djukic, M. (2007). Newly licensed RNs' characteristics, work attitudes, and intentions to work. *American Journal of Nursing, 10*(9), 58–70.

Kramer, M., & Hafner, L. (1989b). Shared values: Impact on staff nurse job satisfaction and perceived productivity. *Nursing Research, 38*(3), 172–177.

Kuhar, P. A., Miller, D., Spear, B. T., Ulreich, S. M., & Mion, L. C. (2004). The meaningful retention strategy inventory: A targeted approach to implementing retention strategies. *Journal of Nursing Administration, 34*(1), 10–18.

Laschinger, H. K., Leiter, M., Day, A., & Gilin, D. (2009). Workplace empowerment, incivility, and burnout: Impact on staff nurse recruitment and retention outcomes. *Journal of Nursing Management, 17*, 302–311. http://dx.doi:10.1111/j.1365-2834.2009.00999.x.

Lee, D. (2008). *Successful onboarding: How to get your new employees started off right.* Retrieved October 6, 2012, from http://humannatureatwork.com/SuccessfulOnboarding.pdf.

Leiter, M. P., Jackson, N. J., & Shaughnessy, K. (2008). Contrasting burnout, turnover intention, control, value congruence, and knowledge sharing between Baby Boomers and Generation X. *Journal of Nursing Management, 16*, 100–109.

Leiter, M. P., Price, S. L., & Laschinger, H. K. (2010). Generational differences in distress, attitudes and incivility among nurses. *Journal of Nursing Management, 18*, 970–980. http://dx.doi:10.111/j.1365-2834.2010.01168.x.

Lipsey, J. (2004). *Targeted selection.* Omaha, NE: Leadership Solutions.

Mackoff, B., & Triolo, P. (2008a). Why do nurse managers stay? Building a model of engagement. Part 1, dimensions of engagement. *Journal of Nursing Administration, 38*(3), 118–124.

Mackoff, B., & Triolo, P. (2008b). Why do nurse managers stay? Building a model of engagement. Part 2, cultures of engagement. *Journal of Nursing Administration, 38*(4), 166–171.

Manion, J., & Bartholomew, K. (2004). Community in the workplace: A proven retention strategy. *Journal of Nursing Administration, 34*(1), 46–53.

May, J. H., Bazzoli, G. J., & Gerland, A. M. (2006). Hospitals' responses to nurse staffing strategies. *Health Affairs, 25*(4), 316–323.

McClure, M. L., Poulin, M. A., Sovie, M. D., & Wandelt, M. A. (1983). *Magnet hospitals: Attraction and retention of professional nurses.* Kansas City, MO: American Nurses Association.

McHugh, M. D., Aiken, L. H., Cooper, R. A., & Miller, P. (2008). The U.S. presidential election and health care workforce policy. *Policy, Politics, & Nursing Practice, 9*(1), 6–14.

Mills, J., & Mullins, A. (2008). The California nurse mentor project: Every nurse deserves a mentor. *Nursing Economic$, 26*(5), 310–315.

Mion, L. C., Hazel, C., & Ca, M. (2006). Retaining and recruiting mature experienced nurses: A multicomponent organizational strategy. *Journal of Nursing Administration, 36*(3), 148–154.

Nall, R. (2012). *Targeted selection interview tips.* Retrieved October 5, 2012, from www.ehow.com/way_5347581_targeted-selection-interview-tips.html.

Nedd, N. (2006b). Perceptions of empowerment and intent to stay. *Nursing Economic$, 24*(1), 13–18.

Palumbo, M. V., McIntosh, B., Rambur, B., & Naud, S. (2009). Retaining an aging nurse workforce: Perceptions of human resource practices. *Nursing Economic$, 27*(4), 221–232.

Park, M., & Jones, C. (2010). A retention strategy for newly graduated nurses. An integrative review of orientation programs. *Journal for Nurses in Staff Development, 26*(4), 142–149. http://dx.doi:10.1097/NND.0b013e31819aa130.

Pierson, M. A., Liggett, C., & Moore, K. S. (2010). Twenty years of experience with a clinical ladder: A tool for professional growth, evidence-based practice, recruitment, and retention. *The Journal of Continuing Education in Nursing, 41*(1), 33–40.

Pine, R., & Tart, K. (2007). Return on investment: Benefits and challenges of a baccalaureate nurse residency program. *Nursing Economic$, 25*(1), 13–18, 39.

PricewaterhouseCoopers. (2007). *What works: Healing the healthcare staffing shortage.* New York: PricewaterhouseCoopers Health Research Institute. Retrieved October 5, 2012, from www.pwc.com/us/en/healthcare/publications/what-works-healing-the-healthcare-staffing-shortage.jhtml.

Sparacio, D. C. (2005). Winged migration: International nurse recruitment—Friend or foe to the nursing crisis? *Journal of Nursing Law, 10*(2), 97–114.

Staiger, D. O., Auerbach, D. I., & Buerhaus, P. I. (2012). Registered nurse labor supply and the recession—Are we in a bubble? *The New England Journal of Medicine, 366*(16), 1463–1465.

Tri-Council for Nursing. (2004). *Joint statement from the Tri-Council for Nursing on recent registered nurse supply and demand projections.* Retrieved October 5, 2012, from www.nln.org/governmentaffairs/pdf/workforce:supply_statement_final.pdf.

Vahey, D. C., Aiken, L. H., Sloane, D. M., Clar, S. P., & Vargas, D. (2004). Nurse burnout and patient satisfaction. *Medical Care, 42*(2), 57–66.

vanWyngeeren, K., & Stuart, T. (n.d.). *Increasing new graduate nurse retention from a student nurse perspective.* Retrieved October 5, 2012, from www.rnjournal.com/journal_of_nursing/increasing_new_graduate_nurse_retention.htm.

Weberg, D. (2010). Transformational leadership and staff retention: An evidence review with implications for healthcare systems. *Nursing Administration Quarterly, 34*(3), 246–258.

Zastocki, D., & Holly, C. (2010). Retaining nurse managers. *American Nurse Today, 5*(12). Retrieved October 5, 2012, from www.americannursetoday.com/article.aspx?id=7322&fid=6856.

Chapter 21

Abdoo, Y. M. (2000). Nurse staffing and scheduling. In L. M. Simms, S. A. Price, & N. E. Ervin (Eds.), *Professional practice of nursing administration* (pp. 264–280). Albany, NY: Delmar.

Aiken, L. H., Clarke, S. P., Cheung, R. B., Sloane, D. M., & Silber, J. H. (2003). Education level of hospital nurses and patient mortality. *Journal of the American Medical Association, 290*, 1617–1623.

Aiken, L. H., Clarke, S. P., Sloane, D. M., Sochalski, J., & Silber, J. H. (2002d). Hospital nurse staffing and patient mortality, nurse burnout, and job dissatisfaction. *Journal of the American Medical Association, 288*(16), 1987–1993.

Aiken, L. H., Xue, Y., Clarke, S. P., & Sloane, D. M. (2007). Supplemental nurse staffing in hospitals and quality of care. *Journal of Nursing Administration, 37*(7–8), 335–342.

American Academy of Ambulatory Care Nursing. (AAACN). (2005). *Ambulatory care nurse staffing: An annotated bibliography.* Pitman, NJ: Author.

American Academy of Pediatrics (AAP) and the American College of Obstetricians and Gynecologists (ACOG). (2007). *Guidelines for perinatal care.* Washington, DC: March of Dimes.

American Association of Colleges of Nursing (AACN). (2003). *White paper on the role of the Clinical Nurse Leader (CNL®).* Washington, DC: Author.

American Association of Colleges of Nursing (AACN). (2007b). *White paper on the education and role of the Clinical Nurse Leader (CNL®).* Washington, DC: Author.

American Nurses Association (ANA). (1999). *Principles for nurse staffing.* Silver Spring, MD: Author.

American Nurses Association (ANA). (2004). *Scope and standards for nurse administrators.* Silver Springs, MD: Author.

American Nurses Association (ANA). (2005b). *Utilization guide for the ANA principles for nurse staffing.* Silver Spring, MD: Author.

American Nurses Association (ANA). (2010c). *Nursing's social policy statement.* (3rd ed.). Silver Spring, MD: Author.

American Nurses Association (ANA). (2010d). *Code of ethics with interpretive statements.* Silver Spring, MD: Author.

American Nurses Association (ANA). (2010e). *Scope and standards of practice.* Silver Spring, MD: Author.

American Organization of Nurse Executives (AONE). (2000). *Staffing management and methods: Tools and techniques for nurse leaders.* Chicago: Author. Retrieved September 8, 2012, from www.josseybass.com/WileyCDA/WileyTitle/productCd-0787955361.html.

American Organization of Nurse Executives (AONE). (2008). *AONE 2008 legislative agenda.* Chicago: Author.

Association of Women's Health, Obstetric and Neonatal Nurses (AWHONN). (2010). *Guidelines for professional registered nurse staffing for perinatal units.* Washington, DC: Author. Retrieved September 8, 2012, from www.awhonn.org/awhonn/content.do;jsessionid=BAECD0D18B545679C75FF84FBA598821?name=04_ConsultingTraining/04_StaffingGuidelines.htm.

Association of periOperative Registered Nurses (AORN). (2005). AORN guidance statement: Perioperative staffing. *AORN Journal, 81*(5), 1059–1066.

Aydelotte, M. K. (1973). *Nurse staffing methodology: A review and critique of selected literature.* U.S. Department of Health, Education and Welfare, Division of Nursing. Publication No. (NIH) 73–433. Washington, DC: Government Printing Office.

Barnum, B., & Mallard, C. (1989). *Essentials of nursing management: Concepts and context of practice.* Rockville, MD: Aspen.

Blegen, M., & Goode, C. J. (1998). Nurse staffing and patient outcomes. *Nursing Research, 47*, 43–50.

Beyers, M. (2000). Foreword. In M. Fralic (Ed.), *Staffing management and methods: Tools and techniques for nursing leaders* (pp. xxi–xxii). San Francisco: Jossey-Bass.

Bogue, R. (2012). Nurses: Key to making or breaking your future margin. *Hospitals and Health Networks*, May 29. Retrieved September 8, 2012, from www.hhnmag.com/hhnmag/HHNDaily/HHNDailyDisplay.dhtml?id=5390002938.

Brooten, D., & Youngblut, J. M. (2006). Nurse dose as concept. *Journal of Nursing Scholarship, 38*(1), 94–99.

Brown, B. (1999). How to develop a unit personnel budget. *Nursing Management, 30*(6), 34–35.

Case Management Society of America (CMSA). (2012b). *What is a case manager?* Little Rock, AR: Author. Retrieved September 8, 2012, from www.cmsa.org/Home/CMSA/WhatisaCaseManager/tabid/224/Default.aspx.

Cho, S. H. (2001). Nurse staffing and adverse patient outcomes: A systems approach. *Nursing Outlook, 49*(2), 78–85.

Cipriano, P., & Cutruzzula, J. (2007). Over-recruiting: Breaking the short staffing and turnover cycle. *Nurse Leader, 5*(6), 28–32.

Clarke, S. P. (2005). The policy implications of staffing-outcomes research. *Journal of Nursing Administration, 35*(1), 17–19.

Dalton, K. (2007). *A study of charge compression in calculating DRG relative weights.* Center for Medicaid and Medicare Services: Contract no. 500-00-0024-TO18.

Dent, R., & Bradshaw, P. (2012). Building the business case for acuity-based staffing. *Nurse Leader*, April 26–28.

Deutschendorf, A. L. (2010). Models of care delivery. In D. L. Huber (Ed.), *Leadership and nursing care management.* (4th ed.), (pp. 441–462). Philadelphia: Saunders.

Emergency Nursing Association (ENA). (2003). *Emergency Nurses Association white paper: Staffing and productivity in the emergency care setting.* Retrieved September 8, 2012, from www.ena.org/SiteCollectionDocuments/Position%20Statements/Staffing_and_Productivity_-_ENA_White_Paper.pdf.

Donabedian, A. (1966). Evaluating the quality of medical care. *Milbank Memorial Fund Quarterly, 44*(3), 166–206.

Eck, S. A. (1999). *The effect of a change in skill mix on patient and organizational outcomes in one teaching hospital.* PhD dissertation, Yale University, New Haven, CT.

Eck Birmingham, S. (2010). Evidenced-based staffing: The next step. *Nurse Leader*, June, 24–26, 35.

Eck Birmingham, S., Nell, K., & Abe, N. (2011). Determining staffing needs based on patient outcomes vs. patient interventions. In P. Cowan & S. Moorhead (Eds.), *Current issues in nursing.* (8th ed, pp. 391–404). St. Louis: Mosby Elsevier.

Edwardson, S. (2007). Conceptual frameworks used in funded nursing health services research projects. *Nursing Economic$, 25*(4), 222–227.

Finkler, S. A., Kovner, C. T., & Jones, C. B. (2007a). *Financial management for nurse managers and executives* (3rd ed.). Philadelphia: Saunders.

Fried, B. J., & Johnson, J. A. (2002). *Human resources in healthcare: Managing for success.* Washington, DC: AUPHA Press.

Frith, K., Anderson, F., Caspers, B., Tseng, F., Sanford, K., Hoyt, N., et al. (2010). Effects of nurse staffing on hospital-acquired conditions and length of stay in community hospitals. *Quality Management in Health Care, 19*(2), 147–155.

Geiger-Brown, J., & Trinkoff, A. (2010). Is it time to pull the plug on 12 hour shifts? Part I. The evidence. *Journal of Nursing Administration, 40*(3), 100–102.

Gurses, A. P., & Carayon, P. (2007). Performance obstacles of intensive care nurses. *Nursing Research, 56*(3), 185–194.

Haas, S., & Hastings, C. (2001). Staffing and workload. In J. Robinson (Ed.), *Core curriculum for ambulatory care nursing* (pp. 133–145). Philadelphia: Saunders.

Hardin, S. R., & Kaplow, R. (2005b). *Synergy for excellence: The AACN Synergy Model for patient care.* Sudbury, MA: Jones & Bartlett.

Hinshaw, A. (2006). Keeping patients safe: A collaboration among nurse administrators and researchers. *Nursing Administrative Quarterly, 30*(4), 309–320.

Huber, D. L. (2008). Testing nurse activity dose. *Journal of Nursing Administration, 38*(5), 212–213.

Institute of Medicine (IOM). (2004c). *Keeping patients safe: Transforming the work environment of nurses.* Washington, DC: National Academies Press.

Institute of Medicine (IOM). (2011e). *The future of nursing: Leading change, advancing health.* Washington, DC: National Academies Press.

Jones, C. B. (2004c). The costs of nurse turnover. Part 1. An economic perspective. *Journal of Nursing Administration, 34*(12), 562–570.

Jones, C. B. (2005). The costs of nurse turnover. Part 2. Application of the nursing turnover cost calculation methodology. *Journal of Nursing Administration, 35*(1), 41–49.

Jones, C. B. (2008). Revisiting nurse turnover costs: Adjusting for inflation. *Journal of Nursing Administration, 38*(1), 11–18.

Jones, C. B., & Gates, M. (2007). The costs and benefits of nurse turnover: A business case for nurse retention. *The Online Journal of Issues in Nursing, 12*(3).

Jones, C. B., & Mark, B. A. (2005). The intersection of nursing and health services research: An agenda to guide future research. *Nursing Outlook, 53*(6), 324–332.

Jones, C. B., Mark, B. A., Gates, M., & Eck, S. A. (2005). *Manager and staff nurse perceptions of vacancy tolerance.* Paper presentation at the National Nursing Administration Research Conference, October, Tucson, AZ.

Kane, R., Shamliyan, T., Mueller, C., Duval, S., & Wilt, T. (2007f). *Nurse staffing and quality of patient care.* U.S. Department of Health and Human Services. AHRQ Publication No. 07-E005. Washington, DC: Author.

Kane, R., Shamliyan, T., Mueller, C., Duval, S., & Wilt, T. (2007g). The association of registered nurse staffing levels and patient outcomes. *Medical Care, 45*(12), 1195–1204.

Kaplow, R., & Reed, K. D. (2008). The AACN Synergy Model for patient care: A nursing model as a force of magnetism. *Nursing Economic$, 26*(1), 17–25.

Kelly, L., McHugh, M., & Aiken, L. (2011c). Nurse outcomes in Magnet and non-Magnet hospitals. *Journal of Nursing Administration, 41*, 428–433.

Kirby, K., & Wiczai, L. (1985). Budgeting for variable staffing. *Nursing Economic$, 3*(3), 160–166.

Koloroutis, M. (Ed.). (2004b). *Relationship-based care: A model for transforming practice.* Minneapolis: Creative Health Care Management.

Kovner, C., & Gergen, P. (1998). Nurse staffing levels and adverse events following surgery in U.S. hospitals. *Image: The Journal of Nursing Scholarship, 30*(4), 315–321.

Lauw, C., & Gares, D. (2005). Resource management: What's right for you? *Nursing Management, 36*(12), 46–49.

Litvak, E., Buerhaus, P., Davidoff, F., Long, M., McManus, M., & Berwick, D. (2005). Managing unnecessary variability in patient demand to reduce nursing stress and improve patient safety. *Journal on Quality and Patient Safety, 31*(6), 330–338.

Manthey, M. (1990). Definitions and basic elements of a patient care delivery system with an emphasis on primary nursing. In G. Mayer, M. Madden, & E. Lawrenz (Eds.), *Patient care delivery models* (pp. 201–211). Rockville, MD: Aspen.

Mark, B. A., Harless, D. W., & Berman, W. F. (2007). Nurse staffing and adverse events in hospitalized children. *Policy, Politics, and Nursing Practice, 8*(2), 83–92.

Mark, B. A., Harless, D. W., McCue, M., & Xu, Y. (2004). A longitudinal examination of hospital registered nurse staffing and quality of care. *Health Services Research, 39*(2), 279–300.

McKinley, J., & Cavouras, C. (2000). Evolving staffing measures. In American Organization of Nurse Executives (AONE). *Staffing management and methods: Tools and techniques for nurse leaders* (pp. 1–33). San Francisco: Jossey-Bass.

Mitchell, P. (2008). *Nurse staffing–A summary of current research, opinion and policy.* The William D. Ruckelshaus Center, pp. 1–37.

Moore, M., & Hastings, C. (2006). The evolution of an ambulatory nursing intensity system: Measuring workload in a day hospital setting. *Journal of Nursing Administration, 36*(5), 241–248.

Moorhead, S., Johnson, M., Maas, M., & Swanson, L. (Eds.). (2008). *Nursing outcomes classification* (4th ed.). St. Louis: Elsevier.

Nash, M., Kniphfer, K., Kuklinski, S., & Sparks, D. (2000). Resource management system design. In M. F. Fralic (Ed.), American Organization of Nurse Executives (AONE) series, *Staffing management and methods: Tools and techniques for nurse leaders* (pp. 35–57). San Francisco: Jossey-Bass.

National Association of Neonatal Nurses (NANN). (1999a). *Minimum staffing in NICU's.* NANN Position Statement No. 3009. Glenview, IL: Author.

National Association of Neonatal Nurses (NANN). (1999b). *Use of assistive personnel in providing care to the high-risk infant.* NANN Position Statement No. 3013. Glenview, IL: Author.

National Labor Relations Board (NLRB). (2102). *National Labor Relations Act.* Washington, DC: Author. Retrieved September 15, 2012, from www.nlrb.gov/national-labor-relations-act.

Needleman, J., Buerhaus, P., Mattke, S., Stewart, M., & Zelevinski, K. (2002a). Nurse-staffing levels and the quality of care in hospitals. *The New England Journal of Medicine, 346*(22), 1715–1722.

Needleman, J., Buerhaus, P. I., Stewart, M., Zelevinsky, K., & Mattke, S. (2006). Nurse staffing in hospitals: Is there a business case for quality? *Health Affairs, 25*, 204–211.

Needleman, J., Buerhaus, P., Pankratz, S., Leibson, C., Stevens, S., & Harris, M. (2011b). Nurse staffing and inpatient hospital mortality. *The New England Journal of Medicine, 364*(11), 1037–1045.

Norrish, B. R., & Rundall, T. G. (2001). Hospital restructuring and the work of registered nurses. *Milbank Quarterly, 79*, 55–79.

Pappas, S. H. (2007a). Describing cost related to nursing. *Journal of Nursing Administration, 37*(1), 32–40.

Person, C. (2004b). Patient care delivery. In M. Koloroutis (Ed.), *Relationship-based care: A model for transforming practice* (pp. 159–182). Minneapolis: Creative Health Care Management.

Pickard, B., & Warner, M. (2007). Demand management: A methodology for outcomes-driven staffing and patient flow management. *Nurse Leader, 4*(2), 30–34.

Porter, C. (2010). A nursing labor management partnership model. *Journal of Nursing Administration, 40*(6), 272–276.

PricewaterhouseCoopers Health Research Institute. (2007). *What works: Healing the healthcare staffing shortage.* Retrieved September 15, 2012, from www.pwc.com/us/en/healthcare/publications/what-works-healing-the-healthcare-staffing-shortage.jhtml.

Robertson, R., & Samuelson, C. (1996). Should nurse patient ratios be legislated? Pros and cons. *Georgia Nursing, 56*(5), 2.

Seago, J. A., Spetz, J., Coffman, J., Rosenoff, E., & O'Neil, E. (2003). Minimum staffing ratios: The California workforce initiative survey. *Nursing Economic$, 21*(2), 65–70.

Sherman, R. (2005). Don't forget our charge nurses. *Nursing Economic$, 23*(3), 125–130, 143.

Simpson, R. (2012). Technology enables value-base nursing care. *Nursing Administration Quarterly, 36*(1), 85–87.

Sullivan, J., Bretschneider, J., & McCausland, M. P. (2003). Designing a leadership development program for nurse managers: An evidence-driven approach. *Journal of Nursing Administration, 33*(10), 544–549.

The Joint Commission (TJC). (2006). *Management of human resources.* Oakbrook Terrace, IL: Author.

Thompson, J. D., & Diers, D. (1985). DRG's and nursing intensity. *Nursing and Healthcare, 6*, 434–439.

Trinkoff, A. M., Johantgen, M., Storr, C. L., Gurses, A. P., Liang, Y., & Han, K. (2011). Nurses' work schedule characteristics, nurse staffing and patient mortality. *Nursing Research, 60*(1), 1–8.

Unruh, L. (2003b). The effect of LPN reductions on RN patient load. *Journal of Nursing Administration, 33*(4), 201–208.

Unruh, L. (2008b). Nurse staffing: Patient, nurse, financial outcomes. *American Journal of Nursing, 108*(1), 62–71.

Unruh, L., & Fottler, M. D. (2004, June 6–8). *Patient turnover and nursing staff adequacy.* San Diego: Academy Health Annual Research meeting. Retrieved September 15, 2012, from www.academyhealth.org/Events/content.cfm?ItemNumber=621.

Warner, M. (2006). Personnel staffing and scheduling. In R. Hall (Ed.), *Patient flow: Reducing delay in healthcare delivery* (pp. 189–209). Los Angeles: Springer.

Watson, J. (2002). *Assessing and measuring caring in nursing and health science.* New York: Springer.

Welton, J. M. (2010). Value-based nursing care. *Journal of Nursing Administration, 40*(10), 399–401.

Welton, J. M., & Harris, K. (2007). Hospital billing and reimbursement: Charging for inpatient nursing care. *Journal of Nursing Administration, 30*(6), 309–315.

Welton, J. M., Zone-Smith, L., & Fischer, M. H. (2006). Adjustment of inpatient care reimbursement for nursing intensity. *Policy, Politics, & Nursing Practice, 7*(4), 270–280.

White, K. M. (2006). Policy spotlight: Staffing plans and ratios. *Nursing Management, 37*(4), 18–22, 24.

Chapter 22

American Association of Colleges of Nursing (AACN). (2011c). *Report on 2011–2012 enrollment and graduations in baccalaureate and graduate programs in nursing.* Retrieved July 18, 2012, from www.aacn.nche.edu/media-relations/fact-sheets/nursing-faculty-shortage.

American Nurses Association. (ANA). (2012). *Nursing shortage.* Retrieved July 17, 2012, from www.nursingworld.org/nursingshortage.

Bureau of Labor Statistics. (2012b). *Economic news release: Table 6. The 30 occupations with the largest projected employment growth, 2010–20.* Retrieved July 19, 2012 from www.bls.gov/news.release/ecopro.t06.htm.

Cho, S., Ketefian, S., Barkauskas, V., & Smith, D. (2003). The effects of nurse staffing on adverse events, morbidity, mortality, and medical costs. *Nursing Research, 52*(2), 71–79.

Dunham-Taylor, J., & Pinczuk, J. Z. (2006). *Health care financial management for nurse managers.* Sudbury, MA: Jones & Bartlett.

Finkler, S. A., Kovner, C. T., & Jones, C. B. (2007b). *Financial management for nurse managers and nurse executives* (3rd ed.). Philadelphia: Saunders.

Health Resources and Services Administration (HRSA). (2010). *The Registered Nurse population. Findings from the 2008 National Sample Survey of Registered Nurses.* Retrieved July 19, 2012, from: http://bhpr.hrsa.gov/healthworkforce/rnsurveys/rnsurveyfinal.pdf.

Kotecki, S., & Schmidt, R. (2010). Cost and effectiveness analysis using nursing staff-prepared thickened liquids vs. commercially thickened liquids in stroke patients with dysphagia. *Nurs Econ. 28*(2):106–109, 113.

Keehan, S., Sisko, A. M., Truffer, C. J., Poisal, J. A., Cuckler, G. A., Madison, A. J., et al. (2011). National health spending projections through 2020: Economic recovery and reform drive faster spending growth. *Health Affairs, 30*(8), 1594–1605.

Lucero, R. J., Lake, E. T., & Aiken, L. H. (2009). Variations in nursing care quality across hospitals. *Journal of Advanced Nursing, 65*(11), 2299–2310.

Murray, M. E. (2012). Economics of the health care delivery system. In J. Zerwekh, & A. Z. Garneau (Eds.), *Nursing Today* (7th ed., pp. 331–350). St. Louis: Elsevier Saunders.

Outten, M. K. (2012). From veterans to nexters: Managing a multigenerational workforce. *Nursing Management, 43*(4), 42–47.

Pappas, S. H. (2007b). Describing costs related to nursing. *Journal of Nursing Administration, 17*(1), 32–40.

Sorbello, B. (2008). Finance: It's not a dirty word. *American Nurse Today, 3*(8), 32–35.

Stanley, D. (2010). Multigenerational workforce issues and their implications for leadership in nursing. *Journal of Nursing Management, 18*(7), 846–852.

Chapter 23

Aiken, L., Clarke, S., Sloane, D., Sochalski, J., & Silber, J. (2002e). Hospital nurse staffing and patient mortality, nurse burnout, and job dissatisfaction. *Journal of the American Medical Association, 288*, 1987–1993.

American Nurses Association (ANA). (1988c). *Peer review guidelines.* Kansas City, MO: Author.

Arnold, E., & Pulich, M. (2003). Personality conflicts and objectivity in appraising performance. *Health Care Manager, 22*(3), 227–232.

Burns, N., & Grove, S. K. (2001). *The practice of nursing research: Conduct, critique & utilization* (4th ed.). Philadelphia: Saunders.

BusinessDictionary.com. (2012). *Performance appraisal.* Retrieved from www.businessdictionary.com/definition/performance-appraisal.html.

Cameron, K. S., & Quinn, R. E. (1999). *Diagnosing and changing organizational culture: Based on the competing values framework.* Reading, PA: Addison-Wesley.

Carroll, J. S., & Edmondson, A. C. (2002). Leading organizational learning in health care. *Quality and Safety in Health Care, 11*, 51–56.

Conlon, M. (2003). Appraisal: The catalyst of personal development. *British Medical Journal, 327*(7411), 389–391.

Detert, J. R., Schroeder, R. G., & Mauriel, J. J. (2000). A framework for linking culture and improvement initiatives in organizations. *Academy of Management Review, 25*(4), 850–863.

Donaldson, M. S., & Mohr, J. J. (2000). *Exploring innovation and quality improvement in health care microsystems: A cross-case analysis.* Retrieved from www.nap.edu/openbook/NI000346/html/65.html.

Duncan, D. (2007). The importance of managing performance processes well. *Kai Tiaki Nursing New Zealand, 13*(10), 25.

Gershon, R. R. M., Stone, P. W., Bakken, S., & Larson, E. (2004). Measurement of organizational culture and climate in health care. *Journal of Nursing Administration, 34*(1), 33–40.

Greguras, G. J., Robie, C., Schleicher, D. J., & Goff, M. (2003). A field study of the effects of rating purpose on the quality of multisource ratings. *Personnel Psychology, 56*(1), 1–21.

Hersey, P., Blanchard, K. H., & Johnson, D. E. (2008d). *Management of organizational behavior: Leading human resources* (9th ed.). Upper Saddle River, NJ: Pearson Education.

Institute of Medicine (IOM). (2000). *To err is human: Building a safer system.* Washington, DC: National Academies Press.

Institute of Medicine (IOM). (2001f). *Crossing the quality chasm: A new health system for the 21st century.* Washington, DC: National Academies Press.

Institute of Medicine (IOM). (2003b). *Priority areas for national action: Transforming health care quality.* Washington, DC: National Academies Press.

Institute of Medicine (IOM). (2004d). *Keeping patients safe: Transforming the work environment of nurses.* Washington, DC: National Academies Press.

Jawahar, M. (2006). Correlates of satisfaction with performance appraisal feedback. *Journal of Labor Relations, 27*, 213–234.

Kelly, L. A., McHugh, M. D., & Aiken, L. H. (2011d). Nurse outcomes in Magnet and non-Magnet hospitals. *The Journal of Nursing Administration, 41*(10), 428–433.

Lundmark, V. A. (2008). Magnet environments for professional nursing practice. In R. G. Hughes (Ed.), *Patient safety and quality: An evidence-based handbook for nurses.* Rockville, MD: Agency for Healthcare Research and Quality. Available from: www.ncbi.nlm.nih.gov/books/NBK2667/.

Meretoja, R., & Koponen, L. (2012). A systematic model to compare nurses' optimal and actual competencies in the clinical setting. *Journal of Advanced Nursing, 68*(2), 414–422.

Merriam-Webster.com (2012). *Performance.* Retrieved from www.merriam-webster.com/dictionary/performance.

Needleman, J., Buerhaus, P., Mattke, S., Stewart, M., & Zelevinsky, K. (2002b). Nurse-staffing levels and the quality of care in hospitals. *The New England Journal of Medicine, 346*, 1715–1722.

Nemeth, L. S., Feifer, C., Stuart, G., & Ornstein, S. M. (2008). Implementing change in primary care practices using electronic medical records: A conceptual framework. *Implementation Science, 3*, 3. http://dx.doi:10.1186/1748-5908-3-3.

Reason, J. (2000). Human error: Models and management. *British Medical Journal, 320*(7237), 768–770.

Robinson, K., Eck, C., Keck, B., & Wells, N. (2003). The Vanderbilt Professional Nursing Practice Program, part 1: Growing and supporting professional nursing practice. *Journal of Nursing Administration, 33*(9), 441–450.

Schein, E. H. (1992). *Organizational culture and leadership* (2nd ed.). San Francisco: Jossey-Bass.

Smith-Trudeau, P. (2008). Culturally sensitive performance appraisals that lead to reenergized managers and employees. *Vermont Nurse Connection, 10*(4), 5 (Nov., Dec. 2007, Jan. 2008).

Stetler, C. B. (2003). Role of the organization in translating research into evidence-based practice. *Outcomes Management, 7*(3), 97–103.

Stone, F. M. (1999). *Coaching, counseling & mentoring: How to choose & use the right technique to boost employee performance.* New York: AMACOM.

Studer, Q. (2003b). *Hardwiring excellence.* Gulf Breeze, FL: Fire Starter Publishing.

Ward, D. (2003). Self-esteem and audit feedback. *Nursing Standard, 17*(37), 33–36.

Wenberg, D. (2010). Transformational leadership and staff retention: An evidence review with implications for healthcare systems. *Nursing Administration Quarterly, 34*(3), 246–258.

Chapter 24

Anderson, C. (2002). Past victim, future victim? *Nursing Management, 33*(3), 26–31.

Beech, B., & Leather, P. (2005). Workplace violence in the health care sector: A review of staff training and integration of training evaluation models. *Aggression and Violent Behavior, 11*, 27–43. http://dx.doi:10.1016/j.aub.2005.05.004.

Beugre, C. D. (2005). Understanding injustice-related aggression in organizations: A cognitive model. *International Journal of Human Resource Management, 16*(7), 1120–1136. http://dx.doi:10.1080/09585190500143964.

Botting, J. M. (2001). Picking up the pieces. *Security Management, 45*(1), 26–39.

Center for American Nurses. (2008). *Position statement: Lateral violence and bullying in the workplace.* Retrieved from www.mc.vanderbilt.edu/root/pdfs/nursing/center_lateral_violence:-and_bullying_position_statement_from_center_for_american_nurses.pdf.

Chapman, R., Styles, I., Perry, L., & Combs, S. (2010). Nurses' experience of adapting to workplace violence: A theory of adaptation. *International Journal of Mental Health Nursing, 19*(3), 186–194. http://dx.doi:10.111/j.1447-0349.2009.00663.x.

Corbo, S. A., & Siewers, M. H. (2001). Hazardous to your health: Don't get burned when tempers ignite. *Nursing Management, 32*(3), 44-c–44-d, 44-s.

Corley, M. C. (2002). Nurse moral distress: A proposed theory and research agenda. *Nursing Ethics, 9*(6), 636–650. http://dx.doi:10.1191/0969733002ne557.oa.

Dolan, J. B. (2000). Workplace violence: The universe of legal issues. *Defense Counsel Journal, 67*(3), 332–341.

Egger, E. (2000). Reasonable and appropriate action important in preventing violent crime. *Health Care Strategic Management, 18*(10), 13–14.

Ginn, G. O., & Henry, L. J. (2002). Addressing workplace violence from a health management perspective. *SAM Advanced Management Journal, 67*(4), 4–10.

Harulow, S. (2000). Ending the silence on violence. *Australian Nursing Journal, 7*(10), 26–29.

Henry, J., & Ginn, G. O. (2002). Violence prevention in health care organizations within a total quality management framework. *Journal of Nursing Administration, 32*(9), 479–486.

Hogh, A., & Viitasara, E. (2005). A systematic review of longitudinal studies of nonfatal workplace violence. *European Journal of Work and Organizational Psychology, 14*(3), 291–313.

Hutchinson, M., Wilkes, L., Jackson, D., & Vickers, M. H. (2010). Integrating individual, work group and organizational factors: Testing a multidimensional model of bullying in the nursing workplace. *Journal of Nursing Management, 18*(2), 173–181. http://dx.doi:10.1111/j.1365-2834.2009.01035.x.

Lanza, M. L., Schmidt, S., McMillan, F., Demaio, J., & Forester, L. (2011). Support our staff-A unique program to help deal with patient assault. *Perspectives in Psychiatric Care, 47*(3), 131–137. http://dx.doi:10.1111/j.1744-6163.2010.00282.x.

Law, T. P., & Petit, F. A. (2007). Insuring for workplace violence. *Risk Management, 54*(11), 14–18.

Matchulat, J. J. (2007). Separating fact from fiction about workplace violence. *Employee Relations Law Journal, 33*(2), 41–122.

McKenna, B. G., Smith, N. A., Poole, S. J., & Coverdale, J. H. (2003). Horizontal violence: Experience of registered nurses in their first year of practice.

Journal of Advanced Nursing, 42(1), 90–96. http://dx.doi:10.1046/j.1365-2648.2003.02583.x.

McKoy, Y. L., & Smith, M. H. (2001). Legal considerations of workplace violence in healthcare environments. *Nursing Forum, 36*(1), 5–14.

McPhaul, K. M., & Lipscomb, J. A. (2004). Workplace violence in health care: Recognized but not regulated. *The Online Journal of Issues in Nursing, 9*(3). Retrieved from www.nursingworld.org/MainMenuCategories/ANAMarketplace/ANAPeriodicals/OJIN/TableofContents/Volume92004/No3Sept04/ViolenceinHealthCare.aspx.

Miller, M., & Hartung, S. Q. (2011). Covert crime at work. *Pennsylvania Nurse, 66*(4), 11–16.

Nachreiner, N., Gerberich, S., McGovern, P. M., Church, T. R., Hansen, H. E., Geisser, M. S., et al. (2005). Relation between policies and work related assault: Minnesota Nurses' Study. *Occupational & Environmental Medicine, 62*(10), 675–681. http://dx.doi:10.1136/oem.2004.014134.

National Institute for Occupational Safety and Health (NIOSH), Centers for Disease Control and Prevention, U.S. Department of Health and Human Services. (2002). *Violence: Occupational hazards in hospitals.* (DHHS, NIOSH Publication No. 2002-101). Retrieved from www.cdc.gov/niosh/docs/2002-101/.

National Institute for Occupational Safety and Health (NIOSH), Centers for Disease Control and Prevention, U.S. Department of Health and Human Services. (2004). *Workplace violence prevention strategies and research needs.* (DHHS, NIOSH Publication No. 2006-144). Retrieved from www.cdc.gov/niosh/docs/2006-144/.

Needham, I., Abderhalden, C., Halfens, R., Fischer, J. E., & Dassen, T. (2005). Non-somatic effects of patient aggression on nurses: A systematic review. *Journal of Advanced Nursing, 49*(3), 283–296. http://dx.doi:10.1111/j.1365-2648.2004.03286.x.

O'Leary-Kelly, A. M., Griffin, R. W., & Glew, D. J. (1996). Organization-motivated aggression: A research framework. *Academy of Management Review, 21*(1), 225–253. http://dx.doi:10.5465/AMR.1996.9602161571.

Occupational Safety and Health Administration (OSHA), U.S. Department of Labor. (2004). *Guidelines for preventing workplace violence for health care and social service workers.* (OSHA publication 3148–01R 2004). Retrieved from www.osha.gov/Publications/osha3148.pdf.

Paetzold, R. L., O'Leary-Kelly, A. M., & Griffin, R. W. (2007). Workplace violence, employer liability, and implications for organizational research. *Journal of Management Inquiry, 16*(4), 362–370.

Romano, S. J., Levi-Minzi, M. E., Rugala, E. A., & Van Hasselt, V. B. (2011). Workplace violence prevention: Readiness and response. *FBI Law Enforcement Bulletin*, Washington DC: Federal Bureau of Investigation, U.S. Department of Justice. Retrieved from www.fbi.gov/stats-services/publications/law-enforcement-bulletin/january2011/workplace_violence_prevention.

Rugala, E. R. & Isaacs, A. R. (Eds.). (2004). *Workplace violence: Issues in response.* Washington, DC: U.S. Department of Justice, Federal Bureau of Investigation (FBI). Retrieved from www.fbi.gov/stats-services/publications/workplace-violence.

Sheehan, J. P. (2000). Protect your staff from workplace violence. *Nursing Management, 31*(3), 24–25.

Smith, A. P. (2001). Removing the fluff: The quality in quality improvement. *Nursing Economics, 19*(4), 183–185.

Spector, P. E., Coulter, M. L., Stockwell, H. G., & Matz, M. W. (2007). Perceived violence climate: A new construct and its relationship to workplace physical violence and verbal aggression, and their potential consequences. *Work and Stress, 21*(2), 117–130.

The Joint Commission. (2010). *Sentinel event alert: Preventing violence in the health care setting.* Retrieved from www.jointcommission.org/sentinel_event_alert_issue_45_preventing_violence:in_the_health_care_setting/.

Tzeng, H., & Ketefian, S. (2002). The relationship between nurses' job satisfaction and inpatient satisfaction: An exploratory study in a Taiwan teaching hospital. *Journal of Nursing Care Quality, 16*(2), 39–49.

Wagner, C., Groenewegen, P. P., de Bakker, D. H., & van der Wal, G. (2001b). Environmental and organizational determinants of quality management. *Quality Management in Health Care, 9*(4), 63–77.

Walrafen, N., Brewer, M. K., & Mulvenon, C. (2012). Sadly caught up in the moment: An exploration of horizontal violence. *Nursing Economics, 30*(1), 6–12, 49.

Weinand, M. (2010). Horizontal violence in nursing: history, impact, and solution. *JOCEPS: The Journal of Chi Eta Phi Sorority, 54*(1), 23–26.

Yang, L. (2009). *Aggression and its consequences in nursing: A more complete story by adding its social context.* Doctoral dissertation, University of South Florida.

Chapter 25

Adams, L. M. (2009). Exploring the concept of surge capacity. *Online Journal of Issues in Nursing, 14*(2). Retrieved from http://www.medscape.com/viewarticle/704505_9.

Agency for Healthcare Research, Quality (AHRQ). (2005a). *Altered standards of care in mass casualty events*. (AHRQ Publication No. 05–0043). Retrieved from http://archive.ahrq.gov/research/altstand/.

Agency for Healthcare Research and Quality. (AHRQ). (2005b). *Surge capacity and health system preparedness.* Retrieved from http://archive.ahrq.gov/news/ulp/btsurgemass/.

American Nurses Association. (2007). *Adapting standards of care under altered conditions.* (Draft document for comment purposes only). New York: Center for Health Policy, Columbia University School of Nursing.

California Hospital Association. (2009). *Emergency preparedness: Hazard vulnerability analysis.* Retrieved from http://www.calhospitalprepare.org/hazard-vulnerability-analysis.

Centers for Disease Control and Prevention (CDC). (2007). *Ethical guidelines in pandemic influenza.* Retrieved from www.cdc.gov/od/science/integrity/phethics/panFlu_Ethic_Guidelines.pdf.

Christian, M. D., Hawryluck, L., Wax, R. S., Cook, T., Lazar, N. M., Herridge, M. S., et al. (2006). Development of a triage protocol for critical care during an influenza pandemic. *Canadian Medical Association Journal, 175*(11), 1377–1381. http://dx.doi.org:10.1503/cmaj.060911.

Coyle, G., Sapnas, K., & Ward-Presson, K. (2007b). Dealing with disaster. *Nursing Management, 38*(7), 24–29. http://dx.doi.org:10.1097/01.NUMA.0000281132.18369.bd.

Danna, D., Bernard, M., Jones, J., & Mathews, P. (2009). Improvements in disaster planning and directions for nursing management. *Journal of Nursing Administration, 39*(10), 423–431.

Department of Homeland Security. (2012). *NTAS public guide.* Retrieved from www.dhs.gov/files/publications/ntas-public-guide.shtm.

Department of Veterans Affairs. (2005). *Emergency management program guidebook 2005.* Retrieved from www1.va.gov/emshg/page.cmp.pg=114.

Drenkard, K., & Rigotti, G. (2002, updated 2011). *Inova Health System survey.* Falls Church, VA: Inova Health System.

Drenkard, K., Rigotti, G., Hanfling, D., Fahlgren, T., & LaFrancois, G. (2002). Healthcare system disaster preparedness, part 1: Readiness planning. *Journal of Nursing Administration, 32*(9), 461–469.

Emergency Medical Services Authority. (2006). *Hospital incident command system guidebook.* Retrieved from www.emsa.ca.gov/HICS/files/Guidebook_glossary.pdf.

Fahlgren, T., & Drenkard, K. (2002). Healthcare system disaster preparedness. Part 2. Nursing executive role in leadership. *Journal of Nursing Administration, 32*(10), 531–537.

Federal Emergency Management Agency. (2010). *FEMA fact sheet: Incident management assistance teams.* Retrieved from http://blog.fema.gov/2012/03/announcing-creation-of-fema-corps.html.

Hick, J. L., & O'Laughlin, D. T. (2006). Concept of operations for triage of mechanical ventilation in an epidemic. *Academic Emergency Medicine, 13*(2), 223–229. http://dx.doi.org:10.1197/j.aem.2005.07.037.

Kaji, A. H., Koenig, K. L., & Lewis, R. J. (2007). Current hospital disaster preparedness. *JAMA, 298*(18), 2188–2190. http://dx.doi.org:10.1001/jama.298.18.2188.

Kraus, C. K., Levy, F., & Kelen, G. D. (2007). Lifeboat ethics: Considerations in the discharge of inpatients for the creation of hospital surge capacity. *Disaster Medicine and Public Health Preparedness, 1*(1), 51–56. http://dx.doi.org:10.1097/DMP.0b013e318065c4ca.

Mahan, B., Lowe, T., & Hughes, N. (2007, June). Teaching the caring professionals to take care. Presentation at the American Nurses Association Quadrennial Pre-Conference. Nursing Care in Life, Death, and Disaster, Atlanta, GA.

Mangeri, A. S. (2006). *Emergency management: Understanding the system.* Retrieved from http://ehstoday.com/fire_emergencyresponse/ehs_imp_13605.

National Advisory Council on Nurse Education and Practice (2009). *Challenges facing the nurse workforce in a changing environment. Part I: Surge capacity: Educating the nursing workforce for emergency and disaster preparedness.* 7th Annual Report. Retrieved from www.hrsa.gov/advisorycommittees/bhpradvisory/nacnep/Reports/seventhreport.pdf.

New York State Department of Health Task Force on Life and the Law. (2007). *Allocation of ventilators in an influenza pandemic.* Albany, NY: Author. Retrieved from www.health.state.ny.us/diseases/communicable/influenza/pandemic/ventilators/.

Phillips, S. J., & Knebel, A. (Eds.). (2007). *Mass medical care with scarce resources: A community planning guide.* (Prepared by Health Systems Research, Inc., an Altarum company, under contract No. 290-04-0010. AHRQ Publication No. 07–0001). Rockville, MD: Agency for Healthcare Research and Quality. Retrieved from http://archive.ahrq.gov/research/mce/mceguide.pdf.

The Joint Commission (TJC). (2012). *Comprehensive accreditation manual for hospitals 2012: Emergency management accreditation standards.* Oakbrook Terrace, IL: Author.

The Joint Commission Resources. (2008). *Emergency management in health care: An all-hazards approach.* Oakbrook Terrace, IL: Author.

Tillman, P. (2011). Disaster preparedness for nurses: A teaching guide. *The Journal of Continuing*

Education in Nursing, 42(9), 404–408. http://dx. doi:10.3928/00220124-20110502-02.

U.S. Department of Defense. (2007). *DOD dictionary of military and related terms.* Retrieved from www. military-dictionary.org/DOD-military-terms.

U.S. Department of Homeland Security. (2008). *National incident management system (NIMS).* Retrieved from www.fema.gov/ national-incident-management-system.

U.S. Department of Homeland Security. (2012). *NTAS public guide.* Retrieved from www.dhs.gov/files/ publications/ntas-public-guide.shtm.

World Health Organization. (2005). *Health action in crisis. Definitions: Emergencies.* Retrieved from www.who.int/ hac/about/definitions/en/index.html.

Chapter 26

American Nurses Association (ANA). (2007). *New criteria for recognition of terminologies supporting nursing practice.* Silver Spring, MD: Author.

American Nurses Association (ANA). (2008). *Nursing informatics: Scope and standards of practice.* Silver Spring, MD: Nursebooks.org.

Austin, C. (1979). *Information systems for hospital administration.* Ann Arbor, MI: Health Administration Press.

Bakken, S., Warren, J., Lundberg, C., Casey, A., Correia, C., Konicek, D., et al. (2001). An evaluation of the utility of the CEN categorical structure for nursing diagnoses as a terminology model for integrating nursing diagnosis concepts into SNOMED. *Studies in Health Technology and Informatics, 84*(Pt 1), 151–155.

Brokel, J. (2007). Creating sustainability of clinical information systems. *Journal of Nursing Administration, 37*(1), 10–13.

Brokel, J. M., Cole, M., & Upmeyer, L. (2011a). Longitudinal study of symptom control and quality of life indicators with patients receiving community-based case management services. *Applied Nursing Research, 25*(3), 138–145. http://dx.doi:10.1016/j.apnr.2011.02.002.

Brokel, J. M., Schwichtenberg, T. J., Wakefield, D. S., Ward, M. M., Shaw, M. G., & Kramer, J. M. (2011b). Evaluating clinical decision support rules as an intervention in clinical workflows with technology. *Computers, Informatics, Nursing, 29*(1), 36–42.

Burnes-Bolton, L. (2009, April 6). SSNI-505-Innovation and trends in technology: Exploring the nursing workflow of the future. In *Nursing Informatics Symposium.* Chicago, IL.

Centers for Medicare & Medicaid Services (CMS). (2011b). *Overview of accountable care organizations (ACOs).* Retrieved from www.cms.gov/ACO/.

Centers for Medicare & Medicaid Services (CMS). (2010). Medicare and Medicaid Programs: Electronic health record incentive program. *Federal Register, 75*(144), 44314–44588.

Clark, J. L., & Lang, N. (1992). Nursing's next advance: An internal classification for nursing practice. *International Nursing Review, 39*(4), 109–111.

Coenen, A., Marin, H., Park, H., & Bakken, S. (2001). Collaborative efforts for representing nursing concepts in computer-based systems: International perspectives. *Journal of the American Medical Informatics Association, 8*(3), 202–211.

DeJong, G. (2007). *Setting the stage: The case for another paradigm.* Washington, DC: Council for the Advancement of Nursing Science Special Topics Conference.

Delaney, C., & Huber, D. (2001). Clinical testing of a national standardized minimum data set designed to capture the management context of health care delivery. In *Proceedings of the AMIA Annual Symposium.* Washington, DC: AMIA.

Donabedian, A. (1986). Criteria and standards for quality assessment and monitoring. *Quarterly Review Bulletin, 12*(3), 99–100.

Englebardt, S. P., & Nelson, R. (2002). *Health care informatics: An interdisciplinary approach.* St. Louis: Mosby.

Fisher, E. S., McClellan, M. B., & Safran, D. G. (2011). Building the path to accountable care. *The New England Journal of Medicine, 365*(26), 2445–2447.

Fuller, R. L., McCullough, E. C., Bao, M. Z., & Averill, R. F. (2009). Estimating the costs of potentially preventable hospital acquired complications. *Health Care Financing Review, 30*(4), 17–32.

Furukawa, M. F., Raghu, T. S., & Shao, B. B. (2011). Electronic medical records, nurse staffing, and nurse-sensitive patient outcomes: Evidence from the national database of nursing quality indicators. *Medical Care Research & Review, 68*(3), 311–331.

Hannah, K., Ball, M., & Edwards, M. (2006). *Introduction to nursing informatics.* New York: Springer.

Hardiker, N., & Rector, A. (2001). Structural validation of nursing technologies. *Journal of the American Medical Informatics Association, 8*(3), 212–221.

Harrington, L., Porch, L., Acosta, K., & Wilkens, K. (2011). Realizing electronic medical record benefits: An easy-to-do usability study. *Journal of Nursing Administration, 41*(7/8), 331–335.

Häyrinen, K., Saranto, K., & Nykänen, P. (2008). Definition, structure, content, use and impacts of electronic health records: A review of the research literature. *International Journal of Medical Informatics, 77*, 291–304.

Horn, S. D., & Gassaway, J. (2010). Practice based evidence: Incorporating clinical heterogeneity and patient-reported outcomes for comparative effectiveness research. *Medical Care, 48*(Suppl. 6), S17–S22.

Huber, D., Schumacher, L., & Delaney, C. (1997). Nursing management minimum data set (NMMDS). *Journal of Nursing Administration, 27*(4), 42–48.

Huber, D. G., Delaney, C., Crossley, J., Mehmert, M., & Ellerbe, S. (1992). A nursing management minimum data set: Significance and development. *Journal of Nursing Administration, 22*(7–8), 35–40.

Ingenerf, J. (1995). *Taxonomic vocabularies in medicine: The intention of usage determines different established structures.* Paper presented at the MEDINFO 95, Vancouver, BC.

Institute of Medicine (IOM) (2004e). *Keeping patients safe: Transforming the work environment of nurses.* Washington, DC: National Academies Press.

Institute of Medicine Committee on Crossing the Quality Chasm: Adaptation to Mental Health and Addictive Disorders, (2006). *Improving the Quality of Health Care for Mental and Substance-Use Conditions: Quality Chasm Series.* (Chap. 7). Washington (DC): National Academies Press.

Institute of Medicine (IOM) Committee on the Robert Wood Johnson Foundation Initiative on the Future of Nursing (2011). *The Future of Nursing: Leading Change, Advancing Health.* Washington, DC.: The National Academies Press.

International Organization for Standardization (ISO) (2002). *Health informatics: Integration of a reference terminology model for nursing.* (Committee Document No. ISO/TC 215/N 142). Geneva: Author.

Jones, S., & Moss, J. (2006). Computerized provider order entry: Strategies for successful implementation. *Journal of Nursing Administration, 36*(3), 136–140.

Kennedy, R. (2003). The nursing shortage and the role of technology. *Nursing Outlook, 51*, S33–S34.

Kopp, B., Erstad, B., Allen, M., Theodorou, A., & Priestley, G. (2006). Medication errors and adverse drug events in an intensive care unit: Direct observation approach for detection. *Critical Care Medicine, 34*(2), 415–425.

Lorenzi, N., & Riley, R. (2003). Organizational issues=change. *International Journal of Medical Informatics, 69*, 197–203.

Minthorn, C., & Lunney, M. (2010). Participant action research with bedside nurses to identify NANDA-International, Nursing Interventions Classification, and Nursing Outcomes Classification categories for hospitalized persons with diabetes. *Applied Nursing Research, 25*(2), 75–80. http://dx.doi:10.1016/j.apnr.2010.08.001.

Moss, J., Andison, M., & Sobko, H. (2007). *An analysis of narrative nursing documentation in an otherwise structured intensive care clinical information system.* In *Proceedings of the American Medical Informatics Association Annual Symposium* (pp. 543–547). Chicago, IL.

Muller-Staub, M. (2009). Study to the implementation of NANDA-1 nursing diagnosis, interventions and nursing sensitive patient outcomes. *Pflegewissenschaft, 11*(12), 688–696.

National Institute of Standards and Testing (NIST). (2011). *Approved test procedures version 1.0.* Retrieved from http://healthcare.nist.gov/use_testing/finalized_requirements.html.

Ochylski, S., McDonald, T. F., Brokel, J., Zimmerman, D., Forzley, G., Banas, C., et al. (2012). Meaningful use and the problem-based medical record. *Journal of Healthcare Information Management, 26*(1), 58–63.

Office of National Coordinator for Health Information Technology (ONC) (2010). *Standards and interoperability framework initiatives.* Posted by: J. Perlin, J. Halamka, Co-Chairs of HIT Standards Committee. Retrieved from http://www.healthit.gov/sites/default/files/pdf/fact-sheets/standards-and-interoperability-framework.pdf.

Osheroff, J. (Ed.). (2009). *Improving medication management, safety and other outcomes with CDS: A Practical Guide.* Chicago: HIMSS.

Ozbolt, J. G. (1991). Strategies for building nursing databases for effectiveness research. *Patient outcomes research: Examining the effectiveness of Nursing Practice.* Bethesda, MD: NIH, NINR.

Pathak, J., Wang, J., Kashyap, S., Basford, M., Li, R., Masys, D. R., et al. (2011). Mapping clinical phenotype data elements to standardized metadata repositories and controlled terminologies: The eMERGE Network experience. *Journal American Medical Informatics Association, 18*, 376–386. http://dx.doi:10.1136/amiajnl-2010-000061.

Petersen, L., Woodard, L., Urech, T., Daw, C., & Sookanan, S. (2006). Does pay-for-performance improve the quality of health care? *Annals of Internal Medicine, 145*(4), 265–272.

Salsberg, E. (2009). *State of the national physician workforce.* Paper presented at Annual Meeting of the Association of American Medical Colleges, Boston, MA.

Sampaio Santos, F. A., de Melo, R. P., & deOliveira Lopes, M. V. (2010). Characterization of health status with regard to tissue integrity and tissue perfusion in patients with venous ulcers according to the nursing outcomes classification. *Journal of Vascular Nursing, 28*(March), 14–20.

Scherb, C. A., Head, B. J., Maas, M. L., Swanson, E. A., Moorhead, S., Reed, D., et al. (2011b). Most frequent nursing diagnoses, nursing interventions, and nursing-sensitive patient outcomes of hospitalized older adults with heart failure, part 1. *International Journal of Nursing Terminologies & Classifications, 22*(1), 13–22.

Schneider, J. S., Barkauskas, V., & Keenan, G. (2008). Evaluating home health care nursing outcomes with OASIS and NOC. *Journal of Nursing Scholarship, 40*(1), 76–82.

Sensmeier, J. (2011). *Are we in the second wave of nursing informatics?* Retrieved from http://blog.himss.org/2011/10/14/.

Sewell, J., & Thede, L. (2013). *Informatics and nursing. Opportunities and challenges* (4th ed.). Philadelphia: Wolters Kluwer, Lippincott Williams & Wilkins.

Staggers, N., Bagley Thompson, C., & Snyder-Halpern, R. (2001). History and trends in clinical information systems in the United States. *Journal of Nursing Scholarship, 33*(1), 75–81.

Stetson, P., McKnight, K., Bakken, S., Curran, C., Kubose, T., & Cimino, J. (2001). *Development of an ontology to model medical errors, information needs, and the clinical communication space.* Paper presented at the AMIA Annual Symposium, Washington, DC.

U.S. Department of Health and Human Services (USDHHS) (2008). *The national alliance for health information technology report to the Office of the National Coordinator for Health Information Technology on defining key health information technology terms.* Retrieved from http://www.healthit.gov/policy-researchers-implementers/technology-standards-certification-glossary.

U.S. Department of Health and Human Services (USDHHS) (2010). *HITECH and funding opportunities.* Retrieved from http://healthit.hhs.gov/portal/server.pt/community/healthit_hhs_gov__hitech_and_funding_opportunities/1310.

U.S. Department of Health and Human Services (USDHHS) (2011). *Partnerships for patients to improve care and lower costs for Americans.* Retrieved from http://www.hhs.gov/news/press/2011pres/04/20110412a.html.

Vogelsmeier, A., Halbesleben, J., & Scott-Cawiezell, J. (2008). Technology implementation and workarounds in the nursing home. *Journal of the American Medical Informatics Association, 15*, 114–119.

Ward, M. M., Jaana, M., Bahensky, J. A., Vartak, S., & Wakefield, D. S. (2006). Clinical information system availability and use in urban and rural hospitals. *Journal of Medical Systems, 30*(6), 429–438.

Ward, M. M., Vartak, S., Schwichtenberg, T., & Wakefield, D. S. (2011). Nurses' perceptions of how clinical information system implementation affects workflow and patient care. *Computers Informatic Nursing, 29*(9), 502–511.

Werley, H., & Lang, N. (Ed.). (1988). *Identification of the nursing minimum data set.* New York: Springer.

Westra, B. L., Subramanian, A., Hart, C. M., Matney, S. A., Wilson, P. S., Huff, S., et al. (2010). Achieving "meaningful use" of electronic health records through the integration of the Nursing Management Minimum Data Set. *Journal of Nursing Administration, 40*(7/8), 336–343.

Chapter 27

American Marketing Association (2011). *Dictionary.* Retrieved July 25, 2012, from www.marketingpower.com/_layouts/Dictionary.aspx.

American Nurses Credentialing Center (2012). *Magnet Recognition Program® FAQ: Data and Expected Outcomes.* Retrieved July 25, 2012, from www.nursecredentialing.org/FunctionalCategory/FAQs/DEO-FAQ.aspx.

American Organization of Nurse Executives (2011). *The AONE nurse executive competencies.* Retrieved July 25, 2012, from www.aone.org/resources/leadership%20tools/PDFs/AONE_NEC.pdf.

Berkow, S., Workman, J., & Aronson, S. (2012). Strengthening frontline nurse investment in organizational goals. *Journal of Nursing Administration, 42*(3), 165–169.

Boyington, A. R., Ferrall, S. M., & Sylvanus, T. (2010). Marketing evidence-based practice: What a CROC™! *Clinical Journal of Oncology Nursing, 14*(5), 653–655. http://dx.doi:10.1188/10.CJON.653-655.

Boyington, A. R., Jones, C. B., & Wilson, D. L. (2006). Buried alive: The presence of nursing on hospital web sites. *Nursing Research, 55*(2), 103–109.

Buerhaus, P. I. (2008b). Current and future state of the U.S. nursing workforce. *The Journal of the American Medical Association, 300*(20), 2422–2424.

Buerhaus, P. I., Auerbach, D. I., & Staiger, D. O. (2009c). The recent surge in nurse employment: Causes and implications. *Health Affairs, 28*(4), w657–w668. http://dx.doi:10.1377/hlthaff.28.4.w657.

Committee on the Robert Wood Johnson Foundation Initiative on the Future of Nursing, at the Institute of Medicine; Institute of Medicine (2011). *The future of nursing: Leading change, advancing health.* Washington, DC: The National Academies Press. Retrieved July 25, 2012, from http://books.nap.edu/openbook.php?record_id=12956.

Epstein, R. M., Fiscella, K., Lesser, C. S., & Stange, K. C. (2010). Why the nation needs a policy push on patient-centered health care. *Health Affairs*, *29*(8), 1489–1495. http://dx.doi:10.1377/hlthaff.2009.0888.

Finkler, S. A., Kovner, C. T., & Jones, C. B. (2007c). *Financial management for nurse managers and executives* (3rd ed.). St. Louis: Saunders Elsevier.

Harvard Business School Press. (2006). *Marketer's toolkit: The 10 strategies you need to succeed.* Boston: Harvard Business School Publishing Corporation.

Karl, K. A., Harland, L. K., Peluchette, J. V., & Rodie, A. R. (2010). Perceptions of service quality: What's fun got to do with it? *Health Marketing Quarterly*, *27*(2), 155–172.

Kotler, P. (2006). Alphabet soup. *Marketing Management*, *15*(2), 51.

Kotler, P., & Armstrong, G. (2011). *Principles of marketing* (14th ed.). Upper Saddle River, NJ: Pearson Prentice Hall.

Kumar, N. (2008). The CEO's marketing manifesto. *Marketing Management*, *17*(6), 24–29.

Lauterborn, B. (1990). New marketing litany; Four P's passe; C-words take over. *Advertising Age*, *61*(41), 26.

McCarthy, E. J. (1964). *Basic marketing: A managerial approach* (rev. ed.). New York: McGraw-Hill.

Millenson, M. L., & Macri, J. (2012, March). Will the Affordable Care Act move patient-centeredness to center stage? Timely analysis of immediate health policy issues. *Urban Quick Strike Series*, 1–10. Retrieved July 25, 2012 from www.rwjf.org/qualityequality/product. jsp?id=74054&cid=XEM_A5765.

Moss, J., & Saba, V. (2011). Costing nursing care: Using the clinical care classification system to value nursing intervention in an acute-care setting. *Computers, Informatics, Nursing*, *29*(8), 455–460.

Peltier, J. W., Pointer, L., & Schibrowsky, J. A. (2008). Internal marketing and antecedents of nurse satisfaction and loyalty. *Health Marketing Quarterly*, *23*(4), 75–108. http://dx. doi:10.1080/07359680802131582.

Planetree. (n.d). *What is Planetree designation?* Retrieved from http://dev.planetree.org/?page_id=89.

Press Ganey Associates, Inc. (2011). *2011 Hospital pulse report: Patient perspectives on American health care.* South Bend, IN: Author.

Wagner, D., & Bear, M. (2008). Patient satisfaction with nursing care: A concept analysis within a nursing framework. *Journal of Advanced Nursing*, *65*(3), 692–701. http://dx.doi:10.1111/j.1365-2648.2008.04866.x.

Welton, J. M., & Dismuke, C. E. (2008). Testing an inpatient nursing intensity billing model. *Policy, Politics, & Nursing Practice*, *9*(2), 103–111. http://dx. doi:10.1177/1527154408320045.

Welton, J. M., Fischer, M. H., DeGrace, S., & Zone-Smith, L. (2006b). Nursing intensity billing. *Journal of Nursing Administration*, *36*(4), 181–188.

Woods, D. K. (2002). Realizing your marketing influence, part 1. *Journal of Nursing Administration*, *32*(4), 189–195.

Woods, D. K., & Cardin, S. (2002). Realizing your marketing influence, part 2. *Journal of Nursing Administration*, *32*(6), 323–330.

INDEX

Note: Page numbers followed by *f* indicate figures, *t* indicate tables and *b* indicate boxes.

523